# THE HUMAN BRAIN

*An introduction to its functional anatomy*

The brain, and the brain alone, is the source of our pleasures, joys, laughter, and amusement, as well as our sorrow, pain, grief, and tears. It is especially the organ we use to think and learn, see and hear, to distinguish the ugly from the beautiful, the bad from the good, and the pleasant from the unpleasant. The brain is also the seat of madness and delirium, of the fears and terrors which assail by night or by day, of sleeplessness, awkward mistakes and thoughts that will not come, of pointless anxieties, forgetfulness and eccentricities.

*Hippocrates, ca. 400 B.C.*

The human mind can be described as a slow-clockrate modified-digital machine with multiple distinguishable parallel processing, all working in salt water.

*Philip Morrison: The mind of the machine, Technology Review 75:17, 1973.*

One of the difficulties in understanding the brain is that it is like nothing so much as a lump of porridge.

*From Eye and brain: The psychology of seeing by R.L. Gregory.* 

# THE HUMAN BRAIN

## *An introduction to its functional anatomy*

JOHN NOLTE, Ph.D.
Professor of Anatomy;
Director, Division of Academic Resources,
The University of Arizona College of Medicine,
Tucson, Arizona

***Third Edition***

*with 524 illustrations and 13 color plates*

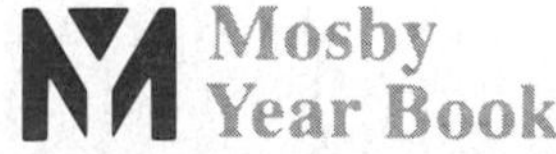


St. Louis Baltimore Boston Chicago London Philadelphia Sydney Toronto

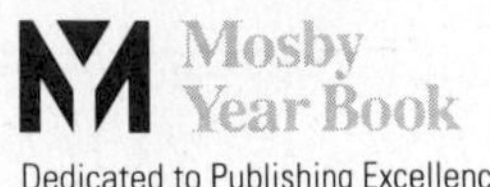

Dedicated to Publishing Excellence

*Publisher:* George Stamathis
*Editor:* Robert Farrell
*Project Manager:* Karen Edwards
*Production Editor:* Rich Barber

Cover: Reproduction of a drawing by Rene Descartes in *De Homine,* 1662, superimposed on a photomicrograph of human cerebral cortex in which a number of its pyramidal neurons had been injected with a fluorescent dye by Dr. Eberhard H. Buhl of the Medical Research Council of the United Kingdom. Descartes thought that the pineal gland was the seat of the soul, monitoring the movement of "animal spirits" in sensory nerves and controlling the movement of animal spirits through motor nerves.

**THIRD EDITION**


Printed in the United States of America

Mosby-Year Book, Inc.
11830 Westline Industrial Drive
St. Louis, Missouri 63146

International Standard Book Number 0-8016-3690-6

95 96 CL/VH/VH 9 8 7 6 5 4

# *Preface to the Third Edition*

The several years since the publication of the second edition of this book have seen unabated growth in our knowledge of neurobiology, which in many ways continues to be one of the most exciting branches of biological science. Indeed, the 1990s have been designated the Decade of the Brain by the scientific and government communities. This, together with dozens of things that were left undone the last time around, provided the incentive for a new edition.

The very kind reception received by the second edition encouraged me to continue following the same principles used since the inception of this book. While the book has grown in length, a minimum of detail has been added. In updating various sections, I tried hard not to include new facts simply for their own sake. Rather, new observations and concepts were added where they help to illuminate function. One new chapter has been added to provide an overview of chemically specified neural pathways, and a brief atlas of forebrain structures has been added at the end of Chapter 17. Since much of our new knowledge has been made possible by new techniques, sections illustrating some of these techniques have been maintained and updated: anatomical labeling and tract-tracing methods, magnetic resonance imaging, positron emission tomography, and studies of regional cerebral blood flow. Finally, many of the illustrations have been revised with the intent of simplification or clarification, and a number of new ones have been added. The bibliographies have been updated, but the same philosophy was retained: recent reviews and research papers are emphasized, with the result that many papers with greater scientific importance or historical priority are omitted.

The challenge of writing a clear, accurate, up-to-date survey of human neuroanatomy continues to be a formidable one, and it is inevitable that I have committed errors of hyperbole, adumbration, and ignorance. I welcome the comments and suggestions of students and colleagues who use this book. They will improve my knowledge and my teaching, and make the next edition that much better.

As in the case of the first two editions, this revision was far from a solitary accomplishment, and I am indebted to many. Thanks to the many colleagues who generously supplied illustrations; to old friends in Colorado and new friends in Arizona for advice and suggestions; and to the students of The University of Arizona College of Medicine, who use the book and offer many helpful comments and suggestions, and who by their curiosity and caring continue to make teaching fun. Many of the illustrations, both new and old, are based on images digitized from a videodisc produced in collaboration with the Educational Services Department of the University of Colorado Health Sciences Center; Bill Blankenship, Chuck Corson, Chuck Courtier, Norm Fringer, Don Redifer, and Clyde Tucker made this adventure a joy. Thanks also to the ever-evolving cast of characters at Mosby – Year Book for their patience and support; to Pam Eller and Ed French, for their helpful comments on Chapter 17, and to Steve Jobs and colleagues for the Macintosh. Finally, my love and thanks to David, Sandi, Pam, Mike, Chris, Erik, Trent, and especially Carol for being with me through a time of transition and triumph.

**John Nolte**

# Preface to the First Edition

The human brain is a marvel in terms of what it allows us to do. Neurologists are fond of saying that the only really important function of the other parts of our bodies is to support the brain. Unfortunately, students often find the brain to be a marvel of complexity as well. I have tried to write a book that will lead beginning students through the basic aspects of the structure and function of their brains. It was designed primarily with students of the health sciences in mind, but I hope others will also find it useful.

In discussing the various parts of the nervous system and its environment, I have tried to restrict myself as much as possible to facts and details that can be correlated with function in some way. To bring home the correlation between structure and function, I have included numerous examples of clinical and experimental findings following damage to or manipulation of the nervous systems of humans and laboratory animals. Because of the difficulty of visualizing the structures and pathways of the brain in three dimensions, a wide variety of diagrams and photographs is also included.

A short and highly selective bibliography accompanies each chapter. The intent in choosing references was not only to document recent findings but also to provide access through those references to the vast neuroscientific literature. For these reasons, the emphasis is on recent reviews and research papers. Many classic and scientifically more important papers have been omitted, although some older or peripherally related articles that make interesting reading are listed.

This book was far from a solitary undertaking and could never have come about without the help and support of many people. I am especially grateful to my friends and colleagues Tom Finger, Claude Selitrennikoff, and Ted Tarby, who read parts (or all) of the manuscript for me and offered many helpful suggestions; to Gary Jenison, Stu Smith, and Jack Willson, who prepared some of the anatomic materials used for illustrations; to Shelley Frisch, Kris McInvaille, and Martha Potter, who watched my gesticulations and somehow came up with drawings; to Betty Aguilar and Sharon Ferdinandsen, who transformed my chicken scratchings into a manuscript; and to all the fellow students of the nervous system, cited in figure captions, who kindly provided illustrations. A very special thanks to Pam Eller, who prepared most of the anatomic materials, did most of the photography, read and commented on the manuscript, and patted me on the head a lot; without her help this would have been a lesser book or no book at all. Most of the photographs in the book depict materials developed for teaching purposes by my just-mentioned colleagues and me; I appreciate the cooperation of the University of Colorado Health Sciences Center in allowing them to be used in this book. Finally, I must acknowledge the students with whom it has been my pleasure to work at the University of Colorado Health Sciences Center; they have made teaching fun, and from the fun arose the notion of writing a book.

**John Nolte**

# Contents

# CHAPTER 1

# *Introduction: The Central Nervous System*

The object of this book is to present and explain some basic anatomical facts about how the brain is put together and to discuss a few aspects of how it works. This introductory chapter describes in a very general way the elements that make up the central nervous system (CNS) and some principles according to which these elements are connected to each other. In addition, there is a discussion of how the relatively simple embryonic nervous system is transformed into the much more complex CNS of the adult.

## WHAT IS IN IT?

The principal cellular elements of the nervous system are *neurons* and *glial cells,* which are both present in enormous numbers. There are around 100 billion neurons in the human brain and several times that many glial cells.

Neurons come in a great variety of sizes and shapes (Figure 1-1); most of them have a long process called an *axon* that conducts information away from the neuronal cell body (or *soma*) and a series of smaller processes called *dendrites* that receive information from other neurons via *synaptic contacts* (or *synapses*). Certain aspects of somatic, dendritic, and axonal morphology give rise to a descriptive terminology for neurons. The vast majority of vertebrate neurons are *multipolar,* meaning that there are multiple dendritic projections from the cell body and almost always an axon as well (Figure 1-1, *C* and *D*). Some are *unipolar* (Figure 1-1, *A*) or *bipolar* (Figure 1-1, *B*), having one or two processes, respectively. There is a wide spectrum not only of neuronal shapes but also of neuronal sizes. Cell bodies range from about 5 to 100 μm in diameter. Many axons are short, only a millimeter or so in length, but some, like those that extend from the cerebral cortex to the sacral spinal cord, measure a meter or more.*

Neurons may also be classified according to their connections. *Sensory neurons* are either directly sensitive to various stimuli (such as touch or temperature changes) or else receive direct connections from nonneuronal *receptor cells. Motor neurons* end directly on muscles or glands. *Interneurons* interconnect other neurons. In a strict sense the nervous system is composed almost entirely of interneurons: there are at most 20 million sensory fibers in all the spinal and cranial nerves combined and no more than a few million motor neurons. Even taking into account the autonomic neurons that innervate muscles and glands (Chapter 7), more than 99% of our neurons are interneurons. However, the words "sensory" and "motor" are often used in a much broader sense to refer to cells and axons that carry information related to sensory stimuli and to the generation of responses, respectively.

There are several types of glial cells in the nervous system. Some of them (*oligodendroglia* in the CNS and *Schwann cells* in peripheral nerves) form *myelin sheaths,* which are spiral wrappings around axons that allow the axons to conduct information more rapidly. Other types of glia are thought to perform a variety of functions, such as regulating the composition of extracellular fluids, complementing neurons in certain metabolic activities, and de-

*Diagrams like Figure 1-1 convey little feeling for the relative sizes of neurons and their parts. If you envision the spinal motor neuron cartooned in Figure 1-1, *C,* as being the size of a tennis ball, then its dendrites would spread out through a room-sized volume, and its axon would correspond to a half-inch garden hose nearly half a mile long. By the same scale, the small interneuron shown in Figure 1-1, *D,* would be little larger than the head of a pin; its axon would be a hair-thin process only a foot or two long.

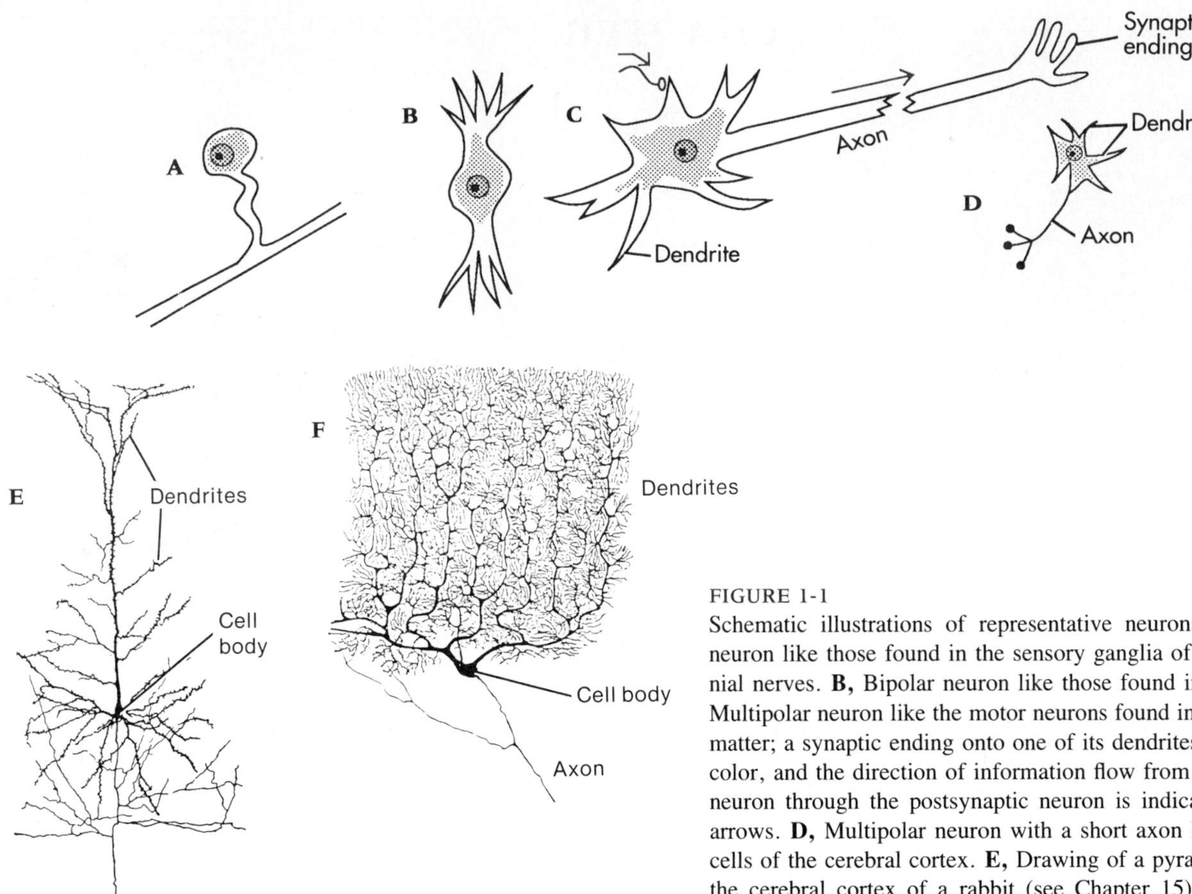


FIGURE 1-1
Schematic illustrations of representative neurons. **A,** Unipolar neuron like those found in the sensory ganglia of spinal and cranial nerves. **B,** Bipolar neuron like those found in the retina. **C,** Multipolar neuron like the motor neurons found in the spinal gray matter; a synaptic ending onto one of its dendrites is indicated in color, and the direction of information flow from the presynaptic neuron through the postsynaptic neuron is indicated by colored arrows. **D,** Multipolar neuron with a short axon like the granule cells of the cerebral cortex. **E,** Drawing of a pyramidal cell from the cerebral cortex of a rabbit (see Chapter 15) stained by the Golgi method. **F,** Drawing of a human cerebellar Purkinje cell (see Chapter 14) stained by the Golgi method.

**E** and **F** from Ramón y Cajal S: Histologie du système de l'homme et des vertébrés, vol. 1, Madrid, 1952, Consejo Superior de Investigaciones Cientificas Instituto Ramon y Cajal.

vouring foreign materials that have gained access to the nervous system.

## HOW IS IT ORGANIZED?

The CNS is composed of the *brain* and the *spinal cord* (Figure 1-2). The brain, in turn, is composed of the *cerebrum,* the *cerebellum,* and the *brainstem*. There is general agreement on what the cerebellum is, but not all authors distinguish the cerebrum from the brainstem in the same way. In this book the cerebrum is treated as being composed of the two massive *cerebral hemispheres* (separated by the *longitudinal fissure*) and the *diencephalon**; in an intact brain most of the diencephalon is hidden from view by the cerebral hemispheres. The brainstem is that part of the CNS, exclusive of the cerebellum, that lies between the cerebrum and the spinal cord. Some authors include the diencephalon with the brainstem, and occasionally small portions of the cerebral hemispheres may be included as well.

For the most part, the CNS is easily divisible into *gray matter* and *white matter* (see Figures 2-18 to 2-24). Gray matter refers to areas where there is a preponderance of cell bodies and dendrites; it is actually a pinkish gray color because of its abundant blood supply. White matter refers to areas where there is a preponderance of myelinated axons; myelin is mostly lipid and therefore has a fatty white appearance.

Specific areas of gray matter are often called *nuclei,* particularly if the contained cell bodies are functionally related to one another. An area where gray matter forms a surface covering on some part of the CNS (and meets certain other technical criteria) is referred to as a *cortex*. The cerebral and cerebellar cortices are two prominent examples. Occasionally, other names such as *body* or *center* are used for areas of gray matter, but these are relatively infrequent.

*Much seemingly arcane neuroanatomical terminology has a Latin or Greek derivation that actually makes sense. In this case, *encephalon* is Greek for "in the head," i.e., "brain." Diencephalon means "in-between-brain," signifying that this part of the CNS is interposed between the cerebral hemispheres and the brainstem.

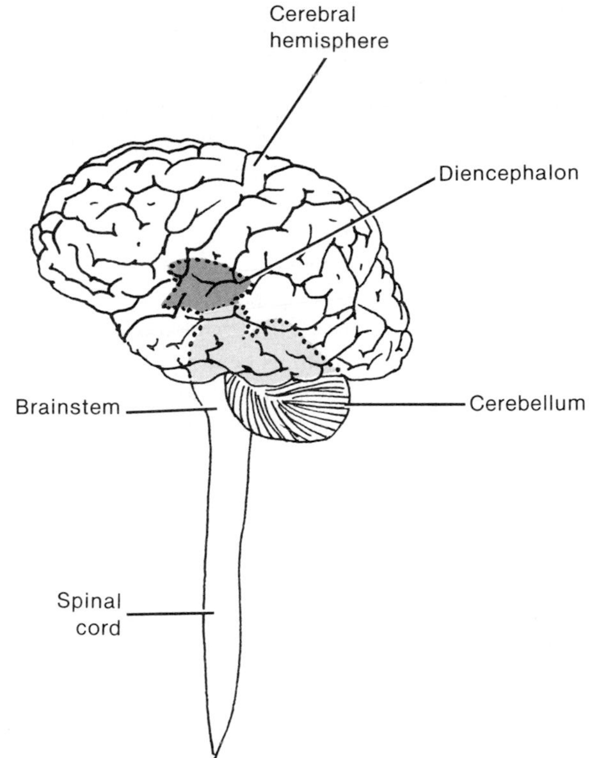


FIGURE 1-2
Major divisions of the central nervous system. Colored areas outlined by dotted lines are normally hidden from view by the massive cerebral hemispheres, but they can be seen in a hemisected brain (Figure 2-3).

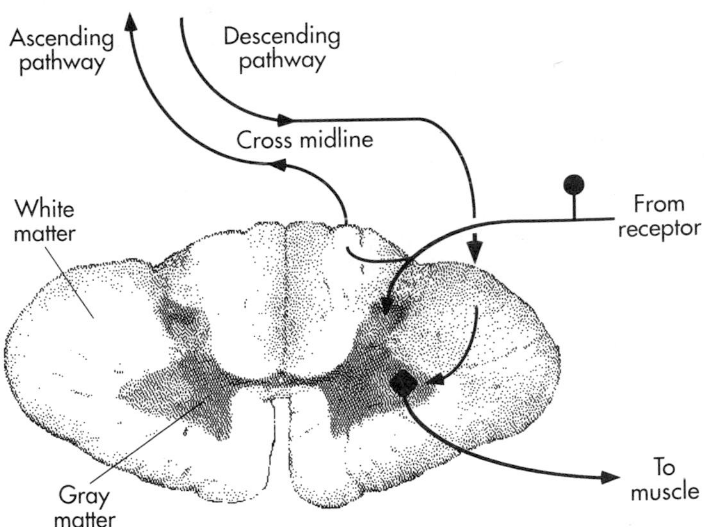


FIGURE 1-3
Division of the CNS into gray matter and white matter, as typified by the spinal cord in cross section. Gray matter contains interneurons, motor neurons, and endings of sensory fibers. White matter contains ascending and descending pathways. One axon in each ascending or descending pathway usually crosses the midline at some point. (Ascending pathways usually include the axons of interneurons, and descending pathways usually end on interneurons, but these links are omitted from this diagram to keep it simple.)

In contrast, subdivisions of white matter (i.e., collections of axons) go by a bewildering variety of names, such as *fasciculus, funiculus, lemniscus, peduncle,* and, used most commonly, *tract*. Many tracts have two-part names that provide some free information about the nature of the tract; the first part of the name refers to the location of the neuronal cell bodies from which these axons originate, and the second part refers to the site where they terminate. Thus a spinocerebellar tract is one that starts in the spinal cord and ends in the cerebellum.

The spinal cord provides a reasonably clear example of the separation of neural tissue into gray matter and white matter (Figure 1-3). Sensory axons, whose unipolar cell bodies are located in the dorsal root ganglia of spinal nerves, enter the spinal cord and divide into a large number of branches, most of which terminate on neuronal processes in the spinal gray matter. Motor axons, whose multipolar cell bodies are located in the spinal gray matter, leave the spinal cord and enter spinal nerves. The white matter contains *long descending tracts* (from the brainstem and cerebrum), *long ascending tracts* (to the brainstem, cerebellum, and cerebrum), and local axons interconnecting different spinal levels. The gray matter, on the other hand, contains motor neurons, the endings of incoming sensory axons and long descending tracts, local interneurons, and tract cells whose axons enter long ascending tracts. This division into white and gray matter is not absolute anywhere in the CNS; for example, axons in long descending tracts obviously must pass through some gray matter before reaching their targets.

Ascending (sensory) pathways usually cross to the opposite side of the CNS at some point before reaching the cerebrum (Figure 1-3). That is, they become *contralateral* to the side on which they originate, so information from the right hand eventually reaches the left cerebral hemisphere.* This crossing of sensory pathways is a curious and unexplained fact of vertebrate evolution. It applies not only to those pathways representing spinal nerves but more or less generally to those representing cranial nerves as well (except for olfaction; see Chapter 16). A number of hypotheses have been advanced to explain this phenomenon, including the notion that it is an early evolutionary mistake still awaiting correction.† Whatever its explana-

*This does not mean that most ascending *axons* cross the midline. The pathway from a peripheral receptor to the cerebral cortex, as will be detailed in subsequent chapters, includes at least three serially arranged neurons; the axon of only one of these crosses the midline.
†Zill, Sasha N: Personal communication, 1977.

tion, it would be even more peculiar if information from the *right* hand reached the left cerebral hemisphere, which in turn controlled the *left* hand. This is not the case, since descending pathways also cross the midline at some point between their origins and their terminations (Figure 1-3).

It follows from this crossing pattern that damage to the relevant regions of one cerebral hemisphere causes sensory and motor deficits on the contralateral side. This is also frequently true of damage at lower levels such as the brainstem. However, different pathways cross at different levels within the CNS. Therefore it is possible for a single lesion to affect one pathway before it crosses and another pathway after it crosses (Figure 1-4). The result would be the curious finding of one type of deficit on one side of the head or body and a second type of deficit on the other side.

As is generally the case, the generalization about crossing pathways has exceptions. Some sensory pathways (for example, auditory) ascend bilaterally, and some motor neurons (for example, trigeminal) are innervated by both cerebral hemispheres. The most glaring exception is the cerebellum. Damage to one side of the cerebellum produces deficits on the same side of the body (that is, the side *ipsilateral* to the lesion). The anatomical bases of this ipsilaterality are discussed in Chapter 14.

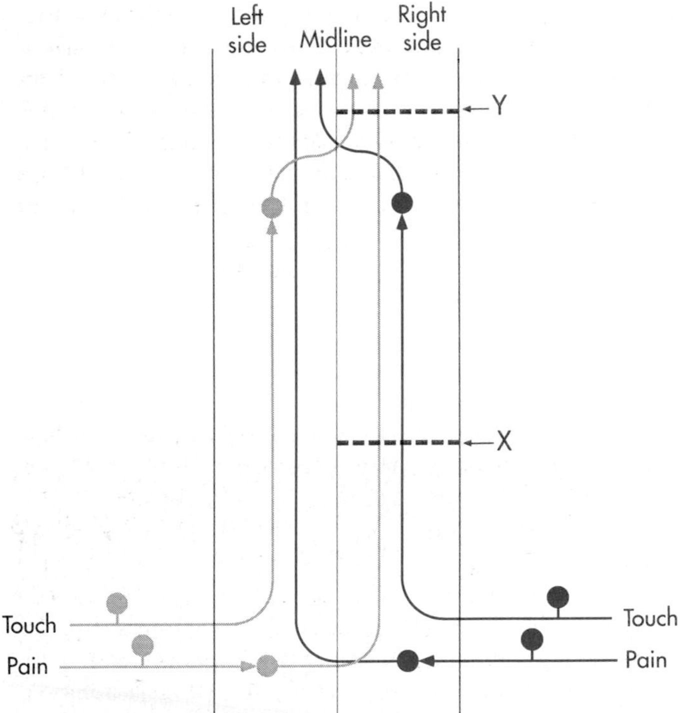


FIGURE 1-4
Different pathways may cross the midline at different points in the CNS. This diagram approximates the actual arrangement in spinal cord pathways, as discussed in Chapter 7. The crossing interneurons for the principal pathway conveying information about pain are located near the level where the primary afferents enter the spinal cord. The crossing interneurons for the principal touch pathway are located more rostrally (in the brainstem). As a result, damage to the right half of the spinal cord (X) could cause a deficit in perceiving pain on the left side of the body and touch on the right side of the body. In contrast, damage to the right half of the brainstem (Y) could cause a deficit in perceiving pain or touch on the left side of the body.

## HOW DO WE KNOW?

Inspection of Plate 1 reveals that gray matter and white matter have fairly uniform appearances, even though in any given section millions of axons interconnect a greater number of neurons. This book is concerned with a description of these connections in some detail. The question arises of how we can know what is connected to what. A number of techniques are available that can help answer this question; some of these are newly devised and are contributing greatly to the current explosive growth of knowledge about the neurosciences.

*Degeneration techniques* have been used since the last century and are based on the reactions of neurons to injury. If an axon is severed, its formerly attached cell body undergoes a characteristic series of cytological changes *(chromatolysis)*. Therefore, examining brain sections for chromatolytic cells can reveal the locations of the cell bodies of origin of the severed axons. While the cell body undergoes chromatolysis, the portion of the axon distal to the cut degenerates *(wallerian degeneration)*. The same distal changes occur if the damage is inflicted at the ultimate proximal location (that is, if the cell body is destroyed). Special staining methods can be used to selectively stain degenerating axons or their synaptic terminals. Therefore, if a particular nucleus is destroyed, the path of axons originating there and the sites of their termination can be determined.

Although a great deal of information has been gained over the years with the aid of degeneration techniques, their use is not without pitfalls. It is technically difficult, and sometimes impossible, to completely destroy a particular structure without also damaging nearby structures. In addition, since the segregation of gray and white matter is not absolute, axons passing through a given nucleus can be destroyed along with the cell bodies forming the nucleus. For these and other reasons, various tracer techniques developed in recent years have been greeted with much enthusiasm. Most of these methods take advantage of the fact that, under normal circumstances, substances are transported from a neuronal cell body down its axon toward its synapses *(anterograde transport)* and in the reverse direction as well *(retrograde transport)*. Appropriate radioactive substances (usually tritiated amino acids) introduced into a nucleus are taken up by the resident neurons, incorporated into macromolecules, and transported down the axons of these neurons. Eventually, the synaptic terminals of these axons become radioactive.

In another method a marker substance (usually a protein) is introduced into selected areas of gray matter, where it encounters synaptic terminals. The terminals take up the protein and transport it back to the parent neurons. A protein commonly used in such experiments is an enzyme called *horseradish peroxidase,* which can be detected with great sensitivity and resolution by appropriate histochemical procedures (Plate 2). While this technique is typically used for retrograde transport studies, it can be used simultaneously for anterograde transport studies, labeling not only the neurons that project to a given area of gray matter but also the targets of axons that leave it (Plate 3). Certain fluorescent dyes can also be used in retrograde transport studies (see Plate 6). By injecting two different dyes at two different sites in the nervous system, it is possible to determine whether any neurons have branching axons that project to both sites.

Other anatomical methods utilize neural tissue that has not been experimentally manipulated before processing. The *Golgi technique* is a staining method that completely stains the cell bodies and processes of a small, random sample of neurons in the tissue (Figure 1-1, *E* and *F*). This is useful for determining the sizes and shapes of the cell types in a given area of the CNS. In addition, different classes of neurons have chemically different interiors, some of which can be distinguished by histochemical or immunocytochemical techniques. For example, neurons that use norepinephrine as the chemical transmitter at their synapses contain this substance throughout their axons and cell bodies. Appropriate fixation and processing causes these neurons to be fluorescent.

Alternatively, it is possible to make a labeled antibody to an enzyme involved in the formation of a neurotransmitter or a labeled antibody to a receptor for a given transmitter. Applying the antibody and then visualizing it by a fluorescence or histochemical technique demonstrates neurons that either manufacture the transmitter in question or are sensitive to it (Plate 4). Such methods have made it possible to map out "chemically coded" neural pathways in recent years (see Chapter 17). Neurons differ chemically from each other not just in terms of their neurotransmitters, and it is possible to detect some of these additional differences using immunocytochemistry (Plate 5). Axoplasmic transport and immunocytochemical techniques can be used together to study the anatomical connections of chemically characterized neurons (Plate 6).

Electrophysiological techniques have also added a great deal of information about pathways and connections, much of which could not have been obtained by strictly anatomical studies. Such experiments range from those in which the electrical activity of various cortical areas is measured after stimulation of peripheral nerves and receptors to those in which the activity and connections of single neurons are measured.

Finally, anatomical and electrophysiological techniques can be used together. For example, a single neuron can be impaled by a micropipette electrode with a very fine tip, allowing measurement of the electrophysiological properties of the neuron. The same electrode can be used as a tiny hypodermic needle to inject a dye or marker substance, allowing study of the anatomy of the same neuron (Plates 7 to 10).

## HOW DID IT GET THAT WAY?*

As complex as the human nervous system is, its embryonic origin is as a simple, tubular, ectodermal structure. An understanding of the development of the nervous system helps make sense of its adult configuration and organization. Similarly, the relatively frequent congenital malformations of the CNS are more easily understood in light of its embryological development; such malformations also provide clues that aid in the understanding of normal development.

### Neural tube formation: the period of dorsal induction

During the third week of embryonic development a longitudinal band of ectoderm thickens to form the *neural plate*. Shortly thereafter the neural plate begins to fold inward, forming a longitudinal *neural groove* in the midline flanked by a parallel *neural fold* on each side (Figures 1-5 and 1-6). The neural groove deepens, and the neural folds approach each other in the dorsal midline. At the end of

*This section was revised by Dr. Theodore J. Tarby.

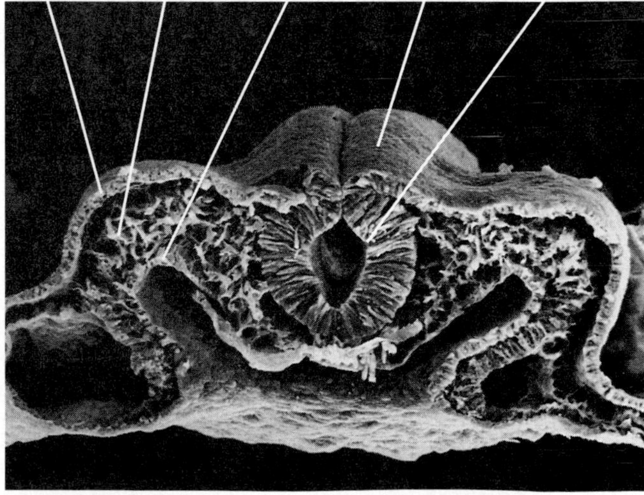


FIGURE 1-5
Scanning electron micrograph of the just-closing neural tube of a chick embryo, fractured at about the level of the future midbrain.
From *Devel* 109(2), 1990. Courtesy of Dr. Gary C. Schoenwolf, University of Utah School of Medicine.

the third week the two folds begin to fuse midway along the neural groove, forming the *neural tube*. As the neural tube closes, it pinches off from the ectodermal (that is, skin) surface and becomes enclosed within the body (Figure 1-6). As this fusion occurs, groups of cells from the crest of each neural fold are pinched off from the neural tube. These *neural crest cells* develop into a variety of cell types, including the sensory neurons of the ganglia of spinal and cranial nerves, the postganglionic neurons of the autonomic nervous system, and the Schwann cells and satellite cells of the peripheral nervous system. The neural tube, on the other hand, develops into virtually the entire CNS*; its cavity becomes the *ventricular system* of the brain.

The area of fusion of the two neural folds, which begins in the cervical region of the future spinal cord, rapidly expands rostrally (toward the future brain) and caudally (toward the sacral end of the future spinal cord). The *rostral neuropore,* the opening at the rostral end of the neural tube, closes completely in the middle of the fourth week;

*The sacral spinal cord forms by a slightly different mechanism. After the neural tube closes, a secondary cavity extends into the mass of cells at its caudal end.

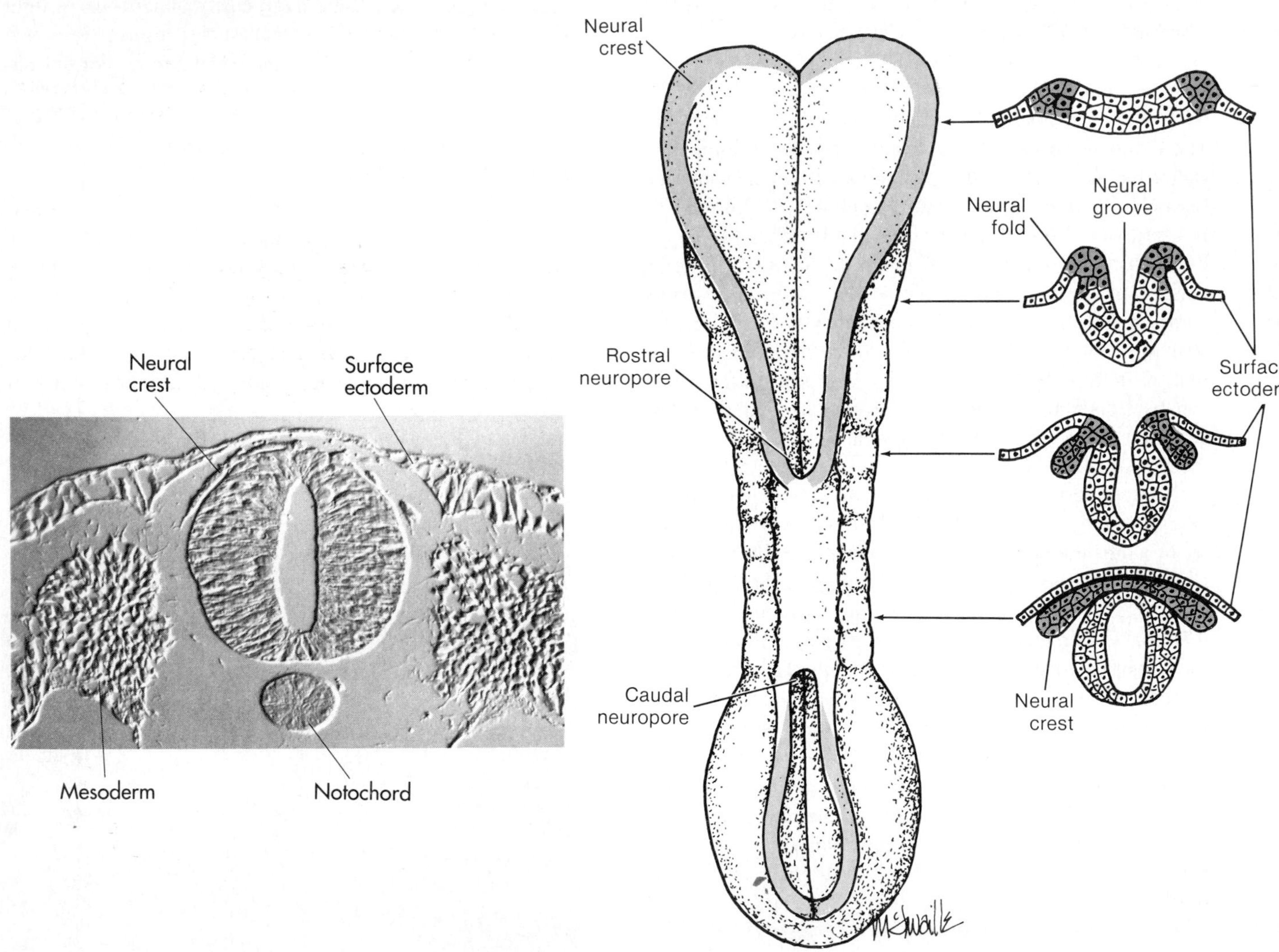


FIGURE 1-6
Neural tube at about the end of the third week. Neural folds have begun to fuse at the cervical level of the future spinal cord. Cross sections of the neural tube at four different levels shown on the right; at any given level the embryonic CNS goes through a series of stages resembling these four cross sections. Total length of neural tube at this time is about 2.5 mm. Photographic inset: section through a chick embryo at the level of the future spinal cord; the notochord is the forerunner of the skeletal axis, helping to form the vertebral column.

Inset from Schoenwolf GC, Smith JL: *Devel* 109:243, 1990. Courtesy of Dr. Gary C. Schoenwolf, University of Utah School of Medicine.

the *caudal neuropore* closes about 2 days later. As each successive bit of neural tube is formed by the progressive fusion of the neural folds, it becomes separated from the overlying ectoderm (Figure 1-6).

Defective closure of the neural tube is a frequent cause of congenital malformations of the nervous system. Since the neural tube forms and closes under the influence of certain dorsal portions of the embryo situated just beneath the neural ectoderm, such defects are referred to as *defects of dorsal induction*. Complete failure of the neural tube to close results in a fatal deformity called *craniorhachischisis* (from the Greek words meaning cleft skull and spine), in which the central nervous system appears as an open furrow on the dorsal surface of the head and body. Failure of the caudal neuropore to close can result in a severe form of *spina bifida* called *myelomeningocele* (from the Greek words meaning *herniated spinal cord* and *meninges*). Vertebrae fail to form over the defect, the caudal walls of the neural tube are still continuous with the skin of the back, and the cord and meninges are displaced into a saclike cavity on the back. Myelomeningocele is accompanied by an *Arnold-Chiari malformation* in which the cerebellum and caudal brainstem are elongated and pushed down into the foramen magnum. Frequently there is obstruction to the flow of cerebrospinal fluid and hydrocephalus results. The reason these two deformities accompany one another is not known with certainty, but it has been proposed that both arise from a single malalignment at the site where the neural tube first begins to close.

If the rostral neuropore fails to close, *anencephaly,* in which much of each cerebral hemisphere is absent, can result. As in spina bifida, the walls of the neural tube then may be continuous with the skin of the head, and the central cavity of the neural tube may be open to the outside.

## Sulcus limitans

During the fourth week a longitudinal groove appears in the lateral wall of the neural tube. This groove, called the *sulcus limitans,* extends throughout the future spinal cord and brainstem and subdivides the gray matter in the walls of the neural tube into a more dorsal *alar plate* and a more ventral *basal plate* (Figures 1-5 and 1-7). This is a distinction of some functional importance, since alar plate derivatives are primarily concerned with sensory processes, whereas motor neurons are located in basal plate derivatives. In the adult spinal cord, even though the sulcus limitans can no longer be found, the central gray matter can be divided into a *posterior horn* and an *anterior horn* on each side (Figure 1-7, *C*). The central processes of sensory neurons (derived from neural crest cells) end mainly in the posterior horn, which contains most of the cells whose axons form ascending sensory pathways. In contrast, the anterior horn contains the cell bodies of motor neurons, whose axons leave the spinal cord and innervate skeletal muscles. The same distinction between sensory alar plate derivatives and motor basal plate derivatives holds true in the brainstem, as discussed briefly in this chapter and in more detail in Chapter 9. The sulcus limitans cannot be followed beyond the brainstem, and the entire cerebrum is considered to be an alar plate derivative. In myelomeningocele the alar and basal plates on each side are visible as four distinct bands on the exposed neural plate. The sulcus limitans on each side and the midline ventral groove between the basal plates also are visible on the body surface (Figure 1-8).

## Cerebral vesicles

Even before the rostral and caudal neuropores close, bulges begin to appear in the rostral end of the neural tube in the region of the future brain. During the fourth week, three bulges, or vesicles, are apparent and are referred to as the *primary vesicles* (Figure 1-9, *B*). From rostral to caudal, these are the *prosencephalon* (forebrain), the *mes-*

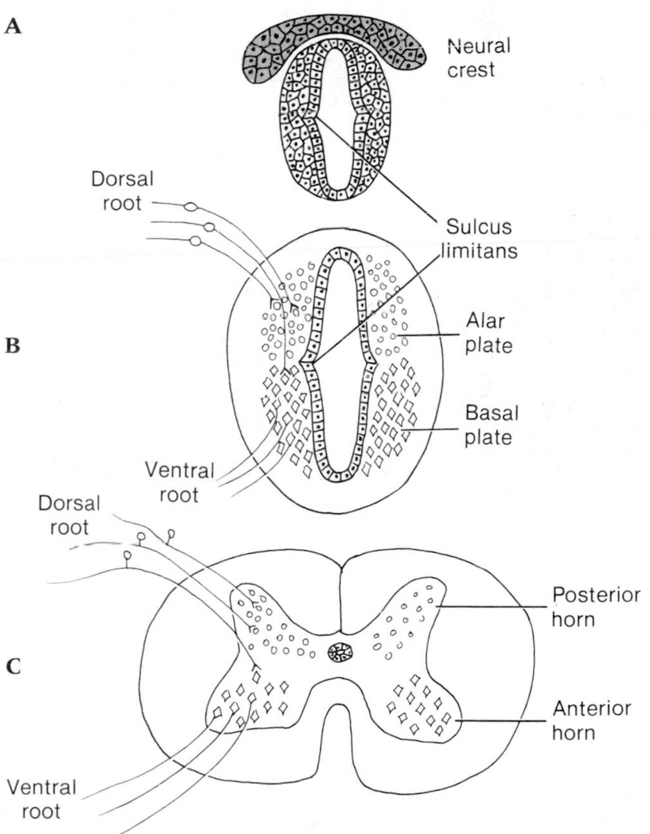


FIGURE 1-7
Sulcus limitans and alar and basal plates. **A,** Neural tube during the fourth week. **B,** Embryonic spinal cord during the sixth week; dorsal root ganglion cells, derived from the neural crest, send their central processes into the spinal cord to terminate mainly on alar plate cells; basal plate cells become motor neurons, whose axons exit in the ventral roots. **C,** Adult spinal cord.

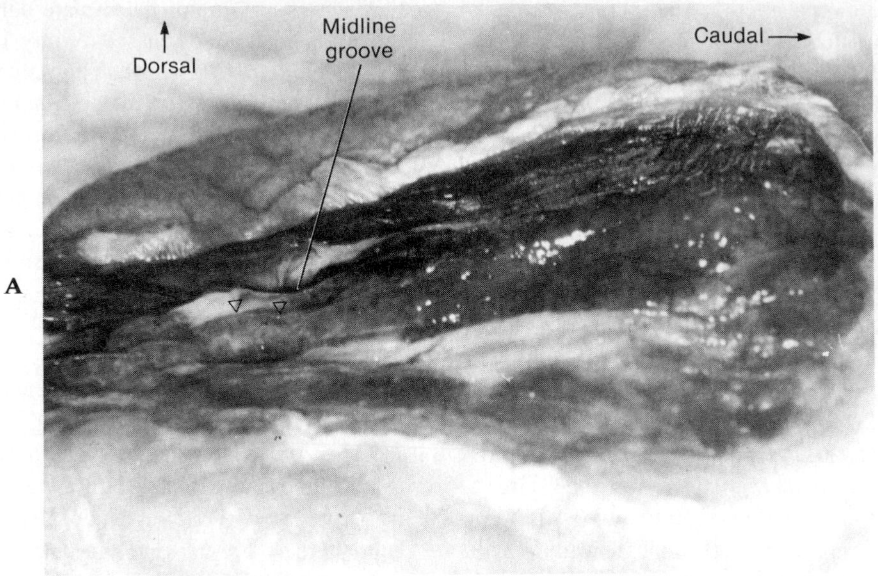


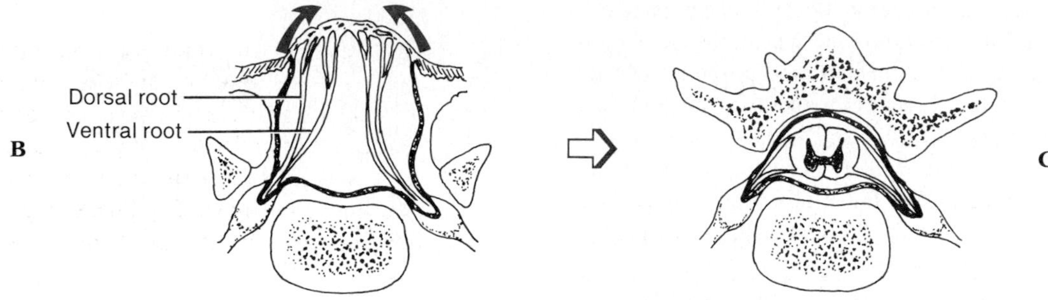


FIGURE 1-8
Myelomeningocele, an embryologic remnant. **A,** Photograph of cystic spina bifida, or myelomeningocele. The patient is in his first day of life, and the spinal defect is about to be closed surgically. The neural placode, representing the unfused spinal part of the embryonic neural tube, is the central element in the myelomeningocele. The midline ventral groove and the sulcus limitans on each side *(arrowheads)* can be seen clearly on the left side of the photograph. More rostrally (to the left and out of the photograph) the spinal cord is normal; more caudally (right side of photograph) the neural placode is more primitive and heavily vascularized. **B,** Within the defect the open spinal cord is exposed at the body surface and is continuous with the skin. Spinal rootlets are attached to the ventral surface of the neural placode. **C,** Rostral to the defect the neural tube has closed, and the spinal cord has a normal appearance in cross section.

**B** and **C** modified from an illustration in Mori K: Anomalies of the central nervous system, New York, 1985, Thieme-Stratton.

*encephalon* (midbrain), and the *rhombencephalon* (hindbrain), which merges smoothly with the spinal portion of the neural tube. The prosencephalon develops into the cerebrum. The mesencephalon becomes the midbrain of the adult brainstem, and the rhombencephalon becomes the rest of the brainstem and the cerebellum (Table 1).

The three primary vesicles are not arranged in a straight line but rather are associated with two bends or flexures in the neural tube (Figure 1-9, *A*). One of these, the *cervical flexure,* occurs between the rhombencephalon and spinal cord but does not persist in the adult CNS. The second, the *cephalic* (or *mesencephalic*) *flexure,* occurs between the mesencephalon and the prosencephalon; it persists in the adult as the bend between the axes of the brainstem and the forebrain (Figure 2-1).

As the brain continues to develop, two of the primary vesicles become subdivided. During the fifth week, five *secondary vesicles* can be distinguished (Figure 1-10, *B*). The prosencephalon gives rise to the *telencephalon* and the *diencephalon;* the mesencephalon remains undivided; the

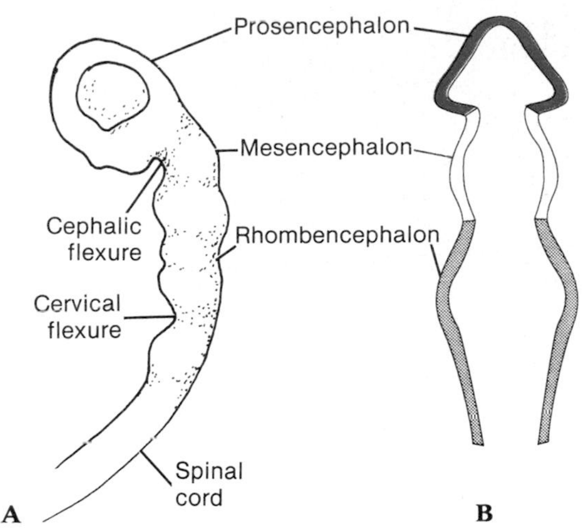


FIGURE 1-9
Primary vesicles at the end of the fourth week.

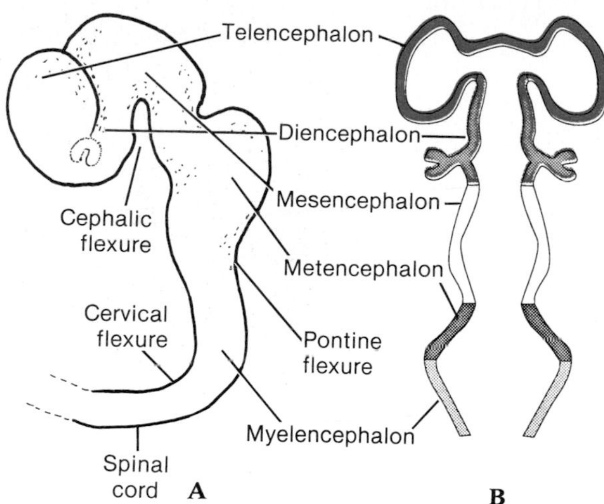


FIGURE 1-10
Secondary vesicles during the sixth week.

rhombencephalon gives rise to the *metencephalon* and the *myelencephalon*. The telencephalon becomes the cerebral hemispheres of the adult brain. The diencephalon gives rise to the *thalamus* (a large mass of gray matter interposed between the cerebral cortex and other structures), the *hypothalamus* (an autonomic control center), the neural part of the eye, and several other structures. These complex changes and subdivisions in the forebrain develop under the influence of more ventrally situated portions of the embryo. Hence malformations in this region are referred to as *defects in ventral induction;* they are typically associated with marked facial abnormalities as well. A spectrum of malformations known as *holoprosencephaly* (from the Greek words meaning *affecting the entire forebrain*) results from partial or complete failure of the prosencephalon to separate into the diencephalon and the paired telencephalic vesicles. Malformations like holoprosencephaly are rare and usually fatal. They sometimes are seen in chromosomal disorders, but the nature of other insults or events responsible for defects of dorsal or ventral induction is obscure in most cases. However, some similar malformations in animals can be produced by viral infections or environmental agents at particular times during gestation.

The metencephalon becomes the *pons* (part of the brainstem) and the cerebellum. The myelencephalon becomes the *medulla* (the part of the brainstem that merges with the spinal cord).

In addition, a *pontine flexure* appears in the dorsal surface of the brainstem between the metencephalon and the myelencephalon (Figure 1-10, *A*). This flexure does not persist as a bend in the axis of the brainstem, but it does have important consequences for the configuration of the caudal brainstem. As the flexure develops, the walls of the neural tube spread apart to form a diamond-shaped cavity (hence the name "rhombencephalon") so that only a thin membranous roof remains over what will become the *fourth ventricle* (Figure 1-11). Thus the alar and basal plates, still separated by the sulcus limitans, come to lie in

**TABLE 1** *Derivatives of vesicles of the neural tube*

| *Primary vesicle* | *Secondary vesicle* | *Neural derivatives* | *Cavity* |
|---|---|---|---|
| Prosencephalon | Telencephalon | Cerebral hemispheres | Lateral ventricles |
| | Diencephalon | Thalamus, hypothalamus, etc. | Third ventricle |
| Mesencephalon | Mesencephalon | Midbrain | Cerebral aqueduct |
| Rhombencephalon | Metencephalon | Pons and cerebellum | Part of fourth ventricle |
| | Myelencephalon | Medulla | Part of fourth ventricle<br>Part of central canal |

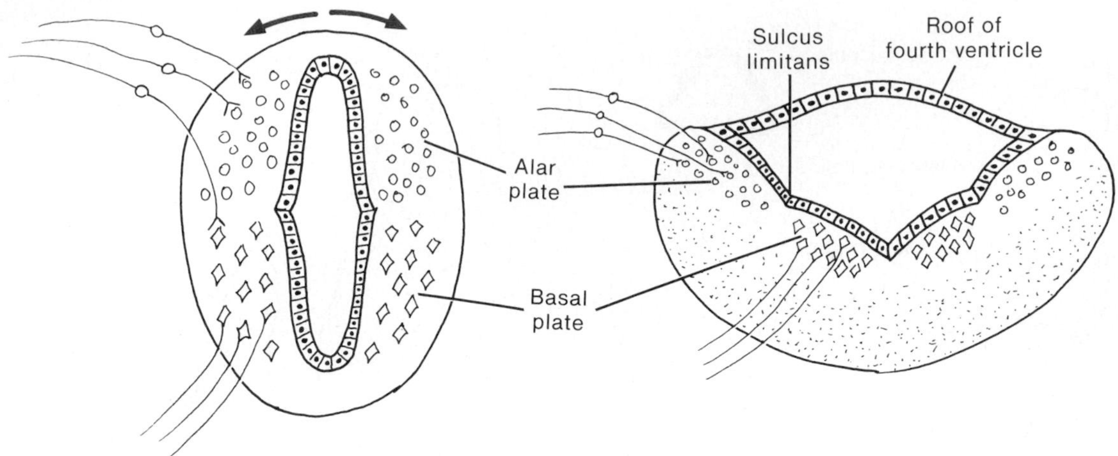


FIGURE 1-11
Formation of the floor of the fourth ventricle. Walls of the neural tube are spread apart by the pontine flexure so that they and the sulcus limitans become the floor of the ventricle and the roof becomes a thin membrane.

the floor of the fourth ventricle. The result is that in the corresponding part of the adult brainstem (rostral medulla and caudal pons) sensory nuclei are located lateral, rather than posterior, to motor nuclei. As discussed further in Chapter 9, this is of some utility in making sense of the arrangement of cranial nerve nuclei.

Lateral portions of the alar plate in the rostral metencephalon thicken considerably and form the *rhombic lips*. These continue to enlarge, finally fusing in the midline to form a transverse ridge that will eventually become the cerebellum.*

## Further development

Subsequent events are dominated by the tremendous growth of the telencephalon. This portion of the neural tube begins as two swellings connected across the midline by a thin membrane, the *lamina terminalis* (Figure 1-10). The basal part of the wall of the telencephalon, adjacent to the diencephalon, thickens to form the primordia of gray masses called the *basal ganglia* or *basal nuclei*. At the same time, the walls of the diencephalon thicken to form the thalamus and hypothalamus, separated by the *hypothalamic sulcus*. With continued growth, the telencephalon folds down alongside the diencephalon until eventually the two fuse (Figure 1-12). The telencephalic surface overlying the area of fusion develops into a portion of the cerebral cortex called the *insula*. The remainder of the telencephalon grows rapidly in all available directions (Figure 1-13) until the insula is completely hidden from view and each cerebral hemisphere has the shape of a great arc encircling the insular cortex (Figure 1-12; compare Figures 2-2 and 2-7). As discussed and demonstrated in the next chapter, knowledge of this growth of each cerebral hemisphere in a great C shape is of considerable importance for understanding the anatomical organization of the forebrain.

## Ventricles and choroid plexus

The cavity of the neural tube persists as the ventricular system of the adult brain (see Figure 4-1). Except for the rudimentary central canal of the spinal cord and caudal medulla, the ventricles comprise a continuous, fluid-filled series of spaces extending through all the major divisions of the CNS. The cavity of the pons and rostral medulla is the fourth ventricle; that of the diencephalon is the *third ventricle;* a large C-shaped *lateral ventricle* occupies each cerebral hemisphere. Each lateral ventricle communicates with the third ventricle through an *interventricular foramen* (Figure 1-12), and the third ventricle communicates with the fourth ventricle through the *cerebral aqueduct* of the midbrain.

Where the walls of the rhombencephalon spread apart to form the fourth ventricle, the roof of the ventricle becomes extremely thin (Figure 1-11). An area covering the roof of the third ventricle and extending onto the surface of the telencephalon becomes similarly thin (Figure 1-14). At each of these locations, tufts of small blood vessels invaginate the ventricular roof to form the *choroid plexus,* which is responsible for the production of most of the *cerebrospinal fluid* that fills the ventricles. As each cerebral hemisphere grows around in a C shape, so too does the choroid plexus, which protrudes into its lateral ventricle.

*Although the cerebellum develops from the alar plate, it is involved in motor functions in the sense that cerebellar lesions cause impairments of posture and movement but not of sensation (see Chapter 14).

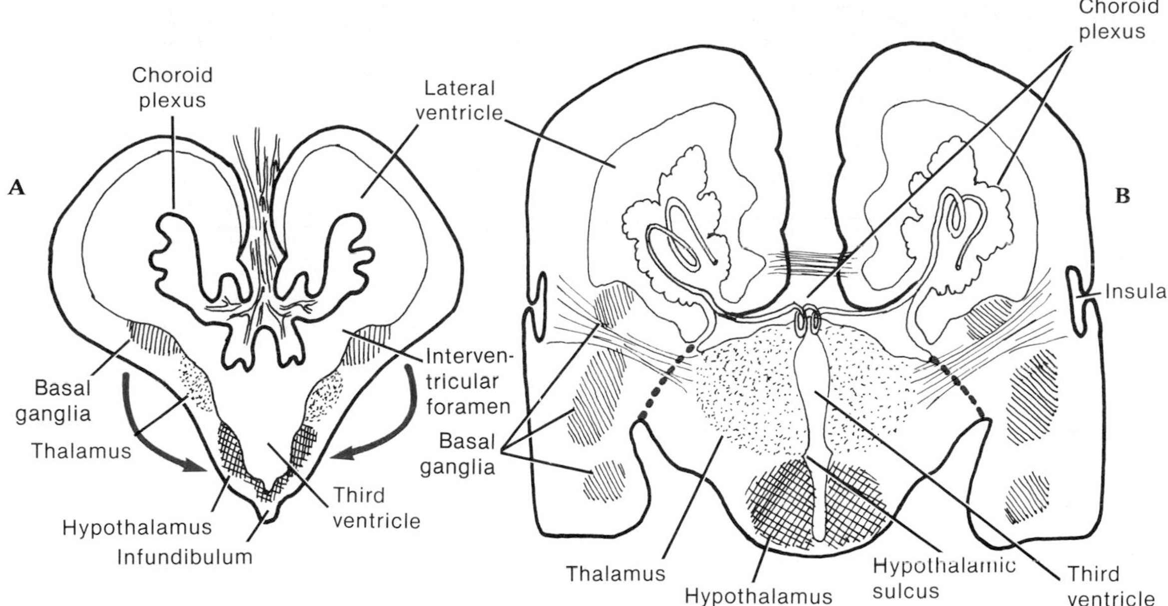


FIGURE 1-12
Formation of choroid plexus and of the fusion between diencephalon and telencephalon. **A,** Condition at the end of the second month; vascular connective tissue has invaginated the third and lateral ventricles to form choroid plexus, and rapid growth of telencephalon begins to fold its basal ganglia down toward diencephalon, as indicated by arrows. **B,** Condition at the end of the third month; telencephalon and diencephalon have fused, as indicated by dashed line, and the insula, overlying the point of fusion, begins to be overgrown by other cerebral cortex.

Modified from Carpenter M: Human neuoroanatomy, ed 7, Baltimore, 1976, Williams & Wilkins.

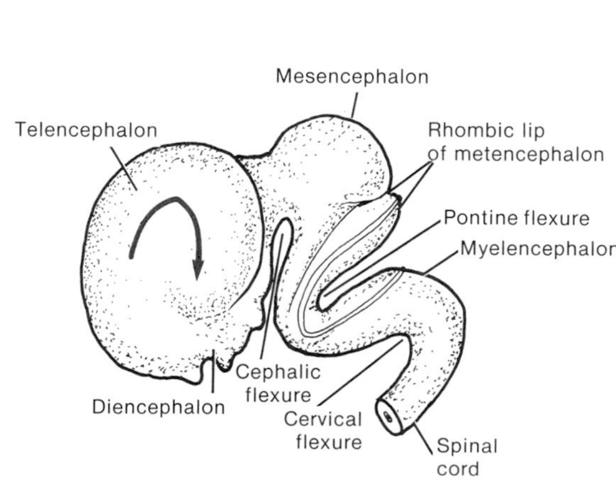


FIGURE 1-13
Neural tube at the end of the second month. Development from this point is dominated by rapid growth of telencephalon in a C shape, as indicated by the arrow.

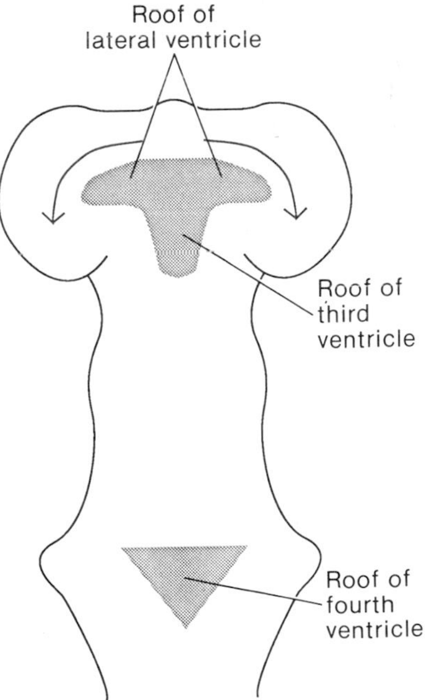


FIGURE 1-14
Sites of formation of choroid plexus. As each cerebral hemisphere grows around in a C shape *(arrows),* so does its choroid plexus.

## ADDITIONAL READINGS


Cherniak C: The bounded brain: toward quantitative neuroanatomy, *J Cog Neurosci* 2:1, 1990. *An interesting account of the widely varying estimates of a number of aspects of the human brain.*

Copp AJ et al: The embryonic development of mammalian neural tube defects, *Prog Neurobiol* 35:363, 1990.

Crelin ES: Development of the nervous system, *CIBA Clin Symp* 26(2), 1974.

Goochee C, Rasband W, Sokoloff L: Computerized densitometry and color coding of [$^{14}$C] deoxyglucose autoradiographs, *Ann Neurol* 7:150, 1980. *A technique for studying the relative levels of activity of different areas of the brain based on the contrasting metabolic requirements of active and inactive neurons.*

Heimer L, Robards MJ: *Neuroanatomical tract-tracing methods,* New York, 1981, Plenum Press.

Heimer L, Záborszky L: *Neuroanatomical tract-tracing methods 2. Recent progress,* New York, 1989, Plenum Press.

Jennings MT et al: Neuroanatomic examination of spina bifida aperta and the Arnold-Chiari malformation in a 130-day human fetus, *J Neurol Sci* 54:325, 1982.

Jones EG, Cowan WM: Nervous tissue. In Weiss L, editor: *Histology: Cell and tissue biology,* ed 5, New York, 1983, Elsevier.

Lemire RJ et al: *Normal and abnormal development of the human nervous system,* New York, 1975, Harper & Row.

Mesulam M-M: Tracing neural connections of human brain with selective silver impregnation: observations on geniculocalcarine, spinothalamic, and entorhinal pathways, *Arch Neurol* 36:814, 1979.

Moore KL: *The developing human,* ed 4, Philadelphia, 1988, WB Saunders.

O'Rahilly R, Müller F: The developmental anatomy and histology of the human central nervous system. In Myrianthopoulos NC, editor: *Handbook of clinical neurology* 6(50): *Malformations,* Amsterdam, 1987, Elsevier.

Paxinos G, editor: *The human nervous system,* San Diego, 1990, Academic Press. *A detailed, extensive, contemporary review of human neuroanatomy.*

Peters A, Palay SL, Webster H deF: *The fine structure of the nervous system: the neurons and their supporting cells, ed 3,* New York, 1991, Oxford University Press.

Robertson RT, editor: *Neuroanatomical research techniques,* New York, 1978, Academic Press.

Schoenwolf GC, Smith JL: Mechanisms of neurulation: traditional viewpoint and recent advances, *Devel* 109:243, 1990. *A contemporary review of the sources of the forces that cause the neural plate to indent and form the neural groove and tube.*

Tuchmann-Duplessis H, Auroux M, Haegel P: *Illustrated human embryology,* vol 3, *Nervous system and endocrine glands,* New York, 1974, Springer-Verlag.

Volpe JJ: *Neurology of the newborn,* Philadelphia, 1987, WB Saunders.

# CHAPTER 2

## *Gross Anatomy*

The human central nervous system is composed of the brain and spinal cord. This chapter briefly discusses the major surface and internal structures of the brain (summarized in Figure 2-25 at the end of the chapter). Together with the following four chapters, it lays the groundwork for the more detailed consideration of the functional anatomy of the CNS in ensuing chapters.

### PLANES AND DIRECTIONS

Before considering the parts of the brain in more detail, it is helpful to discuss the terms used for planes and directions in the nervous system. The *sagittal* plane divides the brain into two symmetrical halves. *Parasagittal* planes are those parallel to the sagittal plane. *Frontal* planes (also called *coronal* planes) are parallel to the long axis of the body and perpendicular to the sagittal plane (for example, a vertical plane passing through both of your ears). These terms are fairly straightforward and have the same meaning with respect to any part of the nervous system. However, directional terms such as *anterior, dorsal,* and *rostral* change their meanings relative to each other in different parts of the nervous system. The reason for this, as indicated in Figure 2-1, is the bend of about 100° between the long axes of the brainstem and the cerebrum. This bend is a consequence of the cephalic flexure, which appears early in the embryological development of the nervous system and persists in the mature brain. Dorsal/ventral terminology ignores this bend, so that the directional meaning of "dorsal" changes by 100° at the midbrain-diencephalon junction. "Anterior" and "superior," in contrast, retain a constant meaning relative to the normal upright orientation of the body as a whole. This means, for example, that the ventral surface of the spinal cord is also its anterior surface, but the ventral surface of the diencephalon is its inferior surface. Rostral/caudal terminology may cause additional confusion because it has a functional connotation for many (implying "toward the telencephalon"), so that the posterior end of the cerebral hemispheres could be considered rostral to all parts of the diencephalon. Use of anterior/posterior and superior/inferior (or dorsal/ventral) terminology in reference to the cerebrum avoids any ambiguity.

### MEDIAL SURFACE

The cerebral hemispheres conceal most of the rest of an intact brain (Figure 2-2). Hemisection reveals many parts of the diencephalon, brainstem, and cerebellum and additional features of the cerebral hemispheres as well (Figure 2-3). The cephalic flexure is visible at the junction between the brainstem and the diencephalon. The brainstem itself is subdivided into (1) the *midbrain,* which is continuous with the diencephalon, (2) the *pons,* and (3) the *medulla,* which is continuous with the spinal cord. The two cerebral hemispheres are joined by a huge fiber bundle, the *corpus callosum,* which has an enlarged and rounded posterior *splenium,* a *body,* and an anterior, curved *genu,* which tapers gently into a ventrally directed *rostrum.*

Finally, the nervous system develops embryologically from a neuroectodermal tube; the cavity of the tube persists in the adult as a system of ventricles (see Figure 4-1), part of which is apparent in the sagittal plane (Figure 2-3). Portions of the medial surfaces of the diencephalon form the walls of the narrow, slitlike *third ventricle,* which opens into the large *lateral ventricle* of each cerebral hemisphere through an *interventricular foramen* (or *foramen of Monro*). Posteriorly the third ventricle is continuous with a narrow channel through the midbrain, the *cerebral aqueduct* (or *aqueduct of Sylvius*). The aqueduct in turn is continuous with the *fourth ventricle* of the pons and medulla, and the fourth ventricle is continuous with the

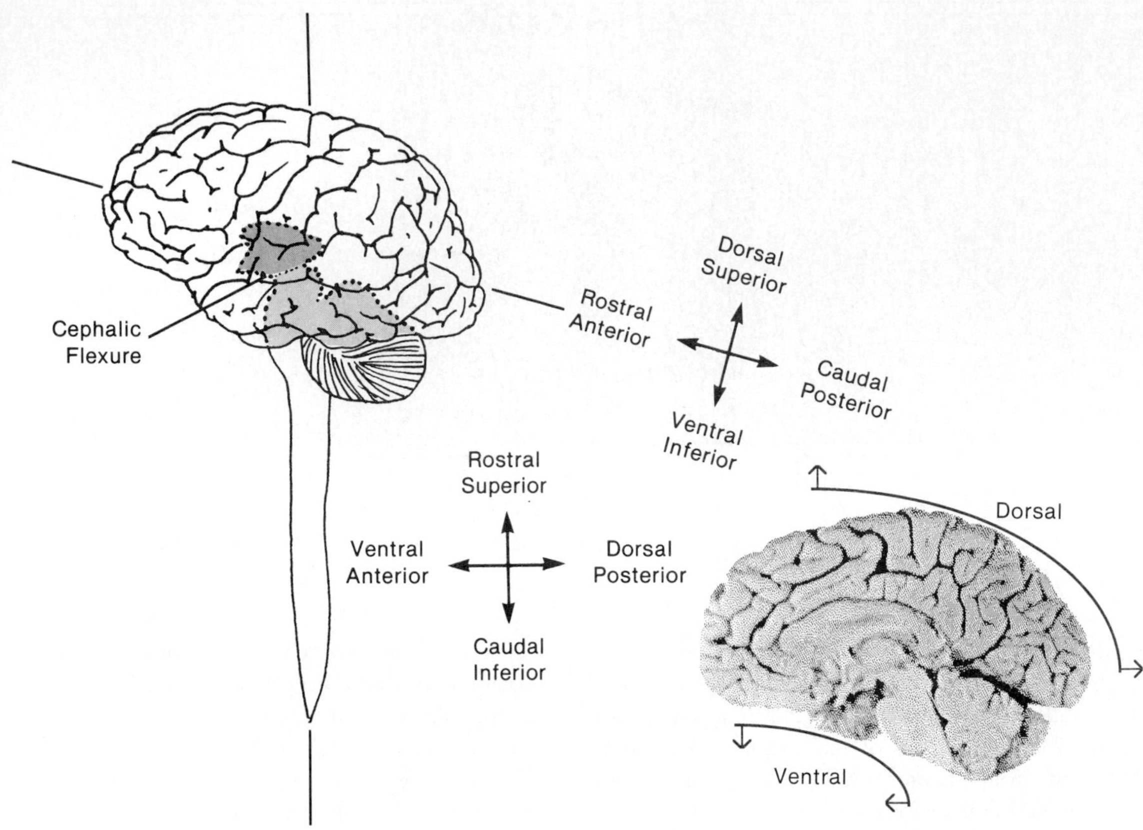


FIGURE 2-1
Various directional terms used when referring to different parts of the CNS. The diencephalon and much of the brainstem, normally hidden from view in an intact brain, are drawn with dashed lines and filled with color. The inset at the lower right indicates the way in which the dorsal and ventral surfaces of the CNS curve around through the cephalic flexure.

microscopically tiny *central canal* of the caudal medulla and the spinal cord.

## SIZE OF THE HUMAN BRAIN

One impressive feature of the human brain is its size, and our distinctively human mental capacities are commonly attributed to this. Our brains weigh about 400 g at birth, and this weight triples during the first 3 years of life (resulting primarily from growth of neuronal processes and addition of myelin, rather than the addition of more neurons). The rate of growth then slows, and the maximum brain weight of around 1400 g is reached by age 18. This weight holds steady until about the age of 50, when a slow decline sets in (Figure 2-4). The weight of 1400 g is only an average figure. Different, normal individuals have brain weights ranging from 1100 g (or less) to around 1700 g. This large range of sizes is surprising and its significance is not well understood, although within this range larger brains do not work better in any obvious way than smaller brains.

Part of the large brain size is simply a reflection of our body size; big animals tend to have big brains. Elephants, for example, have 5000 g brains. Similarly, the size difference between the bodies of human males and females explains, at least to a great extent, the fact that male brains are slightly larger than female brains (Figure 2-4). However, this is not the whole story because many animals that are larger than we nevertheless have smaller brains (Figure 2-5). Overall, then, relative to our body size, humans have larger brains than most other animals. It is tempting to attribute our mental abilities to our relatively large brains, but this is an oversimplification. Relative to body size, dolphins, some small primates and rodents, and even some fish have larger brains than we do. The key differences in our brains appear to lie in an increased complexity of neuronal interconnections and in a selective increase in the size of certain areas of the cerebral cortex thought to be involved in higher functions (see Figure 15-13).

## SURFACE FEATURES OF THE CEREBRAL HEMISPHERES

A striking aspect of human cerebral hemispheres is the degree to which their surface is folded and convoluted. Each ridge is called a *gyrus,* and each groove between

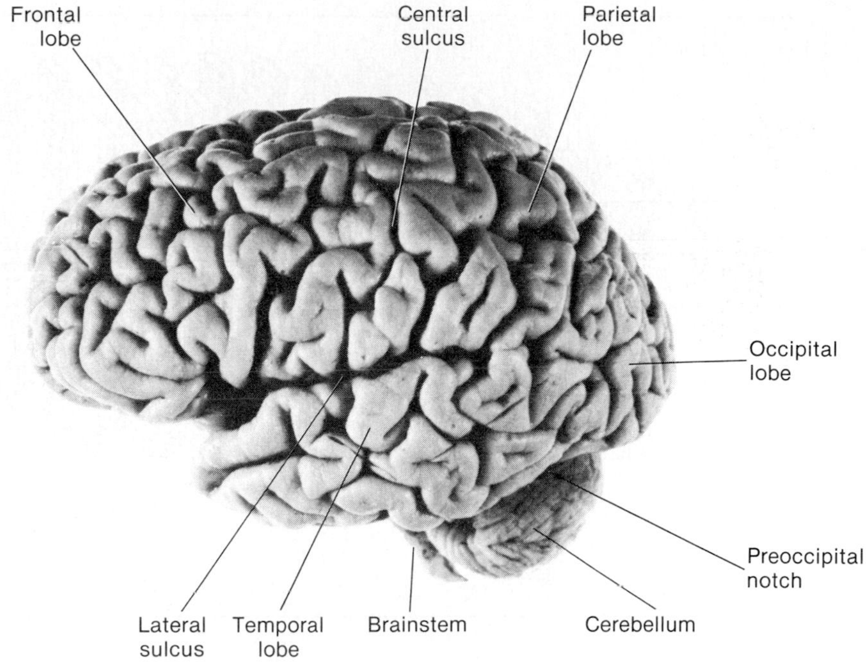


FIGURE 2-2
Major regions of the adult brain as seen in a lateral view.

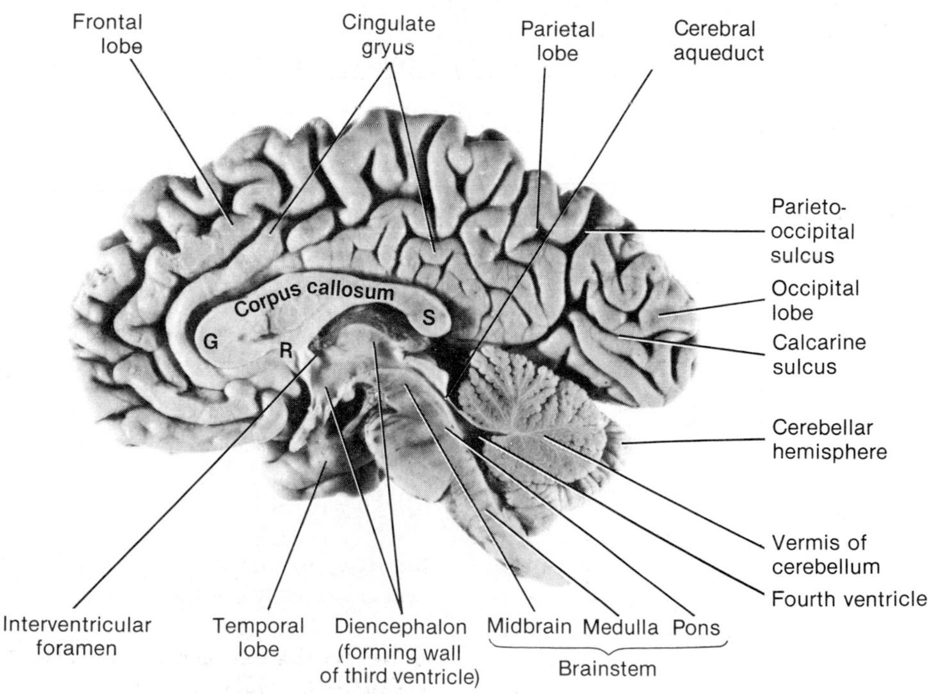


FIGURE 2-3
Major regions of the cerebrum, cerebellum, and brainstem as seen in the sagittal plane. *R*, *G*, and *S* indicate the rostrum, genu, and splenium, respectively, of the corpus callosum.

A

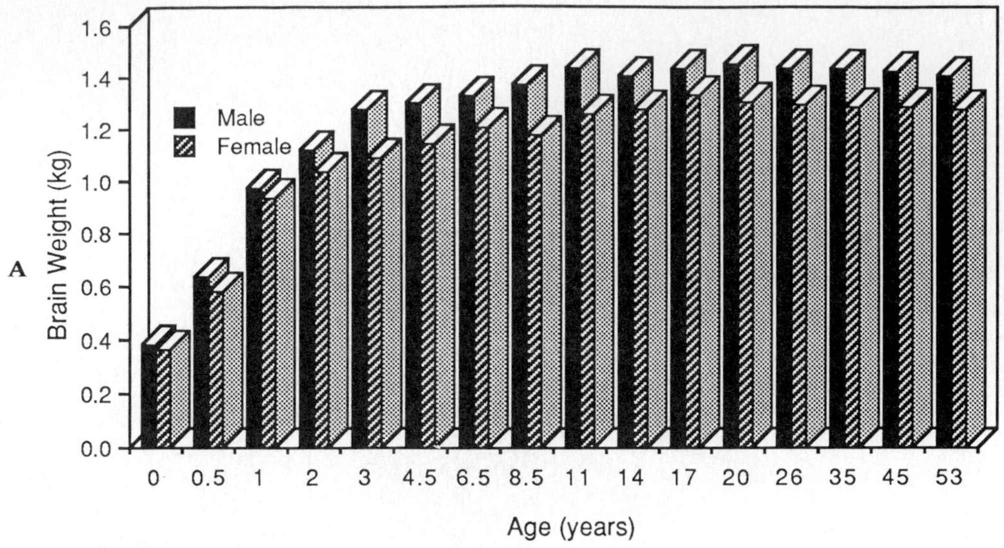


B

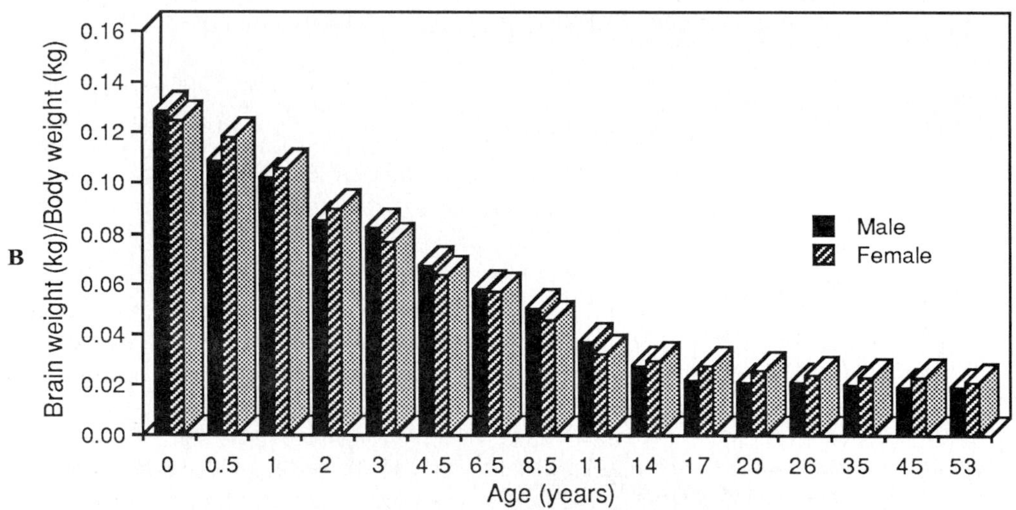


FIGURE 2-4
**A,** Average brain weights of human males and females at different ages. Notice how the brain grows rapidly after birth, doubling in the first year of life, before reaching its full size at about the age of 11. At all ages, male brains have a greater average weight than female brains. However, as indicated in **B,** adult female brains actually account for a greater percentage of body weight than do adult male brains. Brain growth is substantial in utero, and we are born with brains that are very large relative to our bodies. After the brain growth spurt of the first 1 to 3 years of life, body growth takes over and the brain weight/body weight ratio declines progressively until about age 17.

Plotted from the data of Dekaban AS, Sadowsky D: *Ann Neurol* 4:345, 1978.

ridges is called a *sulcus;* particularly deep sulci are often called *fissures*. This folding into gyri and sulci is a mechanism for increasing the total cortical area; each of us has about 2.5 sq ft of cortex, two thirds of which is hidden from view in the walls of sulci. The appearance of various gyri and sulci varies considerably from one brain to another, to the point where they may not even be continuous structures (for example, a particular gyrus may be transected by one or more sulci). Major features are, however, reasonably constant.

In the following account the principal surface features of the hemispheres are described, with some broad generalizations regarding the function of various cortical areas. These functional descriptions are highly oversimplified and are offered merely for purposes of initial orientation. Cortical function is discussed in more detail in Chapter 15.

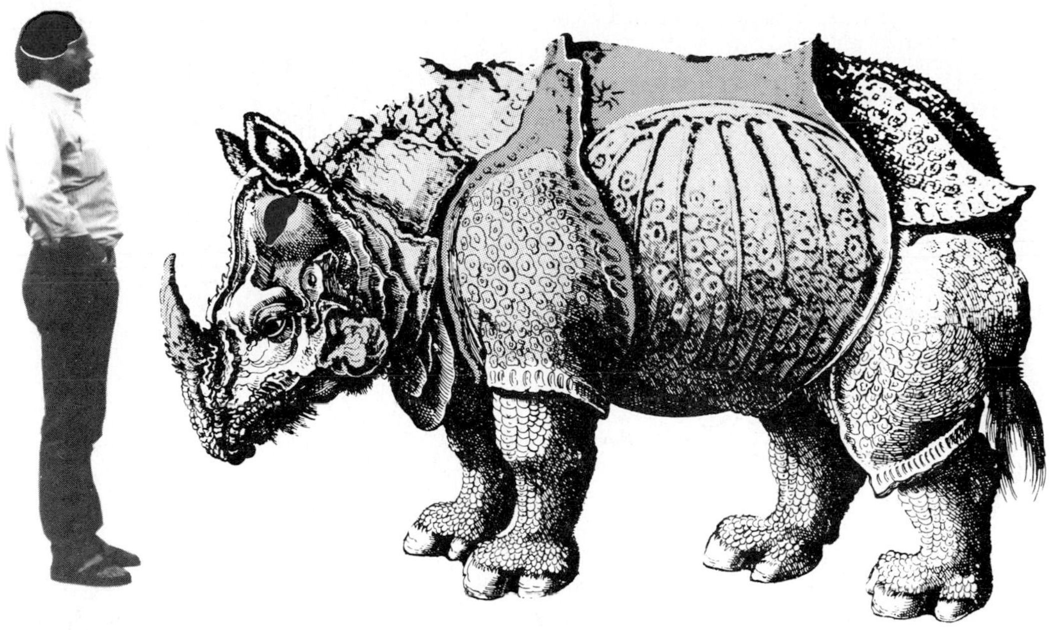

FIGURE 2-5
The relative sizes of the brain of a rhinoceros and the alleged brain of the author. Although the rhino's body weight is about 30 times greater, its brain weight is likely to be only half as great.
Drawing of rhino courtesy of Albrecht Dürer; author courtesy of Mr. and Mrs. Nolte; suggested by an illustration in Cobb, 1965.

## Cerebral lobes

Four prominent sulci—the *central sulcus,* the *lateral sulcus,* the *parietooccipital sulcus,* and part of the *calcarine sulcus*—and the *preoccipital notch* are used to divide each cerebral hemisphere into four lobes (Figures 2-2, 2-3, and 2-6).

1. The *frontal lobe* (see Figure 2-9) extends from the anterior tip of the brain (the *frontal pole*) to the central sulcus (or *sulcus of Rolando*). Inferiorly it ends at the lateral sulcus *(fissure of Sylvius)*. On the medial surface of the brain, it extends posteriorly to an imaginary line from the top of the central sulcus to the corpus callosum.

2. The *parietal lobe* (see Figure 2-10) extends from the central sulcus to an imaginary line connecting the top of the parietooccipital sulcus and the preoccipital notch (see Figure 2-2). Inferiorly it is bounded by the lateral sulcus and the imaginary continuation of this sulcus to the posterior boundary of the parietal lobe. On the medial surface of the brain, it is bounded inferiorly by the corpus callosum and calcarine sulcus, anteriorly by the frontal lobe, and posteriorly by the parietooccipital sulcus.

3. The *temporal lobe* (see Figure 2-11) extends superiorly to the lateral sulcus and the line forming the inferior boundary of the parietal lobe; posteriorly it extends to the line connecting the top of the parietooccipital sulcus and the preoccipital notch. On the medial surface its posterior boundary is an imaginary line from the preoccipital notch to the splenium of the corpus callosum.

4. The *occipital lobe* (see Figure 2-13) is bounded anteriorly by the parietal and temporal lobes on both the lateral and medial surfaces of the hemisphere.

These separations do not correspond to precise functional subdivisions, but they do provide a meaningful basis for discussion and reference.

An additional area of cerebral cortex not usually included in any of the four lobes discussed above lies buried in the depths of the lateral sulcus, concealed from view by portions of the frontal, parietal, and temporal lobes. This cortex, called the *insula,* overlies the site where the telencephalon and diencephalon fused during embryological development (Chapter 1). It can be revealed by prying open the lateral sulcus or by removing the overlying portions of other lobes (Figure 2-7). The portion of a given lobe overlying the insula is called an *operculum* (Latin for lid); there are frontal, parietal, and temporal opercula. The *circular sulcus* outlines the insula and marks its borders with the opercular areas of cortex.

The *cingulate gyrus,* immediately superior to the corpus callosum, can be followed posteriorly to the splenium of the corpus callosum, where it turns inferiorly as the narrow *isthmus* of the cingulate gyrus and continues as the *parahippocampal gyrus* of the temporal lobe. These two gyri give the appearance of encircling the diencephalon and they, together with the *olfactory bulb, olfactory tract,* and certain other small cortical areas, are often referred to separately as the *limbic lobe* (from the Latin word *limbus*

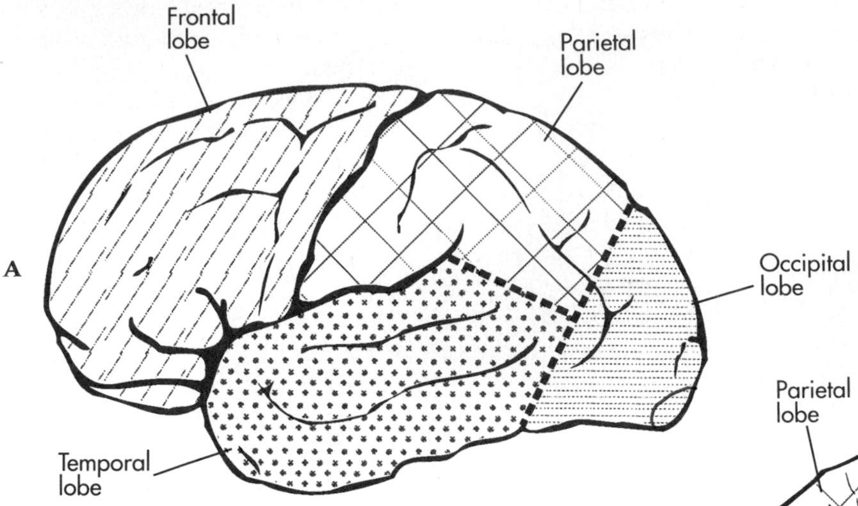

Frontal lobe
Parietal lobe
A
Occipital lobe
Temporal lobe

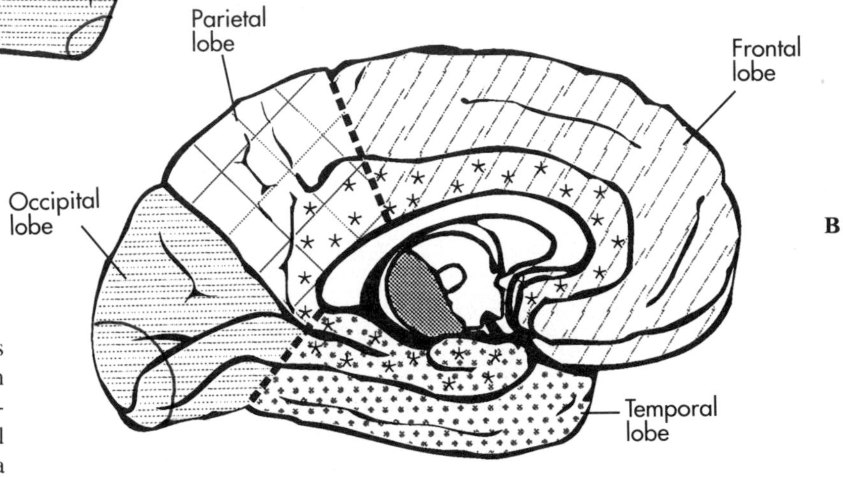

Parietal lobe
Frontal lobe
Occipital lobe
B
Temporal lobe

FIGURE 2-6
Lobes of the cerebral hemisphere. **A,** The boundaries of the frontal, parietal, occipital, and temporal lobes on the lateral surface of the hemisphere. **B,** The boundaries of the frontal, parietal, occipital, and temporal lobes on the lateral surface of the hemisphere; the area covered by stars is considered by many as a separate limbic lobe.

Adapted from Ono M et al, *Atlas of the cerebral sulci,* New York, 1990, Thieme Medical Publishers.

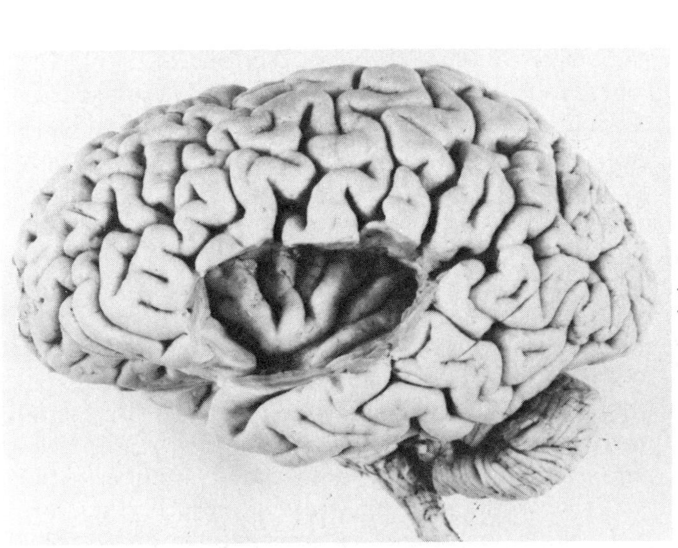

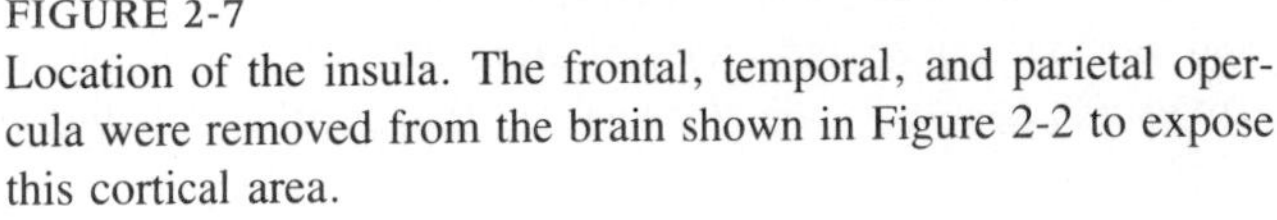

FIGURE 2-7
Location of the insula. The frontal, temporal, and parietal opercula were removed from the brain shown in Figure 2-2 to expose this cortical area.

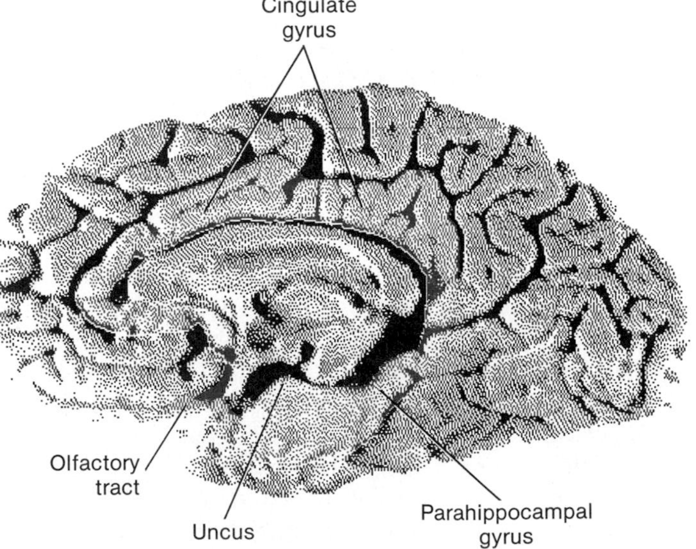


FIGURE 2-8
Limbic lobe as seen on the medial surface of a hemisected brain from which the brainstem and cerebellum were removed.

meaning *border*). As indicated in Figure 2-8, the limbic lobe therefore contains portions of what would otherwise be considered frontal, parietal, and temporal cortex. The limbic lobe and many of the structures with which it is interconnected make up the *limbic system,* which is important in emotional responses and drive-related behavior.

### Frontal lobe

Four gyri make up the lateral surface of the frontal lobe (Figure 2-9). The *precentral gyrus* is anterior to the central sulcus and parallel to it, extending to the *precentral sulcus*. The *superior, middle,* and *inferior frontal gyri* are oriented parallel to one another and roughly perpendicular to the precentral gyrus. The superior frontal gyrus continues onto the medial surface of the hemisphere as far as the *cingulate sulcus*. The inferior frontal gyrus is visibly divided into three parts: (1) the *orbital part,* which is most anterior and is continuous with the inferior *(orbital)* surface of the frontal lobe; (2) the *opercular part,* which is most posterior and forms a portion of the frontal operculum; and (3) the wedge-shaped *triangular part,* which lies between the other two. The inferior or orbital surface of the frontal lobe is mostly occupied by a group of gyri of variable appearance that are collectively called *orbital gyri*. The only named gyrus on this surface is the *gyrus rectus,* which is most medial and extends onto the medial surface of the hemisphere. Between the gyrus rectus and the orbital gyri is the *olfactory sulcus,* containing the olfactory bulb and tract. The medial surface of the lobe contains part of the cingulate gyrus, extensions of the superior frontal gyrus, precentral gyrus, and gyrus rectus, and certain small cortical areas near the rostrum of the corpus callosum that are related to the limbic system.

The frontal lobe contains four general functional areas:

1. The *primary motor cortex* occupies much of the precentral gyrus. It contains many of the cells of origin of descending motor pathways and is involved in the initiation of voluntary movements.
2. The *premotor area* is made up of the remainder of the precentral gyrus together with adjacent portions

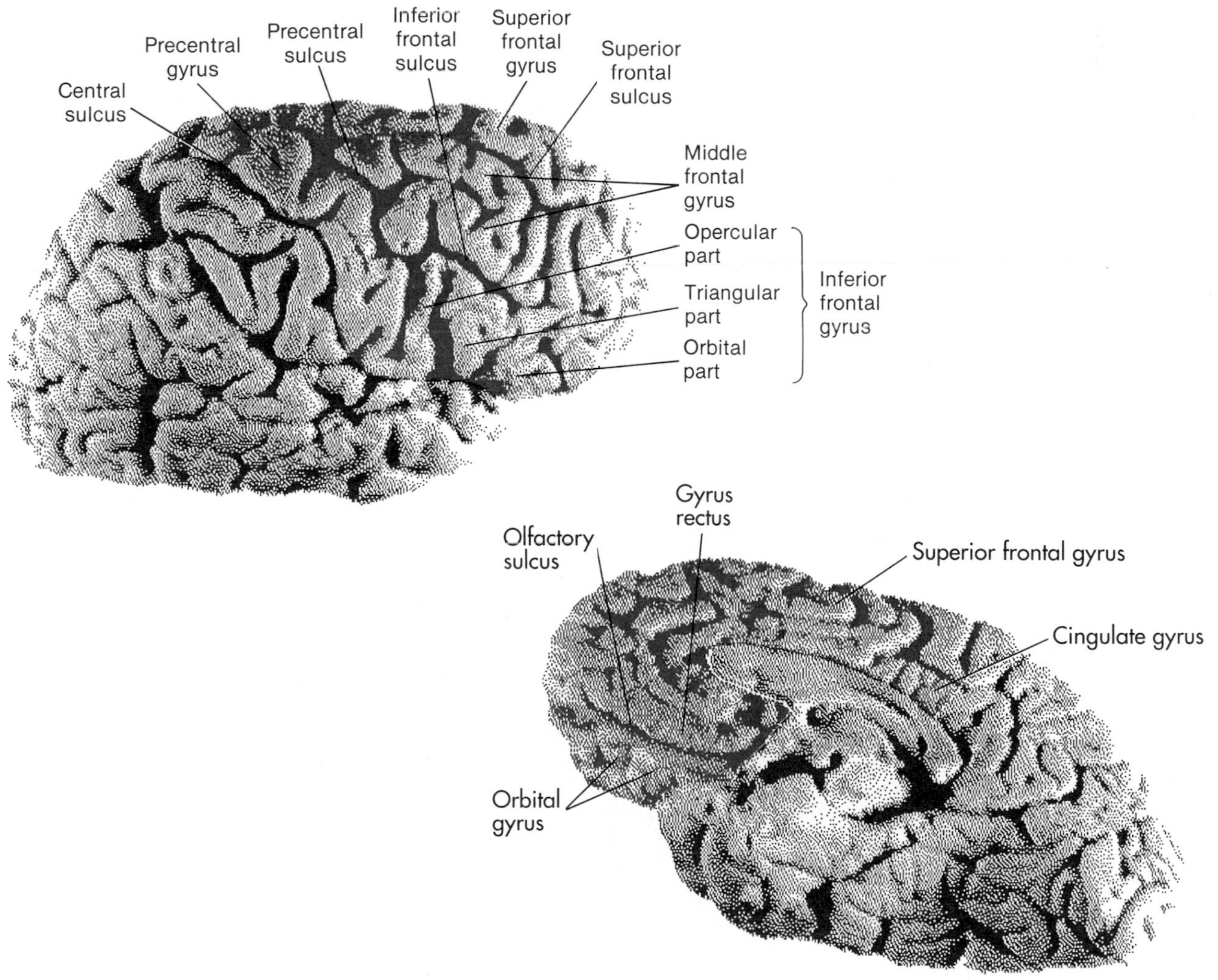


FIGURE 2-9
Lateral, medial, and inferior surfaces of the frontal lobe.

of the superior and middle frontal gyri and also is functionally related to the initiation of voluntary movements.

3. *Broca's area,* the opercular and triangular parts of the inferior frontal gyrus of one hemisphere (usually the left), is important in the production of written and spoken language.
4. The *prefrontal cortex,* a very large and somewhat confusingly named area comprising the remainder of the frontal lobe, is involved with what may very generally be described as personality, insight, and foresight.

### Parietal lobe

The lateral surface of the parietal lobe is divided into three areas: the *postcentral gyrus* and the *superior* and *inferior parietal lobules* (Figure 2-10). The postcentral gyrus is posterior to the central sulcus and parallel to it, extending to the *postcentral sulcus.* The *intraparietal sulcus* runs posteriorly from the postcentral sulcus toward the occipital lobe, separating the superior and inferior parietal lobules. The inferior parietal lobule in turn is composed of the *supramarginal gyrus,* which caps the upturned end of the lateral sulcus, and the *angular gyrus,* which similarly caps the *superior temporal sulcus.* The angular gyrus is typically broken up by small sulci and may overlap the supramarginal gyrus. The medial surface of the parietal lobe contains a portion of the cingulate gyrus and the medial extension of the postcentral gyrus. It is completed by an area called the *precuneus,* which is bounded by the cingulate gyrus, the parietooccipital sulcus, and the *marginal branch* of the cingulate sulcus. The extensions of the precentral and postcentral gyri onto the medial surface of the hemisphere are sometimes referred to together as the *paracentral lobule,* which is partly in the frontal lobe and partly in the parietal lobe.

The parietal lobe is associated, in a very general sense, with three functions:

1. The postcentral gyrus more or less coincides with *primary somatosensory cortex;* that is, it is con-

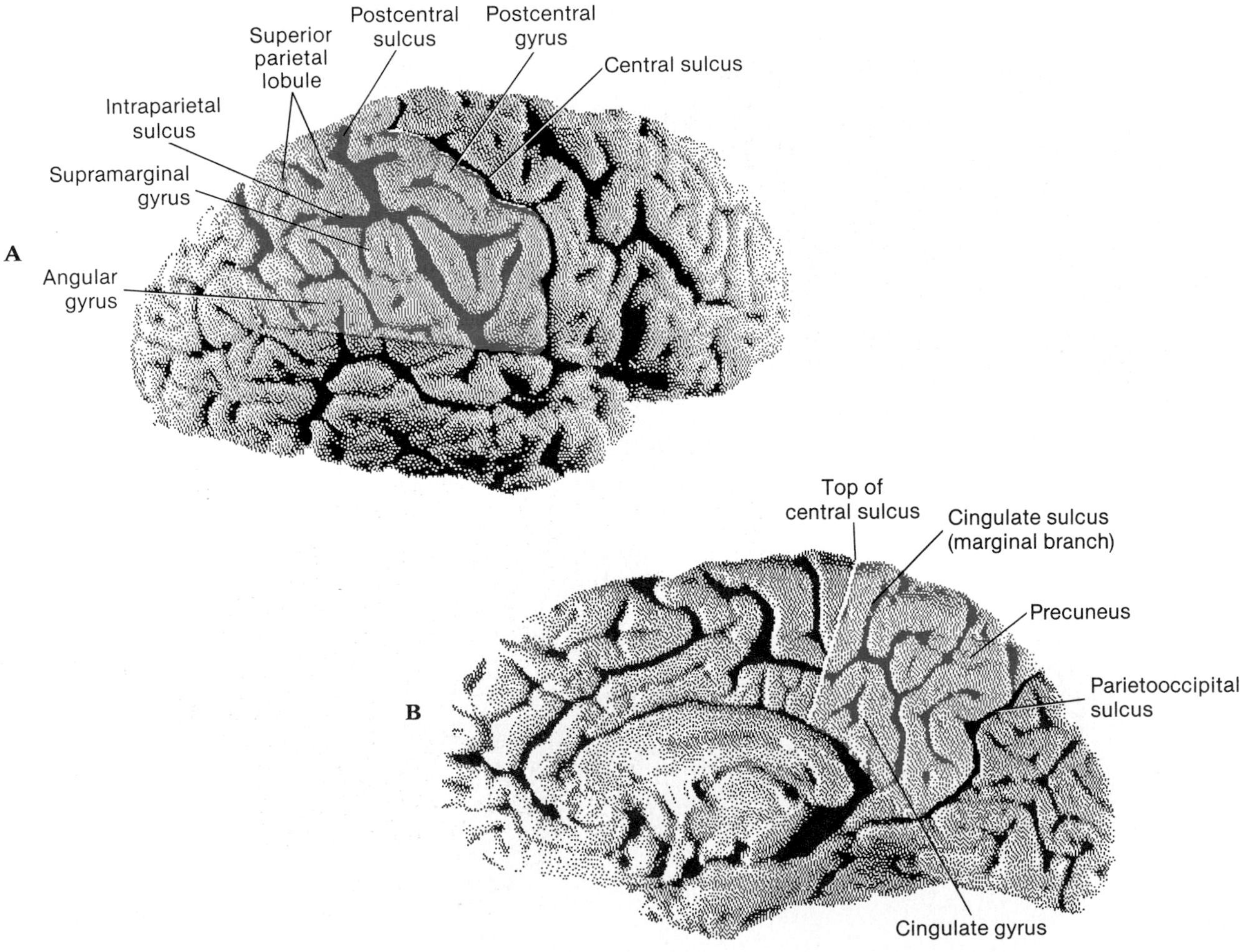


FIGURE 2-10
Lateral and medial surfaces of the parietal lobe.

cerned with the initial cortical processing of tactile and proprioceptive (sense of position) information.

2. Much of the inferior parietal lobule of one hemisphere (usually the left), together with portions of the temporal lobe, is involved in the comprehension of language.
3. The remainder of the parietal cortex subserves complex aspects of spatial orientation and perception.

### *Temporal lobe*

The lateral surface of the temporal lobe is composed of the *superior, middle,* and *inferior temporal gyri* (Figure 2-11). The superior temporal gyrus continues into the lateral sulcus where it forms one of its walls. Thus part of the superior temporal gyrus forms the temporal operculum. The inferior temporal gyrus continues onto the inferior surface of the lobe. The rest of the inferior surface is made up of the broad and often discontinuous *occipitotemporal (fusiform) gyrus* and the *parahippocampal gyrus,* separated from one another by the *collateral sulcus*. The occipitotemporal gyrus, as its name implies, is partly in the occipital lobe and partly in the temporal lobe. The parahippo-campal gyrus is continuous with the cingulate gyrus around the splenium of the corpus callosum by way of the isthmus of the cingulate gyrus. The anterior end of the parahippocampal gyrus turns backward and forms a medially directed bump called the *uncus*. The superior border of the parahippocampal gyrus is the *hippocampal sulcus* (Figures 2-8 and 2-11). Folded into the temporal lobe at the hippocampal sulcus is an area of cortex called the *hippocampus,* which is part of the limbic system. The hippocampus cannot be seen without sectioning or dissecting the brain (Figures 2-12 and 2-21).

The temporal lobe is associated in a general way with three functions:

1. A small area of that portion of the superior temporal gyrus that lies in the lateral sulcus is the *primary auditory cortex*.

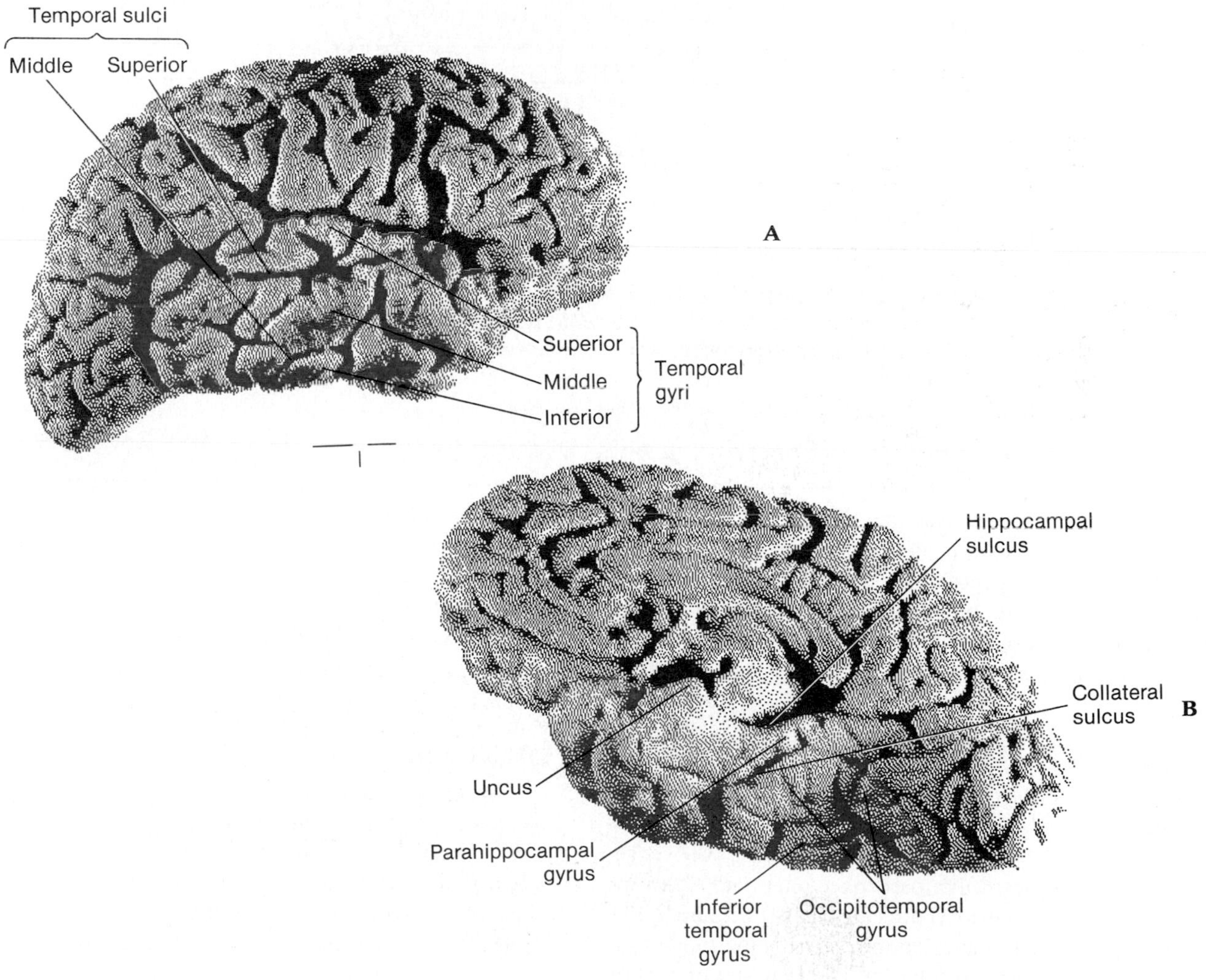


FIGURE 2-11
Lateral, medial, and inferior surfaces of the temporal lobe.

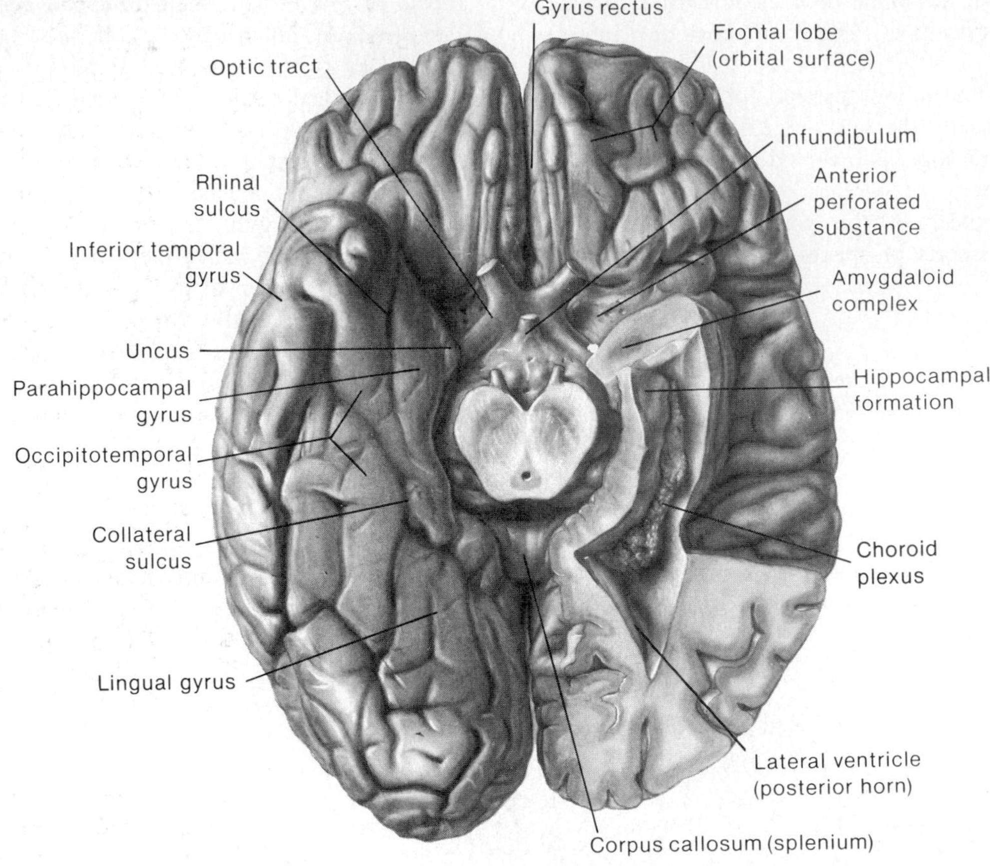


FIGURE 2-12
Dissection of the temporal lobe to demonstrate the hippocampus. The hippocampus is a cortical area that has folded into the inferior horn of the lateral ventricle in the temporal lobe. The anterior perforated substance is an area of the base of the brain where many small blood vessels enter the cerebrum. The rhinal sulcus looks like an anterior continuation of the collateral sulcus, but is acturally a separate landmark.
From Mettler FA: Neuroanatomy, ed 2, St. Louis, 1948, Mosby–Year Book.

2. The parahippocampal gyrus and hippocampus are parts of the limbic system.
3. The temporal lobe is involved in complex aspects of learning and memory.

The second and third functions overlap to some degree. For example, portions of the limbic system, particularly the hippocampus, are important for memory processes.

### *Occipital lobe*

The lateral surface of the occipital lobe is of variable configuration, and its gyri are usually referred to simply as *lateral occipital gyri*. On the medial surface, the wedge-shaped area between the parietooccipital and calcarine sulci is called the *cuneus* (Latin for wedge) (Figure 2-13). The gyrus inferior to the calcarine sulcus is the *lingual gyrus*. The lingual gyrus is adjacent to the posterior portion of the occipitotemporal gyrus, separated from it by the collateral sulcus, and usually continuous anteriorly with the parahippocampal gyrus. The transition from lingual to parahippocampal gyrus occurs at the isthmus of the cingulate gyrus (Figure 2-8).

The occipital lobe is more or less exclusively concerned with visual functions. *Primary visual cortex* is contained in the walls of the calcarine sulcus and a bit of the surrounding cortex. The remainder of the lobe is referred to as *visual association cortex* and is involved in higher order processing of visual information.

## DIENCEPHALON

The diencephalon accounts for only about 2% of the weight of the brain, but nevertheless is extremely important. It has four divisions: *thalamus, hypothalamus, epithalamus,* and *subthalamus*. Portions of three of these divisions can be seen on a hemisected brain (Figure 2-14); the subthalamus is an internal structure that can be seen only in sections through the brain.

The thalamus is an ovoid nuclear mass, part of which borders on the third ventricle. The line of attachment of the roof of this ventricle is marked by a horizontally ori-

A

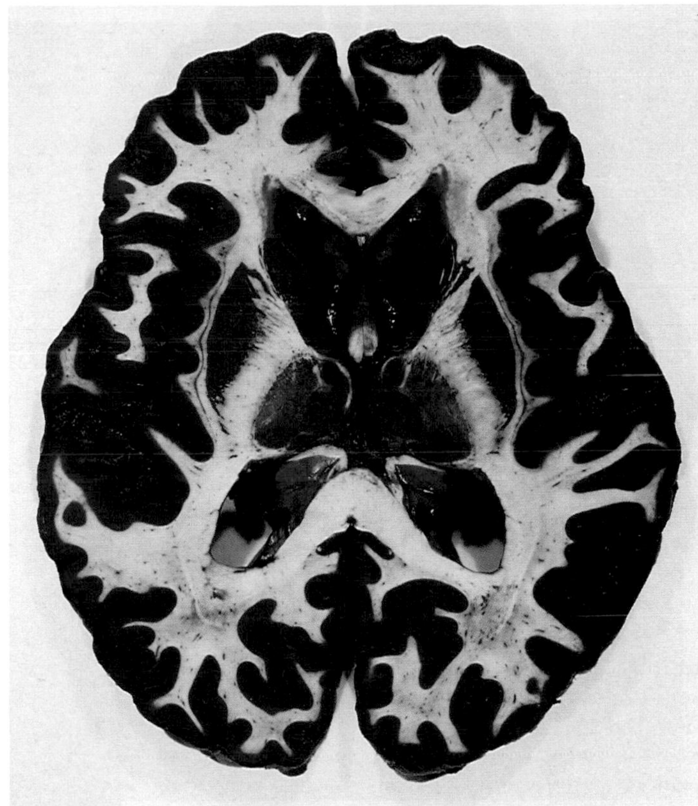

B

PLATE 1

**A,** Slice of a whole human brain, approximately 6 mm thick, stained by a method that differentiates between gray and white matter. Pretreatment with phenol makes the white matter resistant to the blue copper sulfate stain, so white matter appears white and gray matter appears bright blue. **B,** 40 μm section from the central region of the same area shown in **A;** in this case, Luxol fast blue was used to stain myelinated fibers blue-violet, and neutral red was used as a counterstain for neuronal nuclei. Anterior is up in both **A** and **B.**

Courtesy of Pam Eller, University of Colorado Health Sciences Center.

PLATE 9 (below)

Combined use of a neurotransmitter identification technique and intracellular injection of dye. A subset of retinal amacrine cells (see Chapter 11) uses serotonin as a neurotransmitter. These neurons accumulate serotonin from the surrounding medium and also accumulate certain analogs of serotonin. **A,** A flourescent analog (5,7-dihydroxytryptamine) was applied to a living, flat-mounted rabbit retina, which was then viewed using ultraviolet illumination. Serotonin-accumulating amacrine cells fluoresce blue under these conditions, allowing chemically identified neurons to be impaled by dye-filled micropipette electrodes. **B,** A serotoninergic amacrine cell injected with a fluorescent dye (Lucifer yellow). Details of the long, mostly unbranched dendrites of this neuron are readily apparent.

Courtesy of Dr. David I. Vaney, National Vision Research Institute of Australia.

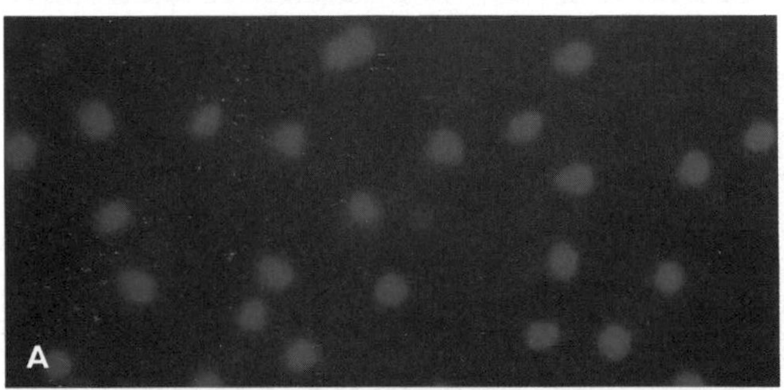


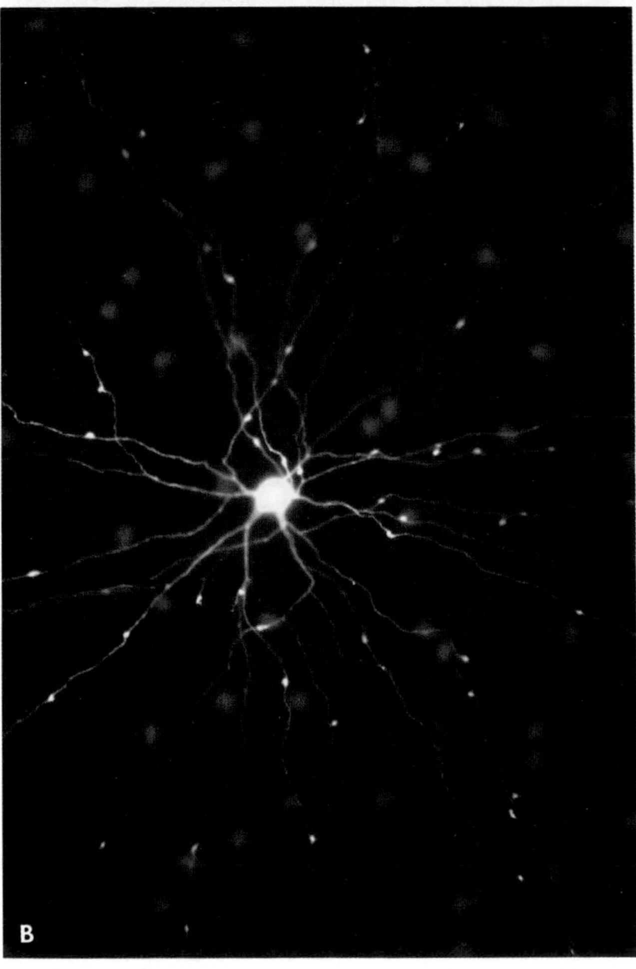


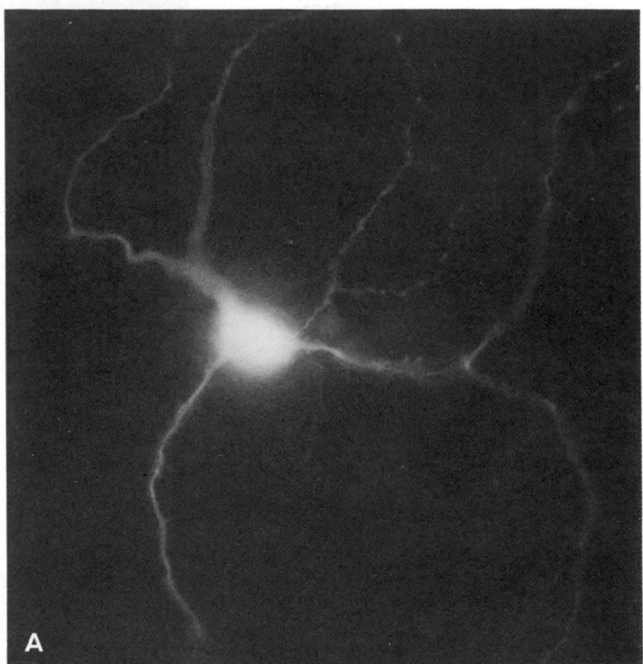


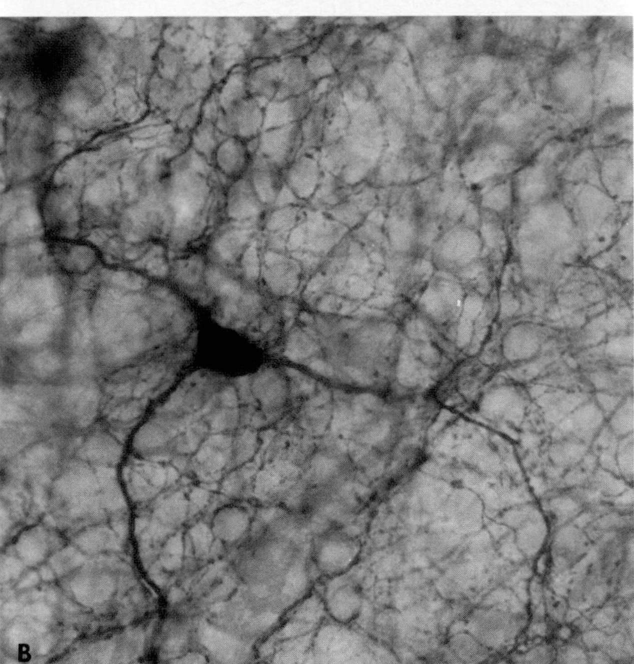


PLATE 10

An additional example of combined use of a neurotransmitter identificaiton technique and intracellular injection of dye. Another subset of retinal amacrine cells uses dopamine as a neurotransmitter. One such ganglion cell was first injected with a fluorescent dye (Lucifer yellow, **A**). The same area of retina was then stained with an antibody to tyrosine hydroxylase (an enzyme involved in the synthesis of dopamine), as shown in **B.** The obvious correspondence between the two images indicates that the injected amacrine cell manufactures dopamine.

Courtesy of Dr. Dennis M. Dacey, University of Washington School of Medicine.

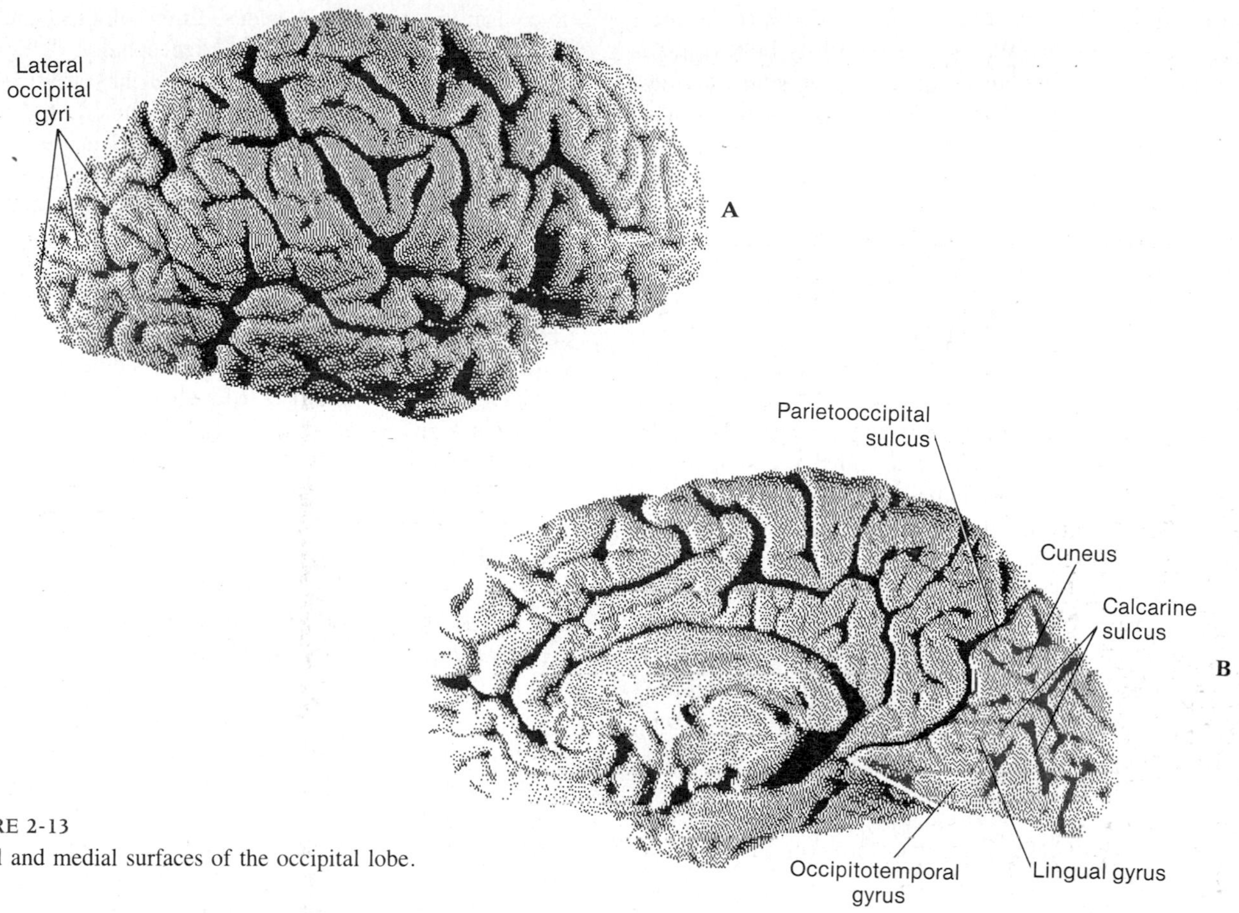

Lateral occipital gyri

A

Parietooccipital sulcus

Cuneus

Calcarine sulcus

B

Occipitotemporal gyrus

Lingual gyrus

FIGURE 2-13
Lateral and medial surfaces of the occipital lobe.

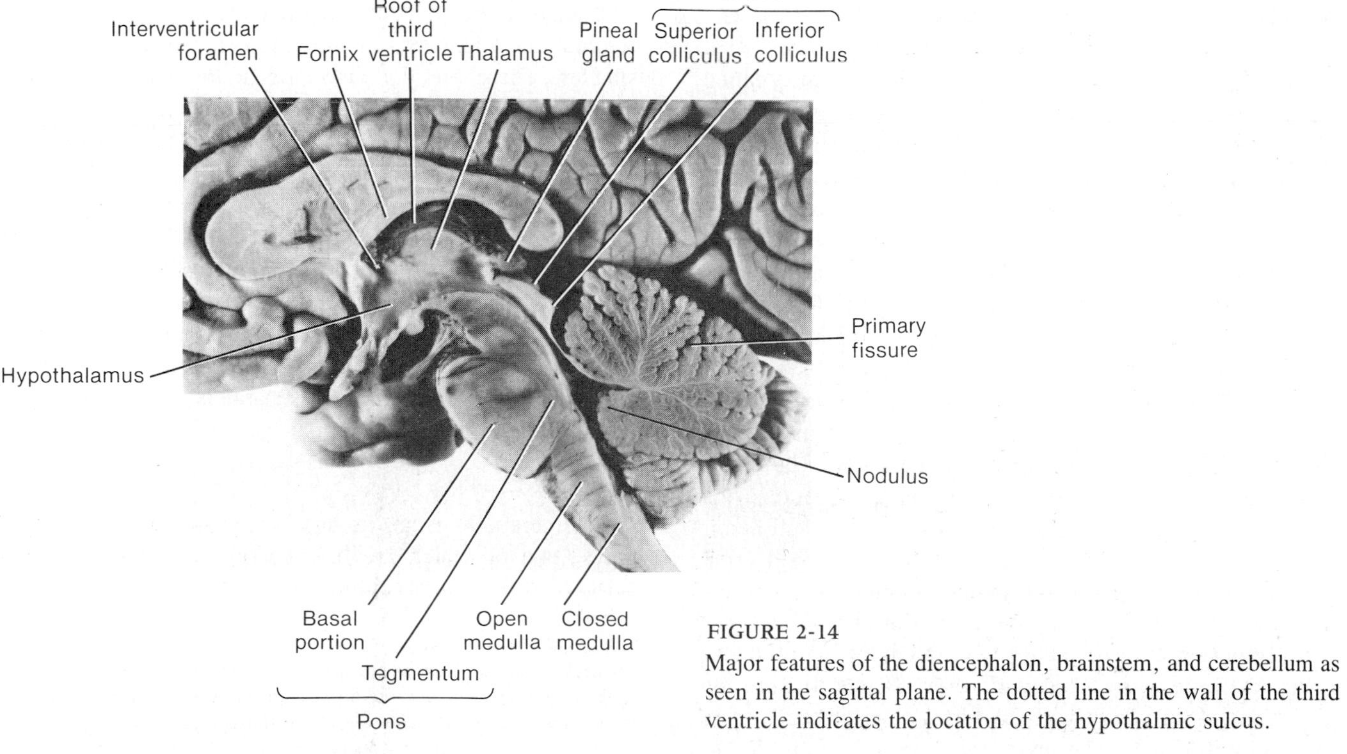


FIGURE 2-14
Major features of the diencephalon, brainstem, and cerebellum as seen in the sagittal plane. The dotted line in the wall of the third ventricle indicates the location of the hypothalmic sulcus.

ented ridge, the *stria medullaris thalami*. Parts of the medial surfaces of the two thalami fuse in many brains, in an area called the *interthalamic adhesion* or *massa intermedia*. Since the massa intermedia is absent in many normal brains (including the one shown in Figure 2-14), it apparently performs no unique function. Posteriorly the thalamus protrudes over the most rostral portion of the brainstem. Anteriorly it abuts the interventricular foramen. The thalamus is a nuclear mass of major importance in both sensory and motor systems. No sensory information, with the exception of olfactory information, reaches the cerebral cortex without prior processing in thalamic nuclei. In addition, the anatomical loops characteristic of motor systems, which involve pathways between the cerebellum and cerebral cortex and between basal ganglia and cerebral cortex, typically involve thalamic nuclei as well.

The hypothalamus is inferior to the thalamus, separated from it by the *hypothalamic sulcus* in the wall of the third ventricle. It also forms the floor of the ventricle, and its inferior surface is one of the few parts of the diencephalon visible on an intact brain. This inferior surface (see Figure 2-16) includes the *infundibular stalk* and two rounded protuberances, the *mammillary bodies*. The hypothalamus is the major visceral control center of the brain and is involved in limbic system functions as well.

The epithalamus comprises the midline *pineal gland* and several small neural structures visible in sections.

## BRAINSTEM

The brainstem plays major roles in cranial nerve functions, in conveying information to and from the cerebrum, and in some special functions of its own. It is divided into the midbrain, the pons, and the medulla (Figure 2-3). The *tectum* (Latin for roof) of the midbrain, that portion dorsal to the cerebral aqueduct, consists of paired bumps called the *superior* and *inferior colliculi* (Latin for little hills). The paired *cerebral penduncles* make up the remainder of the midbrain (see Figures 2-20 and 2-21). The pons consists of a protruding *basal portion,* oval in the sagittal section, and the overlying *pontine tegmentum,* which forms part of the floor of the fourth ventricle. The medulla consists of a rostral *open* portion, containing part of the fourth ventricle, and a caudal *closed* portion, continuous with the spinal cord (Figure 2-14).

The points of attachment of most cranial nerves, as well as additional brainstem structures, can be seen in an inferior view of the brain (Figures 2-15 and 2-16). The olfactory tract is located in the olfactory sulcus, lateral to the gyrus rectus, and is attached directly to the cerebral hemisphere. *Cranial nerve I (olfactory)* is actually a collection of bundles of very fine axons called *olfactory fila* that terminate in the olfactory bulb at the anterior end of the tract. Slightly posterior to the attachment points of the olfactory tracts, the *optic nerves (cranial nerve II)* join to form the *optic chiasm,* in which half the fibers of each nerve cross to the opposite side. The *optic tract* proceeds from the optic chiasm to a thalamic nucleus. Embryologically the optic nerves are outgrowths of the diencephalon (Chapter 1) and properly are tracts of the CNS, but they are treated as cranial nerves because of their course outside the rest of the brain. Considered in this way, cranial nerve II is the only one that projects directly to the diencephalon.

Located farther posteriorly are the cerebral peduncles of the midbrain, each of which contains a massive fiber bundle that carries a great deal of the descending projection from the cerebral cortex to the brainstem and spinal cord. *Cranial nerve III (oculomotor)* emerges into the *interpeduncular fossa* between the cerebral peduncles. *Cranial nerve IV (trochlear)* emerges from the dorsal surface of the brainstem just caudal to the inferior colliculi, then proceeds anteriorly through the space between the brainstem and the cerebral hemisphere.

Caudally the cerebral peduncles disappear into the transversely oriented basal portion of the pons. Dorsolaterally this part of the pons narrows into a large fiber bundle that enters the cerebellum. This is the *middle cerebellar peduncle (brachium pontis),* which carries the major input from the cerebral hemispheres to the cerebellum by way of relays in nuclei of the pons (Figures 2-16 and 2-22). *Cranial nerve V (trigeminal)* emerges from the lateral aspect of the basal portion of the pons. *Cranial nerve VI (abducens)* emerges near the midline at the caudal edge of the pons. *Cranial nerves VII (facial)* and *VIII (vestibulocochlear)* emerge more laterally near the cerebellum, at the caudal edge of the pons. The area of attachment of cranial nerves VII and VIII is called the *cerebellopontine angle* and is a common site of development of tumors, such as tumors of the sheaths of these cranial nerves.

Caudal to the pons are two thick fiber bundles that resemble the cerebral peduncles but are considerably smaller. These are the *pyramids* of the medulla, which carry those fibers of the cerebral peduncles that are directed to the spinal cord. The two pyramids decussate* in the area of transition from brainstem to spinal cord. Dorsolateral to each pyramid is an ovoid protuberance called the *olive*. *Cranial nerve XII (hypoglossal)* emerges from the sulcus between the pyramid and the olive. The more or less continuous series of filaments that will form *cranial nerves IX (glossopharyngeal)* and *X (vagus)* emerge from the sulcus dorsal to the olive. (The most caudal of these filaments are often considered separately as a *cranial part of nerve XI* [*accessory nerve*].)

## CEREBELLUM

The cerebellum can be subdivided in several different ways, two of which are briefly considered here. In one sense the cerebellum comprises a midline *vermis,* which is

*A *decussation* is a site where nerve fibers joining unlike areas of the CNS cross, such as here where fibers cross on their way from one side of the cerebrum to the opposite side of the spinal cord. In contrast, a *commissure* is a crossing site for fibers connecting like areas.

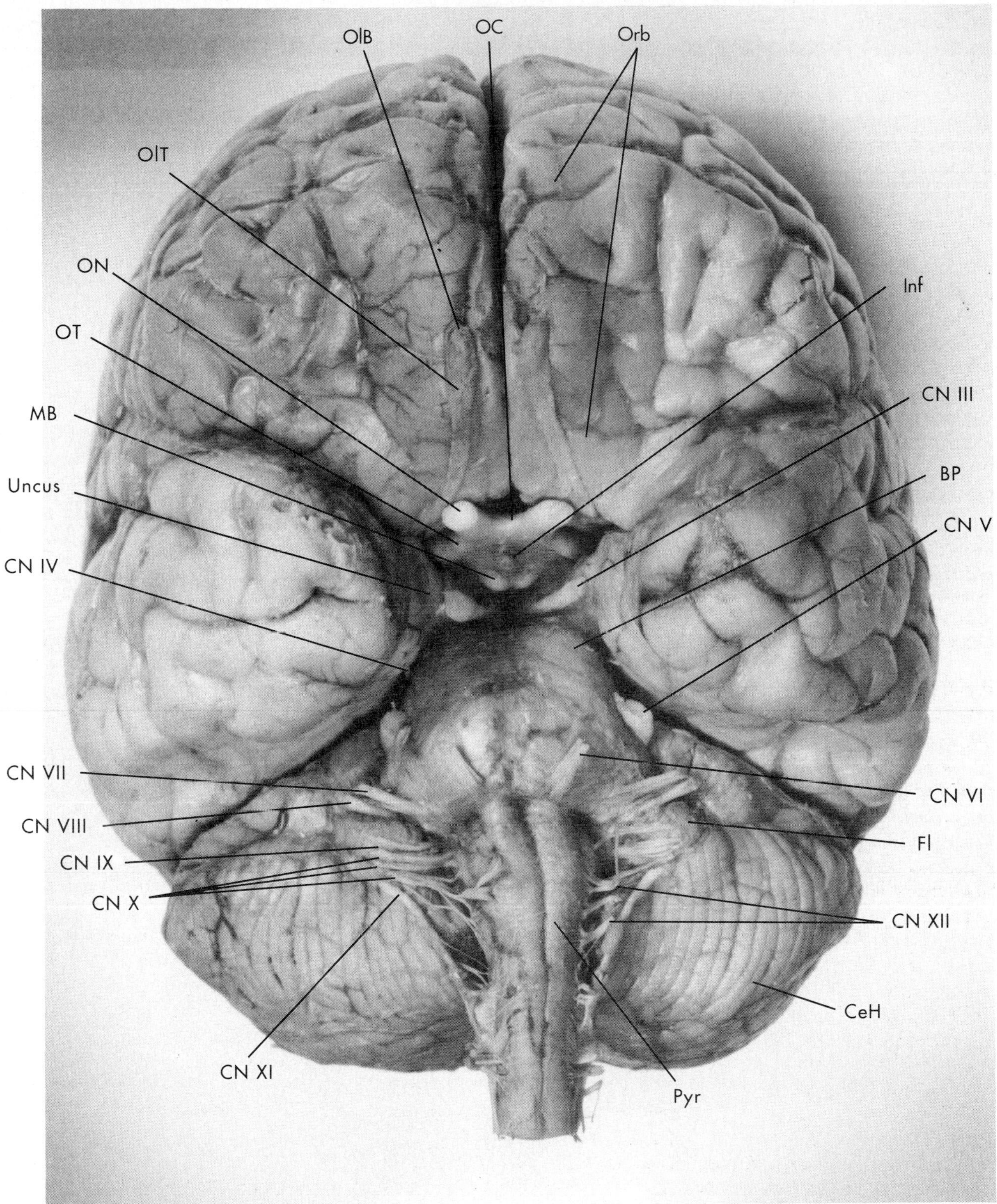


FIGURE 2-15

Inferior surface of a brain, showing the locations of the cranial nerves. Abbreviations: *BP,* basal part of the pons; *CeH,* cerebellar hemisphere; *Fl,* flocculus; *Inf,* infundibular stalk (former attachment of the pituitary gland); *MB,* mammillary body; *OC,* optic chaism; *OlB,* olfactory bulb; *OlT,* olfactory tract; *ON,* optic nerve (cranial nerve II); *Orb,* orbital gyri; *OT,* optic tract; *Pyr,* pyramid.
Dissection courtesy of Norman Koelling, The University of Arizona College of Medicine.

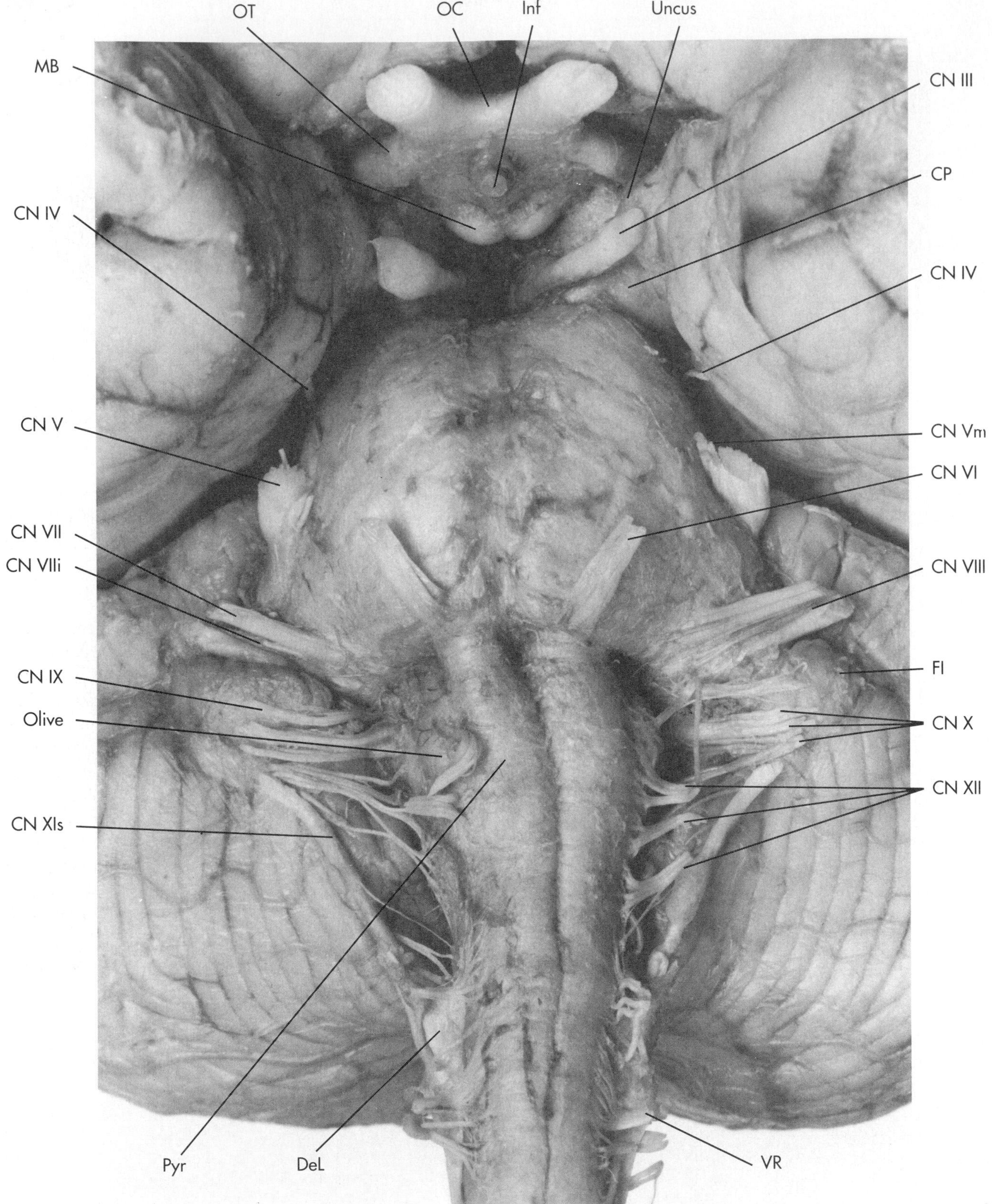


**FIGURE 2-16**

Closeup of the inferior surface of the same brain shown in Figure 2-15. Abbreviations: *CN Vm*, motor root of the trigeminal nerve; *CN VIIi*, intermediate nerve (part of the facial nerve); *CN XIs*, accessory nerve (arises in the cervical spinal cord, often considered separately as the *spinal part* of the accessory nerve); *CP*, cerebral peduncle; *DeL*, dentate ligament (suspensory ligament of the spinal cord); *Fl*, flocculus; *Inf*, infundibular stalk (former attachment of the pituitary gland); *MB*, mammillary body; *OC*, optic chiasm; *ON*, optic nerve (cranial nerve II); *OT*, optic tract; *Pyr*, pyramid; *VR*, cervical ventral root.

Dissection courtesy of Norman Koelling, The University of Arizona College of Medicine.

hemisected in a hemisected brain (Figure 2-3), and a much larger *lateral hemisphere* on each side (Figure 2-2). Using any other method of subdividing the cerebellum, a given division has both a vermal and a hemispheral component.

Lobes of the cerebellum, which roughly correspond to separate functional areas, are also recognized. The *anterior lobe* is that portion anterior to the primary fissure (Figure 2-14). This lobe receives a large proportion of its afferent inputs from the spinal cord and plays a prominent role in postural adjustments. The *flocculonodular lobe* consists of three small components: the *nodulus,* which is the vermal portion of the lobe (Figure 2-14), and a small *flocculus* on each side near the vestibulocochlear nerve (Figure 2-15). The nodulus is actually continuous with the flocculus of each side, but this continuity is difficult to see without dissecting the cerebellum. The flocculonodular lobe receives afferent inputs from the vestibular system and is involved in controlling eye movements and postural adjustments to gravity. All of the cerebellum posterior to the primary fissure, exclusive of the flocculonodular lobe, constitutes the *posterior lobe,* which is the largest of the three. The posterior lobe receives the majority of the afferent input from the cerebral cortex by way of relays in *pontine nuclei* and transmission through the middle cerebellar peduncle. This lobe plays a prominent role in the coordination of voluntary movements. In reality, cerebellar function is not quite so neatly parceled out among the anatomical subdivisions; the details of cerebellar function are considered in Chapter 14.

## INTERNAL STRUCTURES

Before consideration of the internal structures of the brain, it is useful to discuss certain consequences of the shape of the cerebral hemispheres. As a result of the embryological development of the hemispheres (Chapter 1), the cortical lobes are arranged in a C shape from the frontal lobe, through the parietal and occipital lobes, and into the temporal lobe (Figure 2-17). A number of other structures, such as the lateral ventricles (see Figures 4-1 and 4-2), are similarly C shaped, with the result that sections through the brain may cut these structures in two different places. The hippocampus, together with its efferent fiber bundle (the *fornix*) (see Figure 16-9), is another example. The hippocampus is folded into the temporal lobe, forming part of the wall of the lateral ventricle there (see Figure 2-21). It becomes smaller as the temporal lobe curves into the parietal lobe, and it ends near the splenium of the corpus callosum. The fornix continues this curved course (Figure 2-14), arching anteriorly under the corpus callosum, then turning inferiorly and posteriorly toward the hypothalamus, where many of its fibers end in the mammillary bodies.

### Basal ganglia and amygdala

The basal ganglia are a group of nuclei that form part of each cerebral hemisphere. They are internal structures of

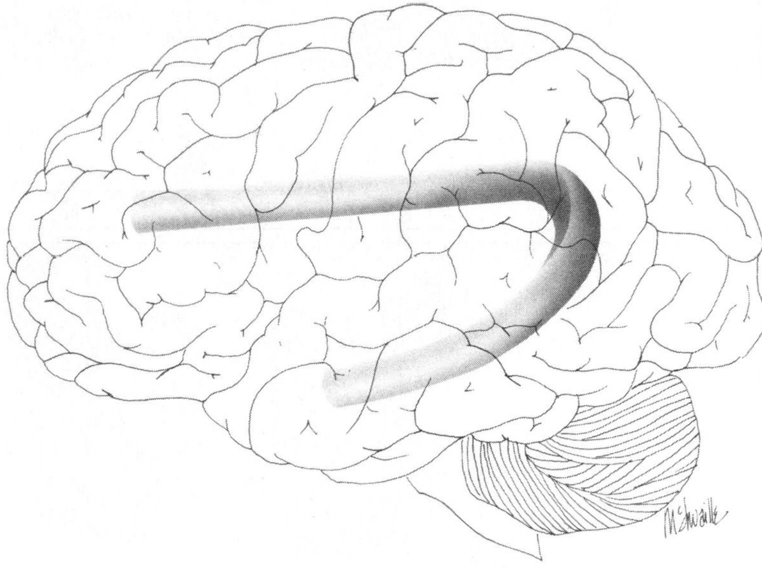


FIGURE 2-17
General configuration of C-shaped structures such as the lateral ventricle, the caudate nucleus, and the hippocampus-fornix system.

the hemisphere, visible only in sections. The major basal ganglia are the *caudate* and *lenticular nuclei* (together with some brainstem structures with which they are interconnected). The *amygdala,* another nucleus contained within each cerebral hemisphere, was historically considered to be one of the basal ganglia as well. However, because it has since been found to be part of the limbic system, the amygdala is now treated separately. The amygdala lies beneath the uncus of the temporal lobe (see Figure 2-20). The caudate nucleus, another example of a C-shaped structure, has an enlarged *head* deep in the frontal lobe, and its increasingly attenuated *body* and *tail* follow the lateral ventricle around into the temporal lobe, where it finally fuses with the amygdala (Figure 13-4). The lenticular nucleus, which is subdivided into the *putamen* and the *globus pallidus,* lies lateral and partially anterior to the thalamus. It is separated from the thalamus and from much of the head of the caudate nucleus by a thick sheet of fibers called the *internal capsule.* The internal capsule contains most of the fibers interconnecting the cerebral cortex and deep structures such as the thalamus and basal ganglia.

Figures 2-18 to 2-24 are intended to introduce the beginning student to the configuration of internal structures of the brain. Each section is in a coronal plane and has been stained with Mulligan's stain, which differentiates gray matter from white matter (Plate 1). In each case the anterior surface of the section is shown, and the plane of this anterior surface is indicated on the right side of each photograph. Only major structures are labeled. Figure 2-25 diagrams the interrelationships (and some of the functions) of the major structures that comprise the central nervous system.

*Text continued on p 32.*

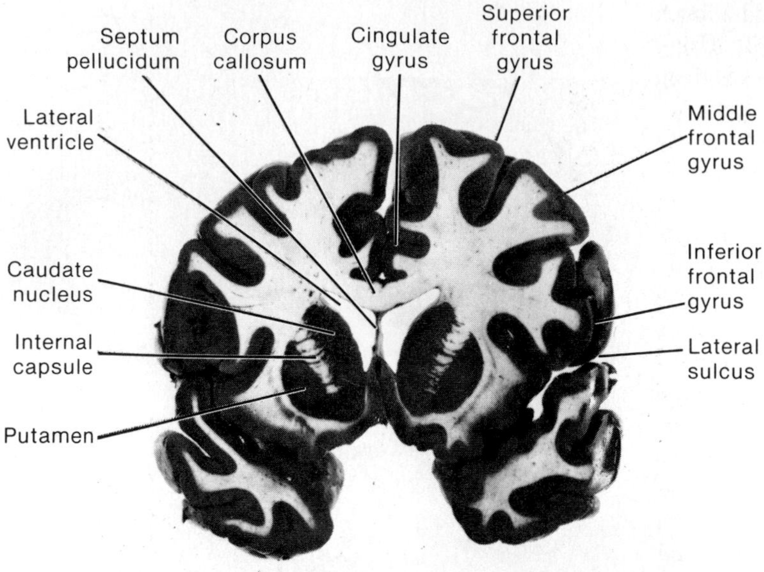


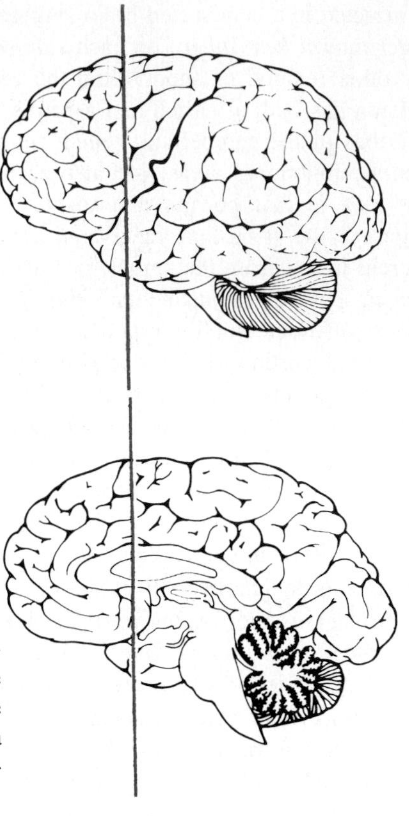

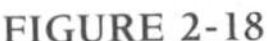

FIGURE 2-18
Section through the frontal lobes, slightly posterior to the genu of the corpus callosum. Inferior to the body of the corpus callosum is the septum pellucidum, a thin paired membrane that intervenes between the corpus callosum and the fornix and separates portions of the two lateral ventricles. At this level, which is anterior to the diencephalon, the basal ganglia are represented by the putamen and the head of the caudate nucleus, with part of the internal capsule between them. Inferiorly, note the continuity between these nuclei.

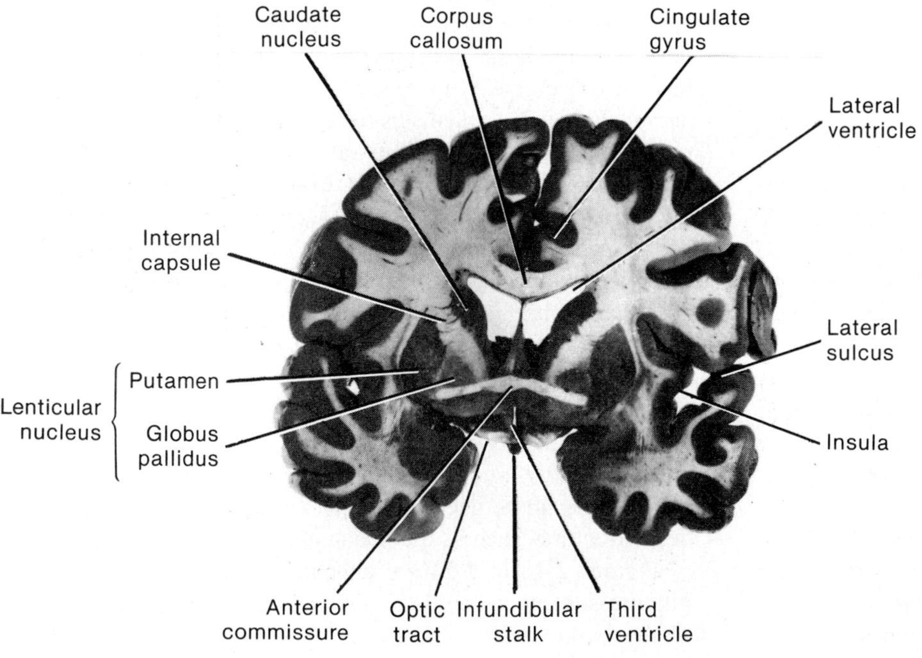


FIGURE 2-19
Section through the anterior commissure, which interconnects portions of the temporal lobes, as well as certain olfactory structures. A small portion of the slit-shaped third ventricle can be seen between the anterior commissure and the optic chiasm. At this level both parts of the lenticular nucleus (the putamen and the globus pallidus) are present. The section is slightly anterior to both the interventricular foramen and the thalamus.

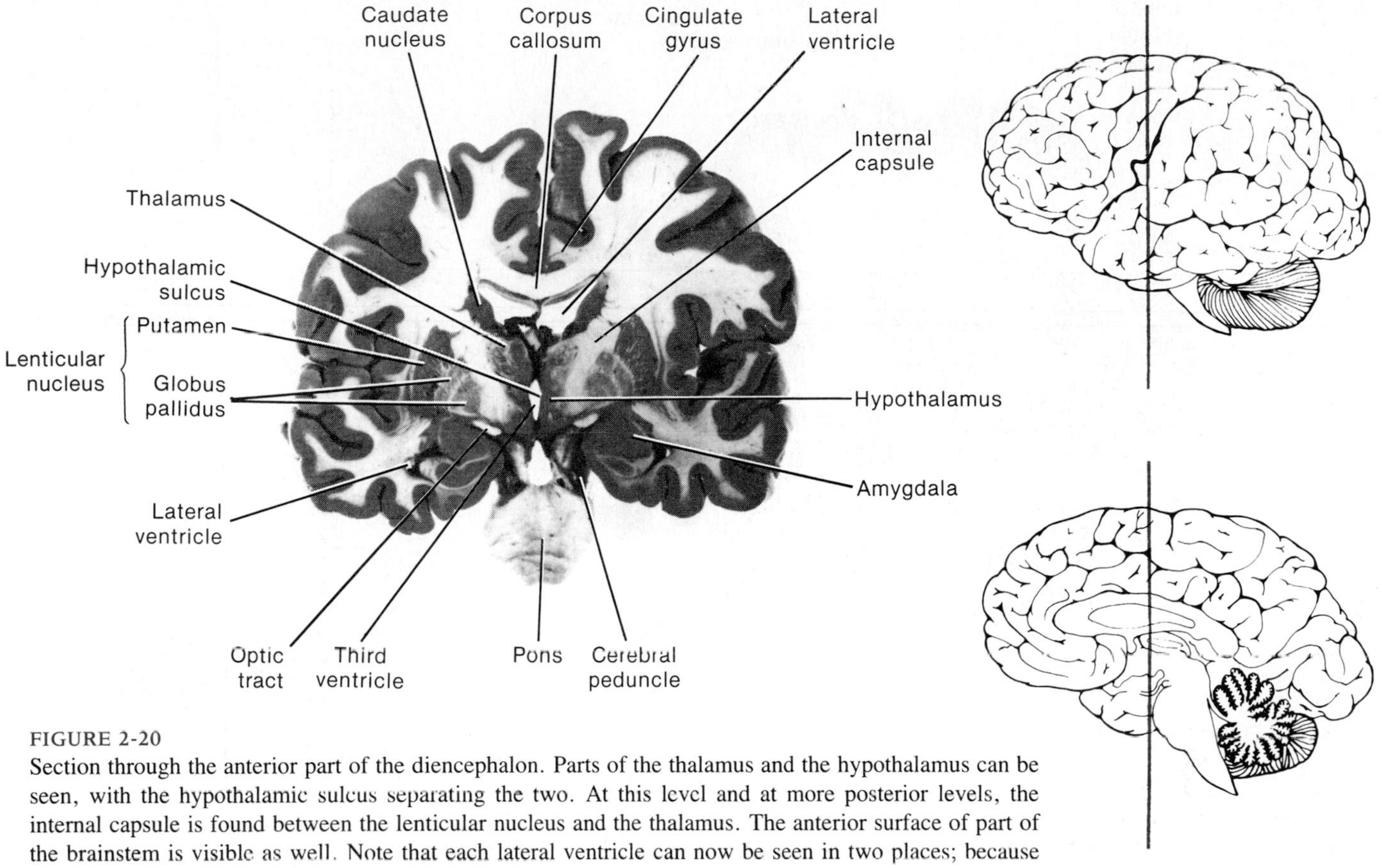

FIGURE 2-20
Section through the anterior part of the diencephalon. Parts of the thalamus and the hypothalamus can be seen, with the hypothalamic sulcus separating the two. At this level and at more posterior levels, the internal capsule is found between the lenticular nucleus and the thalamus. The anterior surface of part of the brainstem is visible as well. Note that each lateral ventricle can now be seen in two places; because of their C shape, they were transected twice in this and the next three sections.

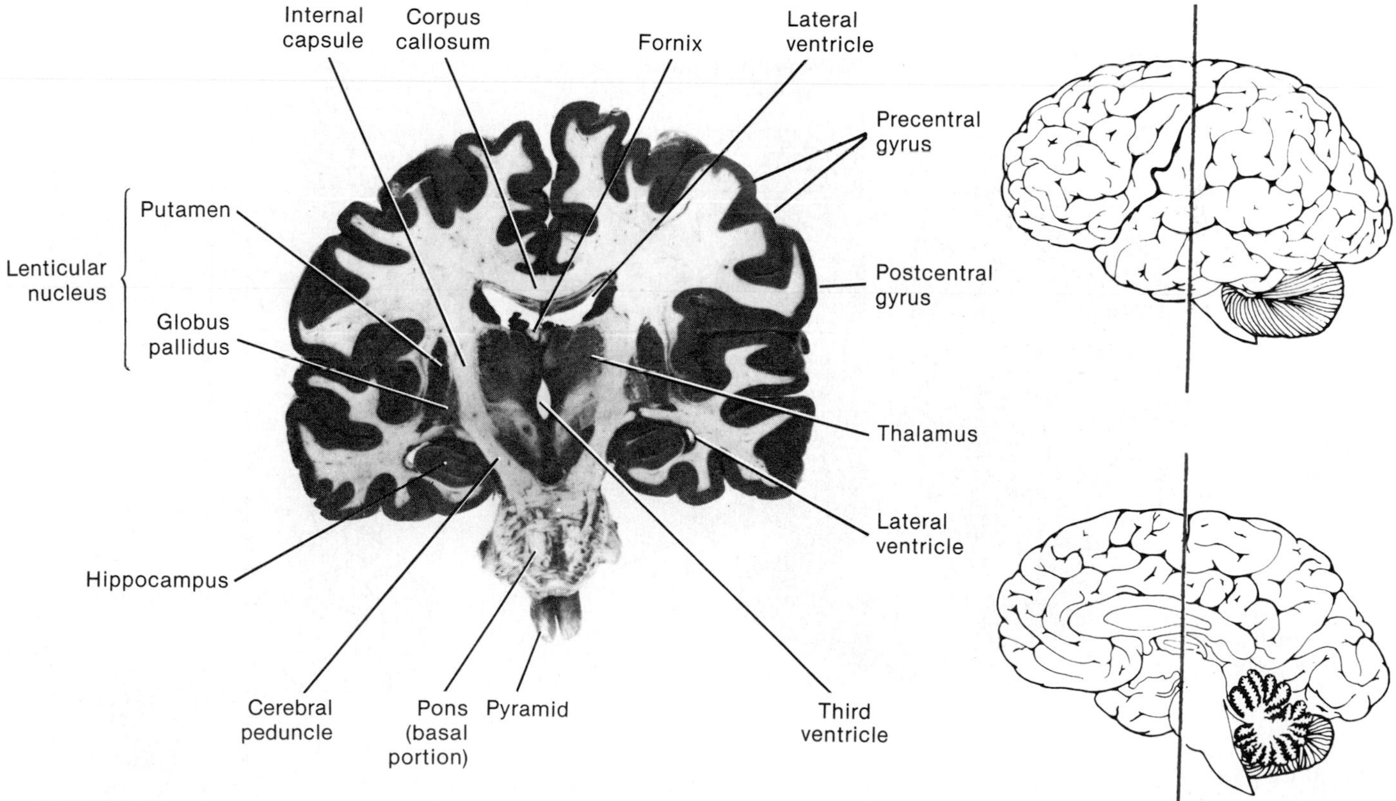

FIGURE 2-21
Section through the thalamus and brainstem. Since the thalamus is partially posterior to the lenticular nucleus, it becomes larger and the lenticular nucleus becomes smaller when proceeding posteriorly from Figure 2-20 to this figure. The anatomical route taken by some axons from the cerebral cortex through the internal capsule and the cerebral peduncle, and thence to terminations in the brainstem or spinal cord, is apparent.

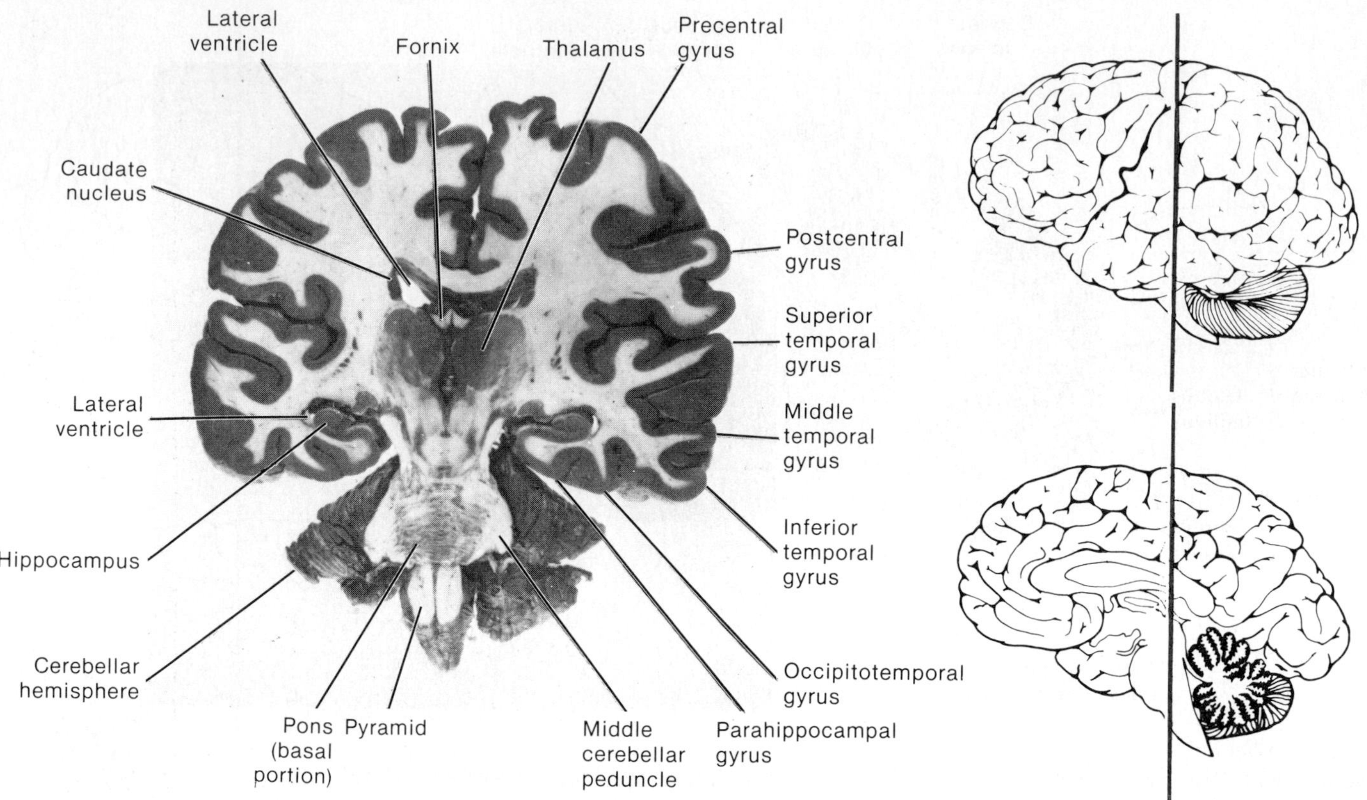


FIGURE 2-22
Section through the brainstem and posterior thalamus. This level is posterior to the lenticular nucleus; the few scattered clumps of gray matter in its former location are bridges of gray matter that extend from the putamen to the caudate nucleus.

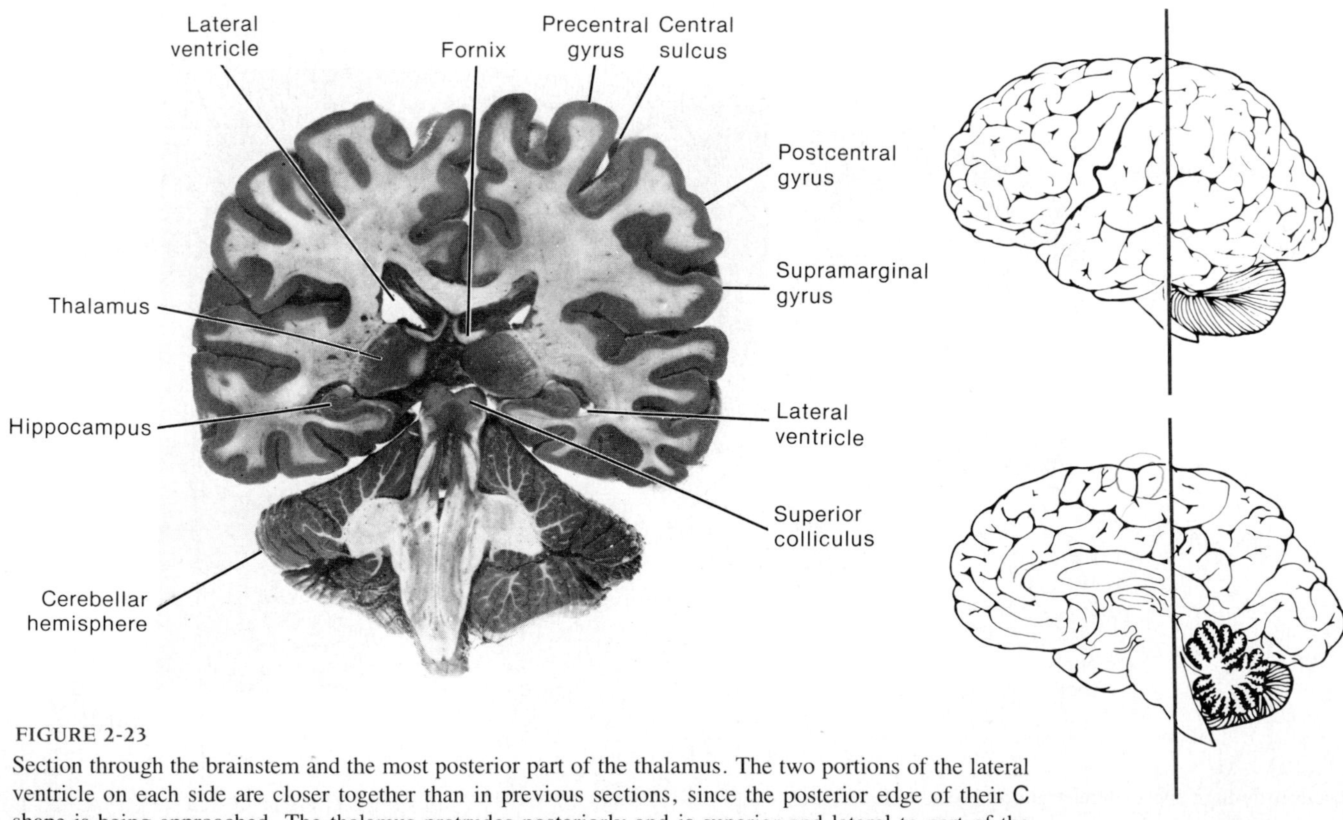


FIGURE 2-23
Section through the brainstem and the most posterior part of the thalamus. The two portions of the lateral ventricle on each side are closer together than in previous sections, since the posterior edge of their C shape is being approached. The thalamus protrudes posteriorly and is superior and lateral to part of the midbrain.

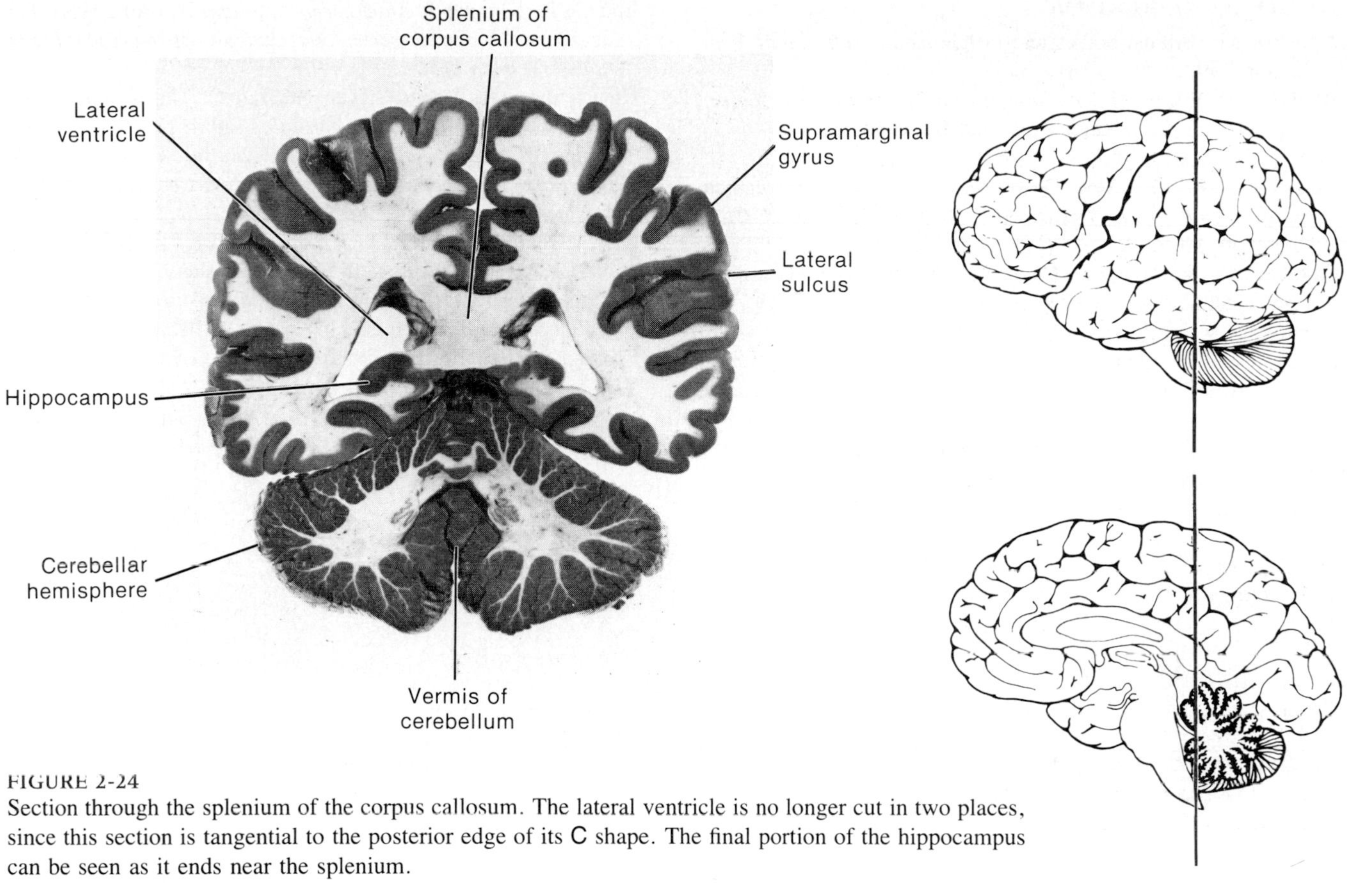

Splenium of corpus callosum
Lateral ventricle
Supramarginal gyrus
Lateral sulcus
Hippocampus
Cerebellar hemisphere
Vermis of cerebellum

FIGURE 2-24
Section through the splenium of the corpus callosum. The lateral ventricle is no longer cut in two places, since this section is tangential to the posterior edge of its C shape. The final portion of the hippocampus can be seen as it ends near the splenium.

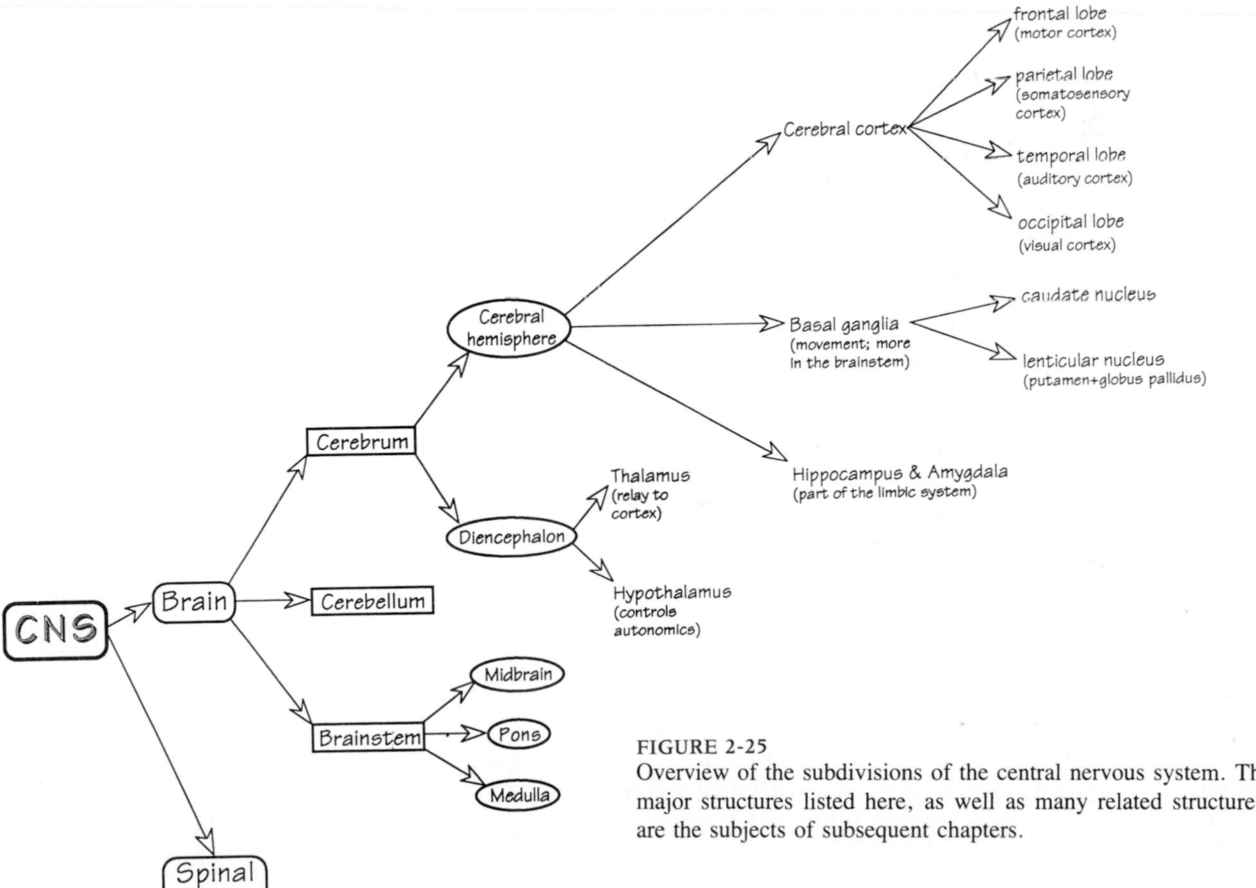


FIGURE 2-25
Overview of the subdivisions of the central nervous system. The major structures listed here, as well as many related structures, are the subjects of subsequent chapters.

## ADDITIONAL READINGS

Armstrong E: Brains, bodies and metabolism, *Brain Behav Evol* 36:166, 1990.

Blinkov SM, Glezer II: *The human brain in figures and tables,* New York, 1968, Plenum Press and Basic Books.

Cobb S: Brain size, *Arch Neurol* 12:555, 1965.

DeArmond SJ, Fusco MM, Dewey MM: *Structure of the human brain: a photographic atlas,* ed 3, New York, 1989, Oxford University Press.

Dekaban AS, Sadowsky D: Changes in brain weights during the span of human life: relation of brain weights to body heights and body weights, *Ann Neurol* 4:345, 1978.

Gluhbegovic N, Williams TH: *The human brain: a photographic guide,* New York, 1980, Harper & Row.

Igarashi S, Kamiya T: *Atlas of the vertebrate brain: morphological evolution from cyclostomes to mammals,* Baltimore, 1972, University Park Press. *Ever wonder what an anteater's brain looks like?*

Ludwig E, Klingler J: *Atlas cerebri humani,* Boston, 1956, Little, Brown & Co. *A series of technically spectacular dissections of human brains.*

Nieuwenhuys R, Voogd J, van Hurjzen C: *The human central nervous system: a synopsis and atlas,* ed 3, New York, 1988, Springer-Verlag. *Includes many beautiful drawings of the brain and various subsystems of the CNS, as well as a brief but thorough text portion.*

Ono M, Kubik S, Abernathey CD: *Atlas of the cerebral sulci,* New York, 1990, Thieme Medical Publishers.

Roberts M, Hanaway J, Morest DK: *Atlas of the human brain in section,* ed 2, Philadelphia, 1987, Lea & Febiger.

Schnitzlein HN, Murtagh FR: *Imaging anatomy of the head and spine. A photographic color atlas of MRI, CT, gross, and microscopic anatomy in axial, coronal, and sagittal planes,* ed 2, Baltimore, 1990, Urban and Schwarzenberg.

CHAPTER

# 3

# *Meningeal Coverings of the Brain and Spinal Cord*

Living brain is on the soft and mushy side. Without support of some kind it would be unable to maintain its shape, particularly as we walk and run around and occasionally bump our heads. The brain and spinal cord are protected from outside forces by their encasement in the skull and vertebral column, respectively. In addition, the central nervous system (CNS) is suspended within a series of three membranous coverings, the *meninges* (from the Greek word *meninx* meaning membrane), that stabilize the shape and position of nerve tissue in two different ways during head and body movements. First, the brain is mechanically suspended within the meninges, which in turn are anchored to the skull so that the brain is constrained to move with the head. Second, there is a layer of *cerebrospinal fluid* within the meninges; the buoyant effect of this fluid environment greatly decreases the tendency of various forces (such as gravity) to distort the brain. Thus a brain weighing 1500 g in air effectively weighs less than 50 g in its normal cerebrospinal fluid environment, where it is easily able to maintain its shape. In contrast, an isolated fresh brain, unsupported by its usual surroundings, becomes seriously distorted and may even tear under the influence of gravity (Figure 3-1).

The three meninges, from the outermost layer inward, are the *dura mater*, the *arachnoid*, and the *pia mater* (Figure 3-2). In common usage the dura mater and pia mater are often referred to simply as the dura and pia. The dura mater is by far the most substantial of the three meninges and for this reason is also called the *pachymeninx* (from the Greek word *pachy* meaning thick, as in thick-skinned pachyderms). The arachnoid and pia mater, in contrast, are thin and delicate. They are similar to and continuous with each other and so are sometimes referred to together as the pia-arachnoid or the *leptomeninges* (from the Greek word *lepto* meaning thin, fine). The dura mater is attached to the inner surface of the skull, and the arachnoid adheres to the inner surface of the dura mater. The pia mater is attached to the brain, following all its contours, and the space between the arachnoid and pia mater is filled with cerebrospinal fluid.

Because of the differences between cranial and spinal meninges, those of the spinal cord are described separately at the end of this chapter.

## DURA MATER

The cranial dura is a thick, tough, collagenous membrane that adheres firmly to the inner surface of the skull (*dura* is the Latin word for hard, as in durable). It is often described as consisting of two layers: an outer layer that serves as the periosteum of the inner surface of the skull and an inner layer, the meningeal dura. Since these two layers are tightly fused with no sharp histological boundary between them, the entire complex is ordinarily referred to as dura mater.

No space exists on either side of the dura under normal circumstances, since one side is attached to the skull and the other side adheres to the arachnoid. However, two *potential* spaces, the *epidural* and *subdural* spaces, are associated with the dura (Figure 3-14). Epidural space refers to the potential space between the cranium and the periosteal layer. Subdural space is commonly described as the potential space between dura and arachnoid and is sometimes said to contain a thin film of fluid. However, electron microscopic evidence indicates that the dura and arachnoid are normally attached to each other, and that when they appear to separate, the splitting actually occurs within the

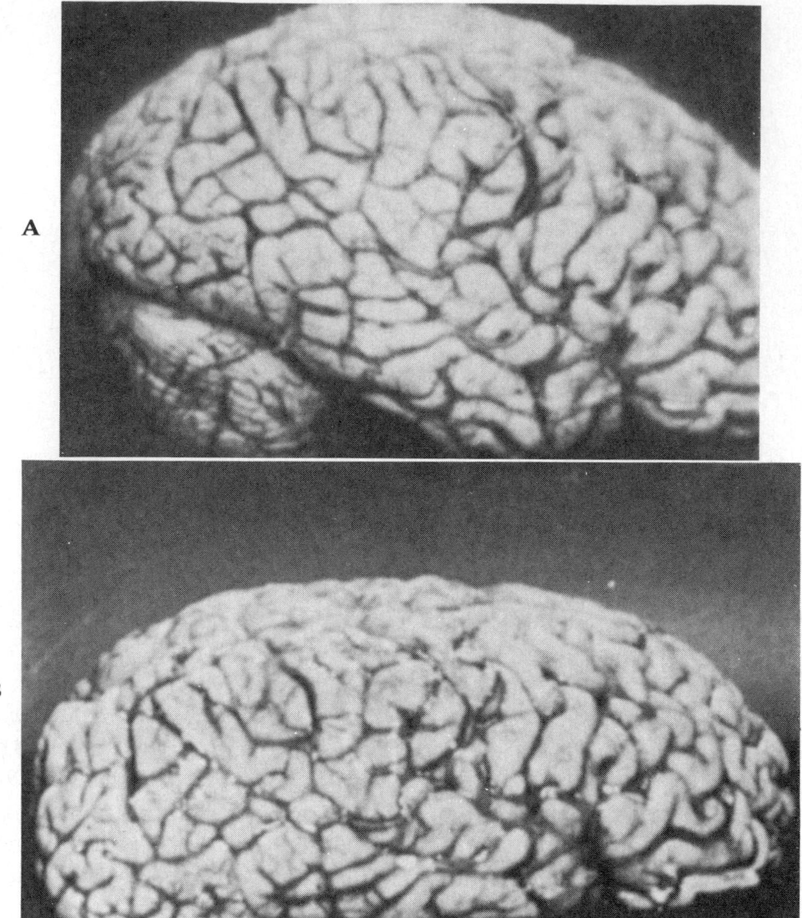


FIGURE 3-1
Effects of gravity and of partial flotation on brain. **A,** An unfixed human brain in a vat of isotonic saline; normal shape is maintained. **B,** The same brain in air, obviously distorted by its own weight.
From Oldendorf W: The quest for an image of brain, New York, 1980, Raven Press.

innermost cellular layers of the dura. Parts of these potential spaces can become actual fluid-filled cavities in certain pathological conditions, most often as a result of hemorrhage.

## Dural reflections

There are several places where the inner dural layer is reflected as sheetlike protrusions, called *dural reflections* or *dural septa,* into the cranial cavity. The principal dural reflections are the *falx cerebri,* which intervenes between the two cerebral hemispheres, and the *tentorium cerebelli,* which intervenes between the cerebral hemispheres and the cerebellum (Figure 3-3). The *falx cerebelli* is a small reflection that partially separates the two cerebellar hemispheres. The *diaphragma sellae,* another small reflection, covers the pituitary fossa, admitting the infundibulum through a small perforation.

The falx cerebri (from the Latin word *falx* meaning sickle) is a long, arched, vertical dural sheet (Figures 3-3 and 3-4) that occupies the longitudinal fissure and separates the two cerebral hemispheres. Anteriorly it is attached to the crista galli of the ethmoid bone. The falx curves posteriorly and fuses with the middle of the tentorium cerebelli at the internal occipital protuberance. The inferior, free edge of the falx generally parallels the corpus callosum, but the falx is somewhat broader posteriorly than it is anteriorly, so this free edge comes closer to the splenium of the corpus callosum than to the genu (Figure 3-3). The anterior portion of the falx is frequently incomplete, containing a number of perforations.

The tentorium cerebelli separates the superior surface of the cerebellum from the occipital lobes, defining *supratentorial* and *infratentorial* compartments. Because the interval between the cerebrum and cerebellum is not horizontal or flat, neither is the tentorium. Rather, it is roughly the shape of a bird with its wings extended in front of it; the bird's body would correspond to the midline region where the falx joins the tentorium, and its wings would corre-

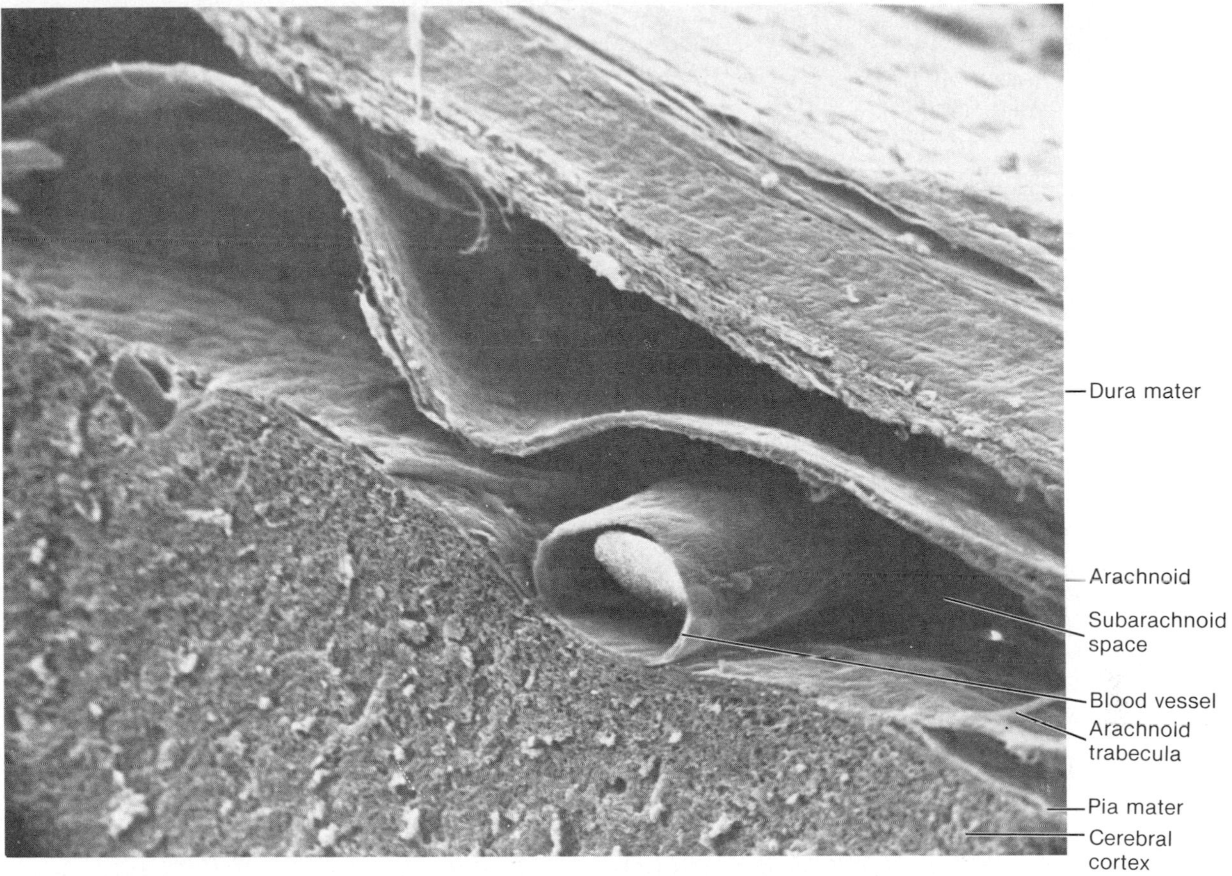


FIGURE 3-2
Scanning electron micrograph of the cranial meninges of a young dog. The apparent space between the dura mater and the arachnoid is an artifact of processing and would not normally be present.
Courtesy of Dr. Delmas J. Allen, Medical College of Ohio.

spond to the rest of the tentorium, which is prolonged anteriorly (Figures 3-3 to 3-5). Posteriorly the tentorium is attached mainly to the occipital bone. This line of attachment continues anteriorly and inferiorly along the petrous temporal bone. The free edge of the tentorium also curves anteriorly on each side, almost encircling the midbrain (Figures 3-5 and 3-6). This space in the tentorium through which the brainstem passes is called the *tentorial notch* (or *tentorial incisure*) and is of great clinical significance, as discussed later in this chapter.

## Dural sinuses

As noted previously, the two layers of the cranial dura are tightly fused, and there are no pathological conditions in which an intradural space (that is, a space between the two layers) develops. However, at some edges of dural reflections (most often attached edges), the two layers are normally separated to form channels, called *dural venous sinuses,* into which the cerebral veins empty. These sinuses are roughly triangular in cross section and are lined with endothelium (Figures 3-7 and 3-8). The locations of the major sinuses can be inferred by considering the lines of attachment of the falx and the tentorium. The *superior sagittal sinus* is found along the attached edge of the falx, the *left* and *right transverse sinuses* are found along the posterior line of attachment of the tentorium, and the *straight sinus* is found along the line of attachment of the falx and tentorium (Figures 3-4, 3-5, and 5-16). All four of these sinuses meet in the *confluence of the sinuses* (also called the *torcular,* or *torcular Herophili*—"the winepress of Herophilus") near the internal occipital protuberance. Venous blood flows posteriorly in the superior sagittal and straight sinuses into the confluence, and from there through the transverse sinuses. Each transverse sinus continues, from the point where it leaves the tentorium, as the *sigmoid sinus,* which proceeds anteriorly and inferiorly through an S-shaped course and empties into the internal jugular vein (Figures 3-6, 3-9, and 5-18).

The confluence of the sinuses is generally not a symmetrical structure. Usually most of the blood from the superior sagittal sinus flows into the right transverse sinus, whereas blood from the straight sinus flows into the left

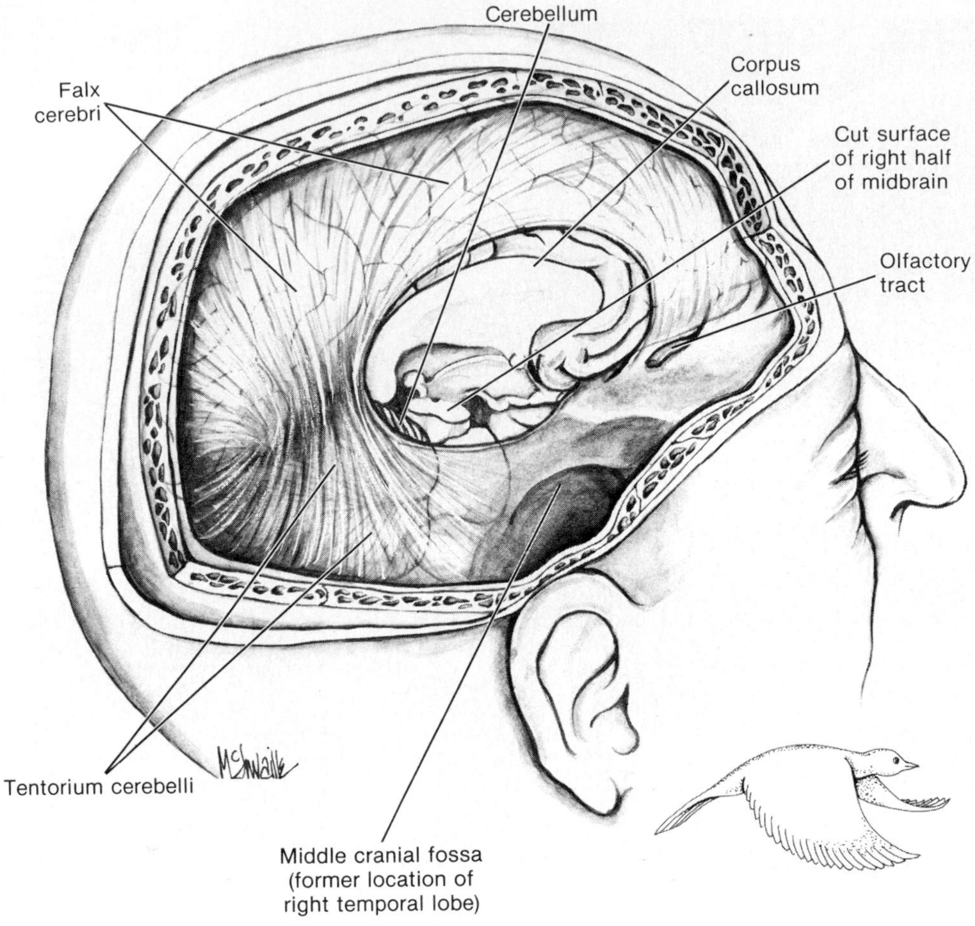


FIGURE 3-3
Shape and spatial relationships of the dural reflections. The cerebellum and part of the left cerebral hemisphere are drawn in on the other side of the falx cerebri and tentorium cerebelli. The small bird in the corner reminds certain individuals of the shape of the tentorium cerebelli.
Drawn from a dissection by Gary Jenison, University of Colorado Health Sciences Center.

transverse sinus (Figures 3-9 and 5-22). Not uncommonly the two transverse sinuses are not interconnected at all.

In addition to receiving cerebral veins, the major dural sinuses mentioned above are connected with several smaller sinuses (Figure 5-16). The *inferior sagittal sinus,* in the free edge of the falx cerebri, empties into the straight sinus. The small *occipital sinus,* in the attached edge of the falx cerebelli, empties into the confluence of the sinuses. The *superior petrosal sinus,* in the edge of the tentorium attached to the petrous temporal bone, carries blood from the cavernous sinus to the transverse sinus at the point where the latter leaves the tentorium to become the sigmoid sinus. The *inferior petrosal sinus* follows a groove between the temporal and occipital bones, carrying blood from the cavernous sinus to the internal jugular vein.

## Dural vasculature and innervation

The arterial supply of the dura comes from a large number of meningeal arteries. These are somewhat misnamed because they travel in the periosteal layer of the dura and function mainly in supplying the bones of the skull; however, many small arterial branches penetrate the dura itself. The largest of the meningeal arteries is the *middle meningeal artery,* a branch of the maxillary artery, which ramifies over most of the lateral surface of the cerebral dura. Anteriorly the dura is supplied by branches of the ophthalmic artery, and posteriorly it is supplied by branches of the occipital and vertebral arteries. Meningeal veins, also located in the periosteal layer, generally parallel the arteries.

Most of the cranial dura, except for that of the posterior fossa, receives sensory innervation from the trigeminal

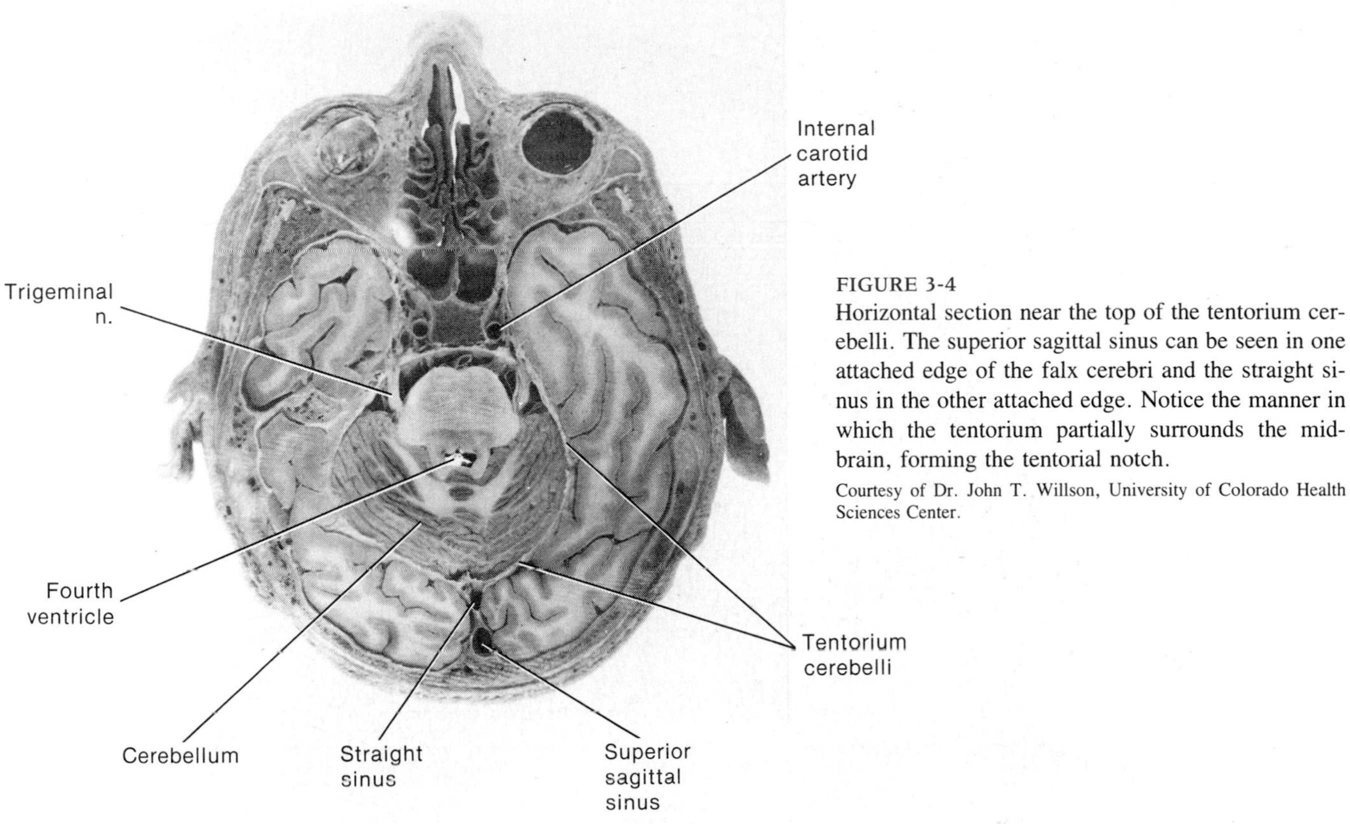


FIGURE 3-4
Horizontal section near the top of the tentorium cerebelli. The superior sagittal sinus can be seen in one attached edge of the falx cerebri and the straight sinus in the other attached edge. Notice the manner in which the tentorium partially surrounds the midbrain, forming the tentorial notch.
Courtesy of Dr. John T. Willson, University of Colorado Health Sciences Center.

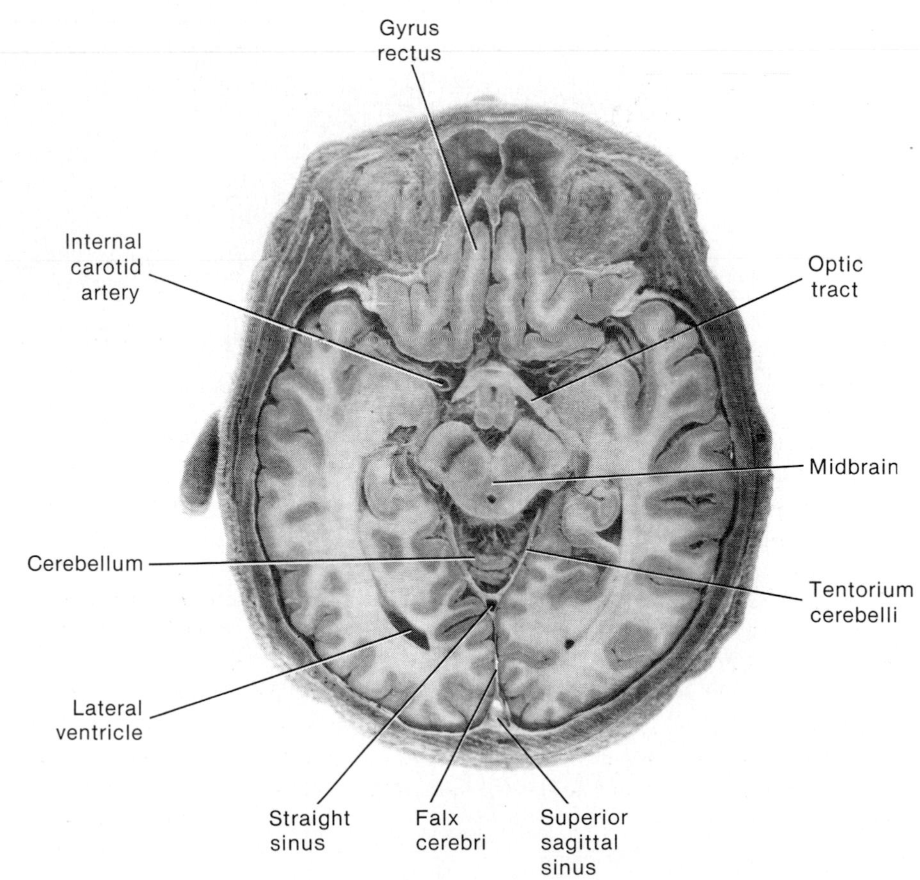


FIGURE 3-5
Horizontal section at a level just above the confluence of the sinuses. The straight sinus is about to join the superior sagittal sinus. Note again how close the brainstem is to the tentorium as it passes through the tentorial notch.
Courtesy of Dr. John T. Willson, University of Colorado Center Health Sciences Center.

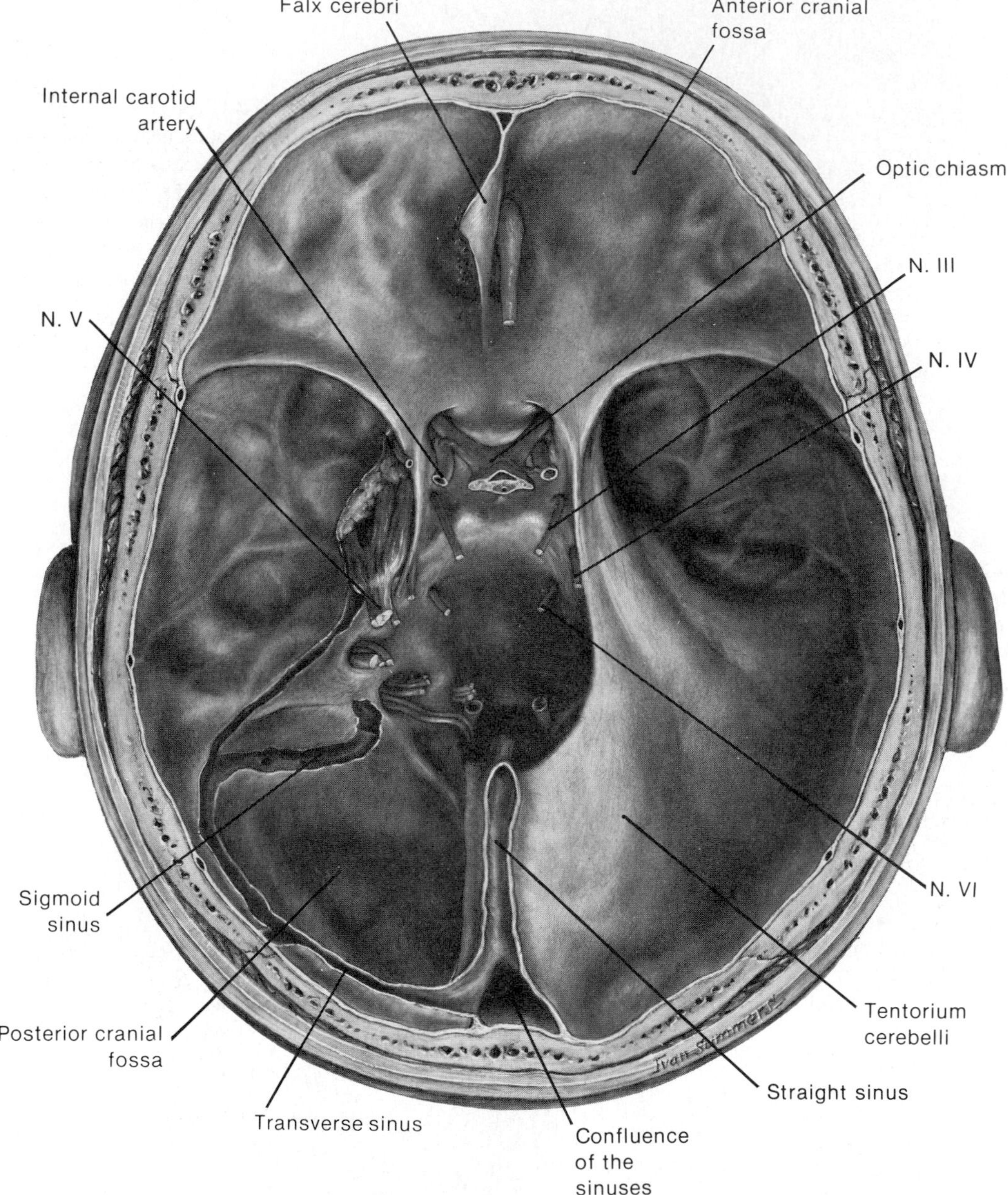


FIGURE 3-6
Dural lining of the base of the skull. The falx has been removed except for a small anterior portion. The left half of the tentorium has also been removed, exposing the posterior fossa (where the cerebellum was). Compare to Figures 3-4 and 3-5.

From Mettler FA: Neuroanatomy, ed 2, St. Louis, 1948, Mosby–Year Book.

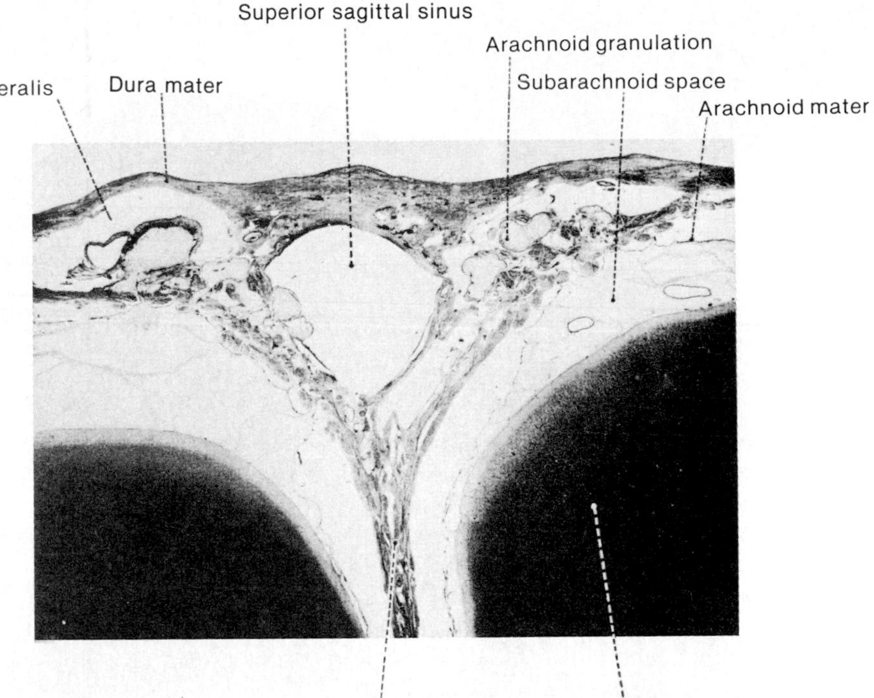


FIGURE 3-7
Cross section of the superior sagittal sinus showing arachnoid granulations. Note the fine arachnoid trabeculae spanning the subarachnoid space. Lacunae laterales are lateral extensions of venous sinuses, particularly the superior sagittal sinus, into which many of the arachnoid granulations protrude.

From Hamilton WJ: Textbook of human anatomy, ed 2, St. Louis, 1976, Mosby—Year Book. By permission of Macmillan Press, London and Basingstoke

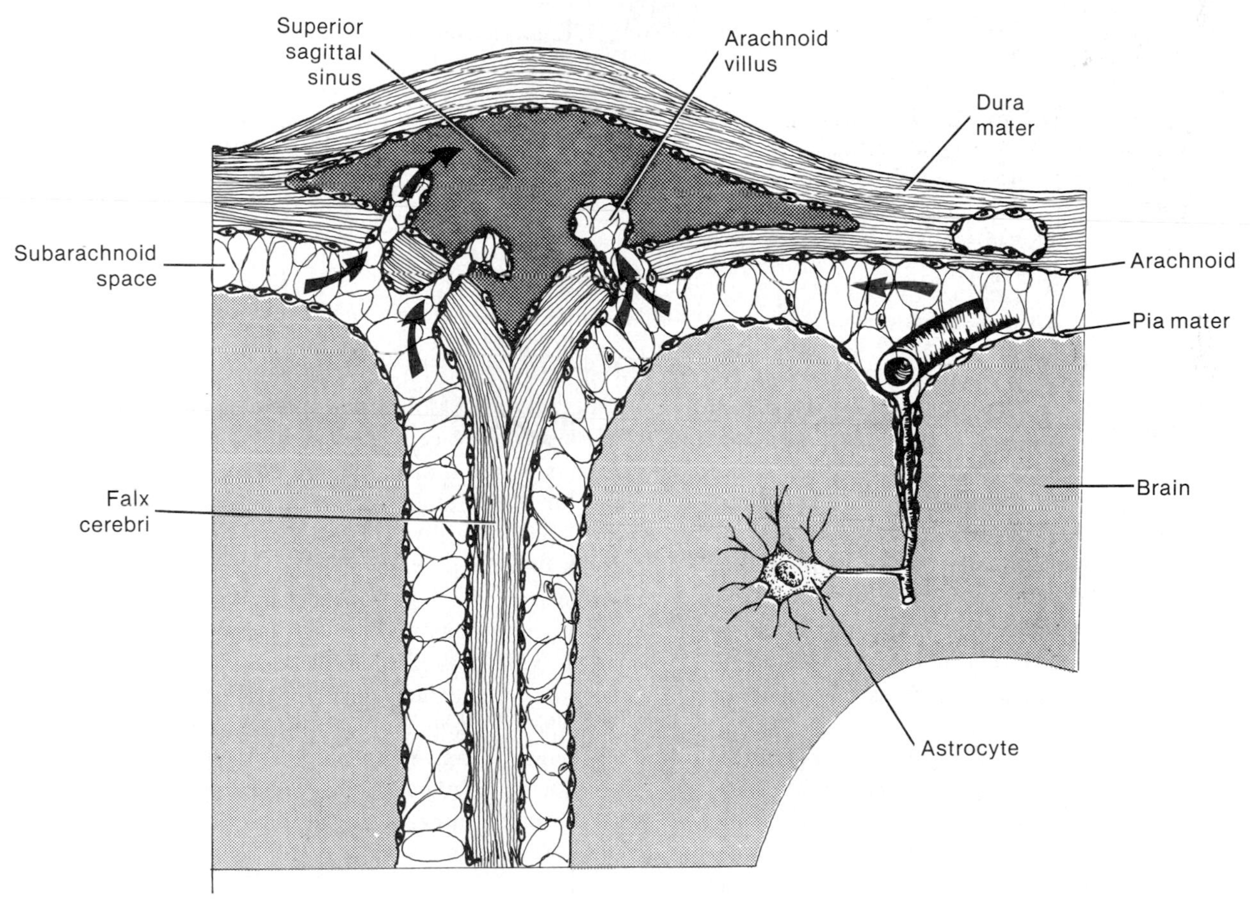


FIGURE 3-8
Section through the superior sagittal sinus showing the movement of cerebrospinal fluid from subarachnoid space, through the arachnoid villi, and into the sinus.

Modified from Hamilton WJ: Textbook of human anatomy, ed 2, St. Louis, 1976, Mosby–Year Book. By permission of Macmillan Press, London and Basingstoke.

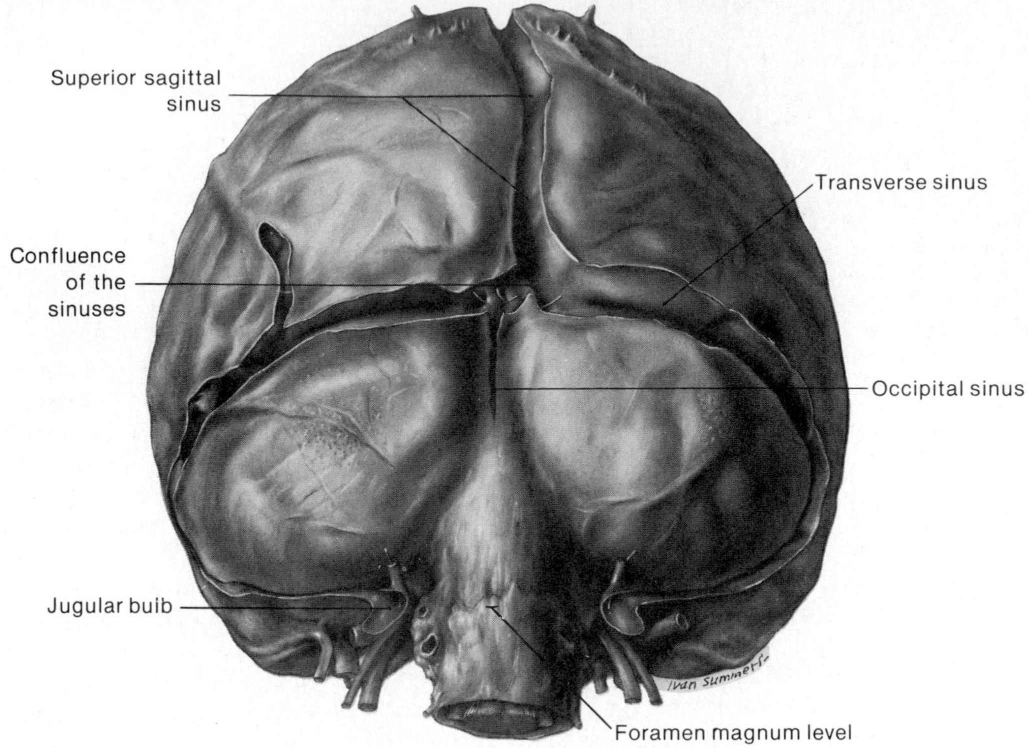


FIGURE 3-9
The brain, still encased in dura, viewed from behind. Note the asymmetry of the confluence of the sinuses (compare to Figure 5-22). Note also the jagged line at the foramen magnum level corresponding to the cut edge of the periosteal layer of the cranial dura. Below this line, a single-layered dural sheath continues around the spinal cord.
From Mettler FA: Neuroanatomy, ed 2, St. Louis, 1948, Mosby—Year Book.

nerve. Dural nerves follow the meningeal arteries and end near either the arteries or the dural sinuses. Areas of dura between branches of meningeal arteries are innervated poorly, if at all. Deformation of these endings causes pain and is presumably the cause of certain types of headache. Interestingly, the way the pain is perceived depends on whether endings near meningeal arteries or endings near dural sinuses are stimulated. In the former case the pain is fairly accurately localized to the area of stimulation; in the latter case the pain is referred to portions of the peripheral distribution of the trigeminal nerve such as the temple or forehead.

The dura of the posterior fossa is supplied primarily by fibers of the second and third cervical nerves.* These fibers travel within the posterior fossa in the sheaths of the vagus and glossopharyngeal nerves. The latter observation probably accounts in part for older reports that these cranial nerves contribute to the innervation of the dura, although there may in fact be a small contribution from the vagus.

*The first cervical nerve rarely has a sensory component.

## ARACHNOID

The arachnoid is a thin avascular membrane composed of a few layers of cells interspersed with bundles of collagen. It is semitransparent and resembles a substantial cobweb, for which it is named (the Greek word *arachne* means spider's web). The outer portion of the arachnoid consists of several layers of flattened cells adhering to the innermost cellular layer of the dura mater. This interface layer of cells, partially dura and partially arachnoid, contains no collagen and is only about 100 μm thick. Small strands of collagenous connective tissue called *arachnoid trabeculae* (Figure 3-10), covered with fibroblast-like arachnoid cells, leave this interface layer and extend to the pia, with which they merge. Arachnoid trabeculae help keep the brain suspended within the meninges, much the way the Lilliputians stabilized Gulliver's position.*

### Subarachnoid cisterns

Because the arachnoid is attached to the inner surface of the dura mater, it, like the dura, conforms to the general

*I thank Dr. Theodore J. Tarby for the analogy.

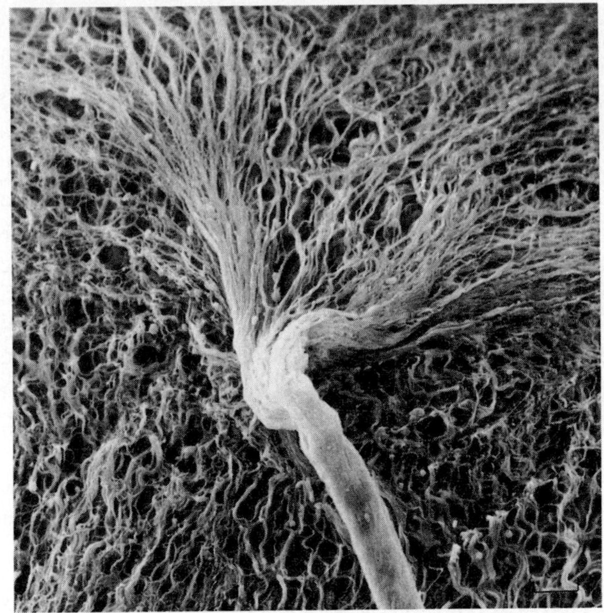

FIGURE 3-10
Scanning electron micrograph of a human arachnoid trabecula. The view is as though you were standing in the lateral sulcus looking out at the overlying arachnoid and dura mater. Collagen bundles spread out from the trabecula and merge with the arachnoid lining of the dura mater. Scale mark = 3 μm.

From Alcolado R et al., *Neuropath Applied Neurobiol* 14:1, 1988. Courtesy of Dr. RO Weller, Department of Pathology, Southampton University Medical School.

shape of the brain but does not dip into sulci or follow the more intricate contours of the surface of the brain. There is therefore a *subarachnoid space,* filled with cerebrospinal fluid, between the arachnoid and the pia mater, since the pia closely covers all the external surfaces of the CNS. This is the only substantial fluid-filled space normally found around the brain. The subarachnoid space is nonexistent over the surfaces of gyri, relatively small where the arachnoid bridges over small sulci, and much larger in certain locations where it bridges over large surface irregularities. An example of such a location is the space between the inferior surface of the cerebellum and the dorsal surface of the medulla. Regions such as this, which contain a considerable volume of cerebrospinal fluid, are called *subarachnoid cisterns*. This particular example is called the *cerebellomedullary cistern* based on anatomical grounds, and since it is the largest cranial cistern, it is also referred to as *cisterna magna*. Other prominent cisterns are indicated in Figure 3-11 and include (1) the *pontine cistern,* around the anterior surface of the pons and medulla, which is continuous posteriorly with the cerebellomedullary cistern; (2) the *interpeduncular cistern,* between the cerebral peduncles, which contains the arterial circle of Willis (Figure 5-2); and (3) the *superior cistern* (also referred to as the *quadrigeminal cistern* and the *cistern of the great cere-*

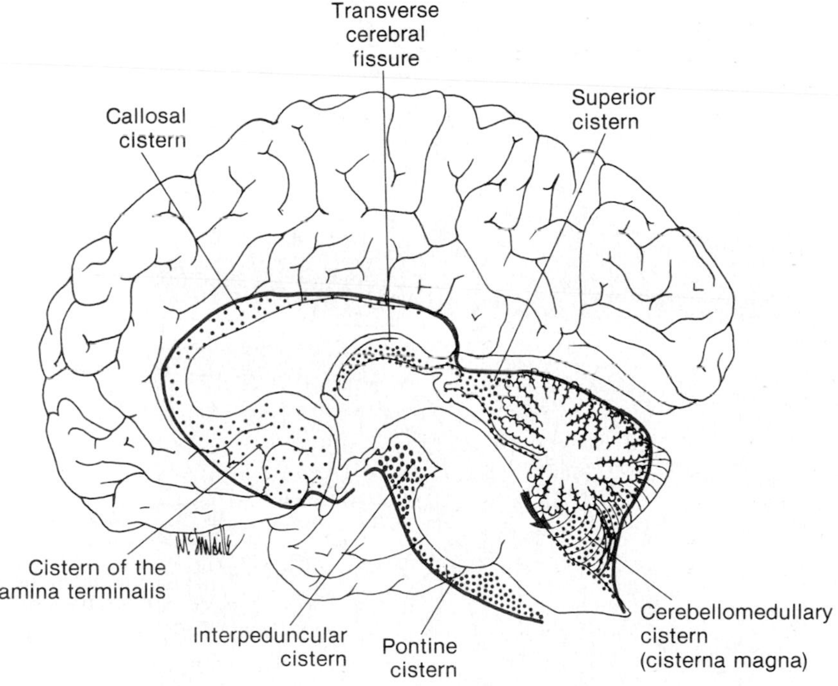


FIGURE 3-11
Hemisected brain in which the falx was split, with the locations of the major subarachnoid cisterns indicated. The density of the dotted pattern is roughly proportional to the amount of fluid in a particular cistern. The heavy line represents the edge of the arachnoid, which would have been cut through during the hemisection. An arrow is shown passing from the fourth ventricle, through its median aperture, and into cisterna magna. This is one of the three routes (discussed in the next chapter) by which cerebrospinal fluid escapes from the ventricles into subarachnoid space.

*bral vein*), a radiological landmark above the midbrain (Figure 4-12, *B*). The superior cistern is continuous laterally with a thin, curved layer of subarachnoid space on each side that partially encircles the midbrain before opening into the interpeduncular cistern. The combination of the superior cistern and these sheetlike extensions is referred to as the *ambient cistern*.

## Arachnoid villi

The cerebrospinal fluid contained in the subarachnoid space generally is separated from the venous blood in dural sinuses by a layer of arachnoid, a thick layer of dura, and the endothelial lining of the sinus. However, at many locations along dural sinuses, particularly along the superior sagittal sinus, small evaginations of the arachnoid, called *arachnoid villi,* protrude into the sinus. At these sites the connective tissue of the dura is lacking, and only a loose layer of arachnoid cells and a layer of endothelium intervene between subarachnoid space and venous blood (Figures 3-8 and 3-12). Large arachnoid villi are called *arachnoid granulations,* and those that become calcified with age are referred to as *pacchionian bodies*. The villi are especially numerous in laterally directed dilations of the superior sagittal sinus, called *venous lacunae* or *lateral lacunae* (see Figure 3-7), but some are found along all the sinuses and even along some cerebral veins.

The arachnoid villi are the major sites of reabsorption of cerebrospinal fluid into the venous system. Function-

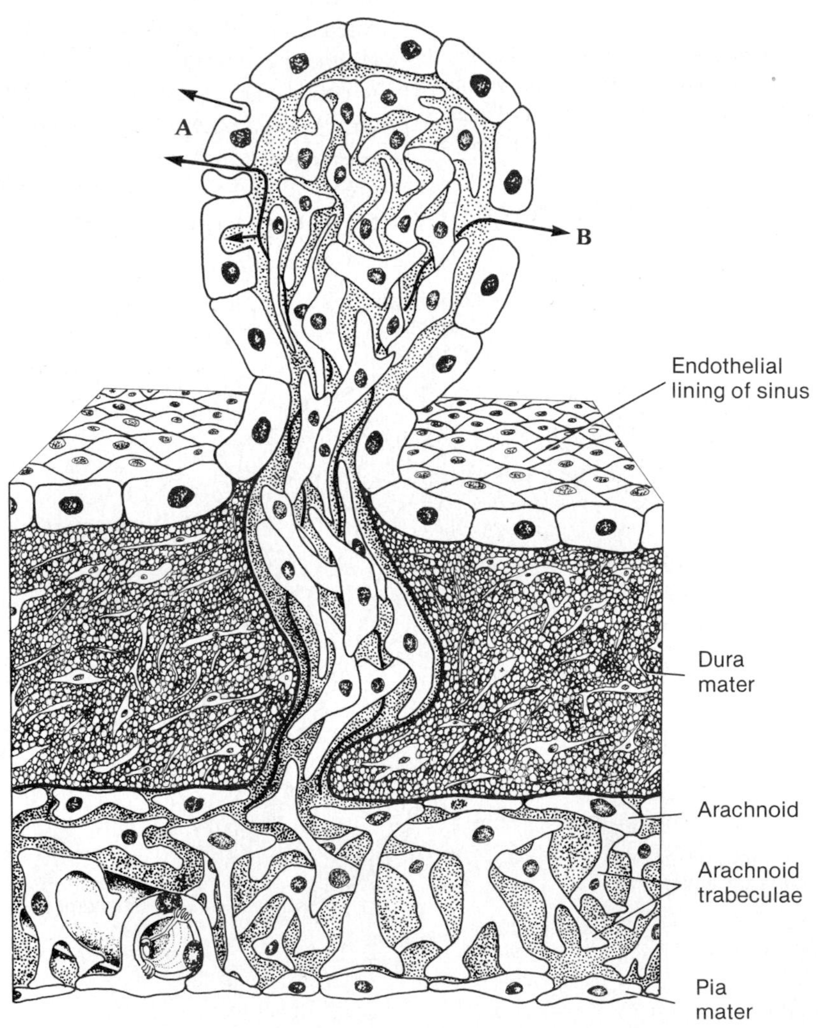


FIGURE 3-12
An arachnoid villus, showing the passage of cerebrospinal fluid from subarachnoid space into a dural venous sinus. **A,** Cerebrospinal fluid movement through large vacuoles in endothelial cells, as described by some workers. **B,** Movement through channels between cells, as described by other workers.
Modified from Shabo AL, Maxwell DS: *J Neurosurg* 29:451, 1968.

ally, they behave like one-way valves, allowing flow from subarachnoid space into venous blood but not in the reverse direction. Since cerebrospinal fluid pressure is ordinarily greater than venous pressure, the villi normally allow continuous movement of cerebrospinal fluid, more or less as though by bulk flow, into the sinuses; however, even if the pressure gradient reverses, the flow does not. The exact mechanism of this flow has been the subject of debate for many years. Some authors have described continuous open channels, micrometers in diameter, through the walls of the arachnoid villi, but others deny their existence. It has recently been suggested that giant vacuoles originating on the subarachnoid side of the endothelial cells, traveling across to the venous side, and sometimes being transiently open to both sides simultaneously, are responsible for the flow.

### Arachnoid barrier layer

The CNS is insulated in some respects from the rest of the body and lives in a tightly controlled environment (discussed in more detail in Chapters 4 and 5). This control is achieved partly by a system of barriers between the extracellular space in and around the nervous system and extracellular space elsewhere. One such barrier is between the cerebrospinal fluid in the subarachnoid space and the extracellular fluids of the dura. Marker substances injected into the middle meningeal artery spread throughout the dura but do not enter the subarachnoid space. The barrier apparently resides in those cellular layers of the arachnoid in the interface layer with the dura, where the cells are connected to each other by a series of tight junctions that occlude extracellular space (Figure 3-14).

## PIA MATER

The pia mater (from the Latin word *pia* meaning tender) is a second delicate membrane that, unlike the arachnoid, closely invests all surfaces, following all the contours of the brainstem and all the folds of the cerebral and cerebellar cortices.

Arachnoid trabeculae span the subarachnoid space and merge with the pia mater so subtly that it is difficult to decide where the arachnoid ends and the pia begins. The area of the pia immediately adjacent to nervous tissue is a very thin layer of cells and collagen and is considered separately, as the *intima pia,* by some authors. The intima pia merges with a more superficial region, which consists of loose connective tissue closely resembling the arachnoid. Those who recognize the intima pia as a separate entity designate this more superficial region the *epipial* layer. Others, however, consider the intima pia to represent the true pia mater and the epipia to be part of the arachnoid. Still others speak of the entire leptomeningeal complex as one entity, the pia-arachnoid.

The pia mater is often referred to as a vascular membrane, but in fact the cranial epipial layer is rather sparse, and the cerebral arteries and veins travel in subarachnoid space before penetrating the brain. The vessels essentially rest on the intima pia, held there by sheets and strands of connective tissue. As each small vessel enters or leaves the brain, it carries with it a sleeve of *perivascular space* (or *space of Virchow-Robin*). This space extends inward, filled with connective tissue and extracellular fluid, to the level at which the vessel becomes a capillary. The actual nature and extent of this microscopic space and the question of whether it provides a functional pathway of communication between the extracellular space around neurons and the subarachnoid space have been matters of controversy for decades. The traditional view holds that the connective tissue elements of the perivascular space arise as an inwardly directed cuff of pia that accompanies each vessel (as in Figure 3-8), but there are indications that in fact the pia may be left behind on the surface of the CNS. Similarly, some claim that perivascular space is small and restricted, although there are indications that it may provide an important route for movement of extracellular fluid that may even be continuous with the cervical lymphatics through the adventitia of larger vessels.

## SPINAL MENINGES

The meningeal coverings of the spinal cord are fundamentally similar to those of the brain, but there are several important differences.

The spinal dura mater is a single-layered membrane, lacking the periosteal component of the cranial dura. The inner layer of the cranial dura is continuous at the foramen magnum with the spinal dural sheath, which is separated from the vertebral periosteum by an epidural space (see Figure 3-9). Thus there are two basic differences between cranial and spinal epidural spaces:

1. Cranial epidural space is a potential space, whereas spinal epidural space is an actual space.
2. Cranial epidural space, when present, is located between periosteum and cranium, whereas spinal epidural space is located between periosteum and dura. This spinal epidural space is filled with fatty connective tissue and a vertebral venous plexus.

The spinal arachnoid, like its cranial counterpart, is closely applied to the inner surface of the dura, leaving a cerebrospinal fluid-filled subarachnoid space between itself and the spinal cord (Figure 3-13). The spinal dural sheath (and its arachnoid lining) ends at about the second sacral vertebra, whereas the spinal cord itself ends at about the level of the disk between the first and second lumbar vertebrae (Figure 7-2). There is therefore a large subarachnoid cistern, the *lumbar cistern,* between these two points. This is the favored site for sampling cerebrospinal fluid, since a needle can be inserted here with relatively little risk of damaging the CNS.

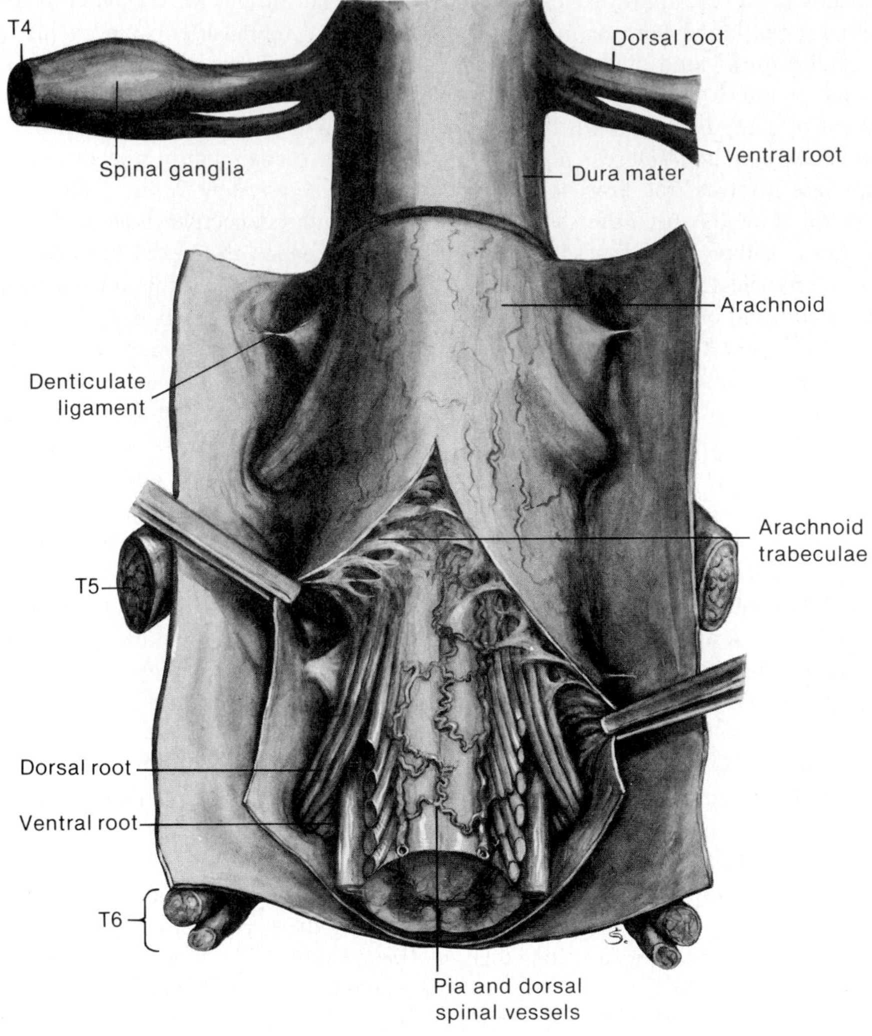


FIGURE 3-13
The spinal meninges, showing how dentate ligaments anchor the spinal cord to its dural sheath through the arachnoid.
From Mettler FA: Neuroanatomy, ed 2, St. Louis, 1948, Mosby–Year Book.

The epipial layer around the spinal cord is relatively thick and gives rise to a toothed longitudinal projection on each side called the *dentate (denticulate) ligament*. The dentate ligament anchors the spinal cord to the arachnoid and through it to the dura. In addition, another pial projection, the *filum terminale,* anchors the caudal end of the spinal cord (the *conus medullaris*) to the caudal end of the spinal dural sheath (Figure 7-2). The caudal end of the dural sheath, in turn, is anchored to the caudal end of the vertebral canal.

## SOME FUNCTIONAL ASPECTS OF THE MENINGES

As discussed previously, the three meningeal coverings of the brain have various real or potential spaces associated with them (Figure 3-14). There is no space between the pia and the brain, but there is a subarachnoid space between the pia and the arachnoid, along with potential subdural and epidural spaces. Both of these potential spaces can become actual fluid-filled spaces under certain conditions.

The meningeal arteries run in the periosteal layer of the dura. If one of these arteries is torn (typically as a result of traumatic skull injury), bleeding occurs between the periosteum and the skull, opening up the potential epidural space and causing an *epidural hematoma*. As the hematoma expands, it compresses and distorts the underlying brain and is almost always fatal unless promptly treated surgically.

Bleeding can also occur into the potential subdural

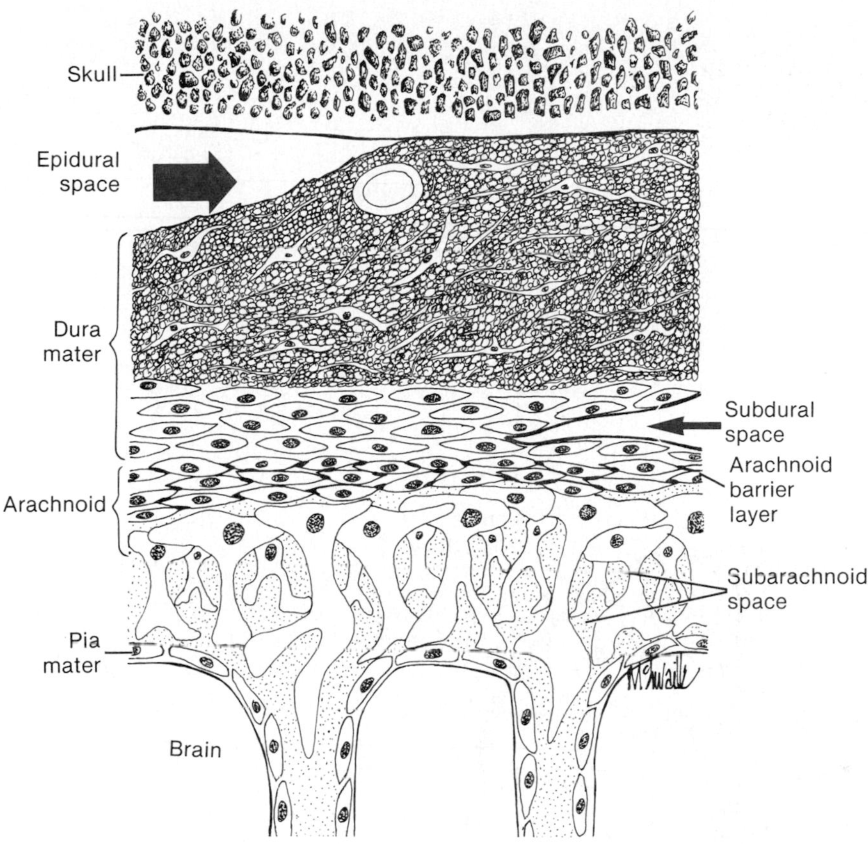


FIGURE 3-14
Spaces and potential spaces in and around the meninges. Epidural space (not normally present) between dura and skull may be opened up by blood from a ruptured meningeal artery. Subdural space (not normally present), typically within the dura near the latter's junction with the arachnoid, may be opened up by blood from a vein that ruptures as it enters a dural sinus. Dark bars joining superficial arachnoid cells represent the tight junctions that are the basis of the barrier properties of this portion of the arachnoid.

space, resulting in a *subdural hematoma*. The most common cause is the tearing of a cerebral vein as it enters a dural sinus. Some subdural hematomas are acute and produce symptoms much like those of an epidural hematoma, while others may progress very slowly and become surprisingly large before producing symptoms.

Dural reflections such as the falx cerebri and the tentorium cerebelli are firmly attached to the cranium. These reflections are stretched rather taut, which allows them to perform their mechanical support function, but this very tautness can result in additional problems in cases of increasing intracranial pressure (for example, subdural hematoma or an expanding tumor). The midbrain may be pushed against the edge of the tentorium while passing through the tentorial notch, causing damage to a cerebral peduncle and one or more cranial nerves. Also, depending on where the expanding mass causing the increased pressure is located, certain portions of the brain may herniate from one side of a dural reflection to another (Figures 3-15 and 3-16). For example, increased pressure on the lateral surface of one cerebral hemisphere can cause the hemisphere to be displaced inferiorly and medially, causing the uncus and adjacent portions of the temporal lobe to herniate through the tentorial notch and compress the midbrain. Such pressure could also cause one cingulate gyrus to herniate under the falx. Similarly, downward pressure can cause portions of the cerebellum to herniate into the foramen magnum and compress the medulla. Herniations that compress the brainstem are likely to have grave consequences.

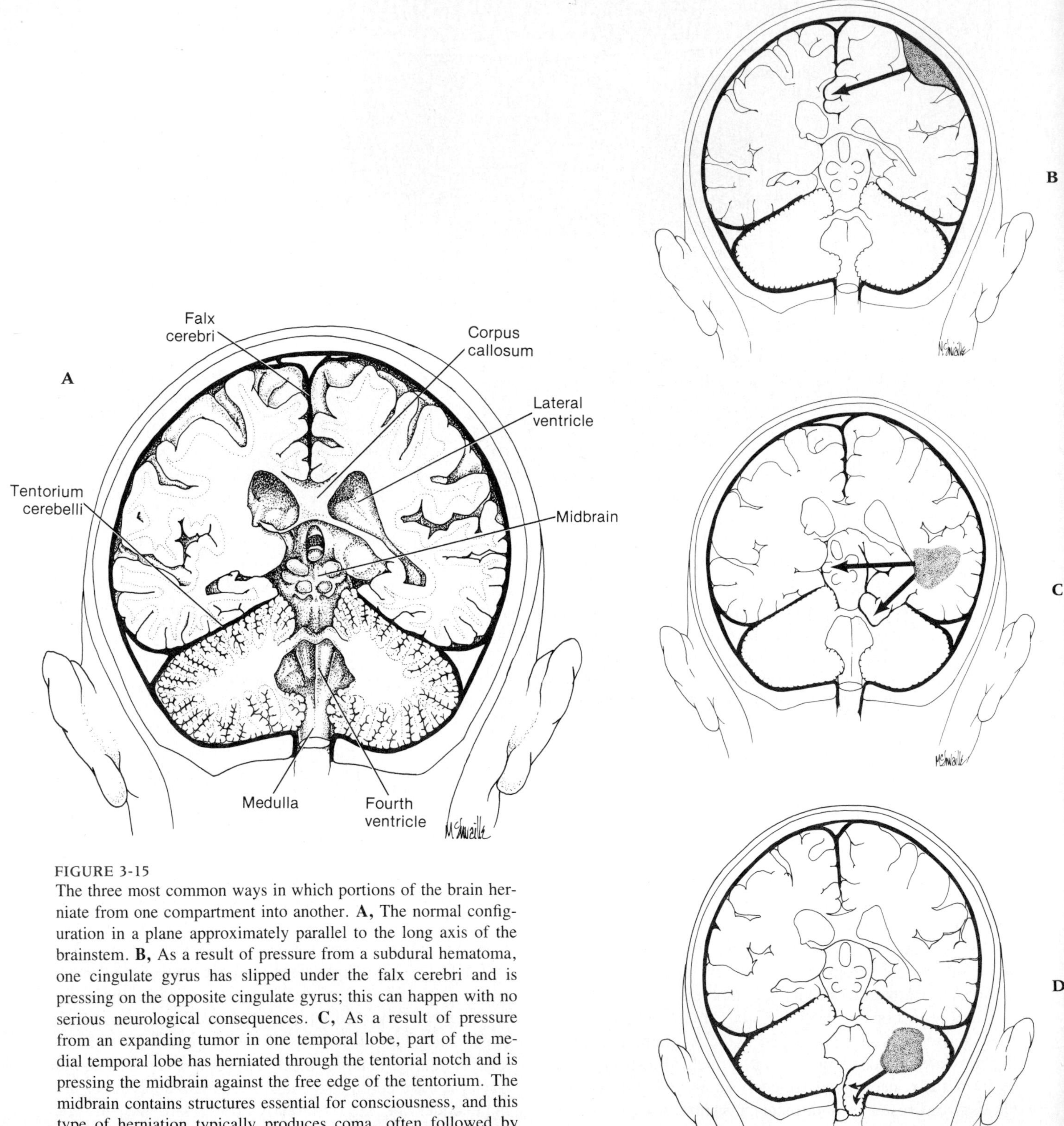


FIGURE 3-15
The three most common ways in which portions of the brain herniate from one compartment into another. **A,** The normal configuration in a plane approximately parallel to the long axis of the brainstem. **B,** As a result of pressure from a subdural hematoma, one cingulate gyrus has slipped under the falx cerebri and is pressing on the opposite cingulate gyrus; this can happen with no serious neurological consequences. **C,** As a result of pressure from an expanding tumor in one temporal lobe, part of the medial temporal lobe has herniated through the tentorial notch and is pressing the midbrain against the free edge of the tentorium. The midbrain contains structures essential for consciousness, and this type of herniation typically produces coma, often followed by death. **D,** As a result of pressure from a cerebellar tumor, one tonsil of the cerebellum has herniated through the foramen magnum, compressing the medulla against the margin of the foramen. The medulla contains respiratory and cardiovascular centers, and pressure on it is usually rapidly fatal.

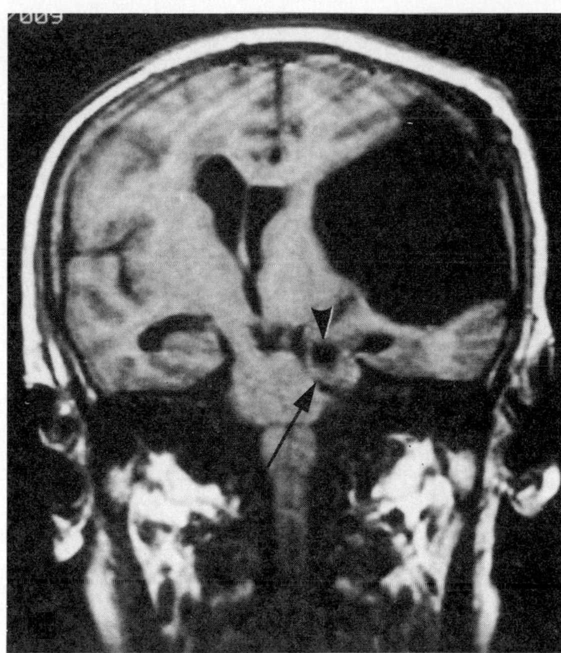

FIGURE 3-16
Magnetic resonance image of uncal herniation; L = left side, R = right side. A 62-year-old woman experienced slowly progressive weakness over a period of 2 years. She was found to have a large cyst that distended the left lateral sulcus. This pushed the left uncus, adjacent portions of the parahippocampal gyrus, and part of the inferior horn of the lateral ventricle *(arrowhead)* through the tentorial notch. Notice how the herniated temporal lobe distorts the midbrain and rostral pons *(arrow)*, and how the large cyst pushed the bodies of both lateral ventricles to the right. Uncal herniation is usually a neurosurgical emergency, so images like this can rarely be obtained.

From Iwama T et al, *Neuroradiology* 33:346, 1991. Courtesy of Dr. T Iwama, Department of Neurosurgery, Prefectural Gifu Hospital.

## ADDITIONAL READINGS


Alcolado R et al: The cranial arachnoid and pia mater in man: anatomical and ultrastructural observations, *Neuropathol Applied Neurobiol* 14:1, 1988. *Argues that cerebral vessels enter the brain beneath the pia, rather than through subarachnoid space.*

Bisaria KK: Anatomic variations of venous sinuses in the region of the torcular Herophili, *J Neurosurg* 62:90, 1985.

Davson H, Hollingsworth G, Segal MB: The mechanism of drainage of the cerebrospinal fluid, *Brain* 93:665, 1970. *Physiological experiments supporting the concept of bulk flow of cerebrospinal fluid through arachnoid villi.*

Esiri MM, Gay D: Immunological and neuropathological significance of the Virchow-Robin space, *J Neurol Sci* 100:3, 1990. *Reviews the evidence for a connection between Virchow-Robin spaces and the lymphatic system, and the idea that this connection can be significant in CNS diseases involving the immune system.*

Keller JT et al: Innervation of the posterior fossa dura of the cat, *Brain Res Bull* 14:97, 1985.

Kimmel DL: Innervation of spinal dura mater and dura mater of the posterior cranial fossa, *Neurology* 11:800, 1961.

Krahn V: The pia mater at the site of the entry of blood vessels into the central nervous system, *Anat Embryol* 164:257, 1982.

Liliequist B: The subarachnoid cisterns: an anatomic and roentgenologic study, *Acta Radiol Suppl* 185, 1959.

Livingston RB: *Mechanics of cerebrospinal fluid*. In Ruch TC, Patton HD, editors: *Physiology and biophysics*, ed 19, Philadelphia, 1965, WB Saunders. *Explains why a brain suspended in cerebrospinal fluid has an effective weight of only 50 grams.*

May PRA et al: Woodpecker drilling behavior: an endorsement of the rotational theory of impact brain injury, *Arch Neurol* 36:370, 1979. *Not closely related to the meninges but an interesting discussion of suspension of the brain within the cranium and protection of the brain from injury. Imagine what would happen to you if you banged your beak on a tree as often and as hard as a woodpecker does.*

Meyer A: Herniation of the brain, *Arch Neurol Psychiatr* 4:387, 1940.

Millen JW, Woollam DHM: On the nature of the pia mater, *Brain* 84:514, 1961. *A lucid discussion of the appearance of the pia at the light microscopic level and of the differences between epipia and intima pia.*

Nabeshima S et al: Junctions in the meninges and marginal glia, *J Comp Neurol* 164:127, 1975. *Ultrastructual appearance of the meninges, the arachnoid barrier layer, and subdural space.*

Pease DC, Schultz RL: Electron microscopy of rat cranial meninges, *Am J Anat* 102:301, 1958.

Penfield W, McNaughton F: Dural headache and innervation of the dura mater, *Arch Neurol Psychiatr* 44:43, 1940. *A long but interesting account of the gross anatomy of dural innervation, headaches resulting from dural distortion, and the surgical relief of such headaches.*

Ray BS, Wolff HG: Experimental studies on headache: pain-sensitive structures of the head and their significance in headache, *Arch Surg* 41:813, 1940.

Schachenmayr W, Friede RL: The origin of subdural neomembranes. I. Fine structure of the dura-arachnoid interface in man, *Am J Pathol* 92:53, 1978.

Shabo AL, Maxwell DS: The morphology of the arachnoid villi: a light and electron microscopic study in the monkey, *J Neurosurg* 29:451, 1968.

Tripathi BJ, Tripathi RC: Vacuolar transcellular channels as a drainage pathway for cerebrospinal fluid, *J Physiol* 239:195, 1974.

Upton ML, Weller RO: The morphology of cerebrospinal fluid drainage pathways in human arachnoid granulations, *J Neurosurg* 63:867, 1985.

Waggener JD, Beggs J: The membranous coverings of neural tissues: an electron microscopy study, *J Neuropathol Exp Neurol* 26:417, 1967.

Zhang ET, Inman CBE, Weller RO: Interrelationships of the pia mater and the perivascular (Virchow-Robin) spaces in the human cerebrum, *J Anat* 170:111, 1990.

Zouaoui A, Hidden G: Cerebral venous sinuses: anatomical variants or thrombosis?, *Acta Anat* 133:318, 1988.

# CHAPTER 4

# *Ventricles and Cerebrospinal Fluid*

The hollow core of the embryonic neural tube develops into a continuous fluid-filled system of ventricles, lined with *ependymal cells,* in the adult; each division of the CNS contains a portion of this ventricular system. Within each cerebral hemisphere is a relatively large *lateral ventricle*. The paired lateral ventricles communicate with the *third ventricle* of the diencephalon through the *interventricular foramina* (or *foramina of Monro*). The third ventricle in turn communicates with the *fourth ventricle* of the pons and medulla through the narrow *cerebral aqueduct* (or *aqueduct of Sylvius*) of the midbrain. The fourth ventricle continues caudally as the tiny *central canal* of the caudal medulla and spinal cord; this canal is usually not patent over much of its extent.

Cerebrospinal fluid is formed within the ventricles, fills them, and emerges from apertures in the fourth ventricle to fill the subarachnoid space.

## VENTRICLES

### Lateral ventricle

The lateral ventricle follows a long C-shaped course through all the lobes of the cerebral hemisphere. It is customarily divided into five parts (Figures 4-1 and 4-2): (1) an *anterior* (or *frontal*) *horn,* in the frontal lobe anterior to the interventricular foramen; (2) a *body,* in the frontal and parietal lobes, extending posteriorly to the region of the splenium of the corpus callosum; (3) a *posterior* (or *occipital*) *horn,* projecting backward into the occipital lobe; (4) an *inferior* (or *temporal*) *horn,* curving down and forward into the temporal lobe; and (5) an *atrium,* or *trigone,* the region near the splenium where the body and the posterior and inferior horns meet.

Various structures form the borders of the lateral ventricle in its course through the cerebral hemisphere; many of them can be easily seen in coronal sections (see Figures 2-18 to 2-24) or in brains dissected from above (Figure 4-3). The *caudate nucleus* is a constant feature in sections through the ventricle. Its enlarged head forms the lateral wall of the anterior horn (see Figure 2-18), its somewhat smaller body is most of the lateral wall of the body of the ventricle (see Figure 2-20), and its attenuated tail lies in the roof of the inferior horn (Figure 4-6, *D*). Proceeding posteriorly, as the caudate nucleus becomes smaller, the thalamus becomes larger and forms the floor of the body of the ventricle (compare Figures 2-18 and 2-22). The *corpus callosum* and *septum pellucidum* give a good indication of the size and location of the anterior horn and body of the ventricle. The body of the corpus callosum forms the roof of these parts of the ventricle, and the genu of the corpus callosum curves down to form the anterior wall of the anterior horn. The septum pellucidum forms the medial wall of the body and anterior horn, and its termination near the splenium marks the site where the bodies of the ventricles diverge from the midline and begin to curve around into the inferior horns (compare Figures 2-21 and 2-24).

The posterior horn is phylogenetically the most recently developed part of the lateral ventricle and is also the most variable in size, sometimes being rudimentary. A number of asymmetries between the cerebral hemispheres of the human brain have been discovered (or rediscovered) in recent years, and it appears that the left posterior horn tends to be longer than the right, particularly in right-handed individuals. The two lateral ventricles are otherwise quite symmetrical.

The *hippocampus* forms most of the floor and medial wall of the inferior horn (Figure 4-6), which ends anteriorly at about the level of the uncus.

## Third ventricle

The narrow, slit-shaped third ventricle occupies most of the midline region of the diencephalon, and so its entire outline can be seen in a hemisected brain (see Figures 2-14 and 4-2). It often looks like a misshapen doughnut in casts of the ventricular system (see Figure 4-1). The hole in the doughnut corresponds to the *interthalamic adhesion,* which crosses the ventricle in most human brains.

Anteriorly the third ventricle ends at the lamina terminalis, the adult remnant of the rostral end of the neural tube. Much of the medial surface of the thalamus and hypothalamus forms the wall of the third ventricle, and part of the hypothalamus forms its floor. It has a thin membranous roof containing choroid plexus (discussed in the next section). At the posterior end of the mammillary bodies, the third ventricle narrows fairly abruptly to become the *cerebral aqueduct,* which traverses the midbrain. The interventricular foramen, in the anterior part of the wall of the third ventricle, is an important radiological landmark since its location can be visualized by several different methods and it bears a known anatomical relationship to a number of deep structures.

An outline of the third ventricle reveals four protrusions, called *recesses* (Figure 4-1), corresponding to structures that have evaginated from the diencephalon. Inferiorly the *optic recess* lies in front of the optic chiasm, at the base of the lamina terminalis; the *infundibular recess* lies just behind the chiasm. Superiorly the *pineal recess* invades the stalk of the pineal gland, and the *suprapineal recess* lies just anterior to this stalk.

## Fourth ventricle

The fourth ventricle is sandwiched between the cerebellum posteriorly and the pons and rostral medulla anteriorly (see Figures 2-14 and 4-2). It is shaped like a tent with a peaked roof, the peak protruding into the cerebellum. The floor is relatively flat, and since it narrows rostrally into the aqueduct and caudally into the central canal, it is somewhat diamond-shaped (Figure 8-3, *A*). For this reason, the floor is sometimes referred to as the *rhomboid fossa*. At the location where the lateral point of the diamond would be expected, the entire ventricle becomes a narrow tube that proceeds anteriorly and curves around the brainstem, ending adjacent to the flocculus of the cerebellum. This tubular prolongation is the *lateral recess* of the fourth ventricle (see Figures 4-1 and 8-8). The portion of the roof of the ventricle rostral to the peak is the *superior medullary velum,* and the portion caudal to the peak is the *inferior medullary velum*. The superior medullary velum is a thin layer of white matter related to the cerebellum, while the inferior medullary velum is a membrane containing choroid plexus, similar to the roof of the third ventricle.

The lateral and third ventricles are closed cavities, communicating only with other parts of the ventricular system. In contrast, there are three apertures in the fourth ventricle through which the ventricular system communicates freely with subarachnoid space. These are the unpaired *median aperture* (or *foramen of Magendie*) and the two *lateral apertures* (or *foramina of Luschka*) of the fourth ventricle

*Text continued on p. 55.*

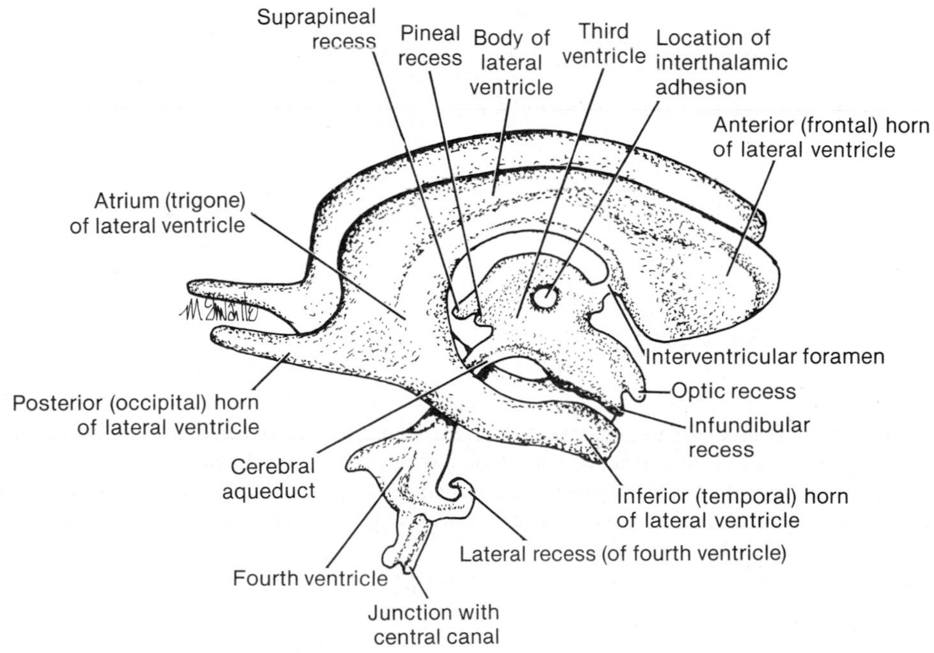


FIGURE 4-1
Drawing of a cast of the ventricular system.

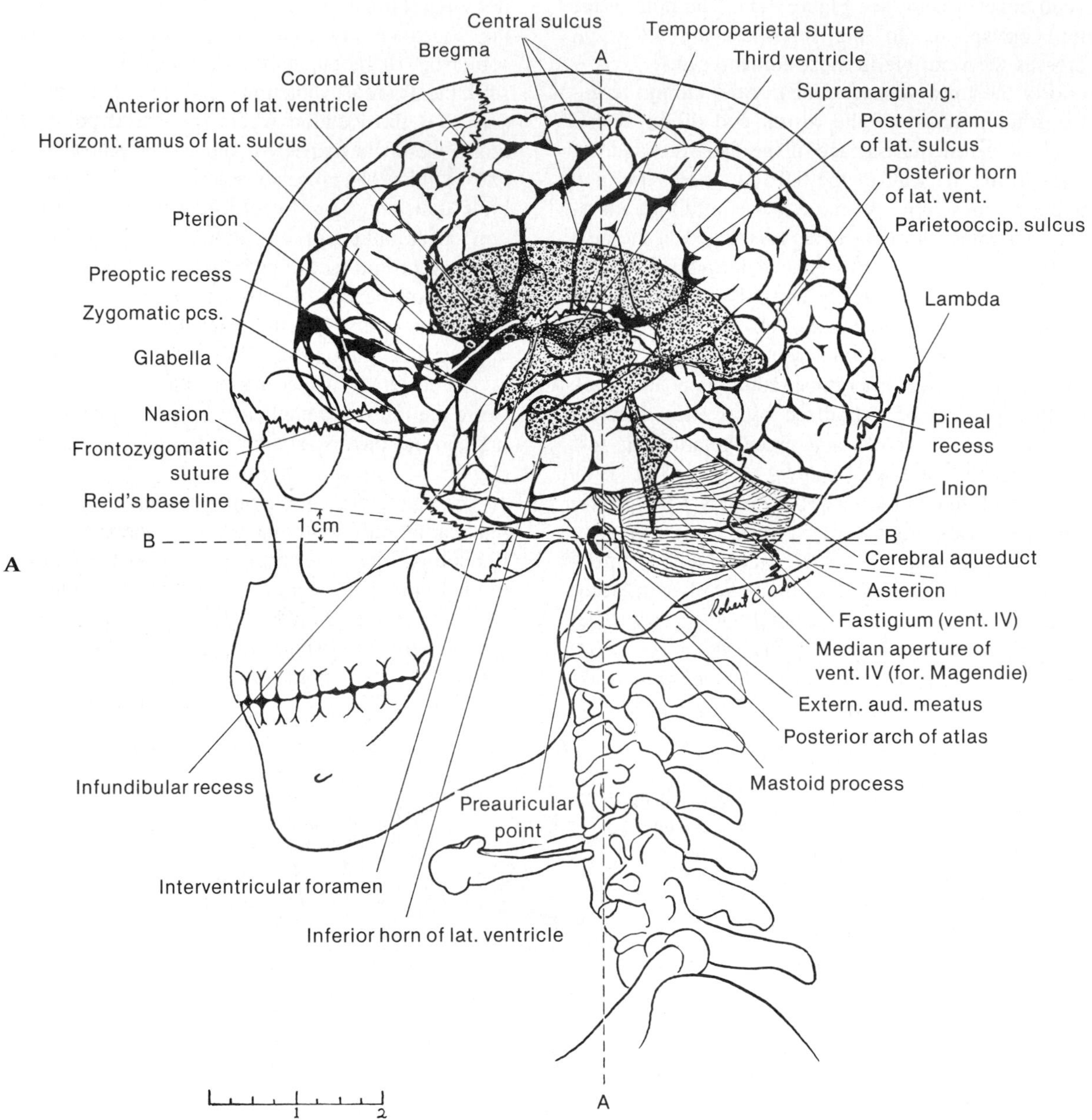


FIGURE 4-2

Spatial relationships of ventricles, brain and skull. **A,** Lateral projection of ventricles within brain and skull; the optical axis for this projection was a line through both external auditory meatuses. A number of gross anatomical features are indicated. The *fastigium* is the apex of the peaked roof of the fourth ventricle. Line A-A indicates the plane of section shown in **D,** and line B-B indicates the optical axis of the projection in **C** and **D.**

From Mettler FA: Neuroanatomy, ed 2, St. Louis, 1948, The CV Mosby Co.

B

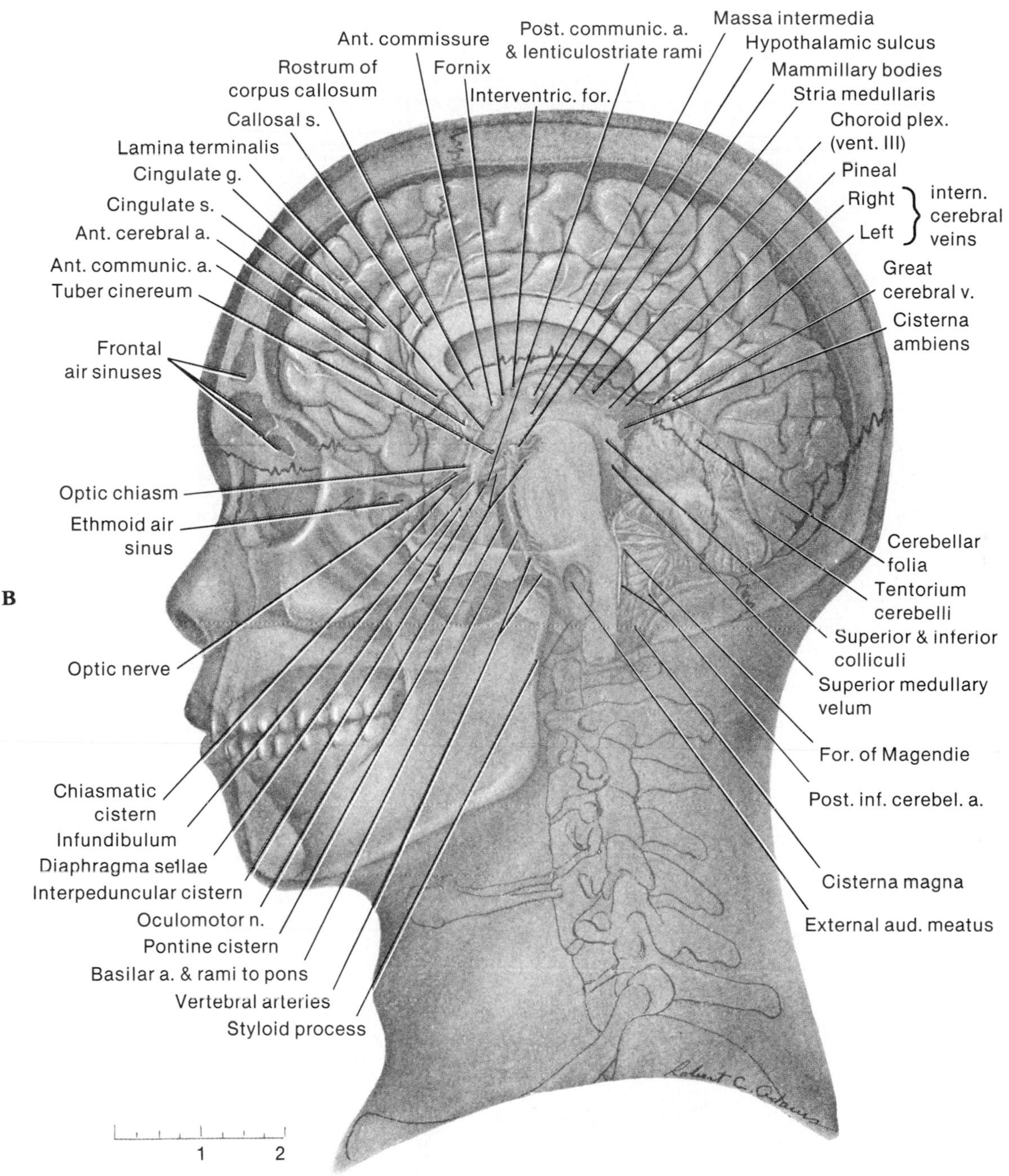


FIGURE 4-2, cont'd

**B,** Medial surface of a hemisected brain, shown as though the skull were transparent. *Superior medullary velum* is a term for the rostral half of the roof of the fourth ventricle.

*Continued.*

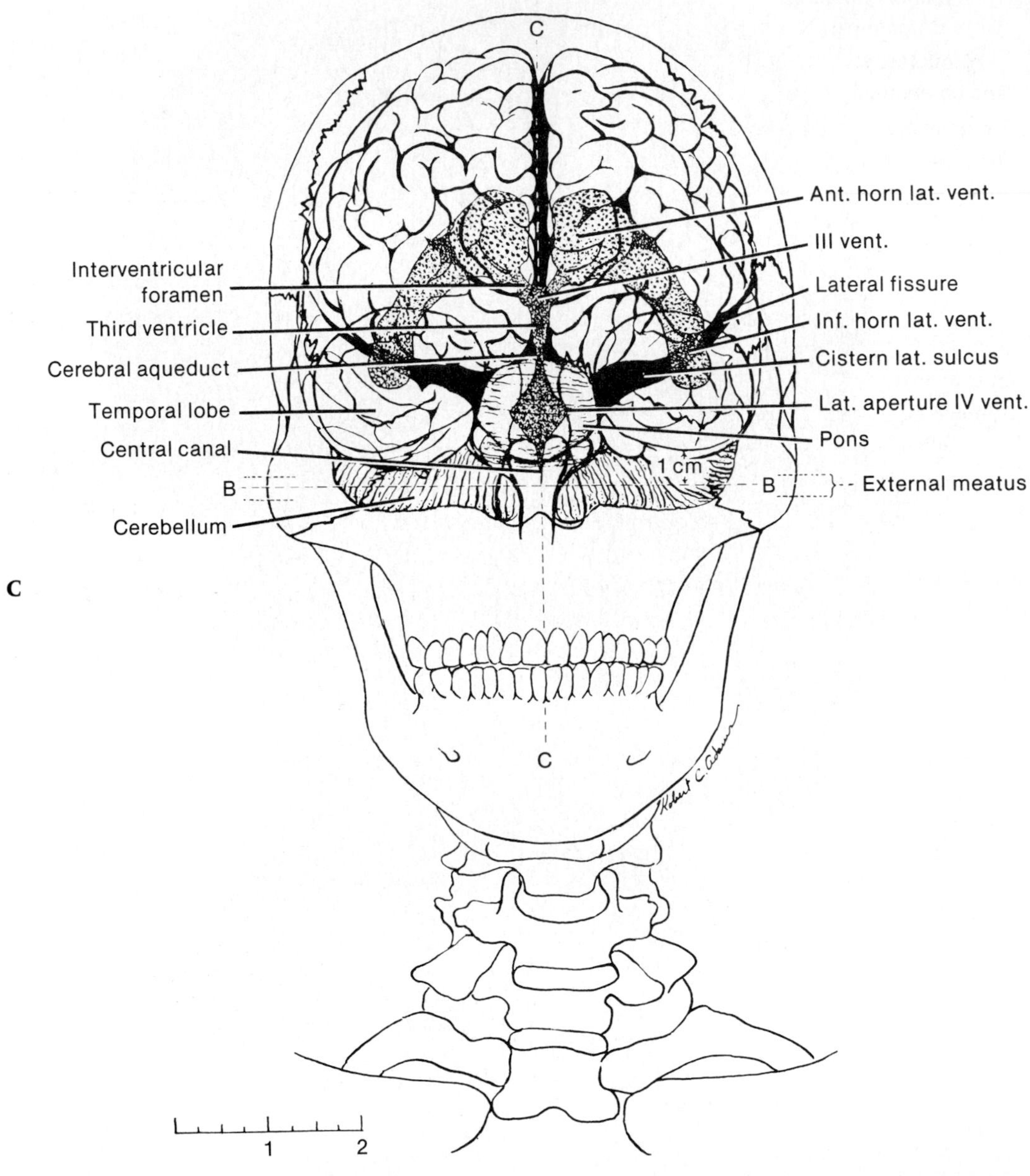


FIGURE 4-2, cont'd

**C,** Frontal projection of ventricles within brain and skull. Line B-B indicates the optical axis of the projection shown in **A** and **B,** and line C-C indicates the plane of section shown in **B.**

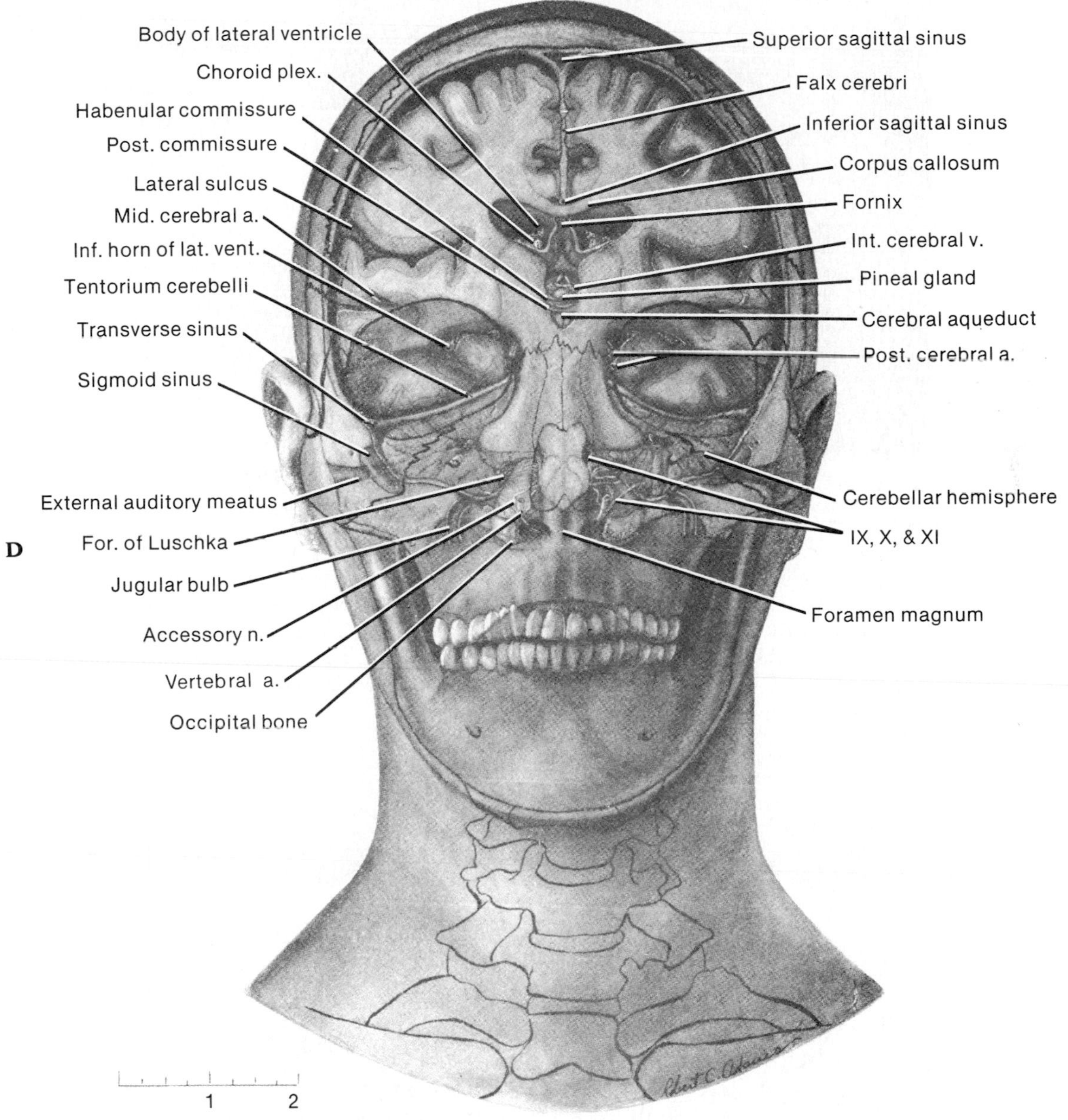


FIGURE 4-2, cont'd

**D,** Coronal section of the brain along line A-A in **A,** as though the skull were transparent. The *habenular commissure* interconnects two small nuclei at the base of the pineal.

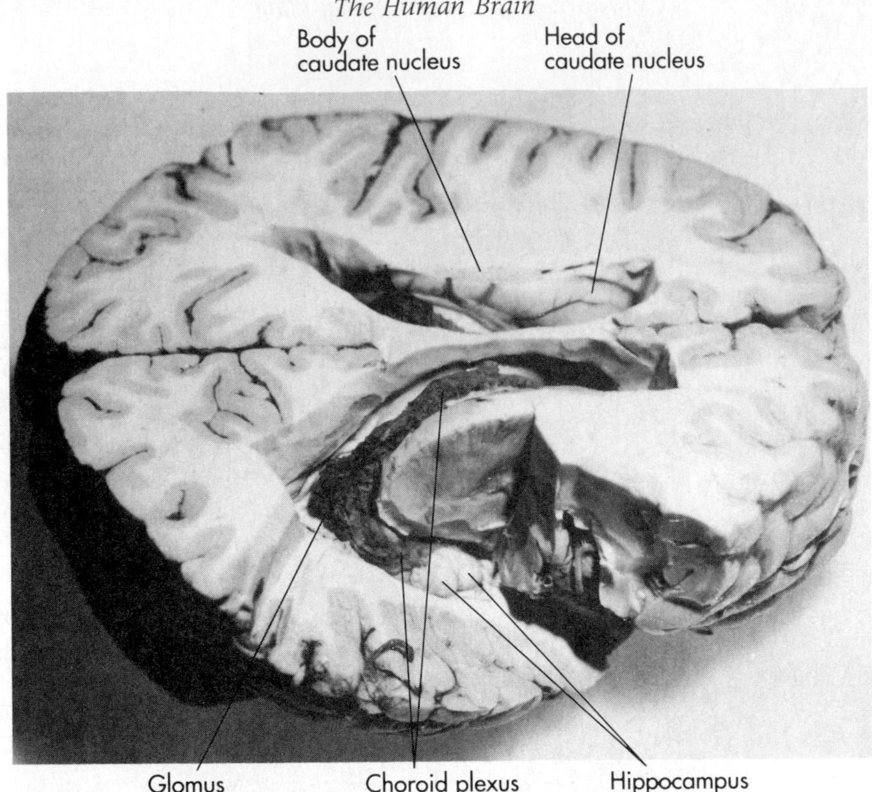


FIGURE 4-3
Dissection demonstrating the lateral ventricles, viewed from above and to the right. A horizontal cut was made to expose the ventricles, and most of the corpus callosum was removed. Some white matter was removed on both sides to expose the posterior horns. The insula and superior portions of the right hemisphere were also removed so that the inferior horn could be seen on that side. Continuous choroid plexus follows a C-shaped course from the inferior horn through the atrium, through the body of the lateral ventricle, and into the interventricular foramen (not visible from this angle). There is no choroid plexus in the anterior or posterior horn.

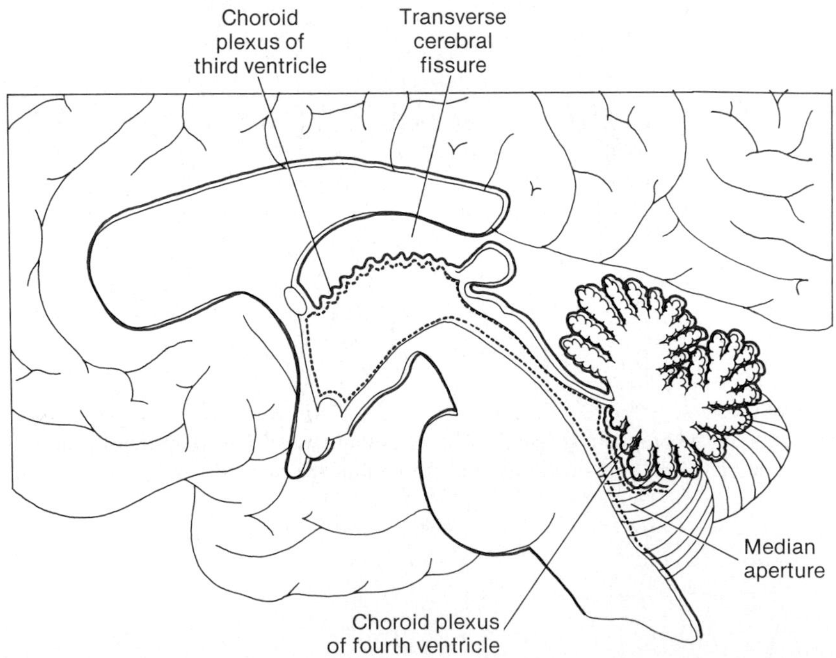


FIGURE 4-4
Disposition of the pia mater and ependyma in and around the third and fourth ventricles. The solid line represents the edge of the pia mater that would have been cut during hemisection. The dashed line represents the cut edge of the ependymal lining. Areas where pia and ependyma are directly applied to one another form part of the choroid plexus.

(Figures 4-8 and 4-9). The median aperture is simply a hole in the inferior medullary velum (Figure 4-4); it is as though the caudal end of the membrane, where it should have closed off the ventricle at its junction with the central canal, had instead been lifted up and attached to the inferior surface of the cerebellar vermis. The result is a funnel-shaped opening from the subarachnoid space (the *cerebellomedullary cistern,* or *cisterna magna*) into the ventricle. The inferior medullary velum also covers the lateral recess, and at the end of each recess is another opening in the velum, the lateral aperture.

### Ventricular size

The ventricles are both smaller and more variable in size than one might expect. Although there is an average total of approximately 130 ml of cerebrospinal fluid within and around the brain and spinal cord, only about 20 ml of this fluid is contained within the ventricles. The rest occupies subarachnoid space. The third and fourth ventricles together have a volume of only about 2 ml, and the volumes of the aqueduct and central canal are negligible, so the lateral ventricles contain nearly all the ventricular cerebrospinal fluid. The total volume of 20 ml is only an average figure, and the ventricles of some apparently normal brains have been found to have total volumes of less than 10 ml or more than 50 ml (however, volumes greater than 30 ml are usually considered suspicious).

## CHOROID PLEXUS

All four ventricles contain strands of highly convoluted and vascular membranous material, *choroid plexus,* that secretes most of the CSF. The composition of choroid plexus can be appreciated by first considering, for example, the anatomy of the roof of the third ventricle (Figures 1-12 and 4-5). This roof is simply a layer of ependymal cells overlaid by a layer of pia. As in all other locations, the pial layer also faces subarachnoid space, where the brain's blood supply is located. At certain locations this pia-ependyma complex invaginates into the ventricle with a collection of arterioles, venules, and capillaries (Figure 4-5). Here the ependymal layer appears as cuboidal epithelium *(choroid epithelium)* and functions as a secretory epithelium; the whole ependyma-pia-capillary complex is the choroid plexus. There is a long, continuous band of choroid plexus in each lateral ventricle, extending from near the tip of the inferior horn, around in a C-shaped course through the ventricle body to the interventricular foramen (see Figures 1-14 and 4-3). There is no choroid plexus in the anterior or posterior horn. The plexus is enlarged in the region of the atrium, and here it is called the *glomus* (Latin for ball of thread). Choroid plexus tends to become calcified with age, and the glomus can often be seen in x-ray studies (Figure 4-12, *C*). The choroid plexus of each lateral ventricle grows through the interventricular foramen, forming part of its posterior wall, and becomes one of the two narrow strands of choroid plexus in the roof of the third ventricle (Figure 4-6). It does not continue through the aqueduct, which is completely surrounded by neural tissue.

The choroid plexus of the fourth ventricle is formed from a similar invagination of the inferior medullary velum into the caudal half of the ventricle. It is T-shaped, with the vertical part of the T consisting of two adjacent longitudinal strands of plexus. These frequently extend as far as the median aperture, where they would be directly exposed to subarachnoid space (see Figure 4-4). The transverse portion of the T consists of one strand of plexus, which extends into each lateral recess. Each end reaches the lateral aperture, where a small tuft of choroid plexus generally protrudes through the aperture and is exposed directly to subarachnoid space (Figure 8-8).

Since one side of pia mater always faces subarachnoid space, choroid plexus must always be adjacent to subarachnoid space on its pial side and to intraventricular space on its choroid epithelial side. Although this may seem contrary to the plexus's apparent location deep within each cerebral hemisphere (see Figure 4-3), it can be easily demonstrated in coronal sections (Figure 4-6). The location of the invagination of choroid plexus into the lateral ventricle is called the *choroid fissure.* The choroid fissure is a C-shaped slit of subarachnoid space that accompanies the fornix system of fibers from the inferior horn to the interventricular foramen. By the same reasoning, the space above the roof of the third ventricle, which continues laterally into the choroid fissure, is also subarachnoid space (see Figures 4-4 and 4-6). This is the *transverse cerebral fissure,* a long finger of subarachnoid space trapped in the middle of the cerebrum by the growth of the cerebral hemispheres posteriorly over the diencephalon and brainstem. The transverse cerebral fissure continues posteriorly into the superior cistern.

A

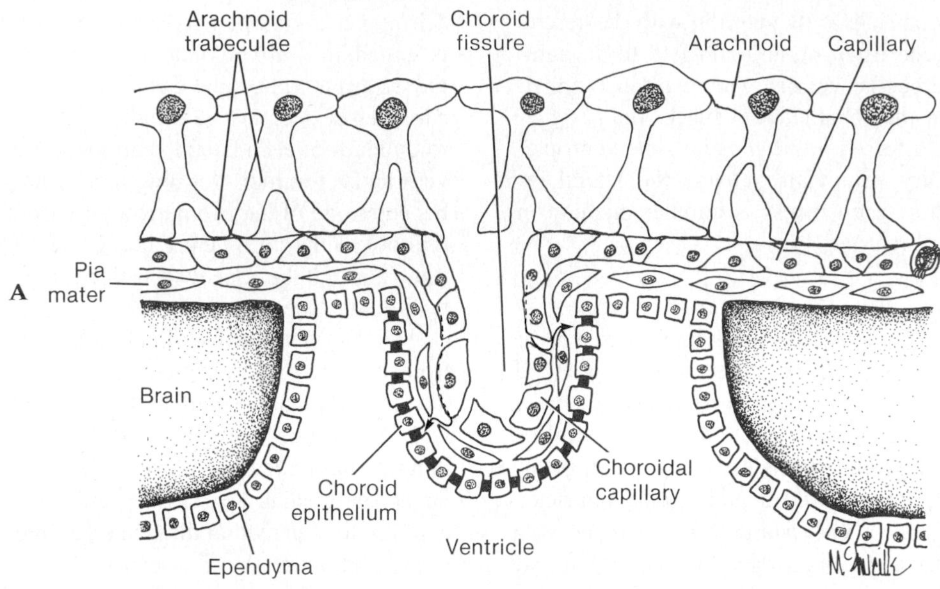


B

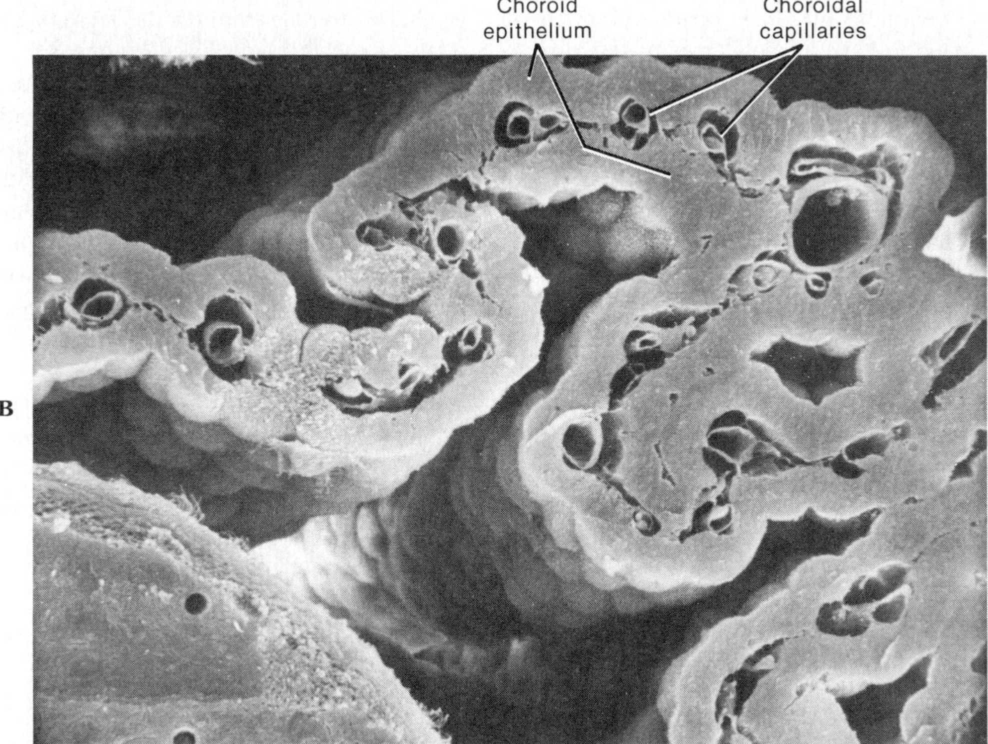


FIGURE 4-5
**A,** Composition of choroid plexus. Spaces are shown between endothelial cells of the choroidal capillary as opposed to those of ordinary cerebral capillaries, indicating that substances can escape from blood into the choroid plexus. However, they are stopped by arrays of tight junctions (represented here as dark bars) between choroid epithelial cells. **B,** Scanning electron micrograph of freeze-fractured preparation of choroid plexus. Note that choroid epithelium almost completely surrounds the choroidal capillaries, being separated from the capillaries only by attenuated pial elements.

**B** from Tissues and organs: a text-atlas of scanning electron microscopy by Richard G. Kessel and Randy H. Kardon. W.H. Freeman & Company. Copyright © 1979.

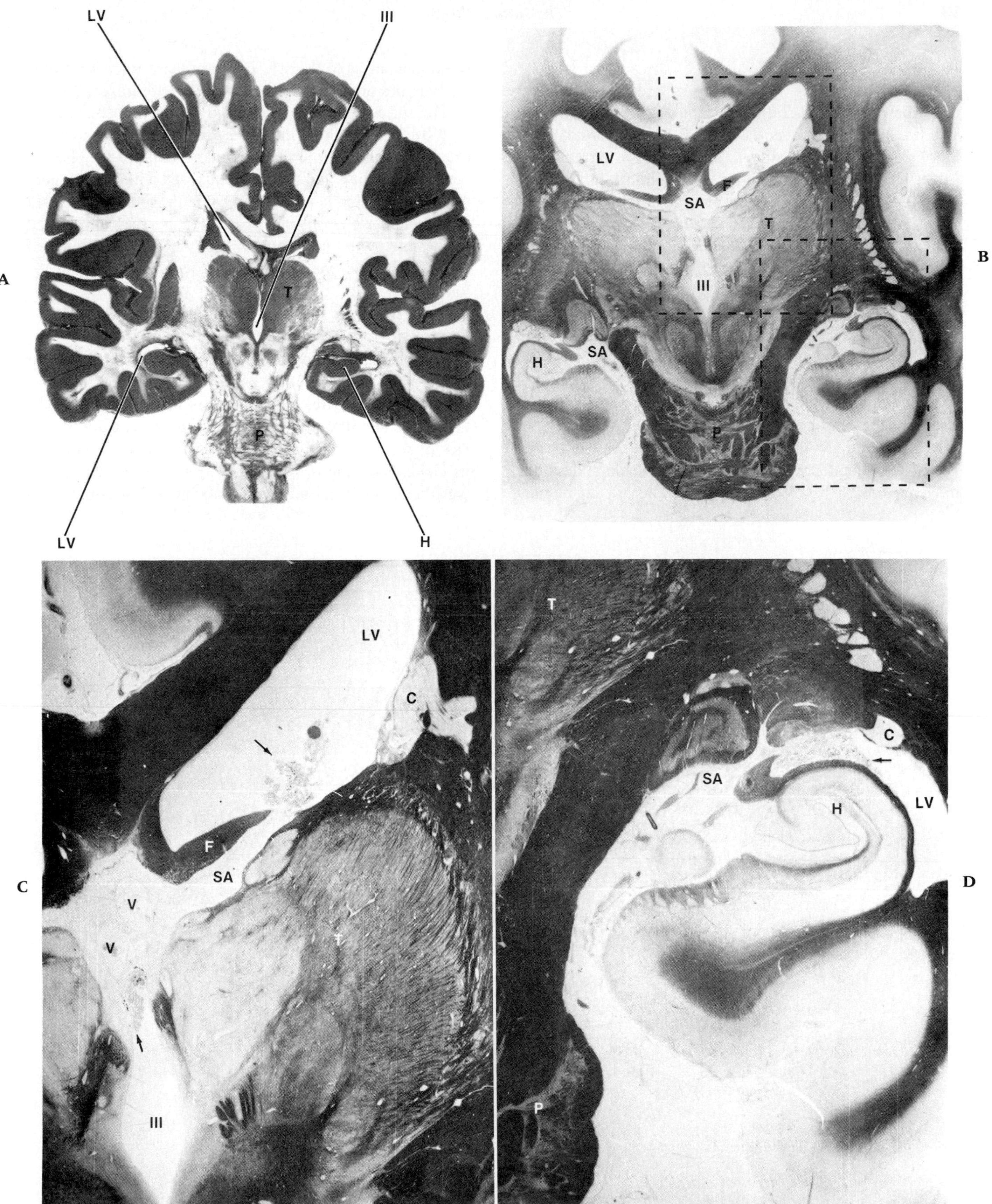


FIGURE 4-6
Coronal sections at different magnifications demonstrating the relationship of choroid plexus to subarachnoid space on one side and ventricular space on the other. *C*, Caudate nucleus; *F*, fornix; *H*, hippocampus; *LV*, lateral ventricle; *P*, pons; *SA*, subarachnoid space; *T*, thalamus; *V*, vein in subarachnoid space; *III*, third ventricle; small arrows point to choroid plexus. The central part of the brain slice in **A** is enlarged in the section shown in **B** (although the planes of section are not quite identical). The areas enclosed in the dotted rectangles in **B** are further enlarged in **C** and **D.**

### Microscopic structure

Choroid plexus is functionally a three-layered membrane between blood and cerebrospinal fluid (Figure 4-7). The first layer is the endothelial wall of the choroidal capillary. This wall is fenestrated, allowing easy movement of substances out of the capillary (in contrast to capillary walls elsewhere in the brain, which, as discussed in Chapter 5, are tightly sealed). The second layer, consisting of scattered pial cells and some collagen, is very incomplete. The third layer, derived from the same layer of cells that forms the ependymal lining of the ventricles, is the choroid epithelium. The choroid epithelial cells look as though they are specialized for secretion because they have many basal infoldings, numerous microvilli on the side facing the cerebrospinal fluid, and abundant mitochondria. In addition, adjacent cells are connected to one another by arrays of tight junctions that occlude the extracellular space around them. As in the case of the arachnoid barrier layer (see Chapter 3), these junctions help to limit the movement of substances across the choroid epithelium; some ions are able to diffuse across these tight junctions, but peptides and other larger molecules are impeded.

The surface area of the choroid plexus is increased not only by the folding of individual cell membranes into microvilli but also by the macroscopic folding of the choroid plexus itself into numerous fronds and villi (see Figure 4-6). This folding is so extensive that the total surface area of the human choroid plexus, neglecting the contribution of the microvilli, is more than 200 sq cm, or about two thirds of the total ventricular surface area.

## CEREBROSPINAL FLUID

### Formation

Cerebrospinal fluid is a colorless liquid, low in cells and proteins, but generally similar to plasma in its ionic composition. For this reason it was considered for some time to be an ultrafiltrate of blood. However, careful analysis of the composition of cerebrospinal fluid reveals that its content of various ions differs from that of plasma in a way that is not consistent with its being an ultrafiltrate. For

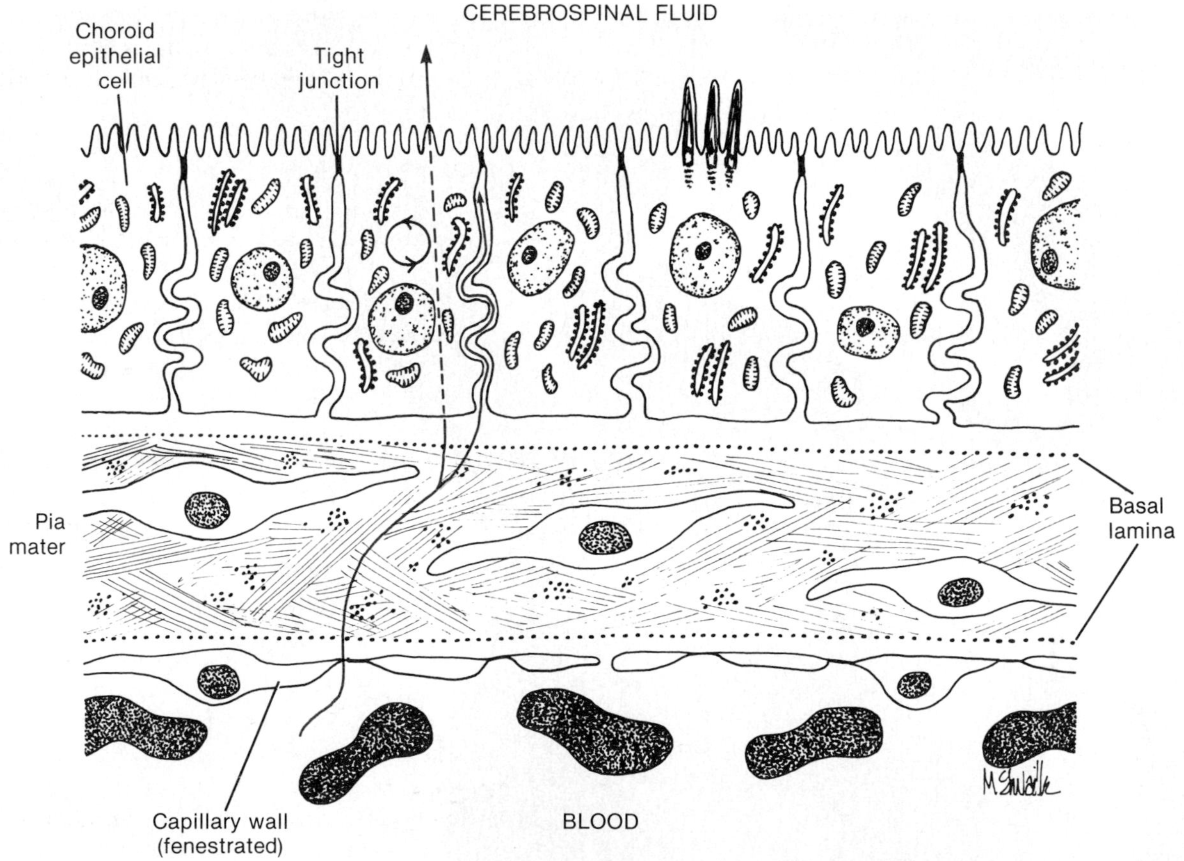


FIGURE 4-7
Microscopic structure of choroid plexus showing the three layers of tissue between blood and cerebrospinal fluid. Substances pass through the fenestrated capillary and through the extracellular space of the pia mater but cannot pass through the bands of tight junctions between choroid epithelial cells. They must pass through these cells by an active transport system.

example, compared to plasma, cerebrospinal fluid contains an excess of magnesium and chloride ions and a deficiency of potassium and calcium ions. Furthermore, these concentrations are maintained at very stable levels in the face of changes in plasma concentrations—a constancy that would not be expected if cerebrospinal fluid were an ultrafiltrate.* Finally, the formation of new cerebrospinal fluid is depressed by certain metabolic inhibitors, as would be expected if it were formed by an active, energy-requiring process. Therefore cerebrospinal fluid is currently considered to be an actively secreted product whose composition is dictated by specific transport mechanisms.

Most of the cerebrospinal fluid is produced within the ventricular system, primarily by the choroid plexus. Production of fluid by the choroid plexus was demonstrated rather directly by the neurosurgeon Cushing early in the twentieth century. During procedures in which it was necessary to open and drain a lateral ventricle, he noted that fluid could be seen accumulating on the surface of the choroid plexus; if he put a small silver clip on the artery supplying the choroid plexus, the fluid stopped appearing. A basically similar procedure has been used since then to study the composition of newly formed cerebrospinal fluid: a micropipette in contact with oil-covered choroid plexus can collect the fluid as it is formed. Chemical analysis has shown that it is identical in composition to bulk cerebrospinal fluid in normal ventricles.

Cerebrospinal fluid apparently is formed by filtration of blood through the fenestrations of the choroidal capillaries, followed by the active transport of substances (particularly sodium ions) across the choroid epithelium into the ventricle. Water then flows passively across the epithelium to maintain osmotic balance. The barrier properties of the choroid epithelium prevent substances from diffusing across it in an uncontrolled manner. The total process is actually more complicated than this and involves a balance between active transport and some passive diffusion of ions and other substances either through or between the choroid epithelial cells. It is also known that some substances are transported in the reverse direction (that is, from cerebrospinal fluid to blood).

Although cerebrospinal fluid seems to be secreted primarily by choroid plexus, there is also evidence that this is not its only source. This has been shown most directly in monkeys from whose lateral ventricles all the choroid plexus had been removed; these ventricles still produced substantial quantities of cerebrospinal fluid, although less than normal. The source of this extrachoroidal cerebrospinal fluid is generally considered to be the parenchyma of the brain, with fluid moving across the ependymal lining into the ventricle. The proportion of cerebrospinal fluid normally arising from this source is not known accurately, but most researchers agree that well over half is made by the choroid plexus.

The rate of formation of new cerebrospinal fluid (an average of about 350 μl/minute in humans) is relatively constant and little affected by systemic blood pressure or intraventricular pressure. This means that the total volume of cerebrospinal fluid is renewed more than three times per day.

One way this rate of formation can be modified is by the autonomic nervous system. Both sympathetic and parasympathetic fibers end not only on choroidal blood vessels, but also near the bases of the choroid epithelial cells. Experimental activation of these fibers can cause substantial changes in cerebrospinal fluid production, mainly through direct effects on the secretory rate of the choroid epithelial cells. Stimulating the sympathetic fibers, for example, causes a reduction of about 30% in the rate of cerebrospinal fluid production. Little is known, however, about the significance of this autonomic innervation under ordinary circumstances.

### Circulation

If the cerebrospinal fluid is turned over several times per day, it must circulate from its site of formation to a site of removal. We have already discussed all the elements of the system involved (Figures 4-8 and 4-9); cerebrospinal fluid formed in the lateral ventricles passes through the interventricular foramina into the third ventricle, from there through the cerebral aqueduct into the fourth ventricle, and thence through the median and lateral apertures into the cisterna magna and the pontine cistern. From the pontine cistern, the fluid slowly moves up over the cerebral hemispheres, through the arachnoid villi, and into the superior sagittal sinus. The flow should not be thought of as slow and steady, since arterial pulsations cause a constant ebb and flow, with a small net movement toward the superior sagittal sinus with each heartbeat. As would be expected from the rate of cerebrospinal fluid formation, it takes several hours for new cerebrospinal fluid to complete the journey.

In addition to this basic pattern of circulation, some cerebrospinal fluid moves from the cisterns around the fourth ventricle into the subarachnoid space around the spinal cord. It slowly makes its way caudally to the lumbar cistern, and then some of it slowly makes its way back rostrally. Along the way, most of this fluid is returned to the venous system through arachnoid villi that are found in the dural sleeves accompanying spinal nerve roots.

*Since the composition of cerebrospinal fluid is so constant in health, changes in its composition can be very helpful in diagnosing neurological disease. For example, meningitis can be either viral or bacterial in origin. In the latter case, the glucose concentration in the cerebrospinal fluid is markedly reduced (the bacteria eat the glucose), and the protein concentration is elevated. In viral meningitis, glucose is normal and protein slightly elevated or normal.

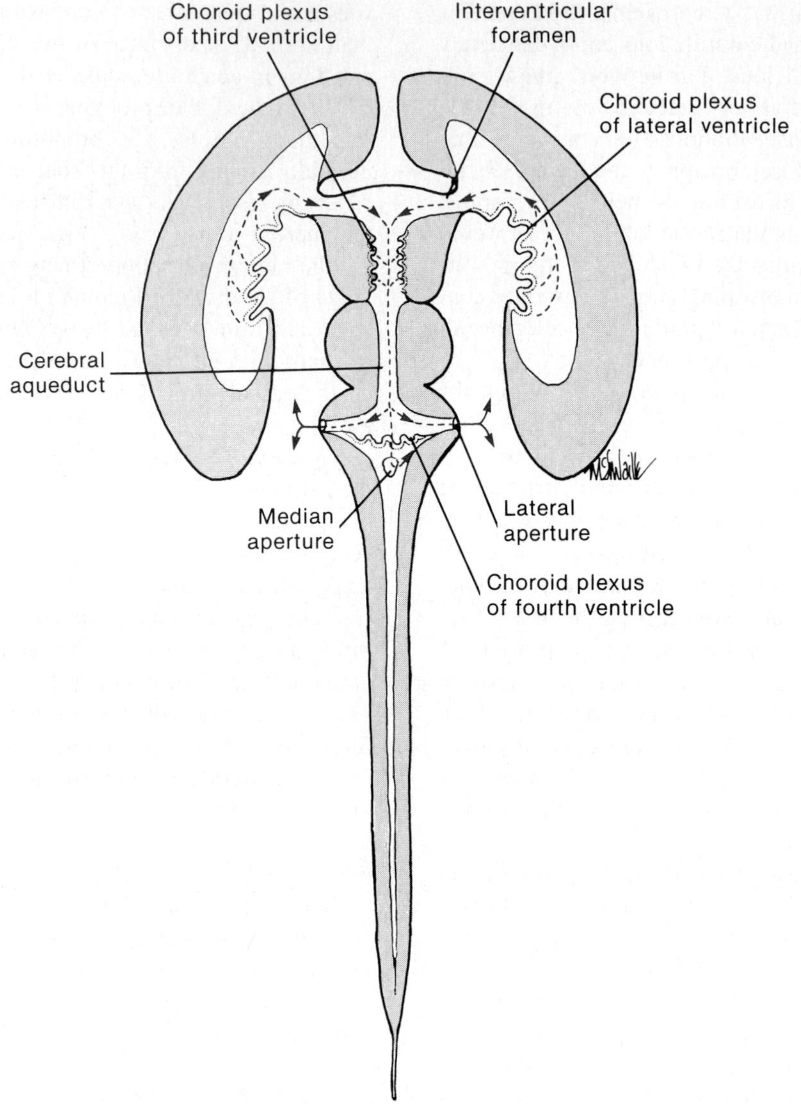


FIGURE 4-8
Path followed by cerebrospinal fluid through the ventricles.

Redrawn from Hamilton WJ, editor: Textbook of human anatomy, ed 2. St. Louis, 1976, Mosby-Year Book. By permission of Macmillan Press, London and Basingstoke.

## Function

The cerebrospinal fluid in the subarachnoid space plays a supportive role because of the buoyant effect discussed previously. However, it seems apparent that an actively secreted, constantly renewed fluid with a closely regulated composition must have other functions as well. Most of the functions that have been suggested involve the regulation of the extracellular environment of neurons. This could happen in either or both of two ways. First, the cerebrospinal fluid is known to be in free communication with the extracellular fluid of the brain, so secretion of controlled cerebrospinal fluid by the choroid plexus will secondarily control, to some extent, the composition of this extracellular fluid. Second, the cerebrospinal fluid system probably exerts a reverse sort of control by acting as a "sink" for substances produced by the brain, which would then be selectively absorbed from cerebrospinal fluid by the choroid plexus or nonselectively removed by flow through arachnoid villi. It is also likely that the cerebrospinal fluid is a route for the spread of neuroactive hormones through the nervous system.

## SOME FUNCTIONAL ASPECTS OF THE VENTRICULAR SYSTEM

Since the rate of production of cerebrospinal fluid is relatively independent of blood pressure and intraventricular pressure, the fluid will continue to be produced even if the path of its circulation is blocked or is otherwise abnormal.

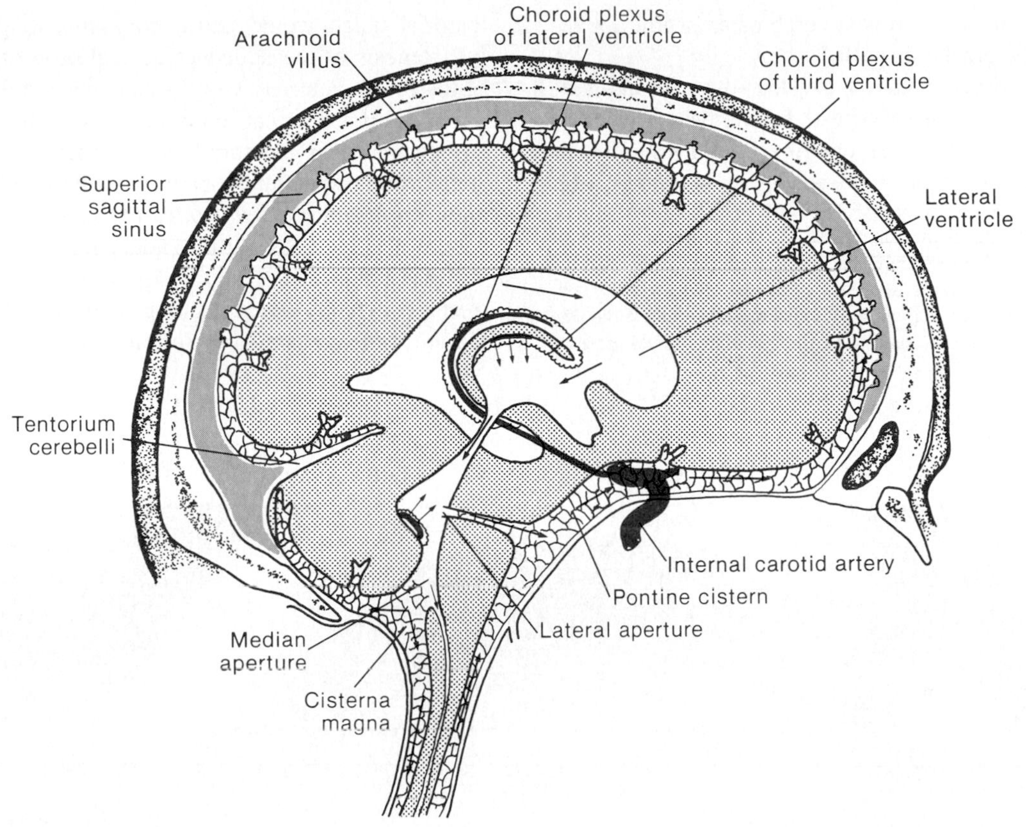


FIGURE 4-9
Path of circulation of cerebrospinal fluid from its formation in the ventricles to its absorption into the superior sagittal sinus.
Redrawn from Hamilton WJ, editor: Textbook of human anatomy, ed 2, St. Louis, 1976, The CV Mosby Co. By permission of Macmillan Press, London and Basingstoke.

When this happens, cerebrospinal fluid pressure rises and ultimately the ventricles expand at the expense of surrounding brain, creating a condition known as *hydrocephalus*. In principle, hydrocephalus can result from excess production of cerebrospinal fluid, from blockage of cerebrospinal fluid circulation, or from a deficiency in cerebrospinal fluid reabsorption. All three types occur, but that caused by a blockage of circulation is by far the most common.

Tumors of the choroid plexus, called *papillomas,* are sometimes associated with hydrocephalus. In some of these cases, a much greater than normal production of cerebrospinal fluid has been shown directly and is believed to be the cause of the hydrocephalus.

Circulation of cerebrospinal fluid can be obstructed at any point in the pathway. A tumor can occlude one interventricular foramen (or both of them), in which case the lateral ventricle involved becomes hydrocephalic, while the remainder of the ventricular system remains normal. Tumors of the pineal gland sometimes push down on the midbrain, squeeze the aqueduct shut, and cause hydrocephalus of the third ventricle and both lateral ventricles (Figure 4-11). In some congenital abnormalities, all three apertures of the fourth ventricle may either fail to develop or be occluded, resulting in hydrocephalus of the entire ventricular system. (Occlusion of only one or two of these apertures apparently has no effect.) Finally, circulation may be obstructed outside the ventricular system in subarachnoid space. For example, meningitis is sometimes followed by meningeal adhesions around the base of the brain that block the flow of cerebrospinal fluid through the tentorial notch. (Since the cerebrospinal fluid passes from the fourth ventricle into the posterior fossa, it must ordinarily pass through the tentorial notch before reaching the arachnoid villi of the superior sagittal sinus.) This too causes hydrocephalus of the entire ventricular system.

Persistent defects in the reabsorption of cerebrospinal fluid are not common, but rare cases have been reported in which apparent congenital absence of arachnoid villi was associated with hydrocephalus. Also there are occasional reports that obstruction of the superior sagittal sinus can cause hydrocephalus, presumably because venous pressure becomes high enough to prevent cerebrospinal fluid movement through the arachnoid villi.*

Clinically, hydrocephalus is divided into *communicating* and *noncommunicating* types, depending on whether or not both lateral ventricles are in communication with subarachnoid space. Thus blockage of flow through the tentorial notch would cause communicating hydrocephalus; stenosis of the aqueduct or occlusion of the apertures of the fourth ventricle would cause noncommunicating hydrocephalus. Note that in both situations the basic cause of hydrocephalus is the same: an obstruction in the cerebrospinal fluid's circulation path. Terminology such as *communicating* and *noncommunicating* is just a partial specification of the location of the blockage.

Once diagnosed, many cases of hydrocephalus can be treated surgically by implanting a shunt that extends from the locus of increased pressure to sites such as the perito-

*The fact that occlusion of the superior saggital sinus is only rarely (if ever) accompanied by hydrocephalus has been taken as evidence that the arachnoid villi are not the sole route by which CSF can leave the subarachnoid space. Possible alternate routes include movement along the adventitia of blood vessels and the sheaths of cranial and spinal nerves.

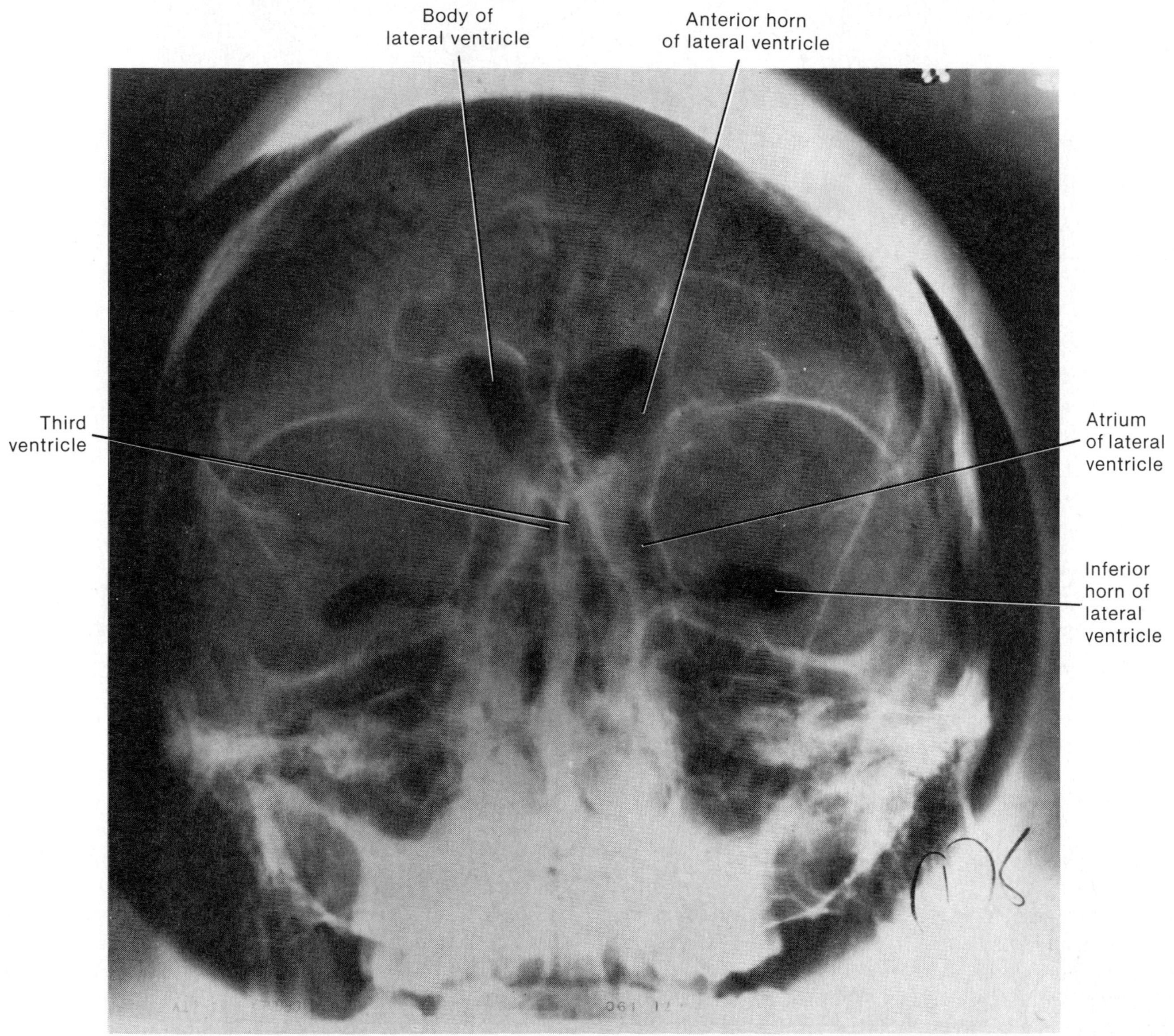


FIGURE 4-10

Normal pneumoencephalogram, anterior-posterior view (as though you were looking into the patient's face). The body and inferior horn of each lateral ventricle are particularly dark because they are viewed approximately end-on, so that the x rays traverse a relatively long path through air.

Courtesy of Dr. John Stears, University of Colorado Health Sciences Center.

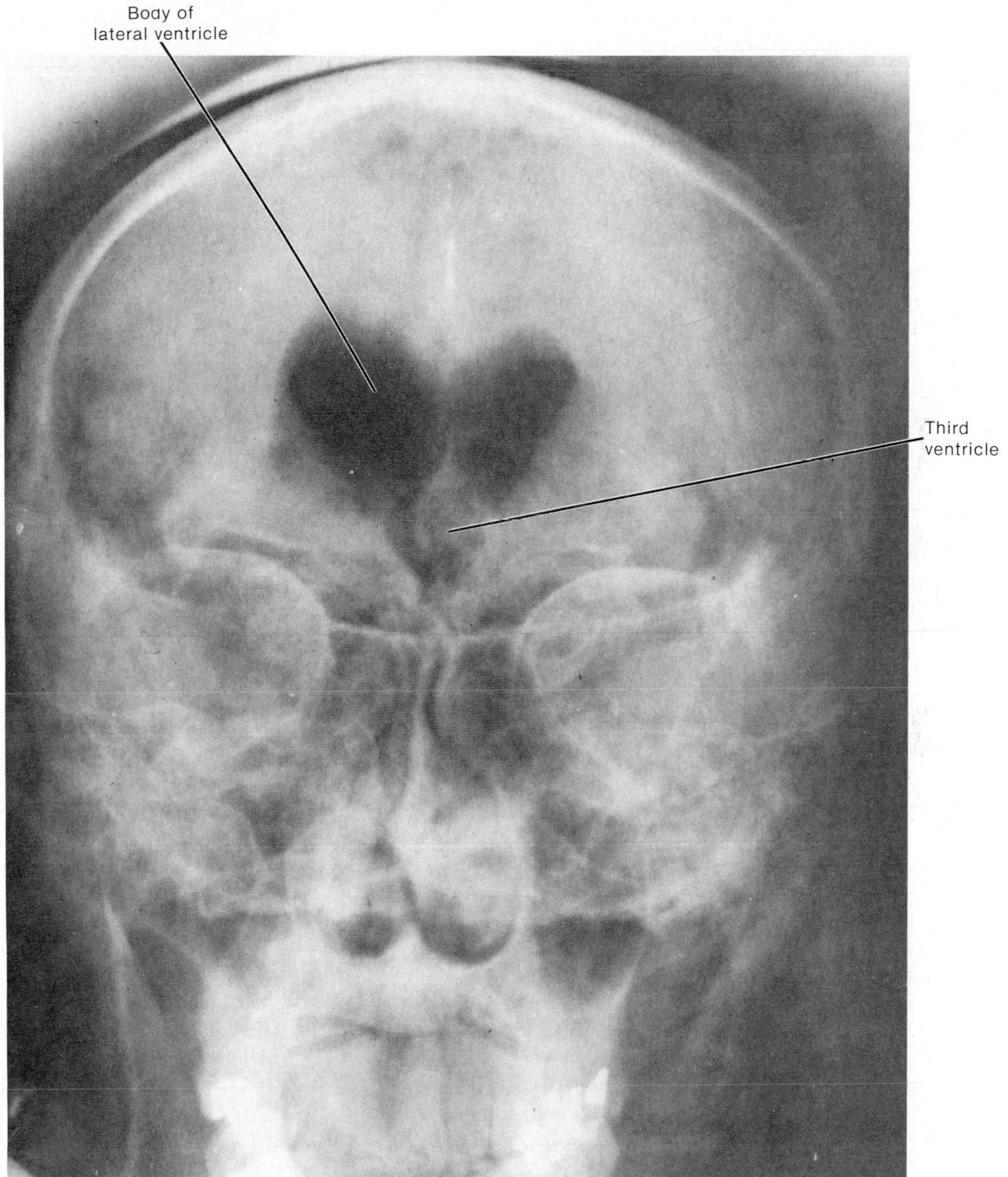


FIGURE 4-11
Pneumoencephalogram of a patient with hydrocephalus, anterior-posterior view. Enlargement of lateral and third ventricles is apparent. This patient had a shunt inserted into one lateral ventricle and improved markedly.

Courtesy of Dr. Michael Earnest, Denver General Hospital and University of Colorado Health Sciences Center.

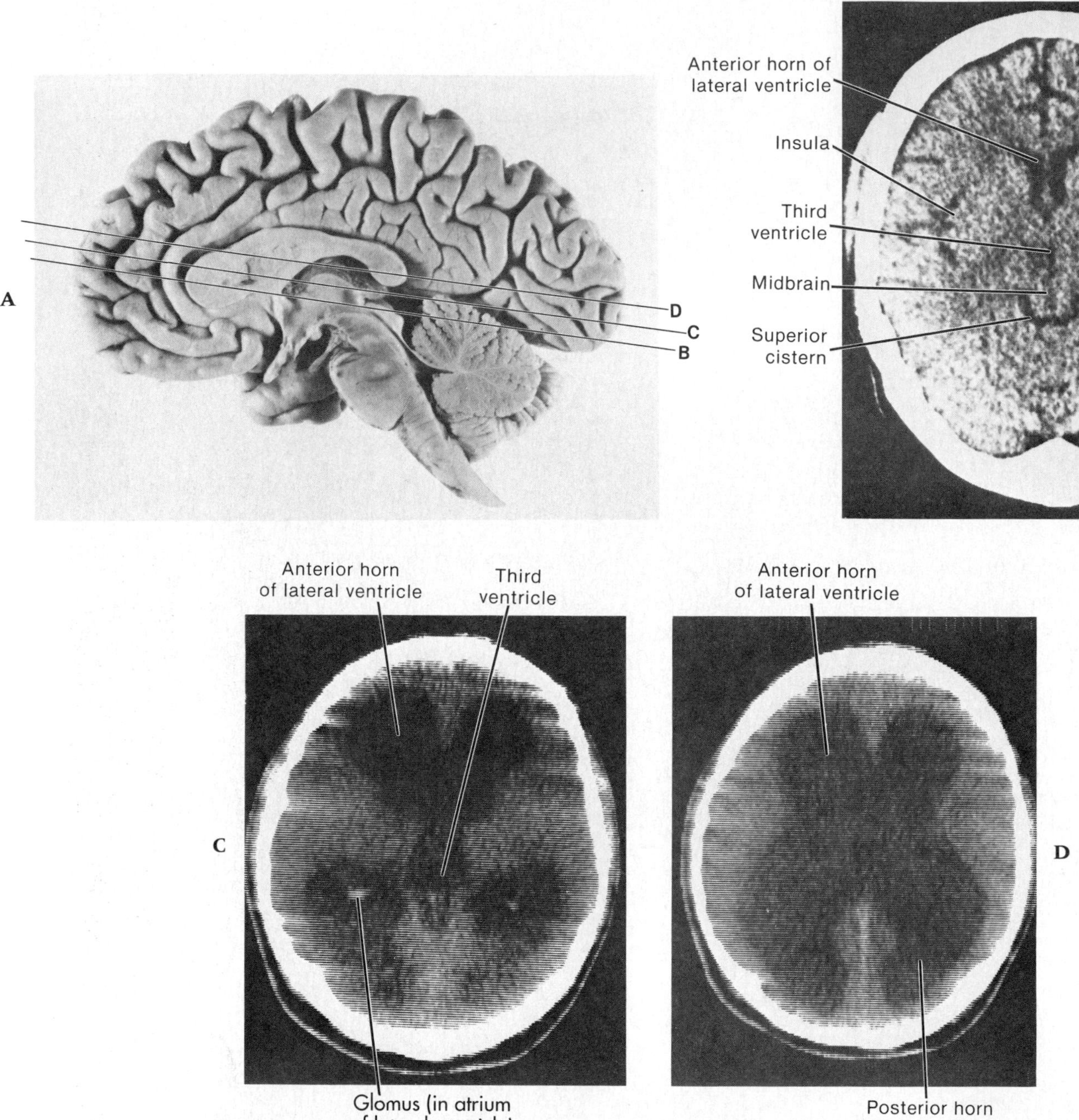


FIGURE 4-12

Examples of CT scans. Cerebrospinal fluid is dark in these scans and fills the ventricular system, subarachnoid cisterns, and cerebral sulci around the edge of the brain. **A,** Planes of section produced by the computer. **B,** Normal CT scan. **C** and **D,** Scans of two different planes from a patient with hydrocephalus; the great enlargement of the lateral and third ventricles is obvious.

**B** courtesy of Dr. John Stears, University of Colorado Health Sciences Center; **C** and **D** courtesy of Dr. Michael Earnest, Denver General Hospital and University of Colorado Health Sciences Center.

neal cavity or the right atrium. The implanted catheter must contain a valve to prevent reverse flow. There were many early attempts to treat hydrocephalus by removing the choroid plexus, but they were generally unsuccessful, probably because of the continued extrachoroidal production of cerebrospinal fluid.

Pneumoencephalography was a clinical test formerly used to diagnose hydrocephalus. This test involved injecting air or oxygen into the lumbar cistern and then maneuvering it into the ventricles. Air is much less dense to x-ray beams than is cerebrospinal fluid, so the shape of the ventricles could be recorded by x-ray photography (Figures 4-10 and 4-11). The shape of the ventricles can yield information not only about the presence and location of hydrocephalus but also about masses pushing against the brain and distorting the ventricles.

Pneumoencephalography was (for the patient) a very unpleasant procedure and has been supplanted by computerized tomography, or CT scanning. This technique involves directing an x-ray beam through the patient's head from a number of different angles and comparing and processing the resulting collection of density profiles with a computer. Small density differences can be detected in this way, and currently available machines can even differentiate between gray and white matter. Since the test is noninvasive and the radiation dosage small, it is ideal for many applications. Examples are shown in Figure 4-12.

A more recent imaging method, *magnetic resonance imaging,* or *MRI,* is another noninvasive technique that allows even greater resolution of anatomical detail in living brains. MRI relies on the fact that atomic nuclei with an odd number of either protons or neutrons behave like tiny magnets, and so tend to align themselves with an externally applied magnetic field. Once in such a field, they preferentially absorb and emit energy at a particular radiofrequency, called the *resonant frequency*. Hence, this phenomenon is called *nuclear magnetic resonance*. The resonant frequency of a given kind of nucleus is specified by the magnitude of the externally applied magnetic field. Therefore an observation of energy emitted at a particular frequency from a particular area of tissue can provide information about the number of atoms of a particular type in that area of tissue. Mapping a given kind of atom's concentration in the brain is the basis for MRI. Since our brains are mostly made of water, and since hydrogen atoms give strong magnetic resonance signals, hydrogen is

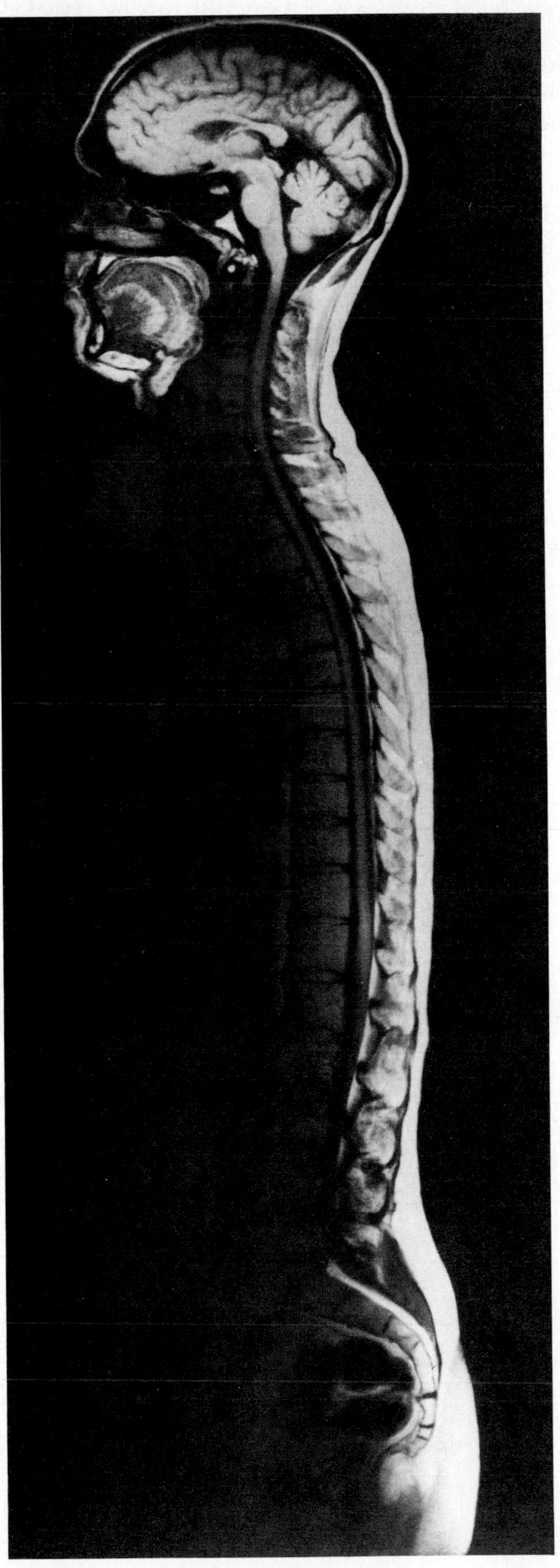

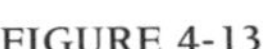

FIGURE 4-13
Midsagittal MRI image, demonstrating the extraordinary anatomical detail possible with this technique. So much can be seen that the figure was left unlabeled (a difficult task for an anatomist). I feared that once I started, the lines and arrows would multiply uncontrollably and obscure the anatomy.

Courtesy of Philips Medical Systems.

the element mapped by current MRI systems. (Other elements can also be mapped, but at much lower resolutions). Gray matter has a higher water concentration than does white matter, so MRI can demonstrate gray and white matter in exquisite detail in computer-generated "slices" of a living brain (Figures 4-13 to 4-17). The water concentrations and other characteristics of pathological areas (such as tumors and hemorrhages) are also distinctive, so images of these can be obtained as well.

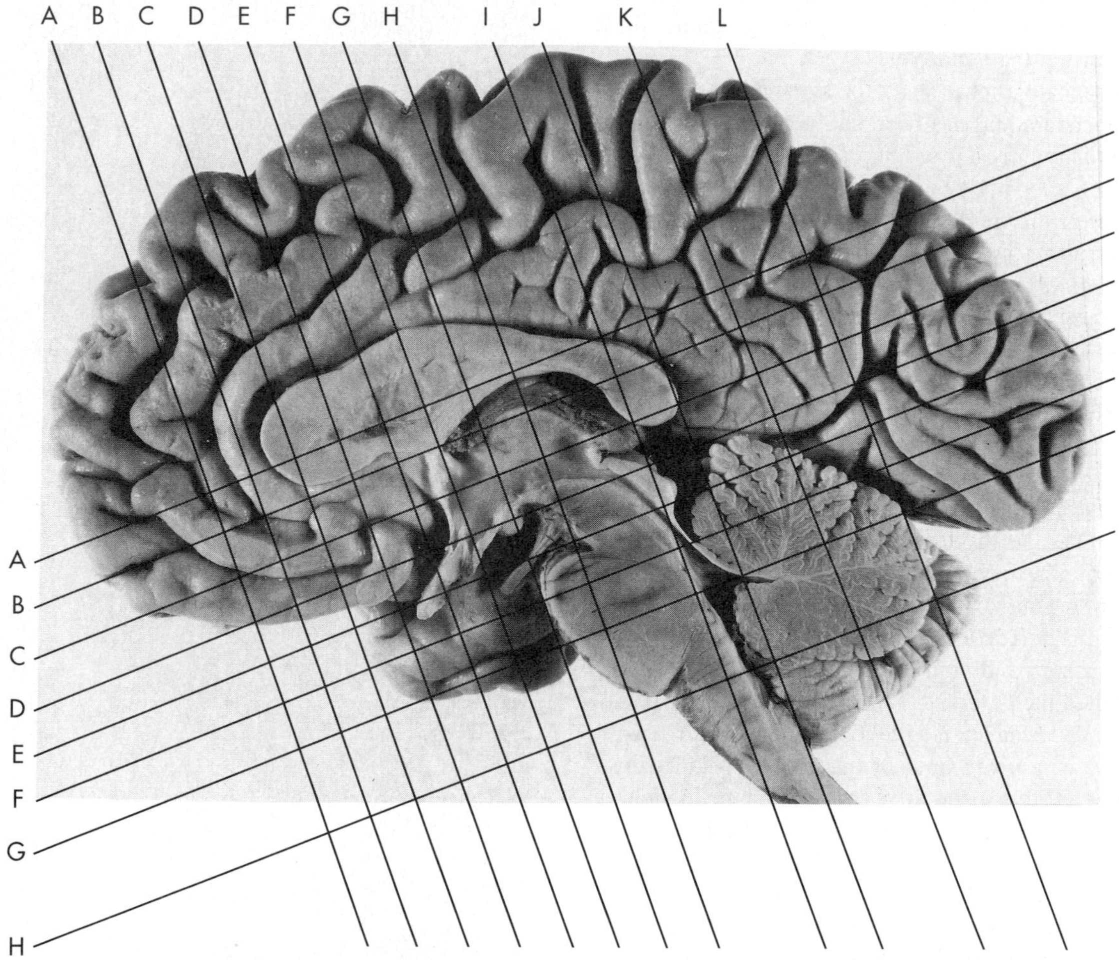


FIGURE 4-14
Planes of the images shown in Figures 4-16 and 4-17 (those in Figure 4-15 are in parasagittal planes and are not indicated here). Figures 4-15–4-17 (kindly provided by Dr. Roger Bird, St. Joseph's Hospital, Phoenix, Arizona) are series of magnetic resonance images of the brain of a single individual shown in three different planes. Most aspects of this individual's brain are quite typical. However, the two sheets of the septum pellucidum are separated by an unusually (though not abnormally) large space, called the *cavum septum pellucidum*. Magnetic resonance parameters can be adjusted to emphasize gray matter, white matter, flowing blood, or (as in these scans) all three. All of the structures indicated in these figures are discussed someplace in this book, although many have not yet been mentioned. My thanks to Dr. Mark Yoshino, The University of Arizona College of Medicine, for helpful discussions of these images.

## ABBREVIATIONS USED IN FIGURES 4-15–4-17

3, third ventricle
4, fourth ventricle
AC, anterior commissure
ACA, anterior cerebral artery (or one of its branches)
Acc, nucleus accumbens
AG, arachnoid granulation
Am, amygdala
AmC, ambient cistern
BA, basilar artery
BP, basal pons
Cal, calcarine sulcus
Caud, caudate nucleus
CCb, body of the corpus callosum
CCg, genu of the corpus callosum
CCr, rostrum of the corpus callosum
CCs, splenium of the corpus callosum
CeFl, flocculus
CeH, cerebellar hemisphere
CeNod, nodulus
CePF, primary fissure of the cerebellum
CeTon, cerebellar tonsil
CeV, cerebellar vermis
ChPl, choroid plexus
ChV, choroidal vein
Cing, cingulate gyrus
Cl, claustrum
CM, cisterna magna (cerebellomedullary cistern)
CmA, callosomarginal artery
CN V, trigeminal nerve
CN VII/VIII, facial and vestibulocochlear nerves
Co, cochlea
ConS, confluens of the sinuses (torcular)
CP, cerebral peduncle
CS, central sulcus
CTT, central tegmental tract
D, diploë
Den, dentate nucleus
EoM, extraocular muscle
F, fornix
FC, falx cerebri
GCV, great cerebral vein (of Galen)
GP, globus pallidus
GR, gyrus rectus
HC, hippocampal formation
Hy, hypothalamus
ICA, internal carotid artery
ICa, anterior limb of the internal capsule
ICg, genu of the internal capsule
ICp, posterior limb of the internal capsule
ICP, inferior cerebellar peduncle
ICV, internal cerebral vein
IF, interventricular formen (of Monro)
IFG, inferior frontal gyrus
Inf, infundibulum
InfC, inferior colliculus
Ins, insula
IpC, interpeduncular cistern
ITG, inferior temporal gyrus
LL, lateral lemniscus
LS, lateral sulcus
LVa, atrium of the lateral ventricle
LVant, anterior horn of the lateral ventricle
LVb, body of the lateral ventricle
LVinf, inferior horn of the lateral ventricle
LVpost, posterior horn of the lateral ventricle
MB, mammillary body
MCA, middle cerebral artery (or one of its branches)
MCP, middle cerebellar peduncle
Med, medulla
MFG, middle frontal gyrus
MLF, medial longitudinal fasciculus
MTG, middle temporal gyrus
MtT, mammillothalamic tract
O, olive
OC, optic chiasm
OlS, olfactory sulcus
ON, optic nerve
OR, optic radiation
Orb, orbital gyri
OT, optic tract
OtG, occipitotemporal gyrus
PAG, periaqueductal gray
PC, posterior commissure
PcA, pericallosal artery
PCA, posterior cerebral artery (or one of its branches)
PCoA, posterior communicating artery
PhG, parahippocampal gyrus
PICA, posterior inferior cerebellar artery
Pit, pituitary gland
PO, parietooccipital sulcus
Post, postcentral gyrus
Pre, precentral gyrus
Put, putamen
Pyr, pyramid
QC, quadrigeminal (superior) cistern
RN, red nucleus
Sc, scalp
SC, semicircular canal
SCP, superior cerebellar peduncle
Sep, septal area
SFG, superior frontal gyrus
SigS, sigmoid sinus
SN, substantia nigra
SP, septum pellucidum
STG, superior temporal gyrus
SupC, superior colliculus
SS, straight sinus
SSS, superior sagittal sinus
TC, tentorium cerebelli
Thal, thalamus
ThalA, anterior division of the thalamus
ThalL, lateral division of the thalamus
ThalM, medial division of the thalamus
TS, transverse sinus
TsV, thalamostriate (terminal) vein
U, uncus
V→SSS, vein entering the superior sagittal sinus
VA, venous angle
Ve, vestibule
VertA, vertebral artery

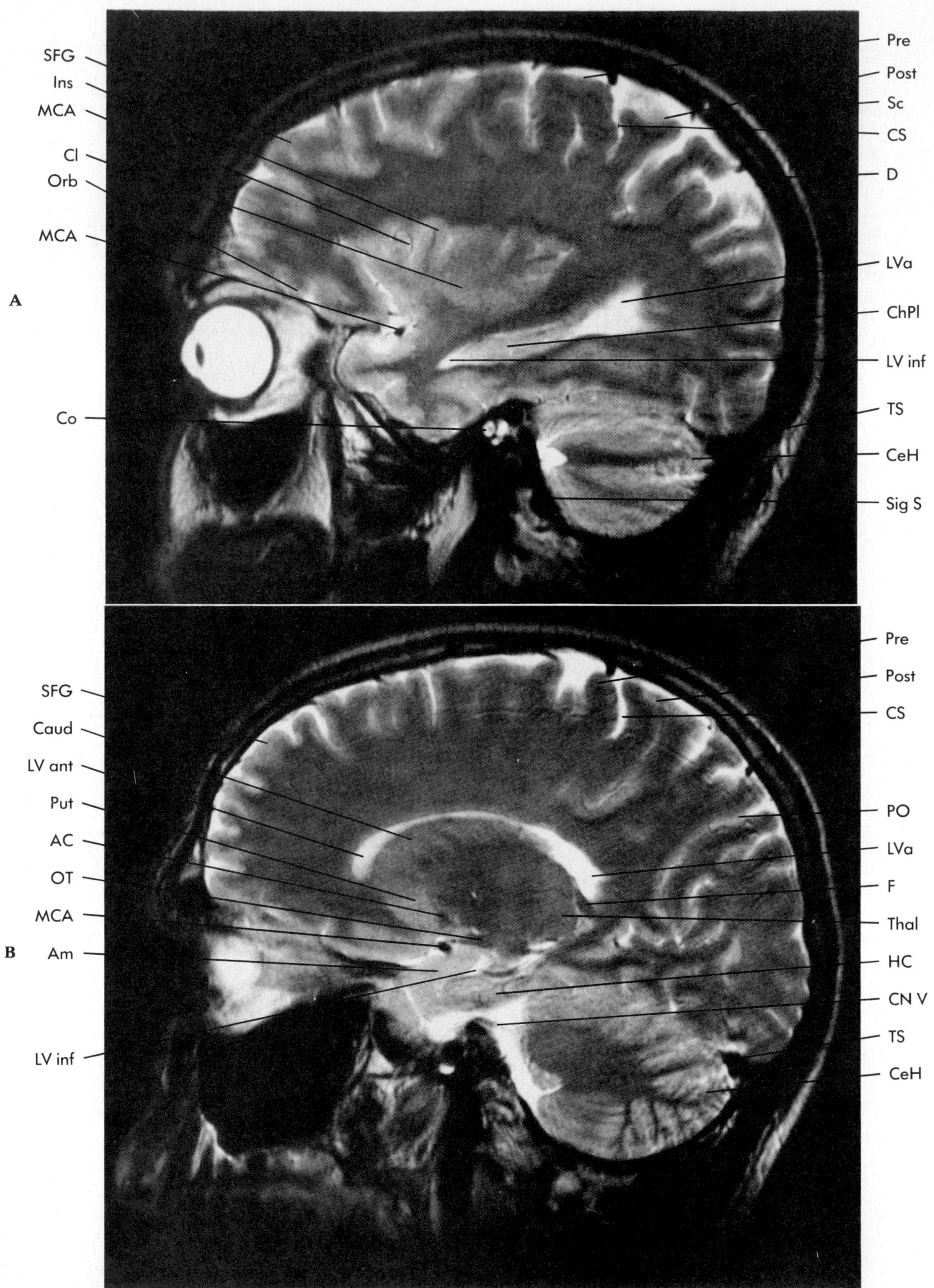


FIGURE 4-15
Magnetic resonance images in sagittal and parasagittal planes.

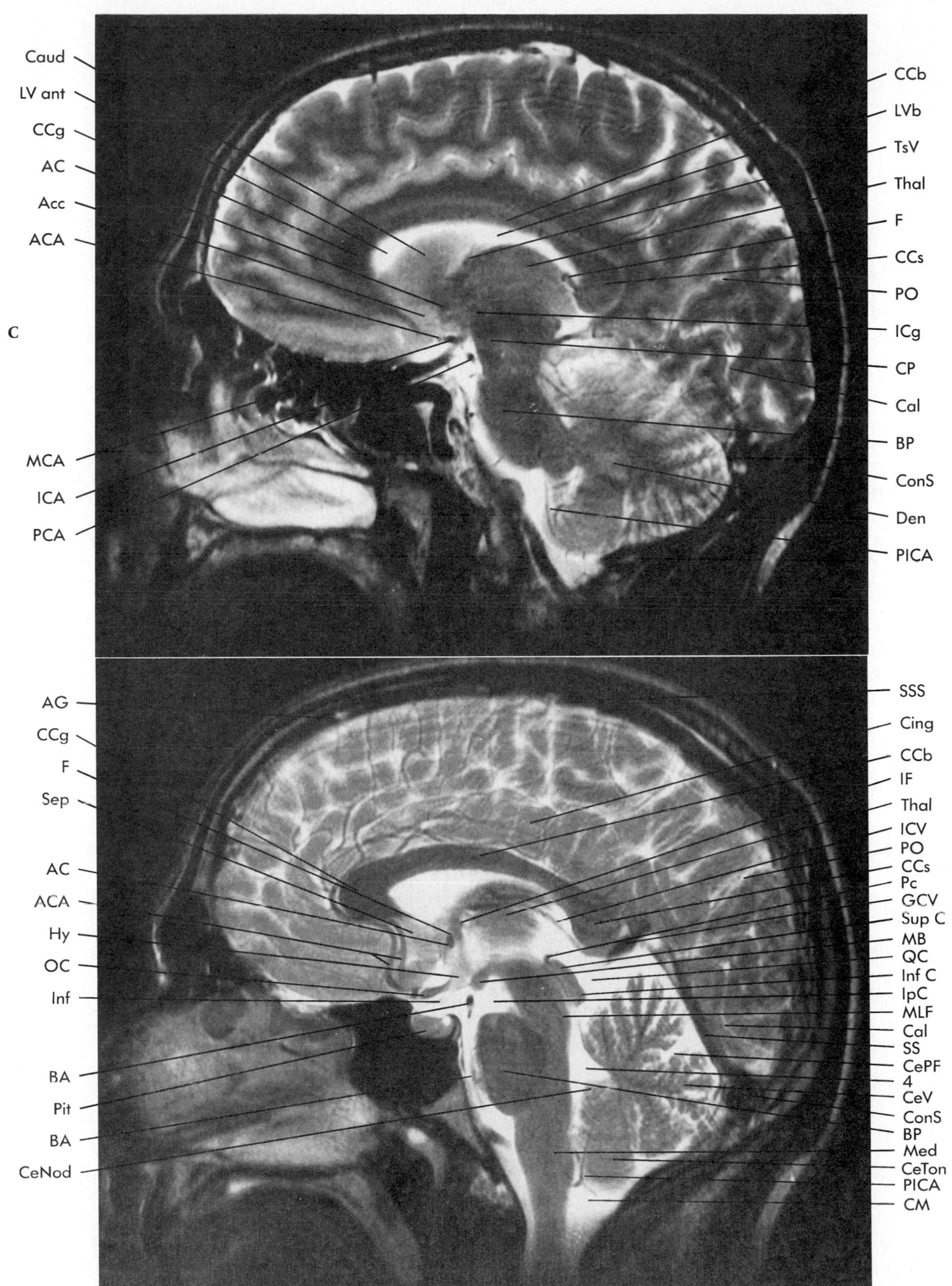


FIGURE 4-15, cont'd
Magnetic resonance images in sagittal and parasagittal planes.

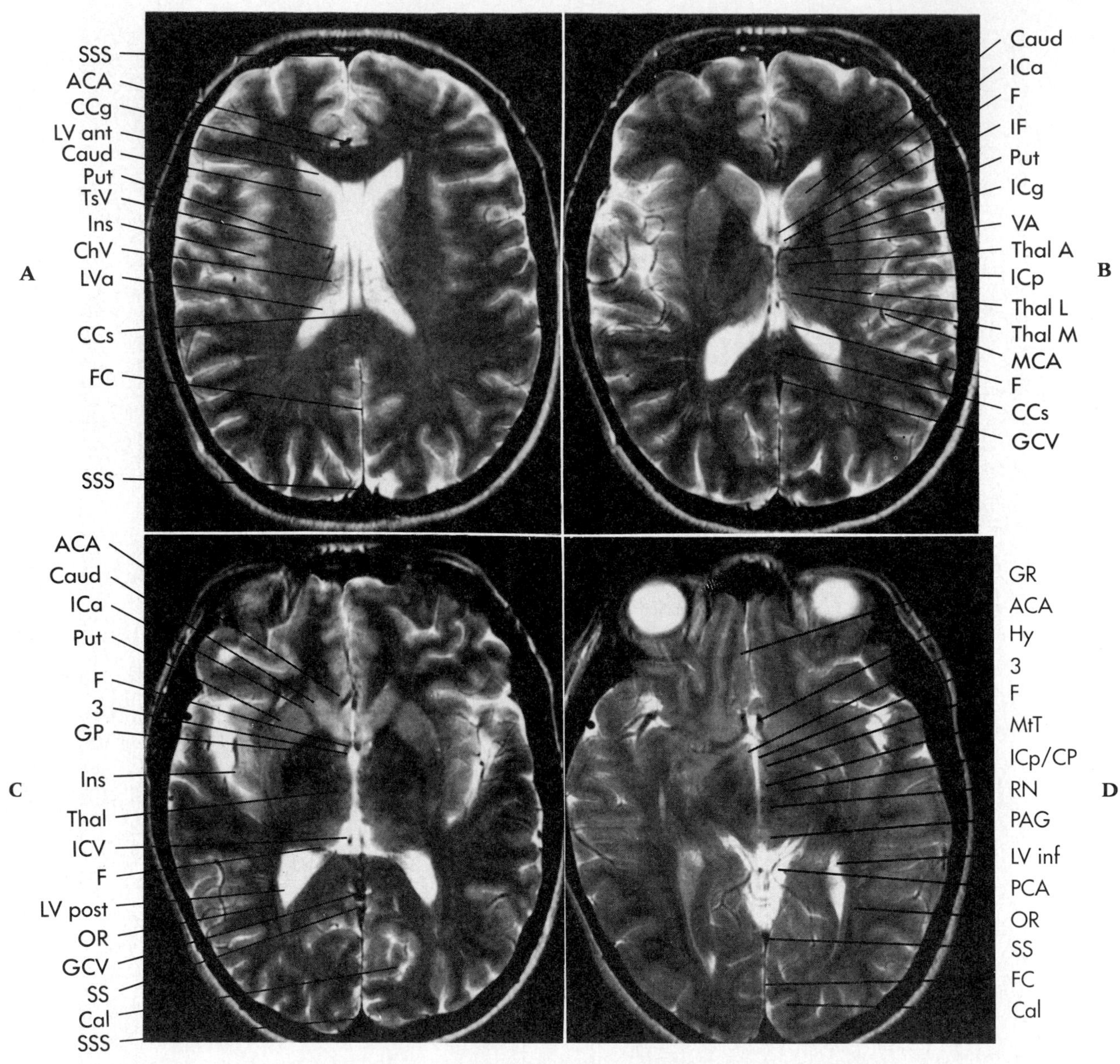


FIGURE 4-16
Magnetic resonance images in approximately horizontal planes.

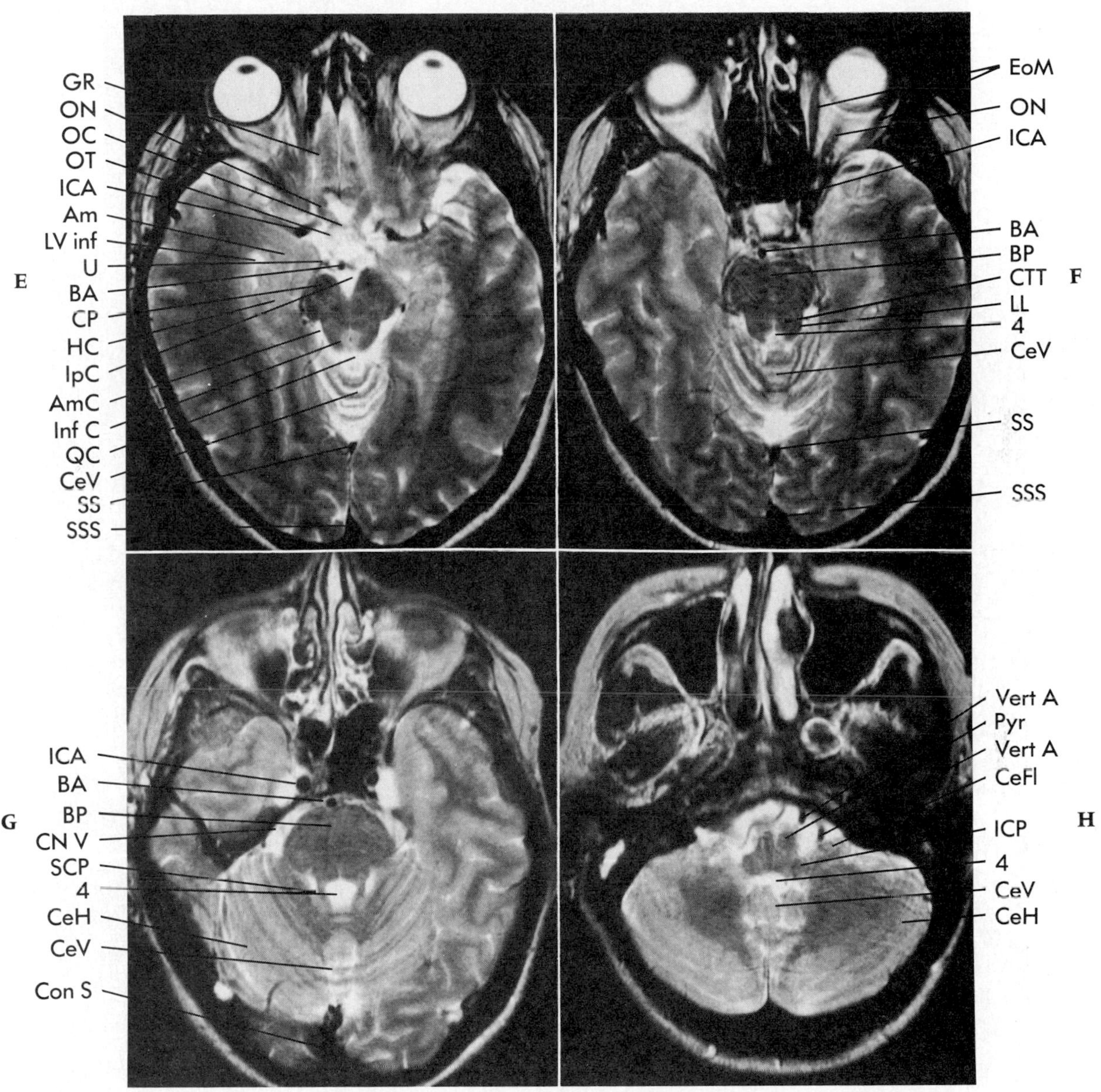


FIGURE 4-16, cont'd
Magnetic resonance images in approximately horizontal planes.

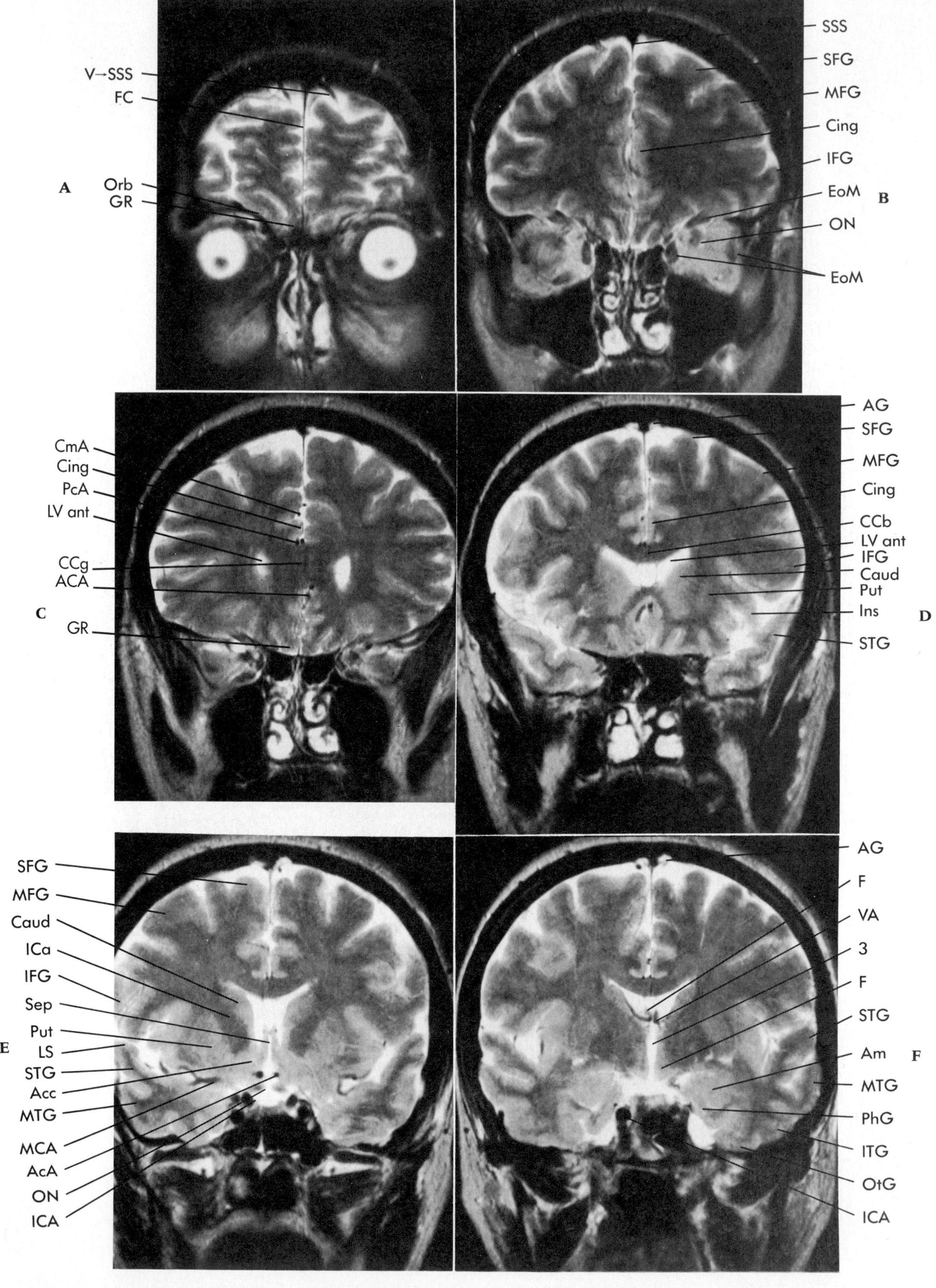


FIGURE 4-17
Magnetic resonance images in coronal planes.

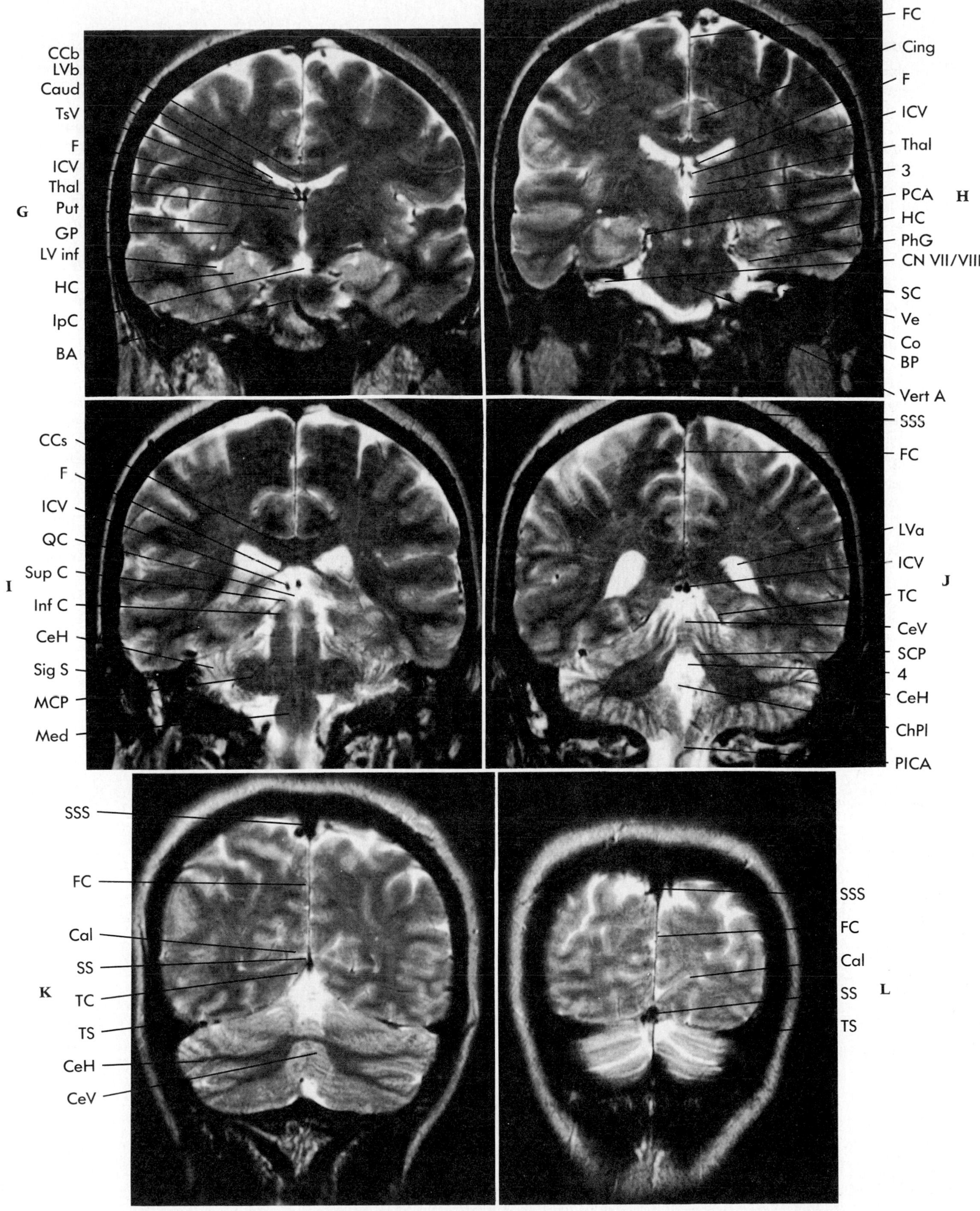


FIGURE 4-17, cont'd
Magnetic resonance images in coronal planes.

## ADDITIONAL READINGS

Brightman MW, Reese TS: Junctions between intimately apposed cell membranes in the vertebrate brain, *J Cell Biol* 40:648, 1969. *An interesting paper that discusses, among other things, the barrier properties of the choroid epithelium.*

Bruni JE, DelBigio MR, Clattenburg RE: Ependyma: normal and pathological—a review of the literature, *Brain Res Rev* 9:1, 1985.

Bull JWD: The volume of the cerebral ventricles, *Neurol* 11:1, 1961.

Cserr HF: Physiology of the choroid plexus, *Physiol Rev* 51:273, 1971.

Cushing H: *Studies in intracranial physiology and surgery,* London, 1926, Oxford University Press. *Contains the classic account of the direct observation of cerebrospinal fluid forming on the surface of human choroid plexus.*

Cutler RWP et al: Formation and absorption of cerebrospinal fluid in man, *Brain* 91:707, 1968. *Direct measurement of the rate of formation of cerebrospinal fluid in humans.*

Dandy WE: Experimental hydrocephalus, *Ann Surg* 70:129, 1919. *The classic description of the production of hydrocephalus by obstruction of an interventricular foramen, the cerebral aqueduct, or subarachnoid space around the base of the brain. It appears in the light of subsequent work that some of the experiments were technically flawed, but the conclusions are basically sound.*

Davson H, Welch K, Segal MB: Physiology and pathophysiology of the cerebrospinal fluid, London, 1987, Churchill Livingstone.

De Rougemont J et al: Fluid formed by choroid plexus, *J Neurophysiol* 23:485, 1960. *Experiments in which droplets of cerebrospinal fluid were collected, under oil, from the surface of the choroid plexus, and their composition analyzed.*

DiChiro G: Observations on the circulation of the cerebrospinal fluid, *Acta Radiol (Diagn)* 5:988, 1966. *Description of the time course and pattern of movement of tracer substances through subarachnoid space on their way toward the venous system.*

Dohrmann GJ: The choroid plexus: a historical review, *Brain Res* 18:197, 1970.

Dohrmann GJ, Bucy PC: Human choroid plexus: a light and electron microscopic study, *J Neurosurg* 33:506, 1970.

Eisenberg HM, McComb JG, Lorenzo AV: Cerebrospinal fluid overproduction and hydrocephalus associated with choroid plexus papilloma, *J Neurosurg* 40:381, 1974.

Fishman RA: *Cerebrospinal fluid in diseases of the nervous system,* Philadelphia, 1980, WB Saunders.

Gudeman SK et al: Surgical removal of bilateral papillomas of the choroid plexus of the lateral ventricles with resolution of hydrocephalus, *J Neurosurg* 50:677, 1979.

Gutierrez Y, Friede RL, Kaliney WJ: Agenesis of arachnoid granulations and its relationship to communicating hydrocephalus, *J Neurosurg* 43:553, 1975.

Haaxma-Reiche H, Piers DO, Beekhuis H: Normal cerebrospinal fluid dynamics: a study with intraventricular injection of $^{111}$In-DTPA in leukemia and lymphoma without meningeal involvement, Arch Neurol 46:997, 1989. *A discussion of the time course of tracer movement out of the ventricles and through subarachnoid space.*

Hewitt W: The median aperture of the fourth ventricle, *J Anat* 94:549, 1960.

Jacobson HG, editor: Fundamentals of magnetic resonance imaging, *JAMA* 258:3417, 1987.

Kean DM, Smith MA: *Magnetic resonance imaging: principles and applications,* Baltimore, 1986, Williams & Wilkins.

Kier EL: *The cerebral ventricles: a phylogenetic and ontogenetic study.* In Newton TH, Potts DG, editors: *Radiology of the skull and brain,* vol. 3: *Anatomy and pathology,* St. Louis, 1977, CV Mosby. *A long but fascinating and beautifully illustrated account.*

Kirkwood JR: *Essentials of neuroimaging,* New York, 1990, Churchill Livingstone.

Lindvall M, Owman C: Autonomic nerves in the mammalian choroid plexus and their influence on the formation of cerebrospinal fluid, *J Cereb Blood Flow Metab* 1:245, 1981.

Matsushima T, Rhoton AL Jr., Lenkey C: Microsurgery of the fourth ventricle, Part 1. Microsurgical anatomy, *Neurosurgery* 11:631, 1982. *Finely detailed and beautifully illustrated.*

McComb JG: Recent research into the nature of cerebrospinal fluid formation and absorption, *J Neurosurgery* 59:369, 1983.

McRae DL, Branch CL, Milner B: The occipital horns and cerebral dominance, *Neurol* 18:95, 1968.

Milhorat TH: Choroid plexus and cerebrospinal fluid production, *Science* 166:1514, 1969. *An account of the continued production of cerebrospinal fluid in the lateral ventricles of monkeys after removal of the choroid plexus.*

Millen JW, Woollam DHM: *The anatomy of the cerebrospinal fluid,* New York, 1962, Oxford University Press.

Oldendorf WH: *The quest for an image of brain,* New York, 1980, Raven Press. *A thoroughly delightful, nontechnical book by one of the founders of computerized tomography, tracing the history of various imaging techniques.*

Pollay M: *Review of spinal fluid physiology: production and absorption in relation to pressure.* In Keener EB, editor: *Clinical neurosurgery,* Baltimore, 1977, Williams & Wilkins. *Well-written, concise review.*

Pollay M, Curl F: Secretion of cerebrospinal fluid by the ventricular ependyma of the rabbit, *Am J Physiol* 213:1031, 1967. *Technically admirable experiments demonstrating the production of cerebrospinal fluid within the aqueduct and rostral fourth ventricle.*

Rodriguez EM: The cerebrospinal fluid as a pathway in neuroendocrine integration, *J Endocrinol* 71:407, 1976.

Timurkaynak E, Rhoton AL, Jr, Barry M: Microsurgical anatomy and operative approaches to the lateral ventricle, *Neurosurgery* 19:685, 1986. *Finely detailed and beautifully illustrated.*

Voetmann E: On the structure and surface area of the human choroid plexus, *Acta Anat suppl* 10, 1949.

Welch K, Pollay M: The spinal arachnoid villi of the monkeys *Cercopithecus aethiops sabaeus* and *Macaca irus, Anat Rec* 145:43:1963.

Wood JH: *Neurobiology of cerebrospinal fluid,* vols. 1 and 2, New York, 1980 and 1983, Plenum Press.

Wright EM: Transport processes in the formation of the cerebrospinal fluid, *Rev Physiol Biochem Pharmacol* 83:1, 1978.

Yamamoto I, Rhoton AL Jr, Peace DA: Microsurgery of the third ventricle. Part 1. Microsurgical anatomy, *Neurosurgery* 8:334, 1981. *Finely detailed and beautifully illustrated.*

# CHAPTER 5

# *Blood Supply of the Brain*

Turtles can walk around for hours with no oxygen supply to their brains. In contrast, our brains are absolutely dependent on a continuous supply of well-oxygenated blood. After just 10 seconds of brain ischemia, we lose consciousness. After 20 seconds, electrical activity ceases; and after just a few minutes, irreversible damage usually begins. Corresponding to this metabolic dependence, blood vessels in the central nervous system (CNS), particularly in gray matter, are arranged in a dense meshwork (Figure 5-1). Obviously, an understanding of the brain's blood supply is essential to an understanding of its normal function. However, the placement of a discussion of the vasculature of the CNS presents a problem in any consideration of neuroanatomy. It is reasonably efficient to treat the arterial supply of individual portions of the brain at the same time the structure and function of that area are treated. This approach requires a prior general overview of the circulatory system, which this chapter attempts to provide.

The arterial supply of the brain is derived from two pairs of vessels, the *internal carotid arteries* and the *vertebral arteries*. The internal carotid system supplies most of the telencephalon and much of the diencephalon. The vertebral system supplies the brainstem and cerebellum, as well as parts of the diencephalon, spinal cord, and occipital and temporal lobes.

Venous drainage occurs by way of a system of *superficial veins* and *deep veins,* which empty into the dural venous sinuses and ultimately into the internal jugular vein.

## ARTERIAL SUPPLY

### Internal carotid system

We begin by considering the internal carotid artery above the cavernous sinus and adjacent to the optic chiasm, assuming that other aspects of its anatomy, such as the carotid siphon and previous branches like the ophthalmic artery, are discussed in most gross anatomy courses. The internal carotid artery proceeds superiorly alongside the optic chiasm (Figure 5-2) and bifurcates into the *middle* and *anterior cerebral arteries*. Before bifurcating it gives rise to two smaller branches, the *anterior choroidal artery* and the *posterior communicating artery*. The anterior choroidal artery is a long, thin artery that can be significant clinically, since it supplies a number of different structures and is not infrequently involved in cerebrovascular accidents. Along its course (indicated in Figure 5-2), it supplies the optic tract, the choroid plexus of the inferior horn of the lateral ventricle, part of the cerebral peduncle, and some deep structures such as portions of the internal capsule, thalamus, and hippocampus. The posterior communicating artery passes posteriorly, inferior to the optic tract and toward the cerebral peduncle, and joins the *posterior cerebral artery* (part of the vertebral artery system).

The anterior cerebral artery runs medially, superior to the optic nerve, and enters the longitudinal fissure (see Figure 5-2). It and its branches then arch posteriorly, following the corpus callosum, to supply the medial aspect of the frontal and parietal lobes (Figure 5-3). Some of the smaller branches extend onto the dorsolateral surface of the hemisphere (Figure 5-4). Along this course, it divides into two particularly prominent branches, the *pericallosal artery,* which stays immediately adjacent to the corpus callosum, and the *callosomarginal artery,* which follows the cingulate sulcus (see Figure 5-3). The two anterior cerebral arteries, near their entrance into the longitudinal fissure, are connected by the *anterior communicating artery*. Since parts of the precentral and postcentral gyri extend onto the medial surface of the frontal and parietal lobes, the occlusion of an anterior cerebral artery causes restricted contralateral motor and somatosensory deficits.

The large middle cerebral artery proceeds laterally into the lateral sulcus (see Figure 5-2). It divides into a number

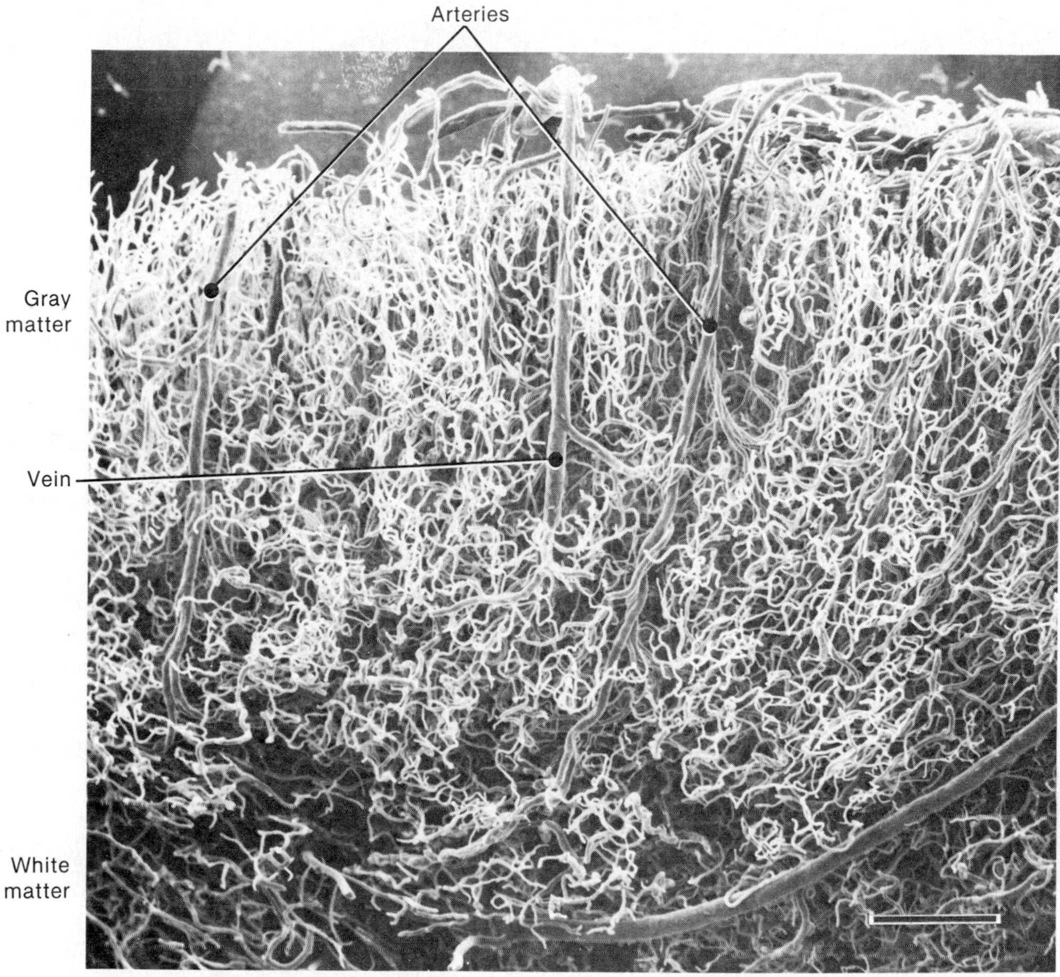


FIGURE 5-1
Arrangement of blood vessels in the cerebral cortex of the temporal pole of a 66-year-old man. The blood vessels were injected with plastic, the surrounding tissues were dissolved away, and the resulting cast was observed with a scanning electron microscope; the scale mark corresponds to 500 μm. Notice that the meshwork of vessels is more dense in gray matter than in white matter, corresponding to the greater metabolic needs of neuronal cell bodies. In gray matter, the vessels are so tightly packed that no neuron is more than 100 μm or so from a capillary.

From Duvernoy HM, Delon S, Vannson JL: *Brain Res Bull* 7:519, 1981. Courtesy of Dr. H.M. Duvernoy, Faculte de Medecine, Universite de Franche-Comte.

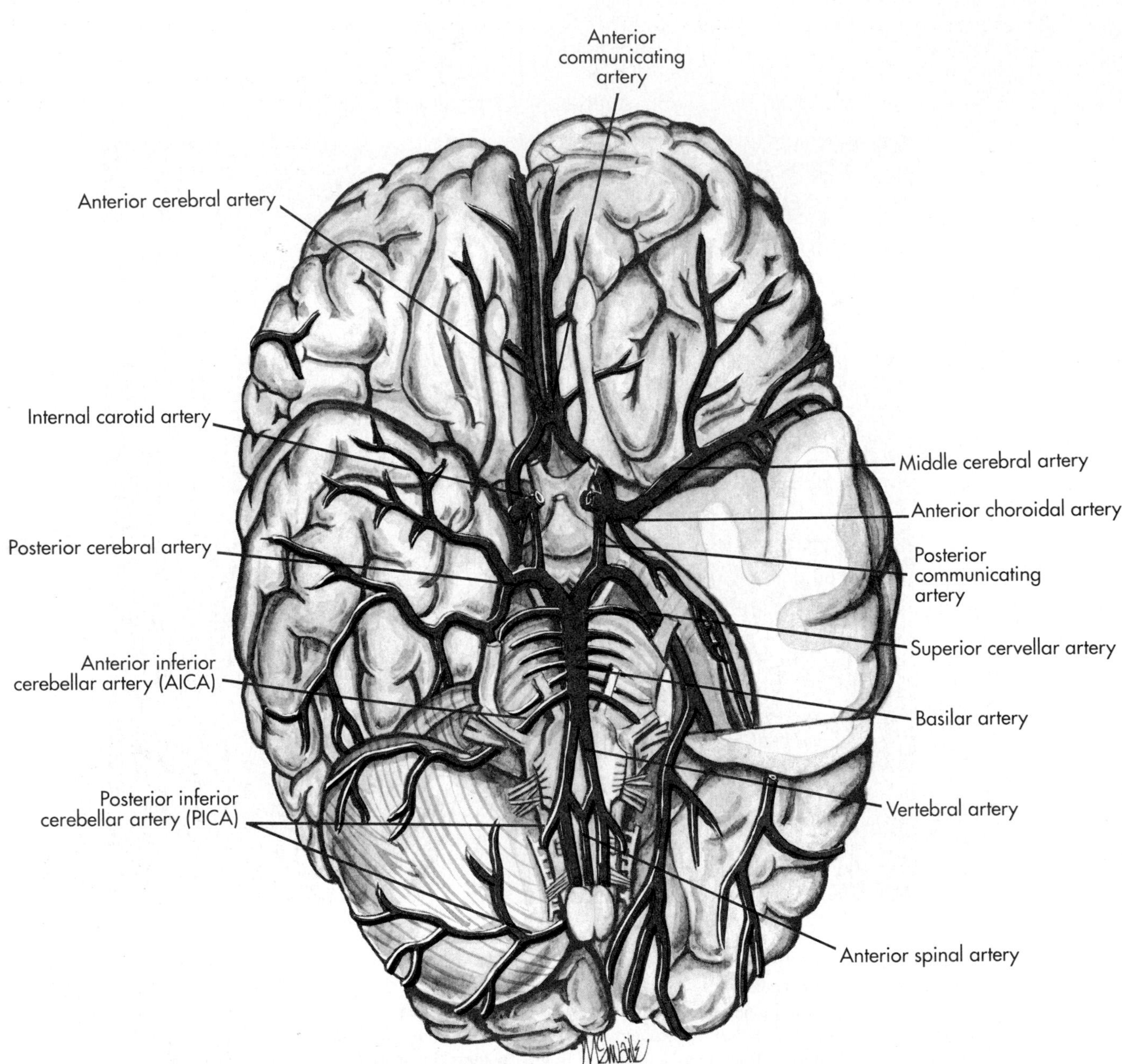


FIGURE 5-2
Arteries on the inferior surface of the brain. The left half of the cerebellum and part of the left temporal lobe have been removed to reveal the courses of the middle and posterior cerebral arteries and the anterior choroidal artery.
Modified from Hamilton WJ, editor: Textbook of human anatomy, ed 2, St. Louis, 1976, The CV Mosby Co.

of branches that supply the insula, emerge from the lateral sulcus, and spread out to supply virtually the entire lateral surface of the cerebral hemisphere. Since most of the precentral and postcentral gyri are within this area of supply, the occlusion of a middle cerebral artery causes major motor and somatosensory deficits. In addition, if the left hemisphere is the one involved, language deficits are almost invariably found.

Along its course toward the lateral sulcus, the middle cerebral artery gives rise to many very small branches that penetrate the brain near their origin and supply deep structures of the diencephalon and telencephalon (Figures 5-5 and 5-6). These particular arteries are called the *lateral striate* (or *lenticulostriate*) *arteries,* but similar small branches arise from all the arteries around the base of the brain. They are referred to collectively as *ganglionic* or *penetrating* branches. Ganglionic arteries are particularly numerous in the area adjacent to the optic chiasm and in

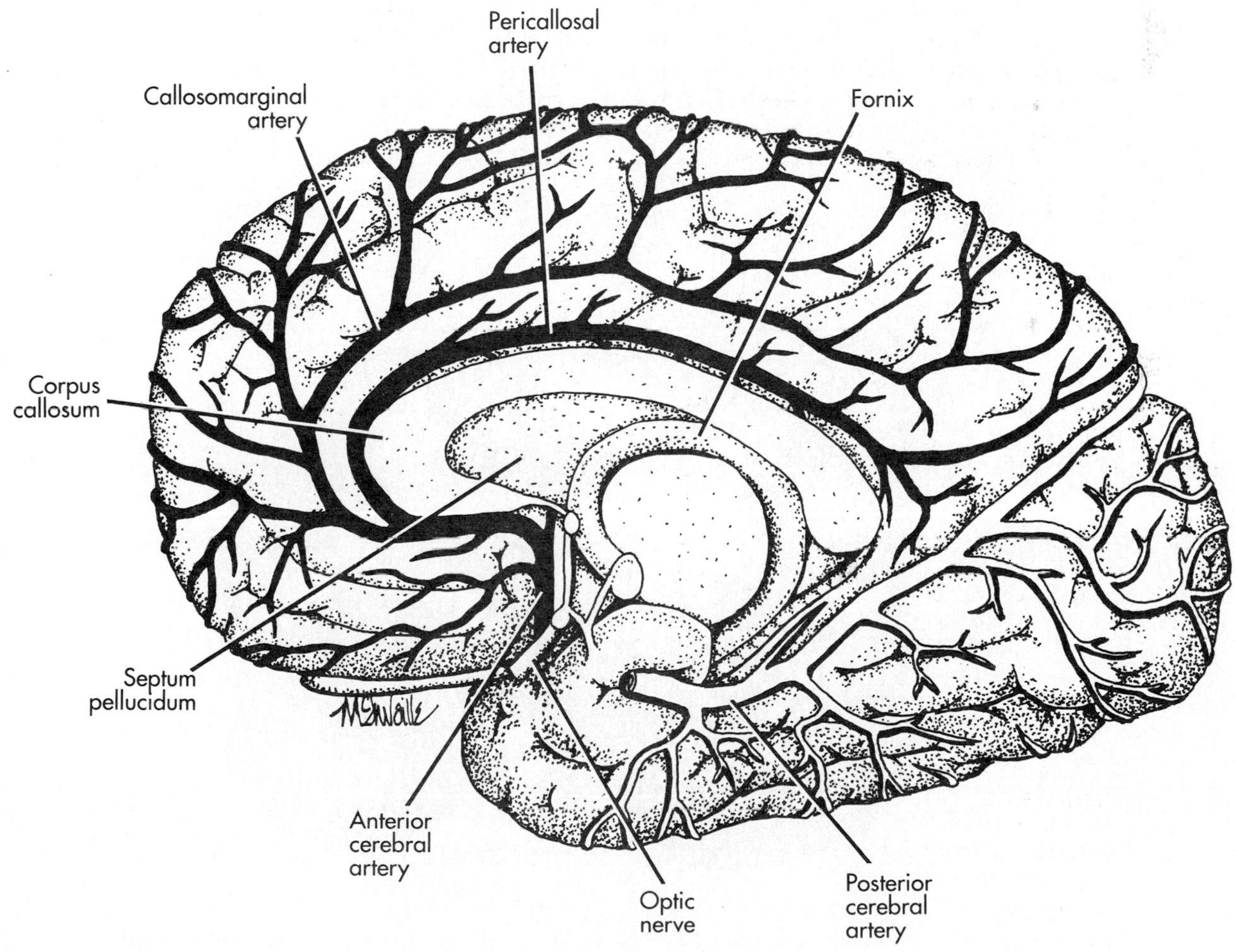


FIGURE 5-3

Arteries of the medial surface of the brain. The anterior cerebral artery and its branches are shown in black, the posterior cerebral artery and its branches are shown in white.

Modified from Hamilton WJ, editor: Textbook of human anatomy, ed 2, St. Louis, 1976, The CV Mosby Co.

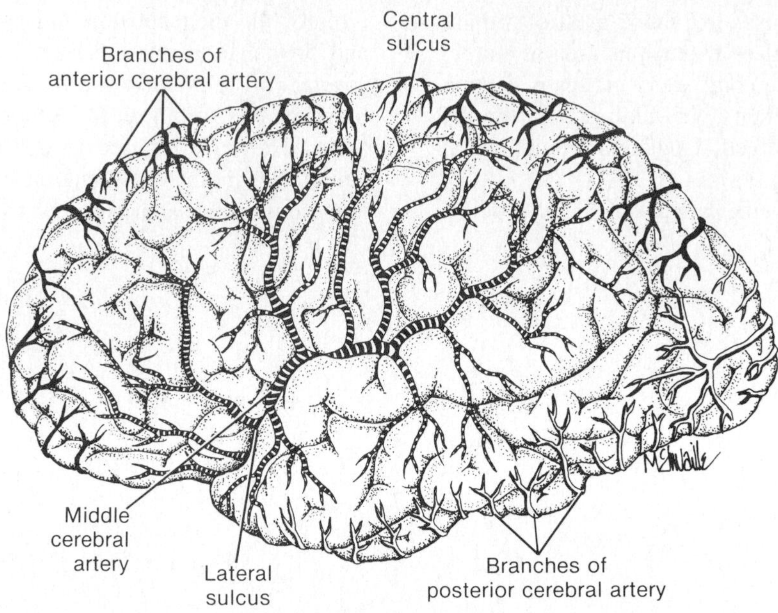


FIGURE 5-4
Arteries of the lateral surface of the brain. The middle cerebral artery and its branches are shown striped. The small branches of the anterior cerebral artery reaching around from the medial surface are shown in black, and those of the posterior cerebral artery are shown in white.
Modified from Hamilton WJ, editor: Textbook of human anatomy, ed 2, St. Louis, 1976, The CV Mosby Co.

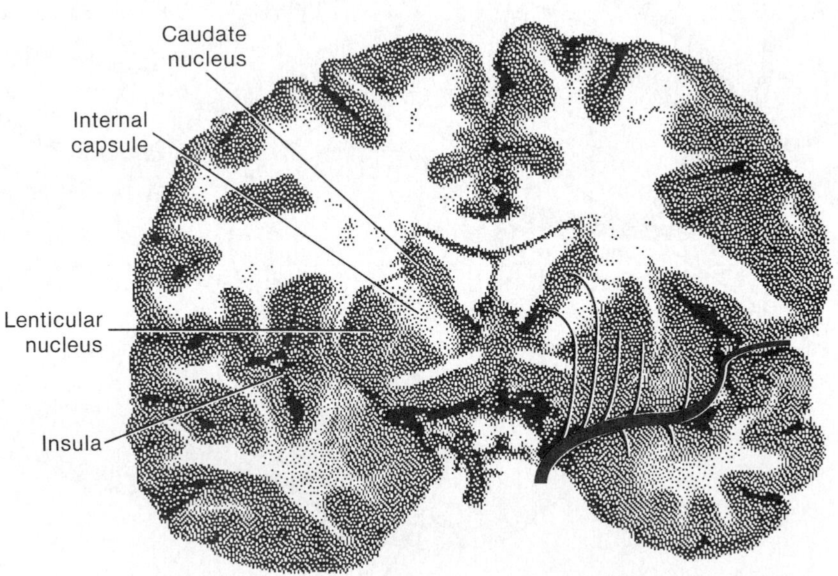


FIGURE 5-5
Lateral striate branches of the left middle cerebral artery as seen in a coronal slice. Similar small branches arise all around the circle of Willis and supply deep structures of the diencephalon and telencephalon.

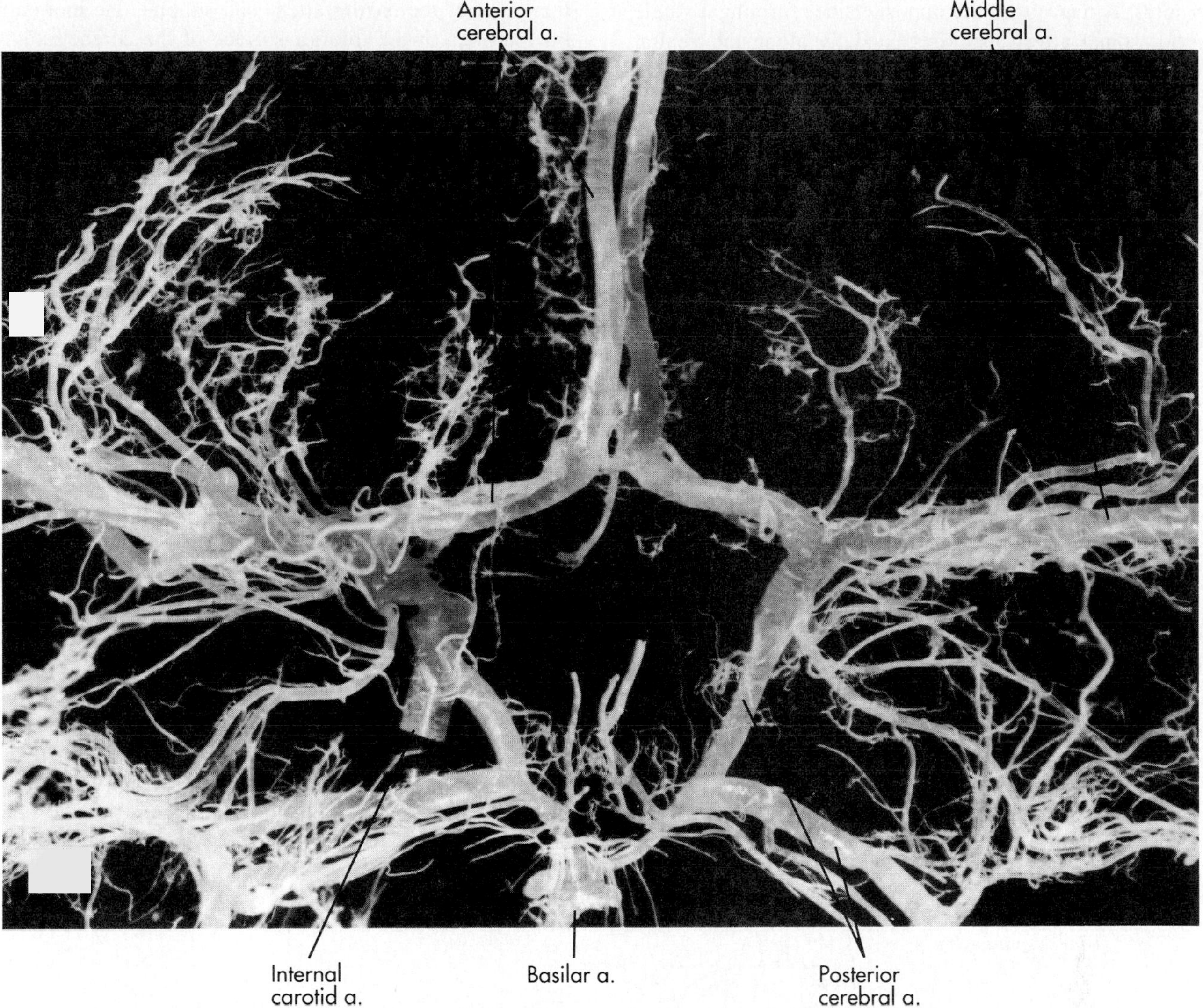


FIGURE 5-6
A cast of a human circle of Willis, demonstrating many of the small ganglionic or penetrating arteries that arise from major vessels in or adjacent to the circle. The internal carotid and basilar arteries were injected with plastic, after which the surrounding tissues were dissolved away. This circle of Willis is somewhat unusual in that both posterior cerebral arteries arise from an internal carotid rather than the basilar artery (see Figure 5-8, *D*).
From Marinković SV et al., *Neurosurg* 26:472, 1990. Courtesy of Dr. S.V. Marinković, Institution of Anatomy, University of Belgrade School of Medicine.)

the area between the cerebral peduncles; for this reason these are called the *anterior* and *posterior perforated substances,* respectively. The narrow, thin-walled vessels of those areas are involved frequently in strokes. The deep cerebral structures they supply are such that damage to these small vessels can cause neurological deficits out of proportion to their size. For example, the somatosensory projection from the thalamus to the postcentral gyrus must pass through the internal capsule; damage to a small part of the internal capsule, from rupture or occlusion of a penetrating artery, can cause deficits similar to those resulting from damage to a large expanse of cortex.

### Vertebral-basilar system

The two vertebral arteries run rostrally alongside the medulla and fuse at the junction between the medulla and pons to form the midline *basilar artery,* which proceeds rostrally along the ventral surface of the pons (see Figure 5-2).

Before joining the basilar artery, each vertebral artery gives rise to three branches, the *posterior spinal artery, anterior spinal artery,* and *posterior inferior cerebellar artery*. The posterior spinal artery runs caudally along the dorsolateral aspect of the spinal cord and supplies the posterior third of that half of the cord. The anterior spinal artery joins its mate from the opposite side, forming a single anterior spinal artery that runs caudally along the ventral midline of the spinal cord, supplying the anterior two thirds of the cord. These spinal arteries cannot carry enough blood from the vertebral arteries to supply more than the cervical segments of the spinal cord and must be reinforced at various points caudal to this (discussed in Chapter 7). The posterior inferior cerebellar artery (often referred to by the acronym "PICA"), as its name implies, supplies much of the inferior surface of the cerebellar hemisphere (Figure 5-7); however, it sends branches to other structures on its way to the cerebellum. As it curves around the brainstem, the artery supplies the choroid plexus of the fourth ventricle and much of the lateral medulla. This is a uniform occurrence in the large named branches of the vertebral-basilar system; on their way to their major area of supply, they send branches to brainstem structures. By knowing the brainstem level at which these branches emerge, one can make reasonably accurate inferences about the blood supply of any given region of the brainstem.

The basilar artery proceeds rostrally and, at the level of the midbrain, bifurcates into the two *posterior cerebral arteries*. Before this bifurcation, it gives rise to numerous unnamed branches and two named branches, the *anterior inferior cerebellar artery* and the *superior cerebellar artery*.

The anterior inferior cerebellar artery (often referred to by the acronym "AICA") arises just rostral to the formation point of the basilar artery and supplies the more anterior portions of the inferior surface of the cerebellum (for example, the flocculus), as well as parts of the caudal pons. The superior cerebellar artery arises just caudal to the bifurcation of the basilar artery and supplies the superior surface of the cerebellum and much of the caudal midbrain and rostral pons. The many smaller branches of the basilar artery, collectively called *pontine arteries* (see Figure 5-2), supply the remainder of the pons. One of these, the *internal auditory* (or *labyrinthine*) *artery* (which often is actually a branch of the AICA), though hard to distinguish from the others by appearance, is functionally important because it also supplies the inner ear. Its occlusion can lead to vertigo and ipsilateral deafness.

The posterior cerebral artery curves around the midbrain and passes through the superior cistern; its branches spread out to supply the medial and inferior surfaces of the occipital and temporal lobes (see Figures 5-2, 5-3, and 5-7). Along the way, it sends branches to the rostral midbrain and caudal diencephalon. It also gives rise to several *posterior choroidal arteries,* which supply the choroid plexus of the third ventricle and of the body of the lateral ventricle. The anterior and posterior choroidal arteries form anastomoses in the vicinity of the glomus. Since the primary visual cortex is located in the occipital lobe, occlusion of a posterior cerebral artery at its origin leads to visual field losses in addition to other deficits referable to the midbrain and diencephalon.

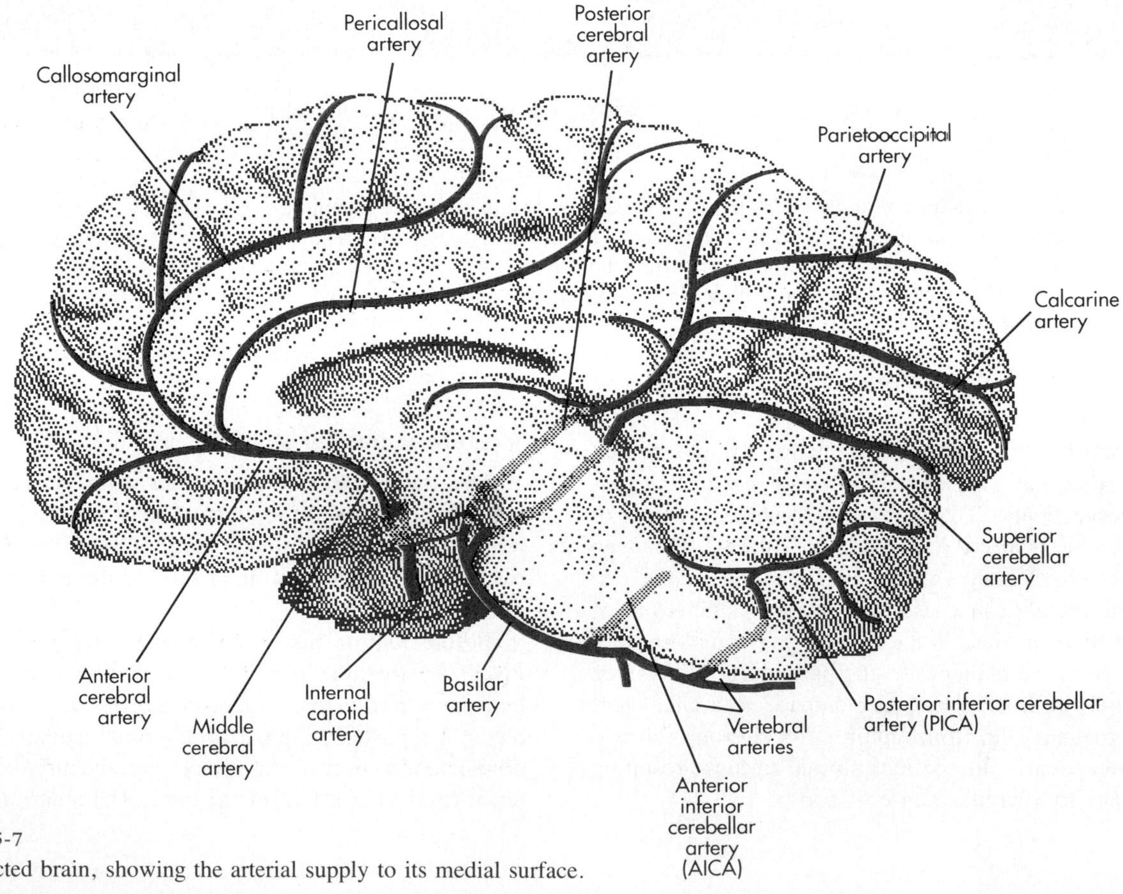


FIGURE 5-7
A hemisected brain, showing the arterial supply to its medial surface.

### Circle of Willis

The posterior cerebral artery is connected to the internal carotid artery by the posterior communicating artery. This completes an arterial polygon called the *circle of Willis,* through which the anterior cerebral, internal carotid, and posterior cerebral arteries of both sides are interconnected. Normally, there is little or no blood flow around this circle, since the appropriate pressure differentials are not present. The arterial pressure in the right internal carotid artery is about the same as that in the right posterior cerebral artery, so little or no blood flows through the right posterior communicating artery. However, if one major vessel becomes occluded, either within the circle of Willis or proximal to it, the communicating arteries may allow critically important anastomotic flow and prevent neurological damage. By such a mechanism it would be theoretically possible (though highly unlikely) for the entire brain to be perfused by just one of the four major arteries that normally supply it. The anterior and posterior communicating arteries are quite variable in size (see below), and so the establishment of effective anastomotic flow in the event of an arterial occlusion may also depend on the time course of the occlusion. A small communicating artery can enlarge slowly to compensate for a slowly developing occlusion, but in such a case an abrupt blockage might cause serious damage.

Designating the circle of Willis shown in Figure 5-2 as "normal" represents to a great extent a nod to an aesthetic need, since fewer than half the circles have this appearance. Some frequently seen "abnormalities" are indicated in Figure 5-8. Asymmetries are common; one or more of the communicating arteries may be very small; one anterior cerebral artery may be much smaller at its origin than the other; one posterior cerebral artery may retain its embryological origin from the internal carotid and may be connected to the basilar artery through a posterior communicating artery. In rare cases one of the communicating arteries may be missing, resulting in an incomplete circle.

Other routes of collateral circulation are available, although the circle of Willis is likely to be the most important. There are anastomoses, at the arteriolar and capillary levels, between terminal branches of the cerebral arteries. These are usually inadequate in the adult for maintaining the entire territory of a major cerebral artery if it becomes occluded, but occasionally they may be sufficient for maintaining a large part of this territory. In addition, well-defined arterial anastomoses may enlarge to a remarkable degree to compensate for slowly developing occlusions. For example, there have been documented cases in which the territory of one posterior cerebral artery was supplied by the internal carotid artery of that side by means of flow through the anterior choroidal artery and from there through a posterior choroidal artery and into the posterior cerebral artery.

### Control of cerebral blood flow

The brain is very active metabolically but has no effective way to store oxygen or glucose. A stable and copious blood supply is therefore required, and the brain, which represents only 2% of the total body weight, uses about 15% of the normal cardiac output and accounts for nearly 25% of the body's oxygen consumption. The overall flow rate is normally maintained at a very constant level, but this rate may increase or decrease in particular regions of the brain, in a pattern correlated with neural activity (Plate 10).

The mechanisms that control cerebral blood flow are not well understood, but at least three factors seem to be involved. The first is a process termed *autoregulation* (Figure 5-9), by which cerebral blood vessels themselves act to maintain constant flow; the vessels constrict (thus increasing their resistance) in response to increased blood pressure, and they relax in response to decreased pressure. The second factor may be generally thought of as a response of the cerebral vessels to metabolites, of which carbon dioxide is the best studied. Increases of carbon dioxide tension in brain extracellular fluid cause dilation of the cerebral vessels and increased blood flow; decreases of carbon dioxide tension have opposite effects. Changes in oxygen tension have reciprocal effects to those of carbon dioxide. Local changes in metabolite concentration may be part of the basis for regional variations in blood flow. Finally, cerebral vessels are innervated, both by standard autonomic fibers and by fibers from several locations within the brain. The evidence concerning the roles of this innervation is incomplete and somewhat conflicting, but the current consensus is that neural control is of relatively minor importance. It may play a part in adaptation to stress of various sorts and in sustaining the extremes of the autoregulation range, but under ordinary circumstances, metabolic and direct autoregulatory mechanisms seem to predominate.

In recent years it has become possible to look fairly directly at the regional blood flow in normal human cerebral hemispheres and, by inference, at the varying levels of metabolic activity of different areas of the brain during different types of mental activity. One such technique involves the injection of a small amount of an inert, radioactive gas (usually $^{133}$Xe, a gamma-emitting isotope of xenon) into the cerebral circulation. After the injection, a bank of gamma-ray cameras records the inflow and washout of the gas while the patient performs various tasks (Plate 10).

A second technique, called *positron emission tomography* (or *PET scanning*), allows an even more direct look at brain metabolism in computer-constructed "slices" of the brain similar to those produced in computed tomography (CT) and magnetic resonance imaging (MRI) scans. PET scanning relies on the fact that certain isotopes decay by

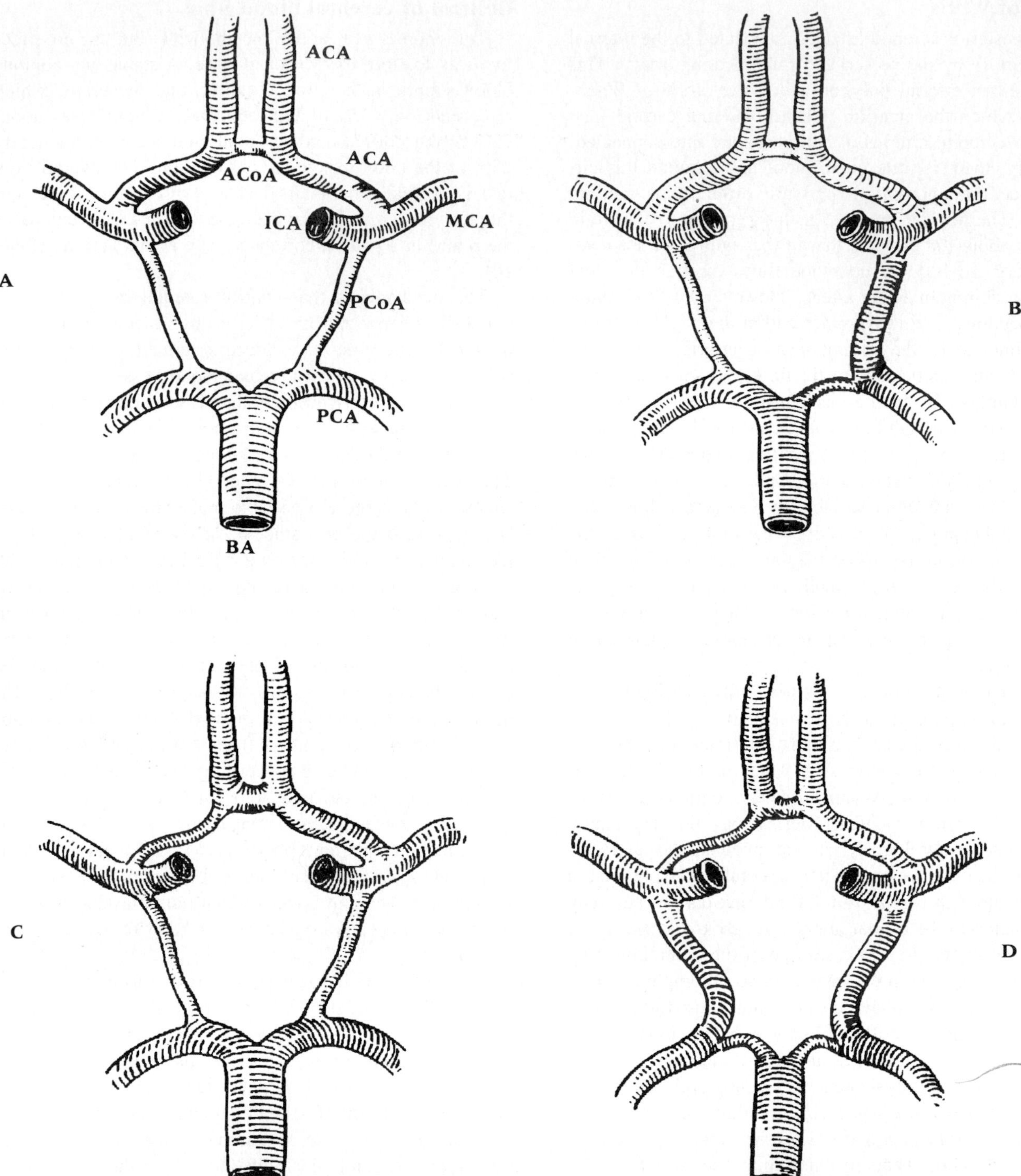


FIGURE 5-8
Normal circle of Willis *(A)* compared to some common "abnormalities" (indicated in color in *B, C, D*). Abbreviations: ACA, anterior cerebral artery; ACoA, anterior communicating artery; BA, basilar artery; ICA, internal carotid artery; MCA, middle cerebral artery; PCA, posterior cerebral artery; PCoA, posterior communicating artery. *B*, One posterior cerebral artery arises from an internal carotid artery in 30-40% of brains. *C*, Both anterior cerebral arteries are perfused primarily from one internal carotid artery in 10-15% of brains. *D*, Various combinations of hypoplastic and asymmetrical arteries are also found, but the circle of Willis is almost always complete.

Adapted from Hodes PJ et al., *Am J Roentgenol* 70;61, 1953.

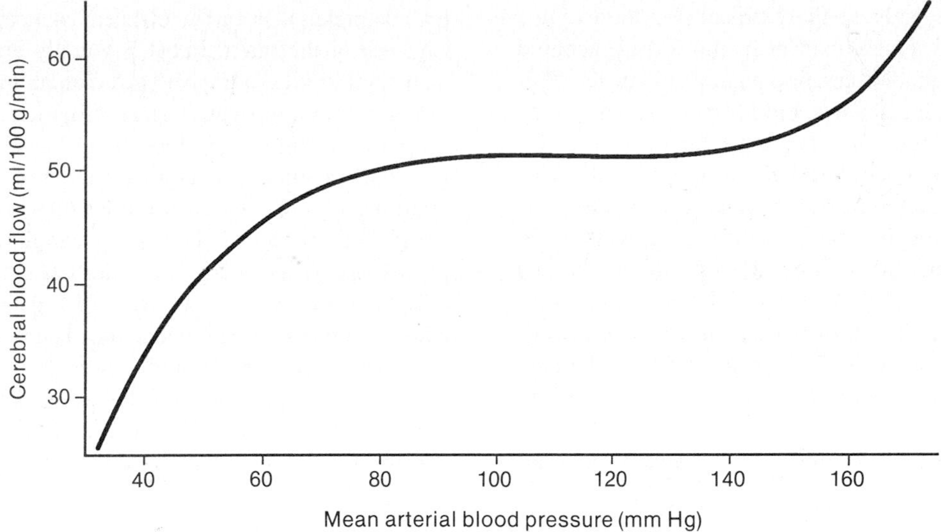


FIGURE 5-9
Autoregulation of cerebral blood flow. Over a broad range of blood pressure, cerebral vessels dilate as pressure decreases, thus keeping flow constant. Outside of the range in which autoregulation functions, increases or decreases in pressure cause increases or decreases in flow.

emitting a positron. The emitted positron quickly combines with a nearby electron, and the two particles are annihilated, producing two gamma rays that travel in opposite directions. By surrounding a patient's head with a ring of gamma-ray detectors, it is possible to localize the positron-emitting isotope within the brain (Figure 5-10). One way to utilize this phenomenon is to label deoxyglucose with the positron emitter $^{18}$F and inject the resulting compound. Active neurons take up deoxyglucose as readily as glucose but metabolize it much more slowly. Therefore the $^{18}$F remains in the active neurons long enough for computer-generated tomographic images to be formed (Plate 11). Although expensive and technologically complex, the potential for PET scanning is exciting (Plate 12). Many different compounds can be labeled with positron-emitting isotopes, making it possible to map out not only glucose metabolism but also oxygen consumption, blood flow, and the locations of receptors for neurotransmitters and hormones.

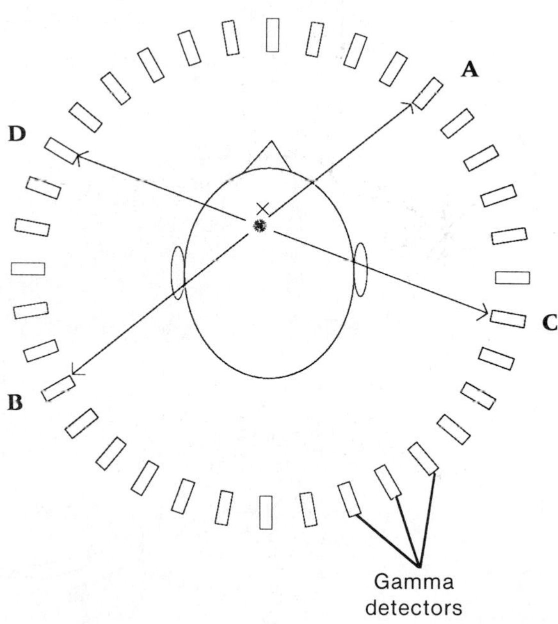


FIGURE 5-10
Localizing positrons in the brain. A positron-electron collision causes two gamma rays to be emitted in exactly opposite directions, so simultaneous registration of gamma rays by detectors *A* and *B* indicates that there is at least one positron source along line AB. Subsequent simultaneous detections by pairs of detectors like *C* and *D* indicate that a positron source must be at *X*. If the gamma detectors are all in one plane, a map of positron sources in that plane can be made. This is the basis for positron emission tomography (PET).

## Blood-brain barrier

The concept of a *blood-brain barrier* arose from the early observation that many substances, when injected into the bloodstream, cannot gain access to the brain. Such a barrier must consist of more than just an impediment at the junction between blood vessels and brain, since this alone would not prevent substances in tissues around the brain from diffusing into it. The term "blood-brain barrier" therefore is commonly used in a more general sense to refer to the anatomical and physiological complex that controls the movement of substances from the general extracellular fluid of the body to the extracellular fluid of the brain. Used in this way, the barrier includes the arachnoid barrier layer and the blood-cerebrospinal fluid barrier (Figure 5-11). It also includes a true blood-brain barrier, which consists of rows of tight junctions between adjacent endothelial cells of cerebral capillaries (Figures 5-12 and 5-13). As in the case of the blood-cerebrospinal fluid barrier, this barrier is selective; glucose can cross it by a process of facilitated diffusion, but other molecules of similar size and solubility cannot. In addition, it appears that various substances can be actively transported in both directions across this endothelial wall. The permeability and transport properties of the barrier are under a degree of neural control.

This complex barrier system can be a mixed blessing. For example, it is rather efficient at keeping microorganisms out of the brain, but it is equally efficient at keeping many antibiotics out. An intracranial infection therefore can be difficult to treat. The development of techniques for reversibly opening the blood-brain barrier and the synthesis of therapeutic agents that can cross an intact blood-brain barrier are both active areas of research.

As discussed in Chapter 4, the capillaries of the choroid plexus are fenestrated, and substances can leave them, only to be stopped by the arrays of tight junctions between adjacent choroid epithelial cells. There are several other locations where the cerebral capillaries are fenestrated and allow free communication between the blood and the brain's extracellular fluid. These additional sites are in contact with the walls of the ventricular system and collec-

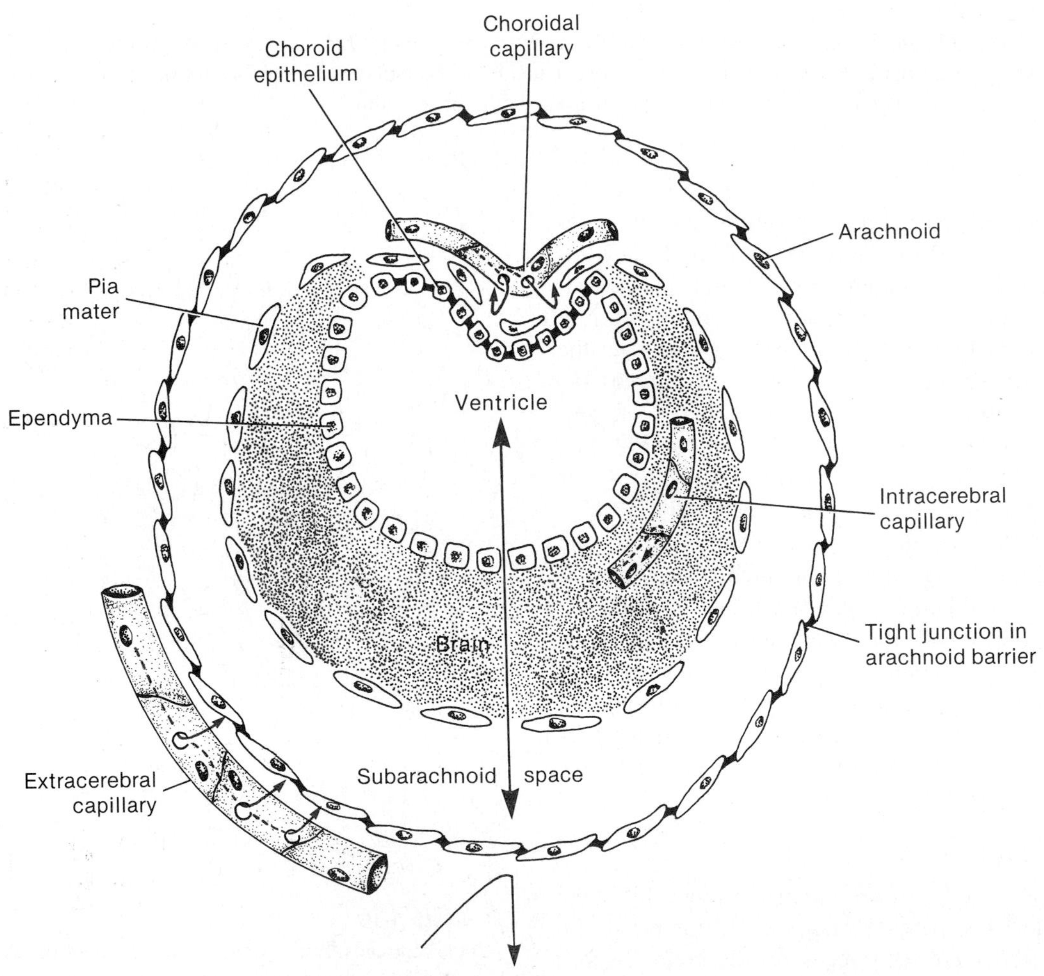


FIGURE 5-11
Barrier systems in and around the brain. Substances can leave extracerebral capillaries but are then blocked by the arachnoid barrier. They can also leave choroidal capillaries but are then blocked by the choroid epithelium. They cannot leave any other capillaries that are inside the arachnoid barrier (except for those in the circumventricular organs). The ventricular and subarachnoid spaces are in free communication with each other, and both communicate with the extracellular space of the brain.

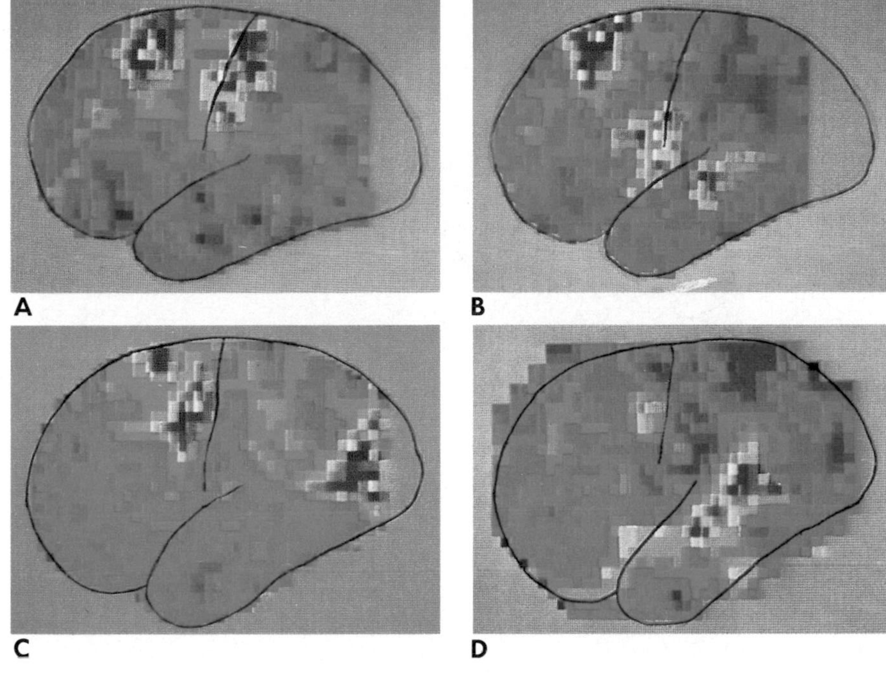

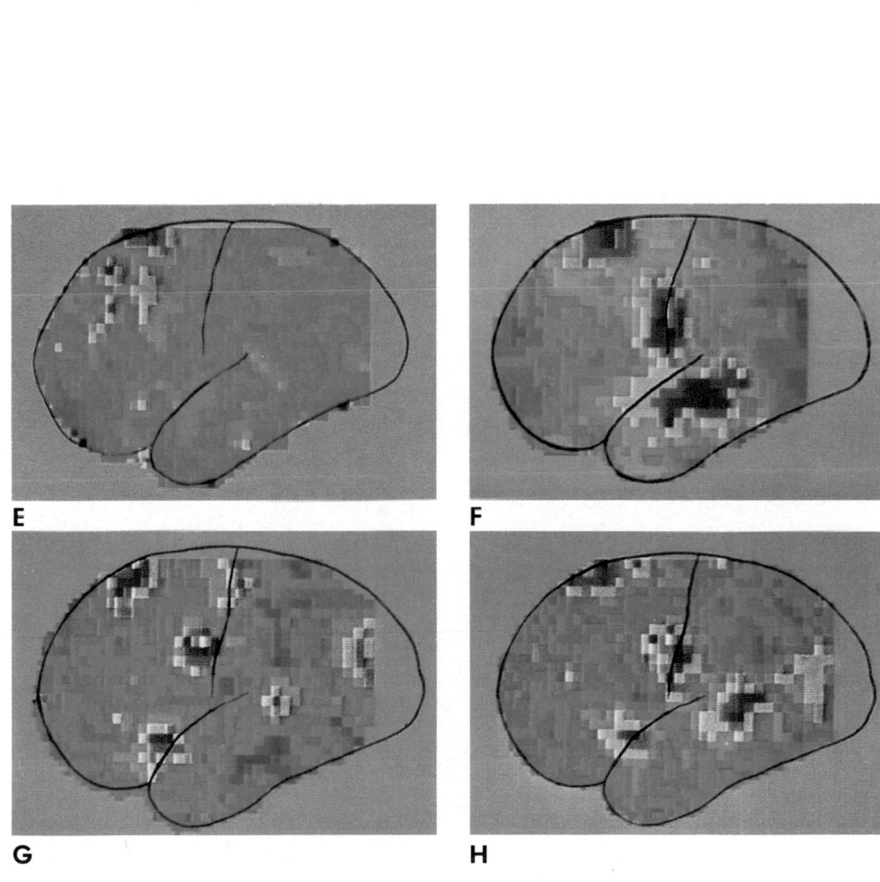

**PLATE 11**

Use of $^{133}Xe$ to map regional changes in cerebral blood flow during different activities. In each case a computer has color coded the blood flow so that green represents no change in flow rate from the resting state, shades of blue indicate decreases in flow rate of up to 20%, and shades of red represent increases of up to 20%. The xenon was injected into the internal carotid artery, so the posterior cerebral circulation (that is, the occipital lobe) is not shown. Pictures from studies involving the right hemisphere were reversed so that all the pictures have the same orientation. **A** and **B,** Use of different parts of motor cortex when moving different parts of the body. **A** was recorded during movement of the contralateral fingers, **B** while counting from 1 to 20 repeatedly. The corresponding somatosensory area in the postcentral gyrus is also activated by the movements. In both cases blood flow also increases in the supplementary motor area (upper, more anterior, increase; see Chapter 12); this area is on the medial surface of the hemisphere above the cingulate gyrus, but the gamma rays pass through the brain and are recorded by the external detectors. **C** and **D,** Use of different sensory systems also causes increased flow to distinctive cortical areas. Following a moving visual target **(C)** activates visual association cortex of the occipital lobe, the supplementary motor area, and the eye-movement part of motor cortex (the frontal eye field; see Chapter 12). In contrast, listening to spoken words **(D)** activates auditory cortex in the superior temporal gyrus and the adjacent Wernicke's area, which is involved in the comprehension of language (see Chapter 15). **E** to **H,** Different kinds of language-related activities are accompanied by distinctive patterns of cortical blood flow increases. While a subject repeatedly counts from 1 to 20 silently **(E),** blood flow increases in the frontal lobes, including the supplementary motor area, but not in Broca's or Wernicke's areas (inferior frontal and superior temporal gyri, respectively). Speaking aloud **(F)** also activates Broca's and Wernicke's areas in the left hemisphere, as well as the auditory cortex and the mouth area of motor and somatosensory cortex. Reading silently **(G)** activates visual association cortex, frontal eye field, Broca's area, the supplementary motor area, and to some extent, Wernicke's area and the mouth area of motor cortex. Reading aloud **(H)** is accompanied by a greater increase in Wernicke's area and the mouth area of motor cortex and by increases in auditory cortex and the mouth area of somatosensory cortex. **E** to **H,** all left hemisphere.

From Lassen NA, et al: Sci Am 239(4):62, 1978.

A

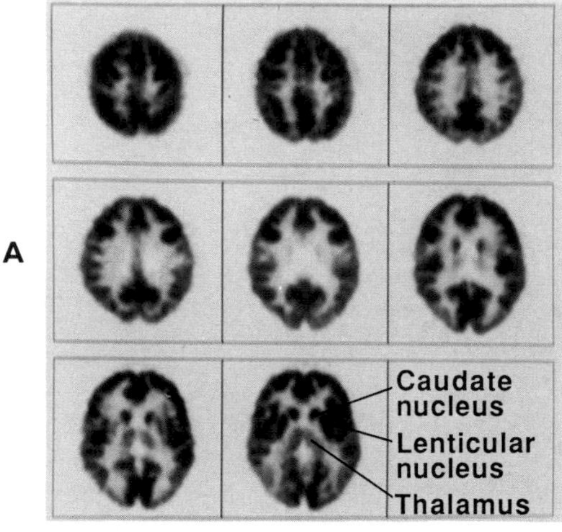
Caudate nucleus
Lenticular nucleus
Thalamus

B

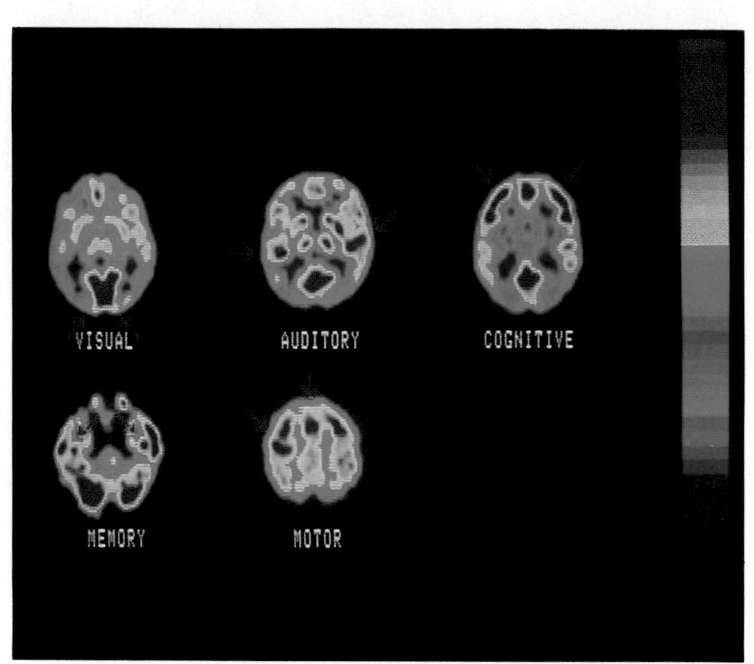
VISUAL
AUDITORY
COGNITIVE
MEMORY
MOTOR

C

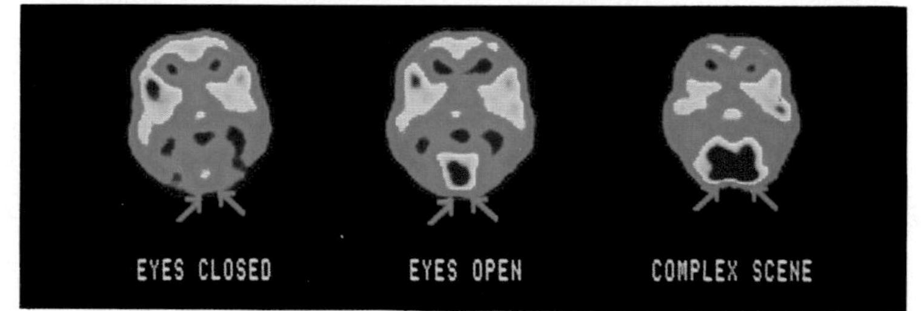
EYES CLOSED
EYES OPEN
COMPLEX SCENE

D

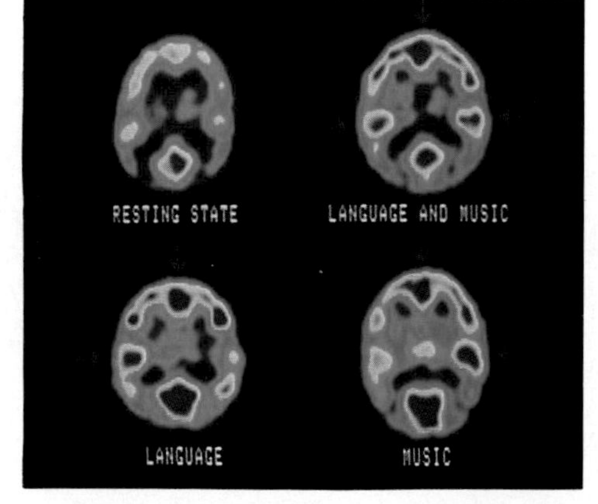
RESTING STATE
LANGUAGE AND MUSIC
LANGUAGE
MUSIC

PLATE 12

Use of PET and $^{18}$F-fluorodeoxyglucose (FDG) to map brain glucose consumption in CT planes (approximately horizontal; parallel to the canthomeatal line). In all images, anterior is at the top. **A,** Series of high-resolution PET images showing the baseline rate of glucose consumption in different areas of the brain; darker shades of gray indicate higher rates of glucose consumption. The upper left image is the most superior "slice" and the lower right image the most inferior. Gray matter obviously has a higher metabolic rate than white matter, and the cerebral cortex, thalamus, caudate nucleus, and lenticular nucleus can all be seen clearly. **B** to **D** demonstrate varying patterns of glucose consumption during different tasks. The color scale in **B** also applies to **C** and **D;** the units are micromoles per minute per 100 grams, and the scale ranges from 2 (violet) to 45 (red). **B,** Different kinds of tasks cause increased glucose consumption in distinctive areas of the brain. A checkerboard visual stimulus activates the medial parts of the occipital lobes. An auditory stimulus causes increased glucose consumption in the superior surfaces of the temporal lobes; the areas of increase have different shapes in the two hemispheres, reflecting the anatomical asymmetry of the surface of the superior temporal gyrus (see Chapter 15). When an individual is engaged in an active, cognitive task rather than passive perception of stimuli, glucose consumption increases in the frontal lobes. Subjects trying to remember information from a verbal stimulus (a story) show increased glucose consumption in the medial parts of the temporal lobes, consistent with increased metabolism in the hippocampal formation and amygdala (see Chapter 16). Sequential movements of the fingers of the right hand activate motor cortex on the left, as well as the supplementary motor are *(vertical arrow).* **C,** Increasing complexity of a particular kind of task causes increased glucose consumption in progressively larger areas of cortex. With the subject blindfolded ("eyes closed"), there is relatively little glucose consumption in the occipital lobes. With eyes open, looking at a plain white light source activates the primary visual cortex on the medial surfaces of the occipital lobes. Looking at an outdoor scene ("complex scene") activates visual association cortex in additional areas of the occipital lobes. **D,** As described in Chapter 15, the left hemisphere usually plays a dominant role in language functions, the right hemisphere in musical and certain other functions. This physiological asymmetry can be demonstrated using auditory stimuli and FDG-PET. When a subject listens simultaneously to a Sherlock Holmes story and a Brandenburg Concerto, both superior temporal lobes (and both frontal lobes) are activated. Listening to just the story activates predominantly the left hemisphere. Musical chords alone activate predominantly the right hemisphere.

Courtesy of Dr. M.E. Phelps and Dr. JC. Mazziotta, University of California School of Medicine. **B** and **D** from Phelps ME, Mazziotta JC: Science 228:799, 1985. 

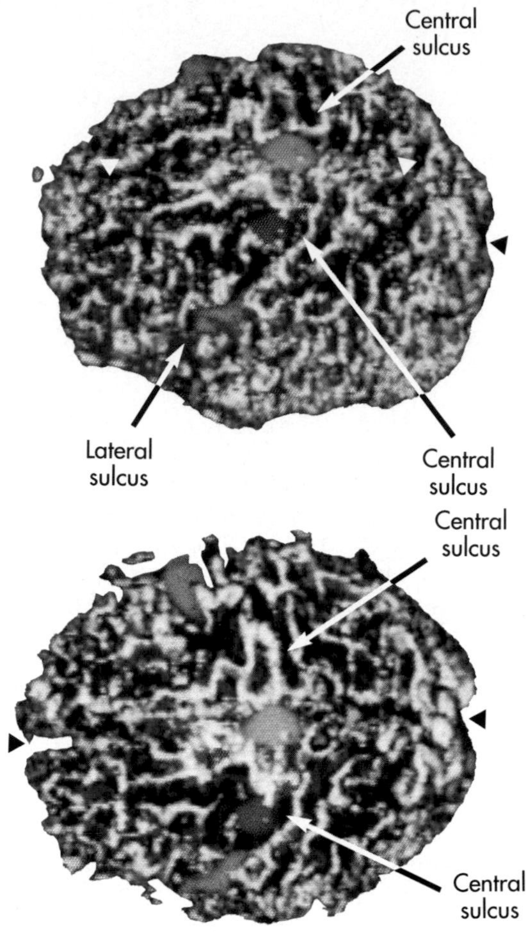


PLATE 13
Combined use of PET scanning and MRI to demonstrate changes in cerebral blood flow. An individual was injected with $H_2{}^{15}O$ before tracking with movements of the right big toe, the right index finger, or the tongue a target moving around on a computer screen. Green, red, and purple areas represent parts of the brain where blood flow increased by at least 15% during toe, finger, or tongue movements, respectively. The images of these areas of increased blood flow were superimposed on a three-dimensional reconstruction (from MRI scans) of the interface between cerebral cortex and white matter; this makes it possible to appreciate the locations of various sulci. The central, lateral, and some other sulci can be seen, and the interhemispheric fissure is indicated by arrowheads. *A* is a view from above and to the left, and *B* is a view from directly above. A systematic mapping of different parts of the body (described further in Chapter 12) is apparent. Note that blood flow increases by more than 15% in only the contralateral motor cortex during finger or toe movements, but bilaterally during tongue movements; this is related to the fact that we can easily move one hand or one foot, but ordinarily cannot contract tongue muscles unilaterally. During all of these tasks, blood flow to the supplementary motor area (see Plate 11) increases by less than 15%, so this increase is not seen in these images.
Courtesy of Dr. John C. Mazziotta, University of California School of Medicine, Los Angeles.

tively are termed the *circumventricular organs* (Figures 5-14 and 5-15). They include the pineal gland, portions of the hypothalamus, and a few other structures. Each circumventricular organ probably has either a secretory function or a role in monitoring the composition of the general extracellular fluid; in both cases, free access to the bloodstream seems reasonable in terms of efficient operation. The ependymal cells overlying each circumventricular organ form a partial barrier between the organ and the ventricular cerebrospinal fluid, but there is no particular barrier between the organs and the surrounding neural tissue. In this sense, the circumventricular organs appear to be small holes in the blood-brain barrier.

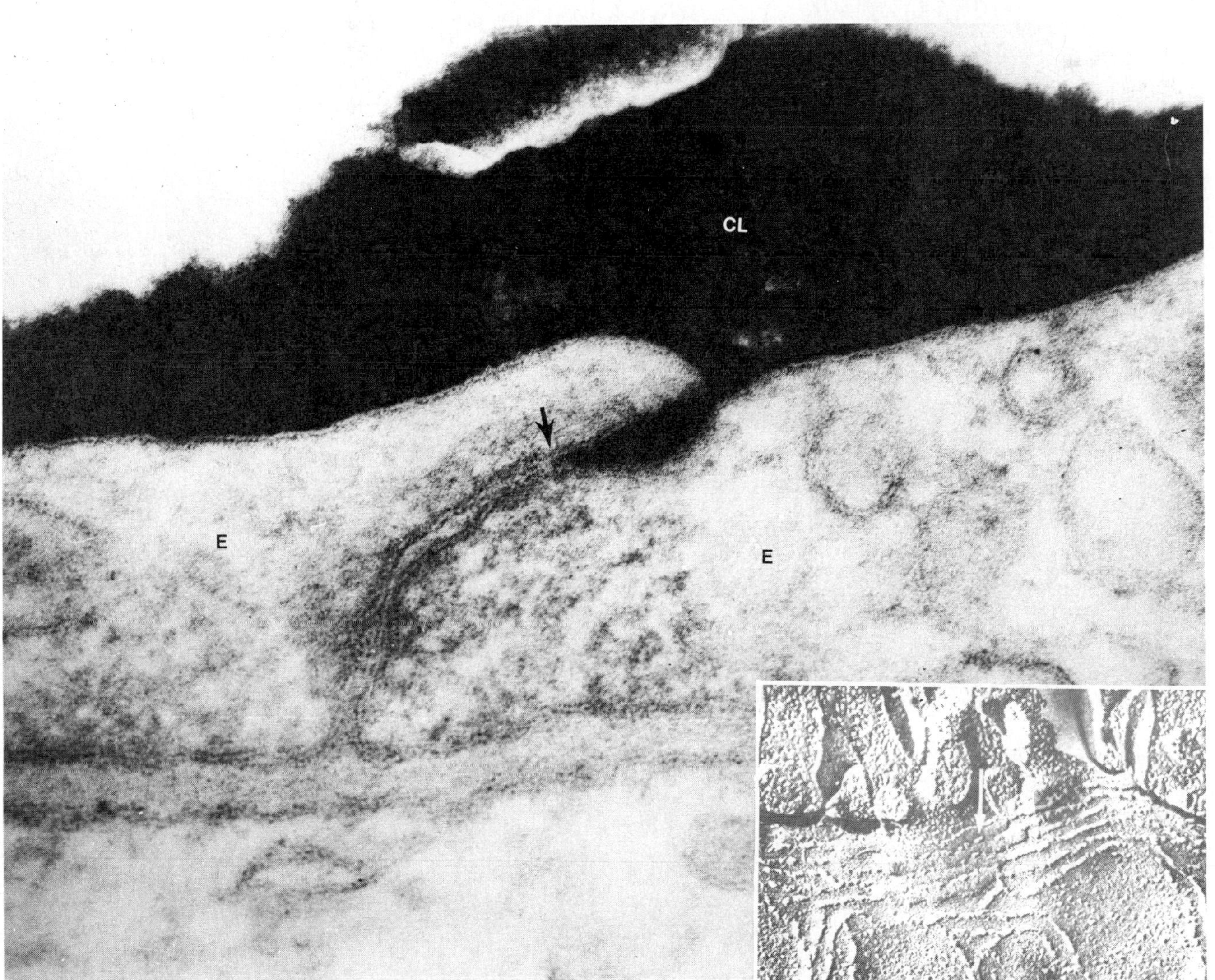


FIGURE 5-12
Endothelial wall of a mouse cerebral capillary. An electron-dense marker (lanthanum hydroxide) that had been injected into the mouse's aorta begins to leave the capillary lumen *(CL)* but is stopped by a tight junction *(arrow)* between two endothelial cells *(E)*. Inset: bands of equivalent tight junctions *(arrow)* between adjacent choroid epithelial cells, revealed by freeze-fracturing. In this technique, the tissue is frozen and then split; the exposed surfaces are then coated with gold or platinum and examined in a scanning electron microscope.

Courtesy of Dr. Milton Brightman, National Institutes of Health.

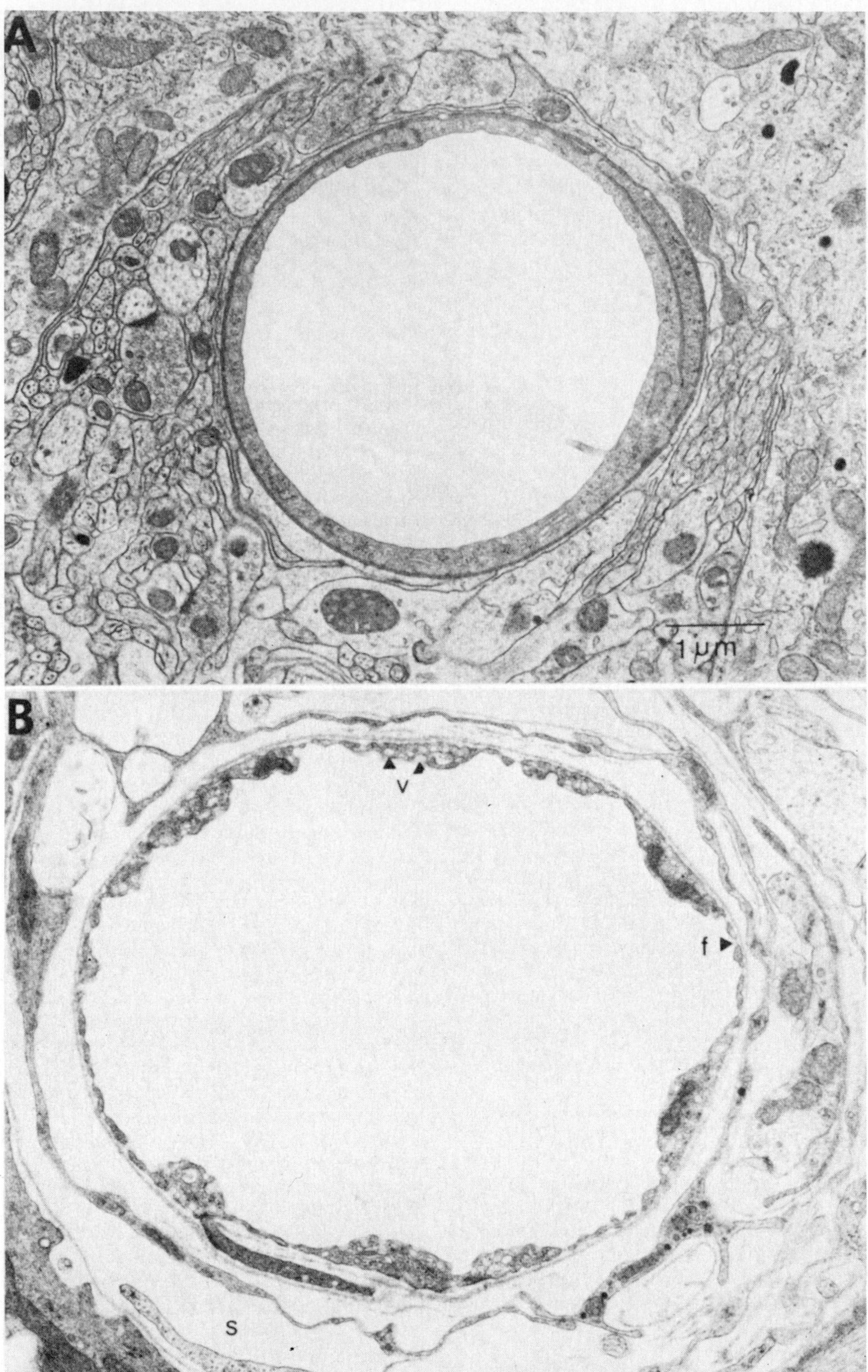


FIGURE 5-13

Capillaries inside and outside the blood-brain barrier. **A,** Capillary in a hypothalamic nucleus (the supraoptic nucleus) of a rat. The continuous endothelial wall and the lack of pinocytotic vesicles are apparent; tight junctions are also present between endothelial cells, but cannot be seen at this magnification. **B,** Capillary in the subfornical organ, which is a circumventricular organ in the roof of the third ventricle near the interventricular foramen. The walls of this capillary are quite permeable, and are characterized by fenestrations *(f)*, pinocytotic vesicles *(v)*, and substantial spaces *(s)* around the capillary.

From Gross PM: *Brain Res Bull* 15:65, 1985. Courtesy of Dr. Paul Gross, Queen's University.

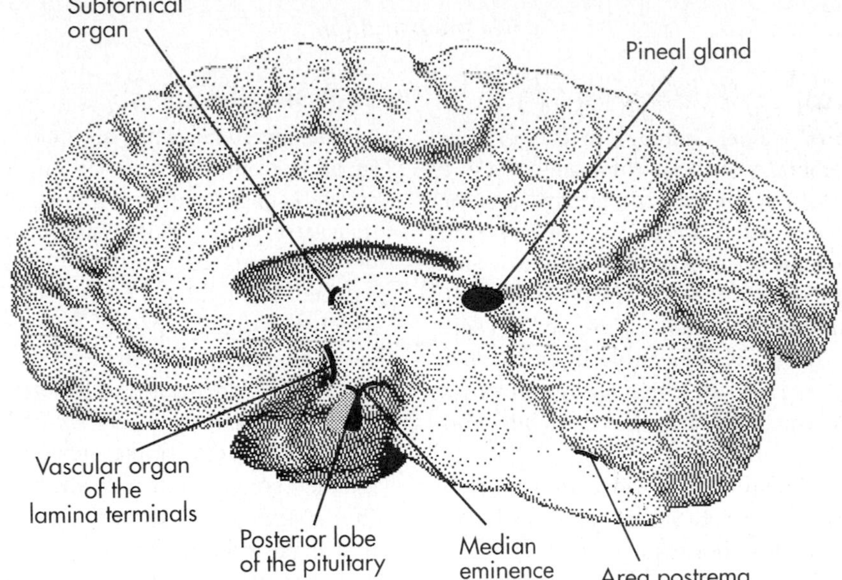


FIGURE 5-14
Locations of human circumventricular organs. The *subfornical organ* is a small nodule in the anterior, superior corner of the third ventricle, adjacent to the interventricular foramina; it has been implicated in the control of fluid balance and drinking behavior. The *vascular organ of the lamina terminalis*, as its name implies, is embedded in the lamina terminalis; it may participate in the control of fluid balance and may be involved in neuroendocrine functions as well. The *median eminence* and the *posterior lobe of the pituitary* are major elements of the neuroendocrine system, and are discussed further in Chapter 10. The *pineal gland* secretes melatonin, which participates in the control of reproductive behavior in many animals; its role in humans is less clear, but dysfunction of this system may be involved in some affective disorders. The *area postrema,* located in the walls of the caudal end of the fourth ventricle, monitors blood for the presence of toxins and triggers vomiting when appropriate. Some authors also include the choroid plexuses of the lateral, third and fourth ventricles in the list of circumventricular organs, since they lack a blood-brain barrier and are located in ventricular walls.

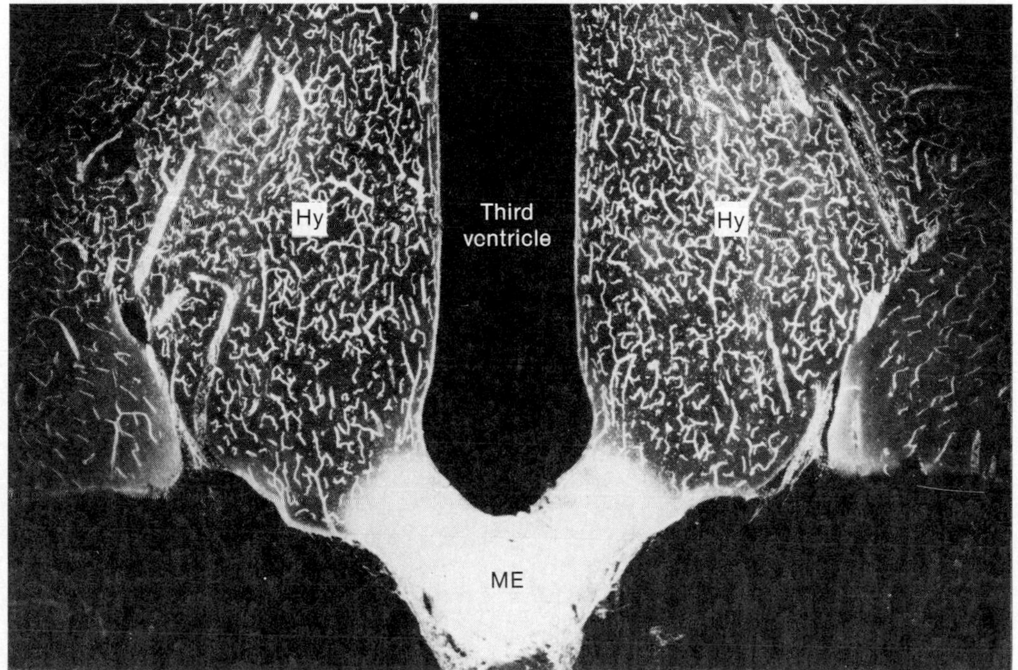


FIGURE 5-15
Macroscopic demonstration of capillaries inside and outside the blood-brain barrier. Horseradish peroxidase was administered intravenously to a monkey, demonstrated histochemically, and viewed in coronal sections using darkfield microscopy. Reaction product fills the median eminence *(ME),* an area of the hypothalamus that has no blood-barrier and is one of the circumventricular organs. However, no reaction product is seen around the numerous capillaries in the remainder of the hypothalamus *(Hy).*

Modified from Broadwell RD et al: *J Comp Neurol* 260:47, 1987. Courtesy of Dr. Richard Broadwell, National Institutes of Health.

## VENOUS DRAINAGE

The principal route of venous drainage of the brain is through a system of cerebral veins that empty into the dural venous sinuses and ultimately into the internal jugular vein (Figure 5-16). There is also a collection of *emissary veins* connecting extracranial veins with dural sinuses and a *basilar venous plexus* around the base of the brain that communicates with the *epidural venous plexus* of the spinal cord. These play a relatively minor role in the normal circulatory pattern of the brain, but emissary veins can be important clinically as a path for the spread of infection into the cranial cavity.

Cerebral veins are conventionally divided into *superficial* and *deep* groups. In general, the superficial veins lie on the surface of the cerebral hemispheres and empty into the superior sagittal sinus, whereas the deep veins drain internal structures and eventually empty into the straight sinus. The *basal vein,* described later in this chapter, does not fit comfortably into this scheme; some consider it a superficial vein because it drains some cortical areas, but most consider it a deep vein because it also drains some deep structures and eventually empties into the straight sinus.

Cerebral veins are valveless and, in contrast to cerebral arteries, are interconnected by numerous functional anastomoses, both within a group and between superficial and deep groups.

### Superficial veins

The superficial veins are quite variable and consist of a superior group that empties into the superior and inferior sagittal sinuses and an inferior group that empties into the transverse and cavernous sinuses (Figure 5-17). Only three of these veins are reasonably constant from one brain to another. These are (1) the *superficial middle cerebral vein,* which runs anteriorly and inferiorly along the lateral sulcus, draining most of the temporal lobe into the cavernous sinus or into the nearby sphenoparietal sinus; (2) the *superior anastomotic vein* (or *vein of Trolard*), which typically travels across the parietal lobe and connects the superficial middle cerebral vein with the superior sagittal sinus; and (3) the *inferior anastomotic vein* (or *vein of Labbé*), which travels posteriorly and inferiorly across the temporal lobe and connects the superficial middle cerebral vein with the transverse sinus.

### Deep veins

The deep veins (Figure 5-18) are more constant in configuration than are the superficial veins. Since they are found deep in the brain in locations where arteries are small, they form clinically useful radiological landmarks.

The major deep vein is the *internal cerebral vein,* which is formed at the interventricular foramen by the confluence of two smaller veins, the *septal vein* (so named be-

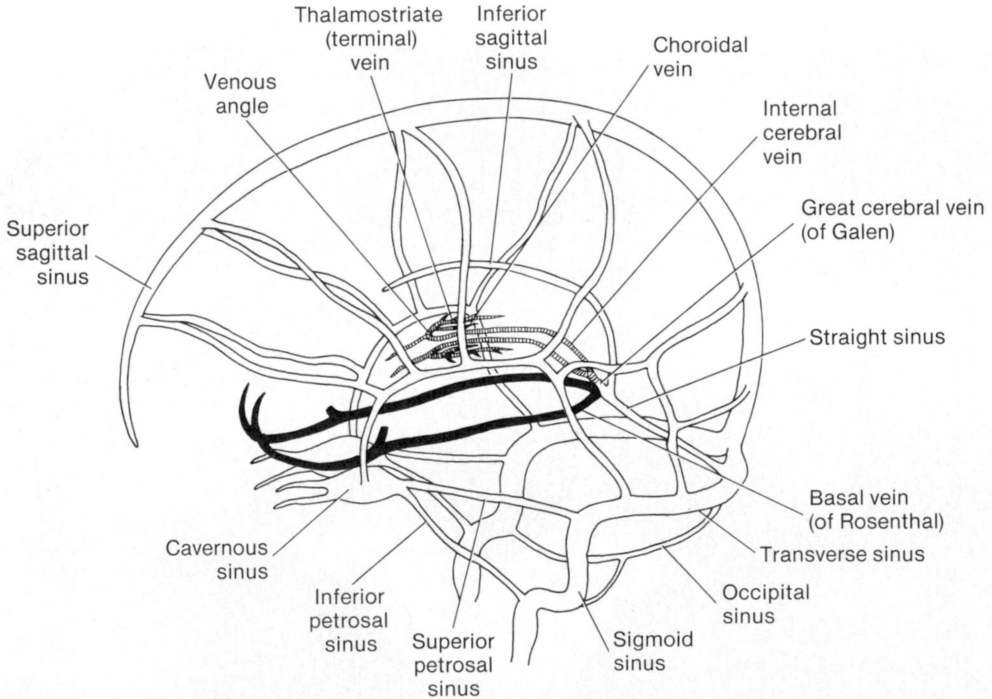


FIGURE 5-16
Venous system of the brain. Dural sinuses and superficial veins are white, deep veins are striped, and the basal vein and its tributaries are colored.
Modified from Warwick R, Williams PL, editors: Gray's anatomy, Br. ed 35, Philadelphia, 1973, WB Saunders.

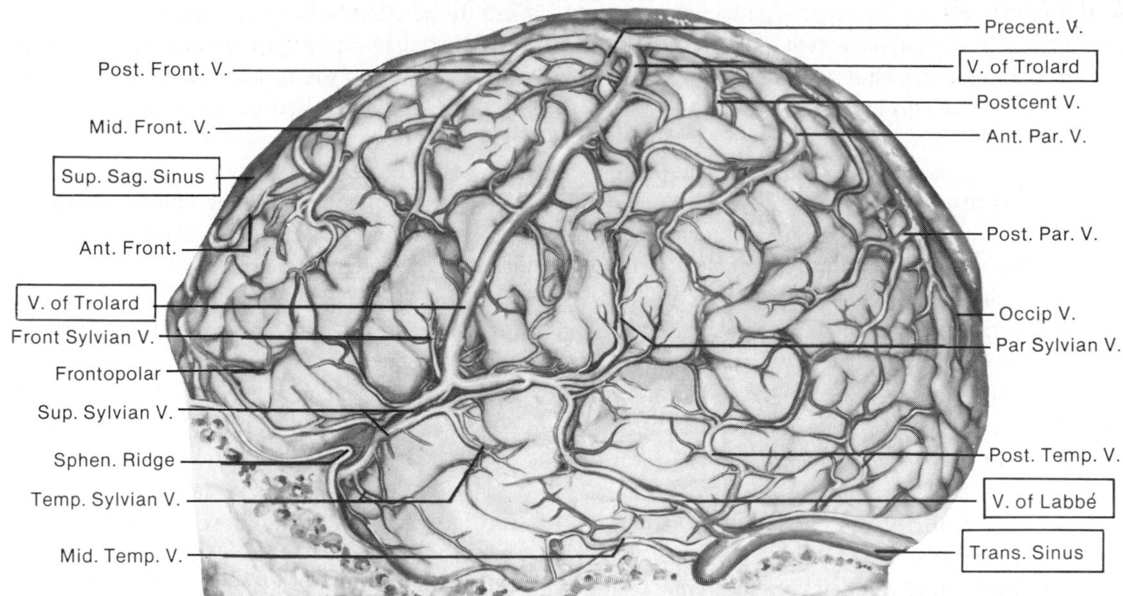


FIGURE 5-17
Superficial veins of the lateral surface of the brain. Anterior is to the left, and the names of the major veins mentioned in the text are outlined in color.

From Oka K et al: *Neurosurgery* 17:711, 1985. Courtesy of Dr. Albert L. Rhoton, Jr, University of Florida College of Medicine.

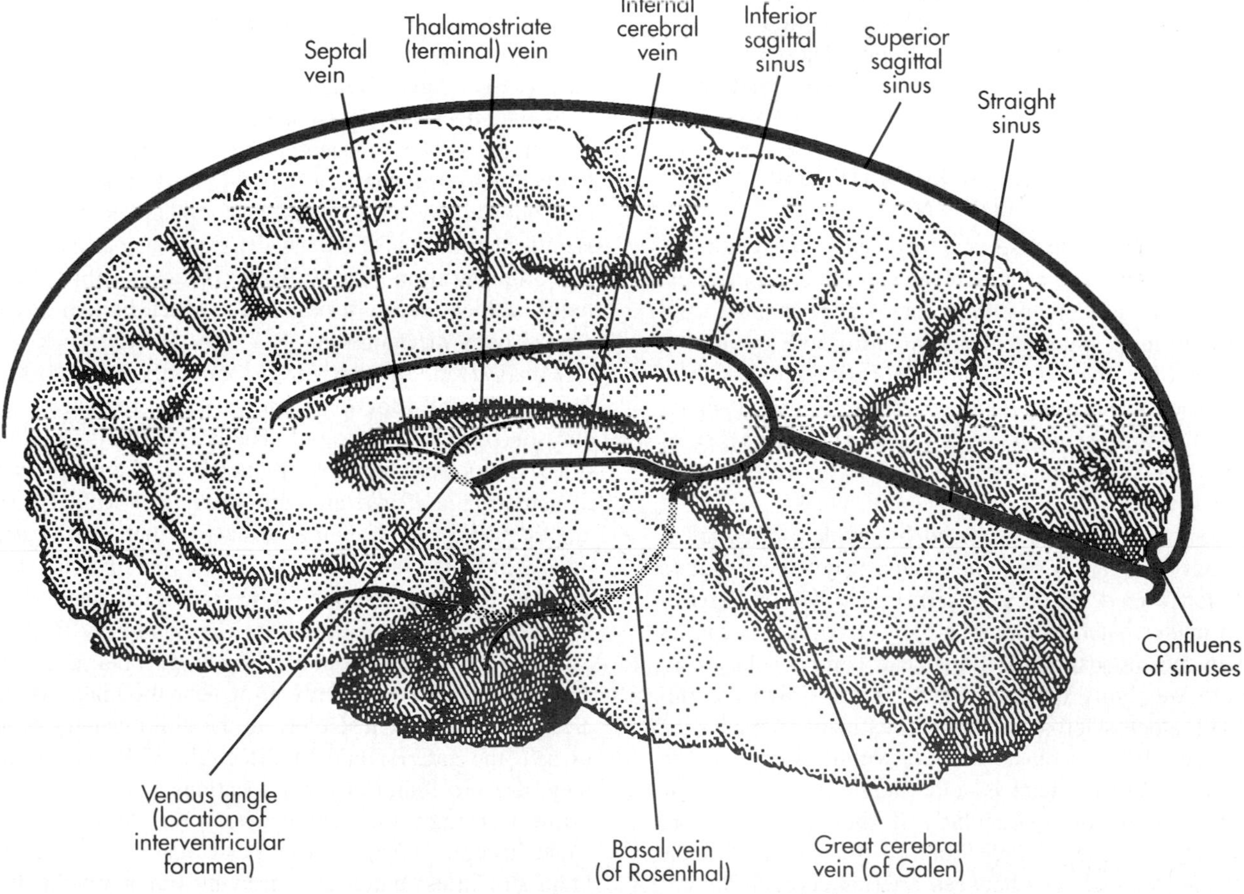


FIGURE 5-18
Deep veins and basal vein, as seen on a hemisected brain.

cause it runs posteriorly across the septum pellucidum) and the *thalamostriate* (or *terminal*) *vein* (which travels in the groove between the thalamus and the caudate nucleus, draining much of both these structures). Near the interventricular foramen, the thalamostriate vein receives the *choroidal vein,* a tortuous vessel that drains the choroid plexus of the body of the lateral ventricle.

Immediately after forming, the internal cerebral vein bends sharply in a posterior direction. This bend is called the *venous angle* and is used in x-ray studies as an indication of the interventricular foramen (Figure 5-21). The paired internal cerebral veins proceed posteriorly through the transverse cerebral fissure and fuse in the superior cistern to form the unpaired *great cerebral vein* (or *vein of Galen*). The great vein turns superiorly and joins the inferior sagittal sinus to form the straight sinus.

Along its short course, the great vein receives the basal veins (or *veins of Rosenthal*). On each side the basal vein is formed near the optic chiasm by the *deep middle cerebral vein,* which drains the insula, and several other tributaries that drain inferior portions of the basal ganglia and the orbital surface of the frontal lobe. It then proceeds along the medial surface of the temporal lobe, curves around the cerebral peduncle, and enters the great vein.

In addition to the superficial and deep veins already described, there is a separate, complex collection of veins that serves the cerebellum and brainstem. These drain into the great vein and into the straight, transverse, and petrosal sinuses.

## SOME FUNCTIONAL ASPECTS OF THE BLOOD SUPPLY OF THE CNS

Cerebrovascular disease and accidents constitute the most common cause of neurological deficits. Since the brain, compared to other organs, has a very high demand for oxygen and glucose, vascular insufficiency lasting more than a few minutes results in necrosis of the involved brain tissue. A necrotic region of tissue is called an *infarct*. An abrupt incident of vascular insufficiency or of bleeding into, or immediately adjacent to, the brain is called a *stroke*.

*Ischemic strokes* (those caused by sudden vascular insufficiency) are most commonly caused by a *thrombus* (a blood clot formed within a vessel) or an *embolus* (a bit of foreign matter, such as part of a blood clot, that is carried along in the bloodstream). Either can cause occlusion of an artery supplying the brain, and both are highly correlated with atherosclerosis (although this is by no means the only cause). If the occlusion occurs within or proximal to the circle of Willis, there is some possibility of adequate collateral circulation, particularly if the involved artery had slowly become occluded before the stroke. On the other hand, anastomoses between arteries distal to the circle of Willis are variable and collateral circulation is less likely to be adequate, so occlusion of one of these vessels typically results in an infarct. The size of the infarct is obviously related to the size of the occluded vessel, ranging from tiny lesions (called *lacunes*) caused by occlusion of a small ganglionic artery to infarcts that affect large expanses of a cerebral hemisphere. However, as pointed out earlier in this chapter, the magnitude of a neurological deficit is not necessarily related to the size of the infarct causing it. A very small lesion in the brainstem or internal capsule can have a much more devastating effect than damage to certain relatively large areas of the cerebellum or cerebral hemispheres.

The exact mechanism whereby ischemia causes neuronal death is not known. Given the brain's metabolic needs, one might expect that total ischemia would be more detrimental than partial ischemia and that increased blood glucose during partial ischemia would be helpful. In fact, exactly the opposite is observed. Apparently, neurons are damaged less by total ischemia and a total halt of metabolism than they are by lactic acidosis and other consequences of anaerobic metabolism and the inability of the vasculature to remove waste products. The fact that neurons are more tolerant of anoxia than was believed previously has given rise to some hope for treatments that can ameliorate the effects of stroke.

Another vascular problem with symptoms somewhat similar to an ischemic stroke is the *transient ischemic attack* (TIA). The crucial difference between a transient ischemic attack and an ischemic stroke is that the deficits associated with a transient ischemic attack (as the name implies) persist for only a few minutes to a few hours and are followed by an essentially complete recovery. Transient ischemic attacks are usually caused by minute emboli that originate from atherosclerotic plaques or thrombi, partially occlude brain arteries, and are then broken down by normal body mechanisms.

*Hemorrhagic strokes* most commonly result from the rupture of small ganglionic arteries or the rupture of an aneurysm (see next paragraph). The lateral striate (lenticulostriate) arteries are the most frequent site of the former type of hemorrhage. These are particularly thin-walled vessels, and the likelihood of their spontaneous rupture is increased greatly in individuals suffering from hypertension. The lateral striate arteries supply some important deep cerebral structures, and hemorrhage here can be rapidly fatal.

*Aneurysms* are balloonlike swellings of arterial walls. They occur most frequently at or near the place where an artery bifurcates. Those close to the brain usually occur in or near the anterior half of the circle of Willis, although they also are found at other locations. An aneurysm can cause neurological deficits in two ways. As it grows (and some become huge), it can push against and compress brain structures, much as a growing tumor would. It also can rupture and, depending on its size and location, have

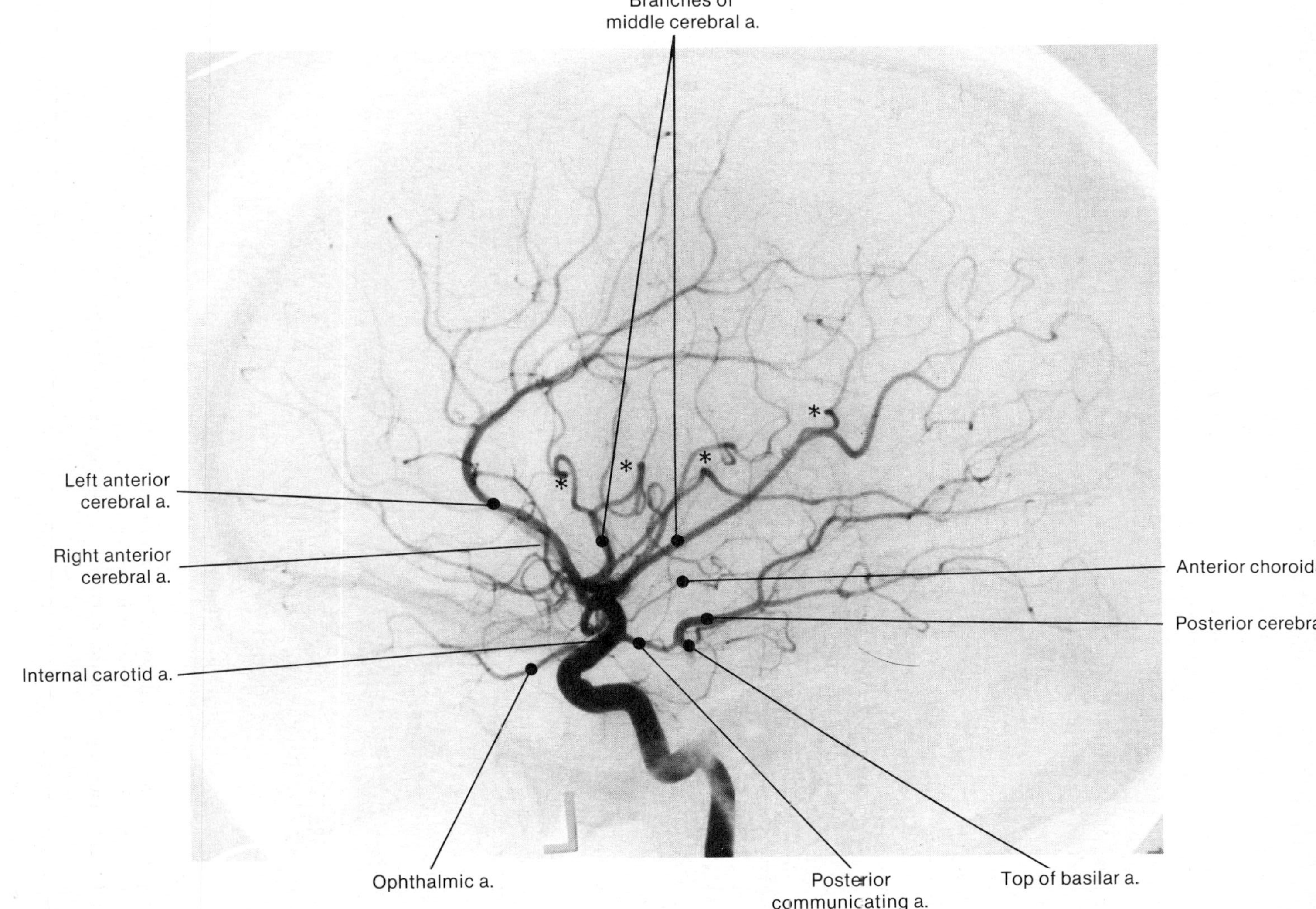


FIGURE 5-19
Lateral projection of the arterial phase of an internal carotid angiogram. Anterior is to the left. This particular individual had relatively large communicating arteries so that contrast medium traveled from the left internal carotid artery into both anterior cerebral arteries and into the left posterior cerebral artery. The small astericks indicate sites where middle cerebral branches are seen end-on (and so look especially dense) as they turn toward the veiwer to emerge from the lateral fissure.
Courtesy of Dr. Roger Bird, St. Joseph's Hospital, Phoenix, Arizona.

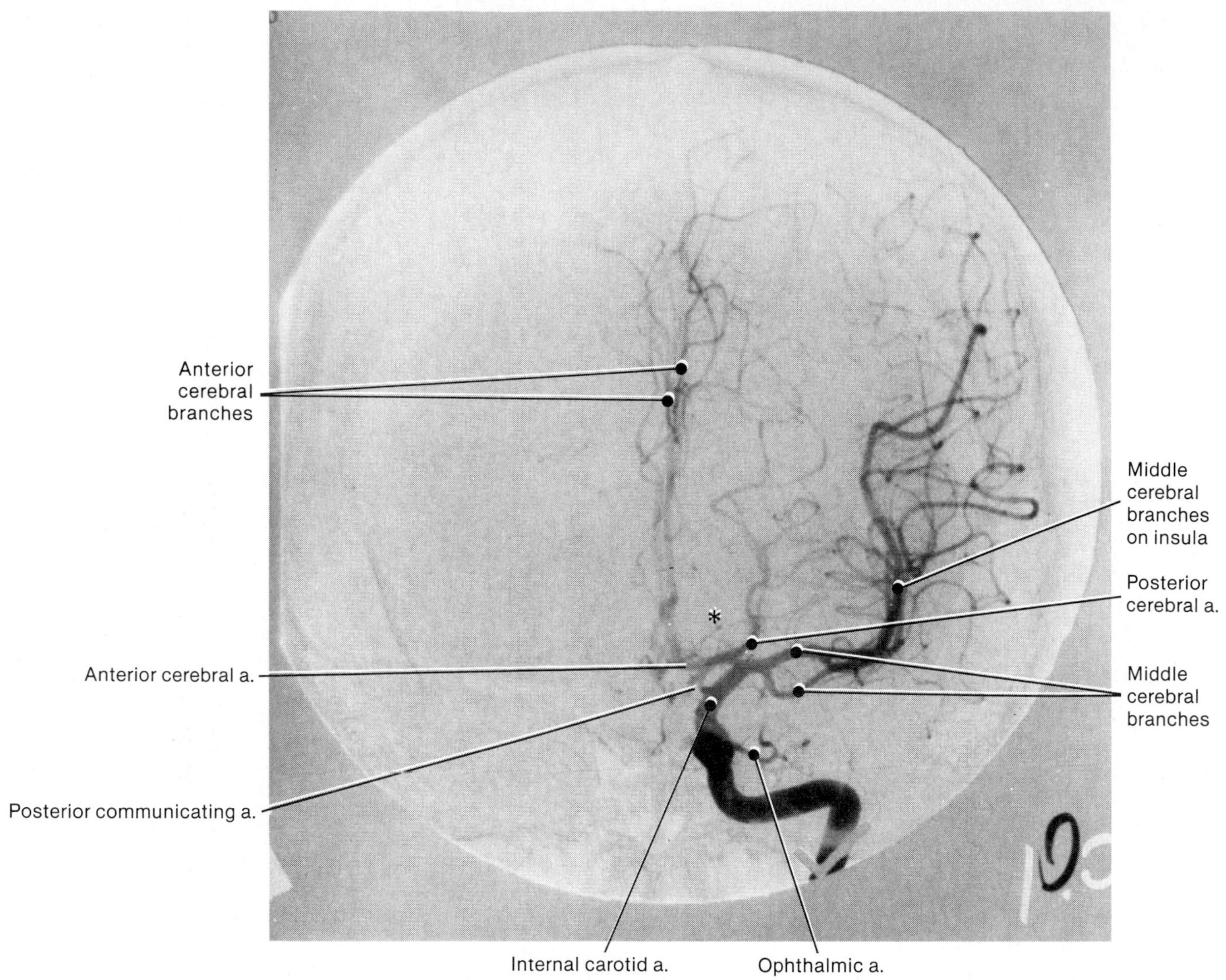


FIGURE 5-20
Anteroposterior projection of the arterial phase of an internal carotid angiogram from the same individual pictured in Figure 5-19. The view is as if you were looking into the patient's face. The asterisk indicates the location of the midbrain, with the posterior cerebral artery wrapping around it.
Courtesy of Dr. Roger Bird, St. Joseph's Hospital, Phoenix, Arizona.

disastrous consequences. Many aneurysms, particularly if they are detected before they become too large, can be corrected surgically.

Another type of vascular problem is an *arteriovenous malformation (AVM)*. This is a congenital malformation in which large anastomoses exist between arteries and veins in a relatively circumscribed area. These malformations may become larger with age and can cause neurological problems, either by "stealing" blood from adjacent normal brain tissue as a result of their low resistance or by hemorrhaging.

Vascular problems involving the venous system are not seen nearly as often as those involving the arterial supply. This is partly because occlusions and hemorrhages occur less often in the venous system and partly because of the large number of functional anastomoses. Thus a slowly developing occlusion of the anterior portion of the superior sagittal sinus probably would be asymptomatic. Even if such an occlusion developed rapidly, the symptoms might be no more than a transient headache. However, if the occlusion were in a more critical location, such as the posterior portion of the superior sagittal sinus, the consequences would be much more serious and might include seizures, motor problems, and even coma and death.

Conditions such as thrombosed arteries, aneurysms, and arteriovenous malformations can be detected by a technique called *cerebral angiography*. This involves injecting a radiopaque dye into the carotid or vertebral circulation and then taking a rapid series of x-ray photographs. Early photographs demonstrate the arterial circulation (Figures 5-19, 5-20, 5-23, and 5-24), and later ones show the venous circulation (Figures 5-21, 5-22, and 5-25).

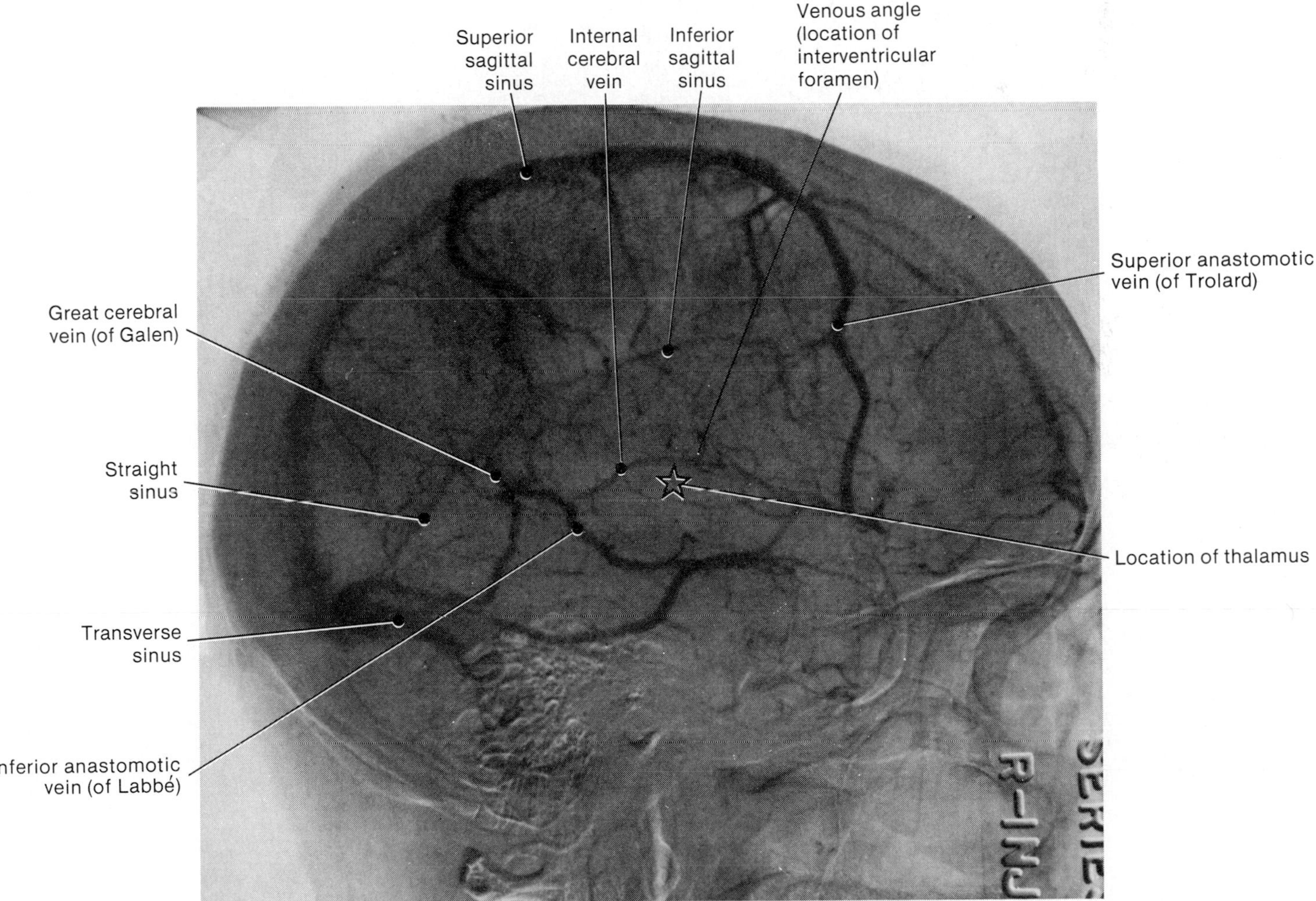


FIGURE 5-21
Lateral projection of the venous phase of an internal carotid angiogram. Anterior is to the right.
Courtesy of Dr. John Stears, University of Colorado Health Sciences Center.

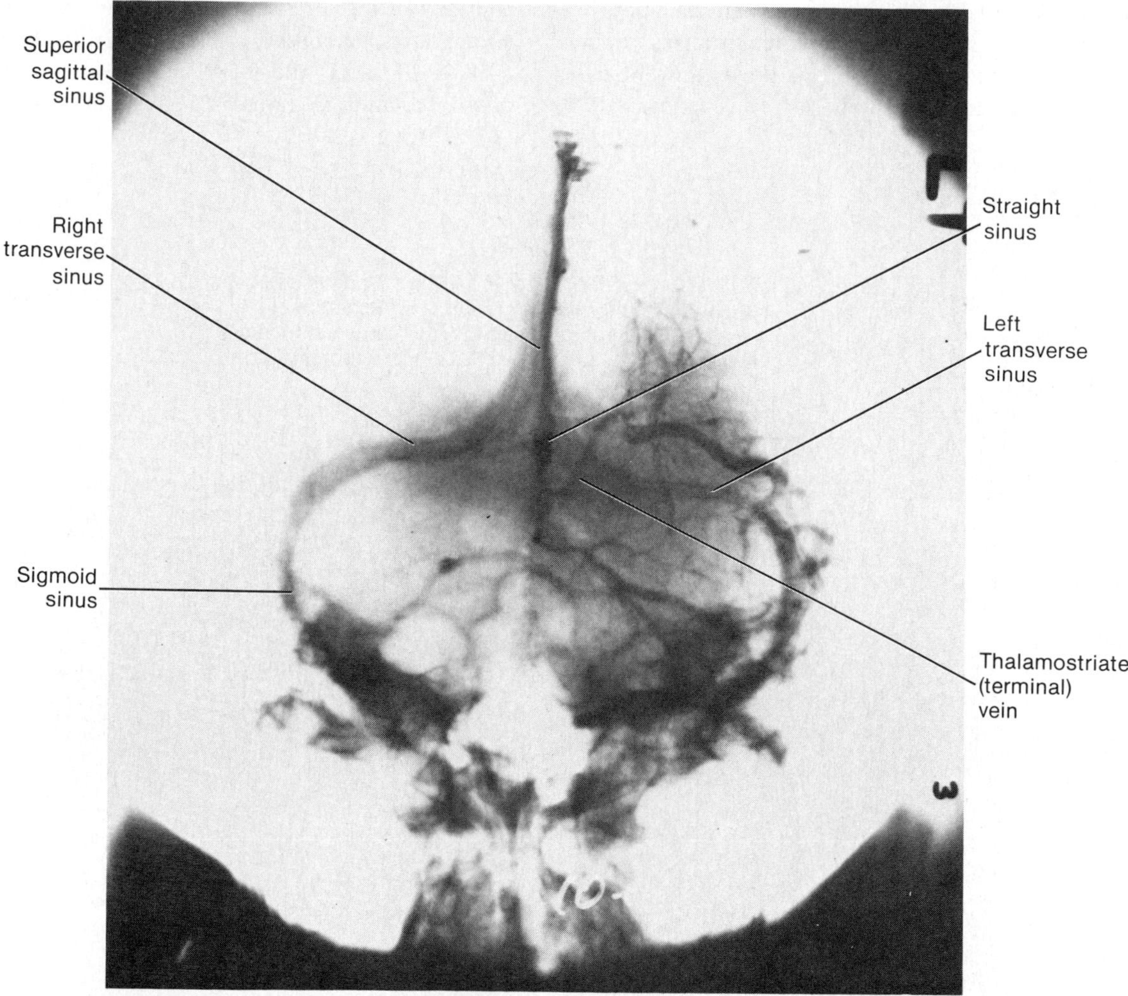


FIGURE 5-22
Anterior-posterior projection of the venous phase of an angiogram. The superior sagittal sinus drains into the right transverse sinus. The straight sinus, seen end-on, drains into the left transverse sinus.
Courtesy of Dr. John Stears, University of Colorado Health Sciences Center.

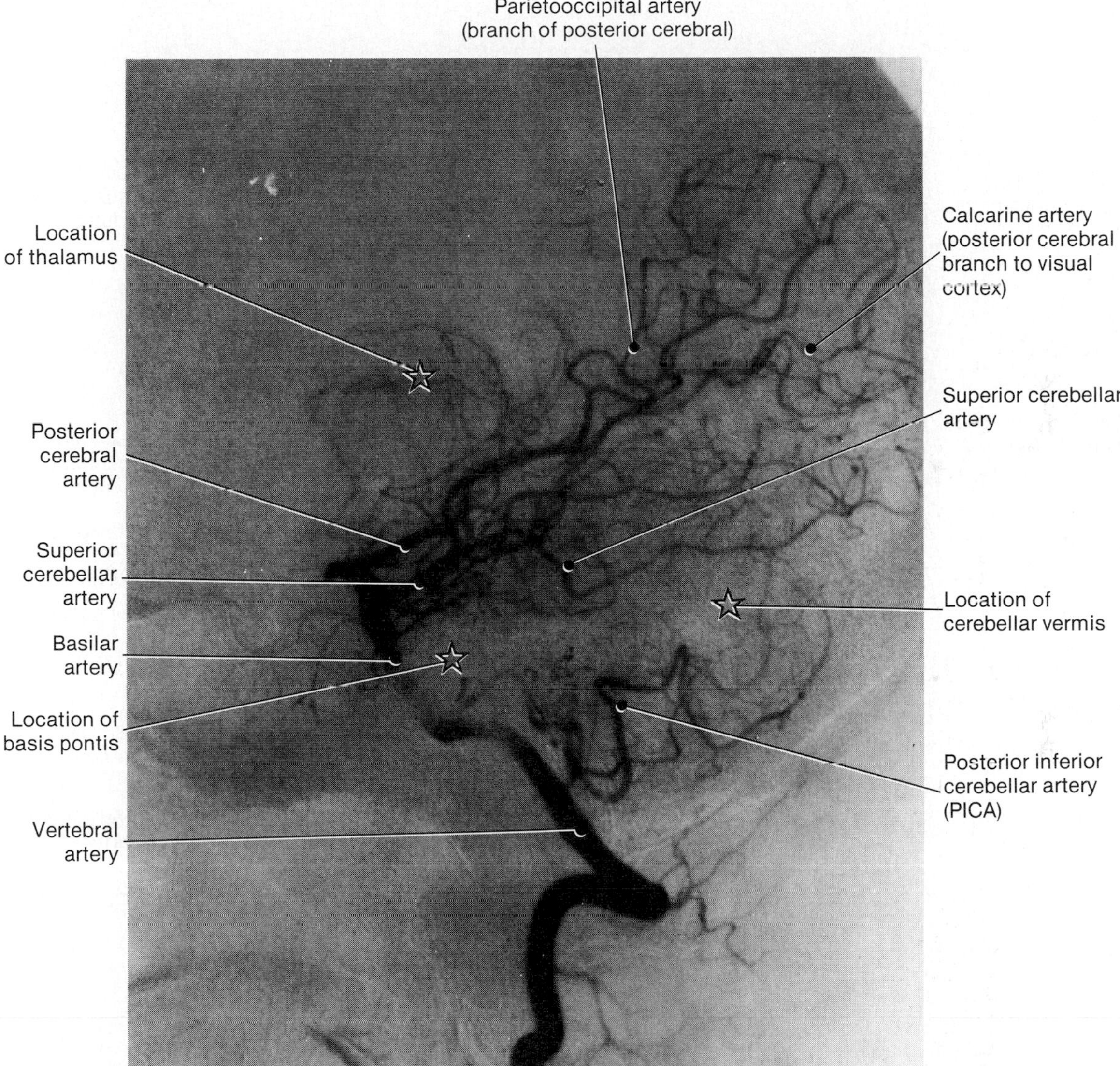


FIGURE 5-23
Lateral projection of the arterial phase of a vertebral angiogram. Anterior is to the left.
Courtesy of Dr. John Stears, University of Colorado Health Sciences Center.

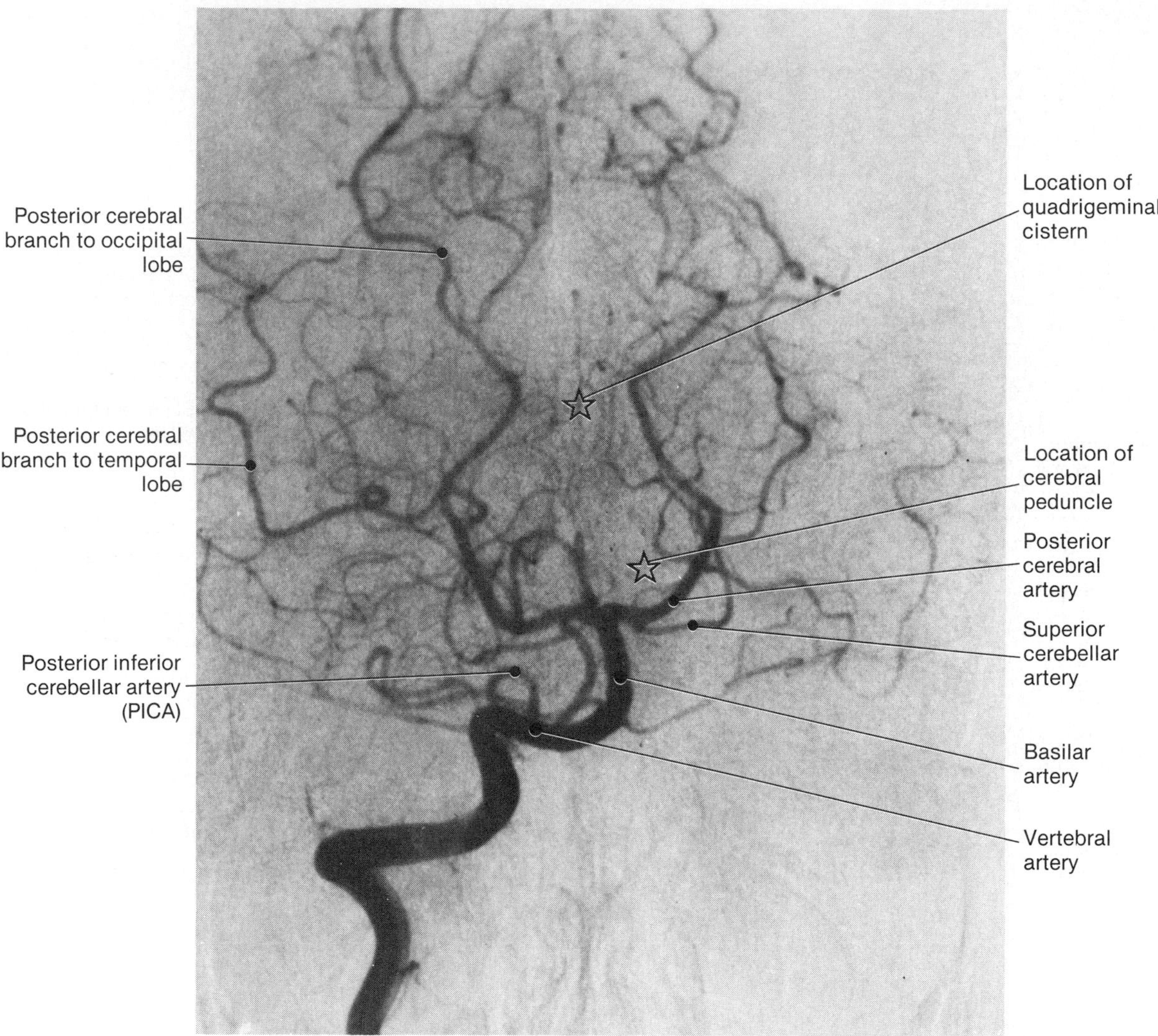


FIGURE 5-24
Anterior-posterior projection of the arterial phase of a vertebral angiogram. Notice how the two posterior cerebral arteries separate to encircle the rostral midbrain, then move back toward the midline to supply the medial surfaces of the occipital lobes.
Courtesy of Dr. John Stears, University of Colorado Health Sciences Center.

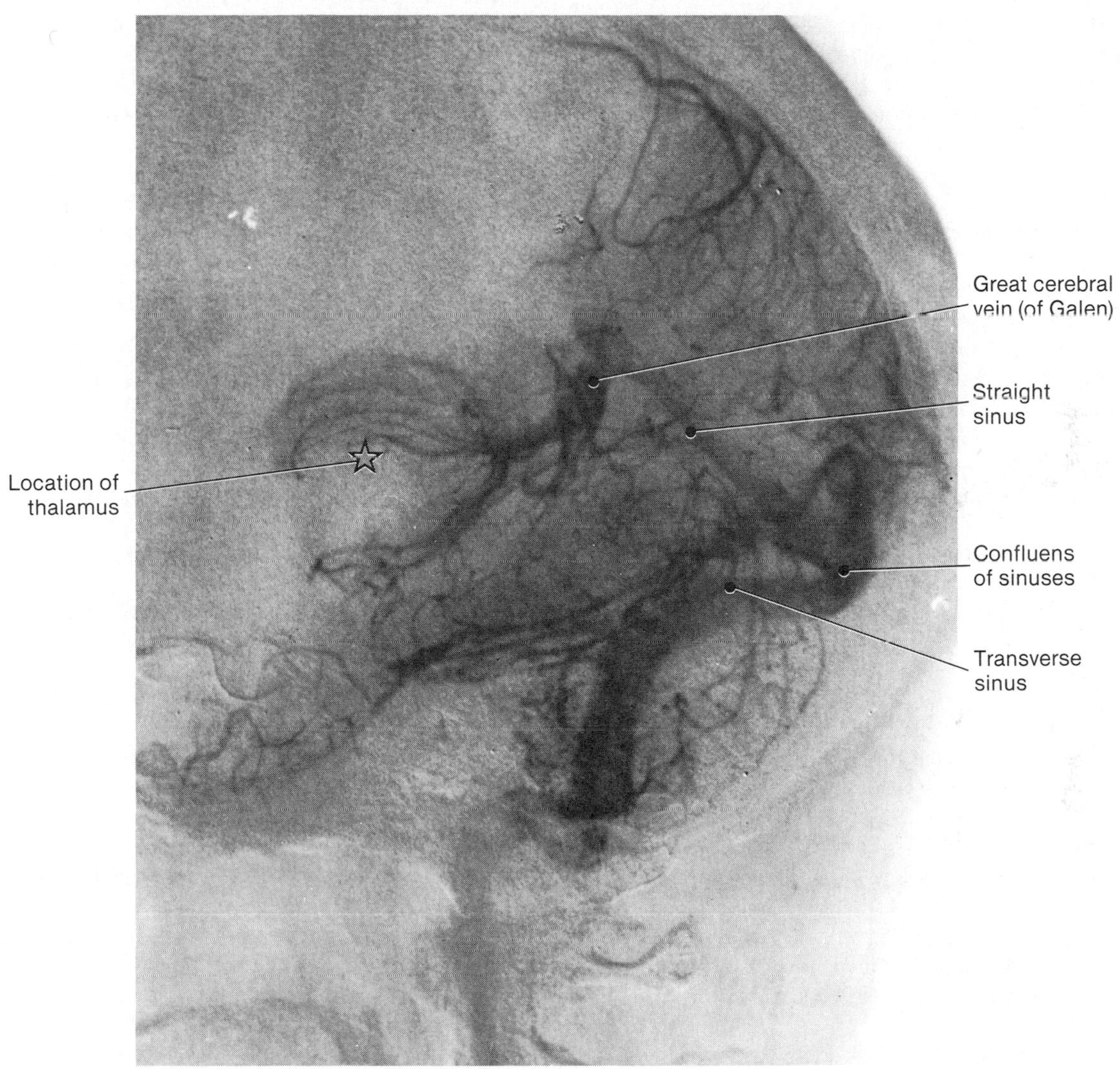


FIGURE 5-25
Lateral projection of the venous phase of a vertebral angiogram. Anterior is to the left. Since the vertebral-basilar system supplies the brainstem, cerebellum, occipital lobes, and much of the diencephalon, only veins in those parts of the CNS are filled.
Courtesy of Dr. John Stears, University of Colorado Health Sciences Center.

## ADDITIONAL READINGS


Balin BJ et al: Avenues for entry of peripherally administered protein to the central nervous system in mouse, rat and squirrel monkey, *J Comp Neurol* 251:260, 1986. *A discussion of the possible significance of circumventricular organs, peripheral nerve sheaths, endothelial transport, and other potential ways of circumventing the blood-brain barrier.*

Bradbury M: *The concept of a blood-brain barrier,* New York, 1979, John Wiley & Sons.

Brightman MW, Reese TS: Junctions between intimately apposed cell membranes in the vertebrate brain, *J Cell Biol* 40:648, 1969.

Brooks DJ: PET: its clinical role in neurology, *J Neurol Neurosurg Psych* 54:1, 1991.

Candelise L et al: Prognostic significance of hyperglycemia in acute stroke, *Arch Neurol* 42:661, 1985.

Choi D: Cerebral hypoxia: some new approaches and unanswered questions, *J Neurosci* 10:2493, 1990. *A brief review of some of the exciting recent research indicating it may some day be possible to treat directly the damage caused by strokes.*

Chorobski J, Penfield W: Cerebral vasodilator nerves and their pathway from the medulla oblongata: with observations on the pial and intracerebral vascular plexus, *Arch Neurol Psychiatr* 28:1257, 1932.

Cobb S, Finesinger JE: Cerebral circulation. XIX. The vagal pathway of the vasodilator impulses, *Arch Neurol Psychiatr* 28:1243, 1932. *While not all subsequent investigators agree with the findings, this paper provides a straightforward and convincing demonstration of a pathway through the vagus nerve into the brainstem and out through the facial nerve, causing dilation of cortical vessels.*

Damasio H: A computed tomographic guide to the identification of cerebral vascular territories, *Arch Neurol* 40:138, 1983.

Duvernoy HM: *Human brainstem vessels,* New York, 1978, Springer-Verlag. *A painstakingly detailed, magnificently illustrated, fabulously expensive book.*

Fisher CM: Lacunes: small, deep cerebral infarcts, *Neurol* 15:774, 1965.

Galatius-Jensen F, Ringberg V: Anastomosis between the anterior choroidal artery and the posterior cerebral artery demonstrated by angiography, *Radiol* 81:942, 1963.

Harik SI: Blood-brain barrier sodium/potassium pump: modulation by central noradrenergic innervation, *Proc Nat Acad Sci U.S.* 83:4067, 1986.

Helgason C et al: Anterior choroidal artery-territory infarction: report of cases and review, *Arch Neurol* 43:681, 1986.

Kapp JP, Schmidek HH: *The cerebral venous system and its disorders,* Orlando, Fla., 1984, Grune & Stratton.

Lassen NA, Ingvar DH, Skinhøj E: Brain function and blood flow, *Sci Am* 239(4):62, 1978. *An exciting technique for studying the activity of different areas of the brain by measuring, with an external gamma-ray camera, the amounts of radioactive isotope delivered to different areas through the arterial circulation.*

Long JB, Holaday JW: Blood-brain barrier: endogenous modulation by adrenal-cortical function, *Science* 277:1580, 1980.

McCulloch J: Perivascular nerve fibers and the cerebral circulation, *Trends Neurosci* 7:135, 1984.

McKinley MJ, Oldfield BJ: *Circumventricular organs.* In Paxinos G, editor: *The human nervous system,* San Diego, 1990, Academic Press.

Millen JW, Woollam DHM: Vascular patterns in the choroid plexus, *J Anat* 87:114, 1953.

Newelt EA, editor: *Implications of the blood-brain barrier and its manipulation,* vol 1: *basic science aspects,* vol 2: *clinical aspects,* New York, 1989, Plenum Publishing.

O'Connell JEA: Some observations on the cerebral veins, *Brain* 57:484, 1934. *A lucid description of the developmental patterns of the superficial cerebral veins and their relationship to the superior sagittal sinus.*

Oka K et al: Microsurgical anatomy of the superficial veins of the cerebrum, *Neurosurg* 17:711, 1985.

Ono M et al: Microsurgical anatomy of the deep venous system of the brain, *Neurosurg* 15:621, 1984.

Reese TS, Karnovsky MJ: Fine structural demonstration of a blood-brain barrier to exogenous peroxidase, *J Cell Biol* 34:207, 1967.

Reivich M: *Embryology, anatomy and pathophysiology of the cerebral circulation.* In Goldensohn ES, Appel SH, editors: *Scientific approaches to clinical neurology,* Philadelphia, 1977, Lea & Febiger. *A fine review with a good bibliography covering the clinical manifestations of various vascular problems.*

Rhoton AL, Jr., Fujii K, Fradd B: Microsurgical anatomy of the anterior choroidal artery, *Surg Neurol* 12:171, 1979. *Finely detailed and beautifully illustrated.*

Riggs HE, Rupp C: Variation in form of circle of Willis, *Arch Neurol* 8:8, 1963.

Robin ED: The evolutionary advantages of being stupid, *Perspect Biol Med* 16:369, 1972/73. *Turtles may not be very smart, but they don't need much oxygen either and they've been around for a long, long time.*

Saeki N, Rhoton AL, Jr.: Microsurgical anatomy of the upper basilar artery and posterior circle of Willis, *J Neurosurg* 46:563, 1977.

Scheinberg P: Transient ischemic attacks: an update, *J Neurol Sci* 101:133, 1991.

Sengupta RP, McAllister VL: *Subarachnoid haemorrhage,* Berlin, 1986, Springer-Verlag. *A recent account including discussions of normal anatomy and its variations, aneurysms, and arteriovenous malformations.*

Sochurek H: Medicine's new image, *Nat Geographic* 171:2, 1987. *A nontechnical article, loaded with impressive color photographs, that conveys some of the sense of excitement engendered by new imaging techniques.*

Sokoloff L: *Brain imaging and brain function,* vol. 63, *Research publications: association for research in nervous and mental disease,* New York, 1985, Raven Press.

Stephens RB, Stilwell DL: *Arteries and veins of the human brain,* Springfield, Ill., 1969, Charles C Thomas. *A well-photographed series of dissections of brains in which the arteries or veins had been injected.*

Toole JF: *Cerebrovascular disorders,* ed 4, New York, 1990, Raven Press.

Van den Bergh R, Vander Eecken H: Anatomy and embryology of cerebral circulation, *Prog Brain Res* 30:1, 1968.

Vander Eecken HM, Adams RD: The anatomy and functional significance of the meningeal arterial anastomoses of the human brain, *J Neuropathol Exp Neurol* 12:132, 1953.

Wackenheim A, Braun JP: *The veins of the posterior fossa,* New York, 1978, Springer-Verlag.

Welch K et al: The collateral circulation following middle cerebral branch occlusion, *J Neurosurg* 12:361, 1955. *Discussion of two cases in which much of the middle cerebral artery filled through the anterior cerebral artery.*

# CHAPTER 6

# *Sensory Receptors and Peripheral Nervous System*

The ongoing activity and output of the central nervous system are greatly influenced, and sometimes more or less determined, by incoming sensory information. An example is our constant awareness of the position of our limbs in space and the use of this awareness in guiding our movements. This chapter considers the functional organization of the general receptors of the body as a prelude to the discussion of how sensory information is routed and processed within the nervous system. Specialized receptors, such as those of the eye and the ear, are described in later chapters.

## RECEPTORS

### Classification

There are many types of receptors on and within the human body and several different systems for classifying them. One system subdivides them into *interoceptors, proprioceptors,* and *exteroceptors*. Interoceptors monitor events within the body, such as distention of the stomach or changes in the pH of the blood. Proprioceptors respond to changes in the position of the body or its parts; examples are the receptors in muscles and in joint capsules. Vestibular receptors of the inner ear are commonly classified as proprioceptors, since they signal movement and changes in the orientation of the head in space. Exteroceptors respond to stimuli that arise outside the body, such as the receptors involved in touch, hearing, and vision. Exteroceptors are sometimes subdivided into *teloreceptors* (from the Greek word *tele,* meaning distant, as in television), which respond to stimuli or objects separated from the body (for example, visual receptors and auditory receptors), and *contact receptors* (for example, tactile receptors and pain receptors). Interoceptor-proprioceptor-exteroceptor terminology is not used as commonly as it was in the past, partly because some receptors do not fit neatly and uniquely into one of these categories. For example, heat-sensitive receptors respond to both radiant heat and to contact with a warm object, so to classify them as either teloreceptors or contact exteroceptors is somewhat arbitrary. Also, some vestibular receptors respond to gravity, an external force, but are classified as proprioceptors; on the other hand, the visual system is very much involved in our perception of motion and body position, but visual receptors are considered exteroceptors.

A more commonly used classification system subdivides receptors on the basis of the type of stimulus to which they are most sensitive (called the *adequate stimulus*). *Chemoreceptors* include those for smell, taste, and many internal stimuli such as pH and metabolite concentrations. *Photoreceptors* are the visual receptors of the retina. *Thermoreceptors* respond to temperature and its changes. *Mechanoreceptors,* the most varied group, respond to physical deformation. They include cutaneous receptors for touch, receptors that monitor muscle length and tension, auditory and vestibular receptors, and others. Pain receptors are a bit difficult to classify, since the physical mechanism by which they are actually stimulated is not understood. This problem is commonly finessed by classifying them separately as *nociceptors* (from the Latin word *noci* meaning hurt, as in noxious or obnoxious).

### General organization

The basic task of a receptor is to monitor some aspect of its environment by converting and amplifying part of the stimulus energy into an electrical signal that is meaningful to the nervous system. This process is called *trans-*

*duction*. Receptors do this by producing relatively slow potential changes called *receptor potentials* in response to an appropriate stimulus. The magnitude of the receptor potential is related in a systematic way to the magnitude of the stimulus. The duration of the receptor potential is typically the same as that of the stimulus, although in some cases the receptor potential is a transient event at the beginning of the stimulus (and sometimes at the end of the stimulus as well). If a particular receptor (a *short receptor*) contacts the next cell in its neuronal pathway close to the site of transduction, then the receptor potential itself can adequately modulate the receptor's rate of transmitter release and thereby cause either changes in spike frequency or slow potential changes in the second cell (Figure 6-1). However, some receptors *(long receptors)* must convey information over long distances (for example, from a big toe to the spinal cord), and the receptor potential dies out in a relatively short distance. In such cases, most of the receptor, beginning near the site of transduction, is capable of propagating action potentials. The spike frequency is then modulated by the receptor potential (Figure 6-1). Receptor potentials that directly cause changes in spike frequency are also called *generator potentials*. All general receptors of the body are long receptors. Short receptors are found in some special sense organs of the head, such as the eye and ear.

Although their morphology varies widely, all receptors seem to have three general parts: a receptive area, an area rich in mitochondria (near the receptive area), and a synaptic area where the receptor's message is passed toward or into the CNS (Figure 6-2). The receptive area may have specializations suited to the adequate stimulus, as in the

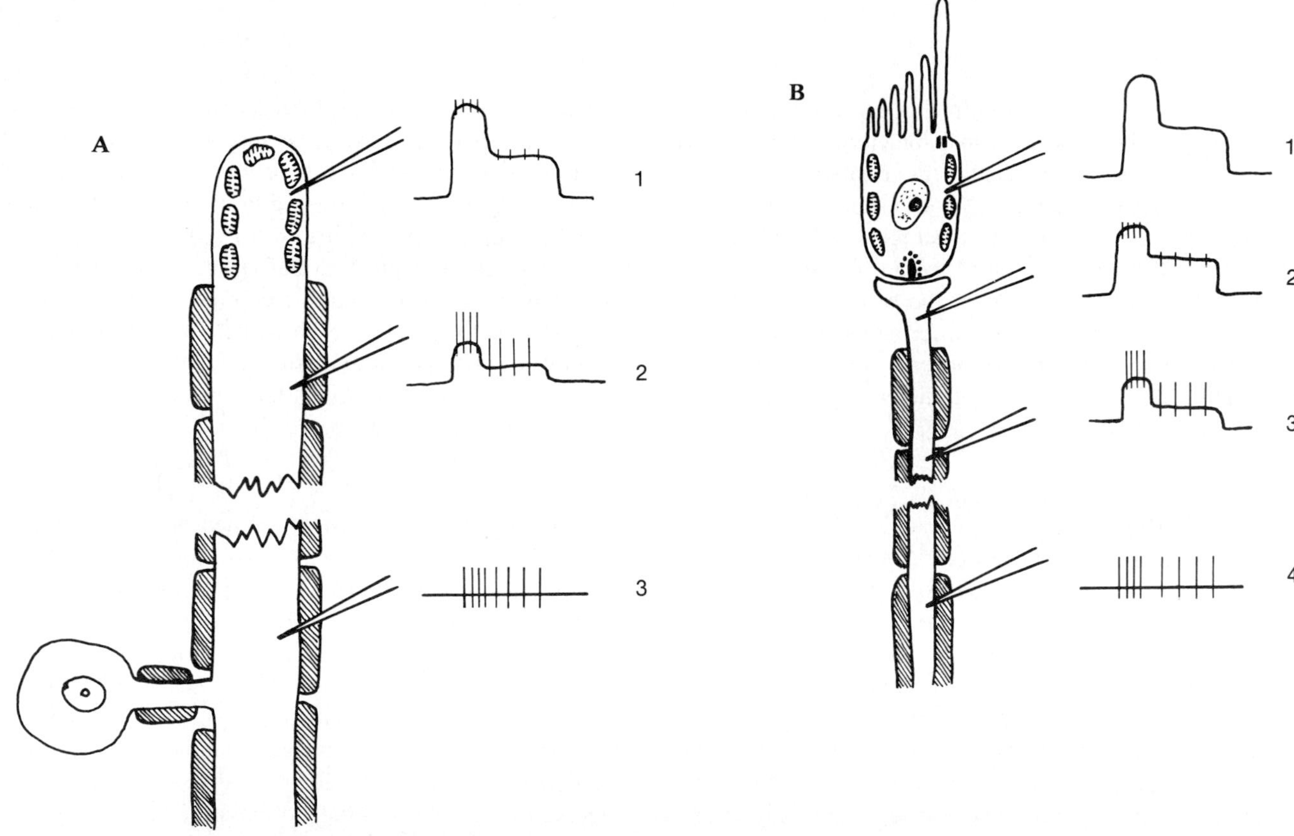


FIGURE 6-1
Organization of long and short receptors. **A,** A long receptor, such as a mechanoreceptor with its cell body in a dorsal root ganglion. Stimulation of the sensory ending causes a generator potential, recorded at *1*, with small passively conducted action potentials superimposed on it. The generator potential decays with distance from the ending *(2)*, until at distances of more than a few millimeters from the ending, it has died out completely *(3)*. Action potentials, however, are conducted without decrement from a point near the ending all the way to the CNS *(2* and *3)*. **B,** A short receptor, such as a hair cell in a semicircular canal. Stimulation of the hair cell causes a receptor potential *(1)*. This in turn causes a postsynaptic potential in an eighth nerve fiber *(2)*. Subsequent events are similar to those in the long receptor: the postsynaptic potential decays, but action potentials are conducted to the CNS *(3* and *4)*.

case of photoreceptors, which have an elaborately folded array of photopigment-bearing membrane; in other cases, there are no obvious specializations in this area. The area rich in mitochondria is either immediately adjacent to the receptive membrane or nearby and is presumed to supply the energy needs of the transduction process. In long receptors, the synaptic area may be far removed from the other two.

All receptors show some *adaptation,* which means they become less sensitive during the course of a maintained stimulus. Those that adapt relatively little are called *slowly adapting* and are suitable receptors for such things as static position. Those that adapt a great deal are called *rapidly adapting* and can only indicate change and movement of stimuli (Figure 6-3). Adaptation is generally a property of one or more parts of the receptor's membrane: a maintained stimulus may cause less and less receptor potential with time, or (in long receptors) a given value of the receptor potential may generate progressively fewer action potentials. In addition, accessory structures such as cellular capsules may modify the physical stimulus before it reaches the sensory ending.

## Cutaneous receptors

The skin and adjacent subcutaneous tissues are richly innervated by a wide variety of sensory endings. These endings may be divided conveniently into *encapsulated* and *nonencapsulated* receptors, depending on whether an accessory structure surrounds the ending. A bewildering variety of encapsulated receptors have been described in the past, and a bewildering variety of mostly eponymous names have been attached to them. These classifications seem to be merely variations on two common themes: receptors with lamellated capsules and receptors with thin capsules. This chapter describes only the best known of these. The function of the capsule is not known for all en-

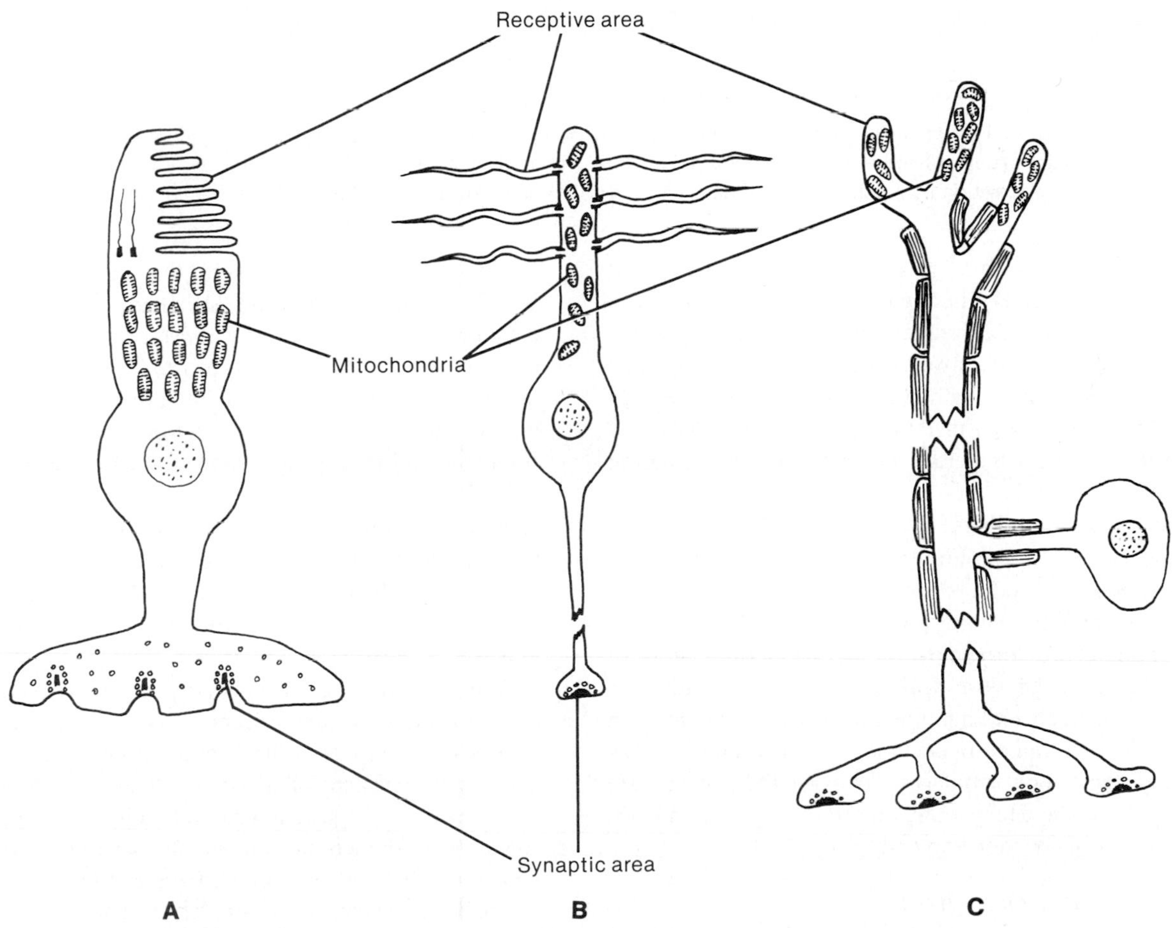


FIGURE 6-2
General features of receptor anatomy. **A,** A retinal cone (photoreceptor). **B,** An olfactory receptor cell (chemoreceptor). **C,** A mechanoreceptor or pain receptor from skin. All have a specialized area for the reception of stimuli, a nearby area rich in mitochondria, and a synaptic area that may be some distance away.

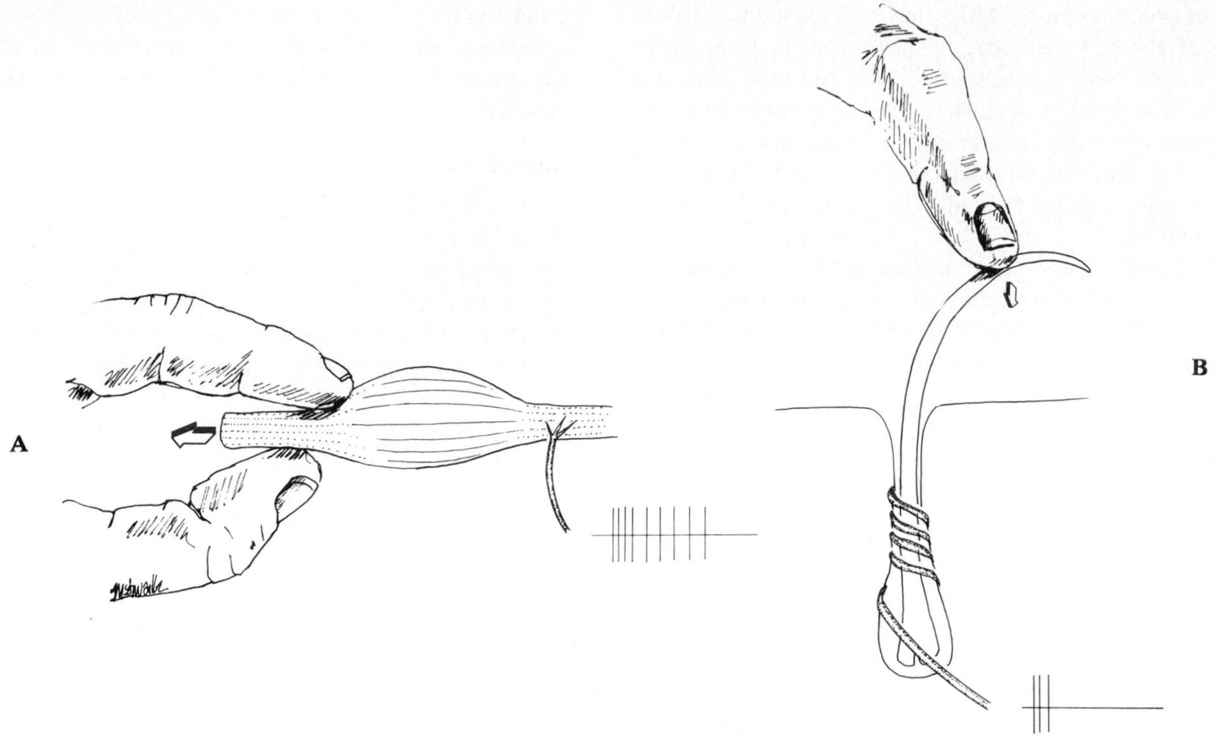


FIGURE 6-3
Slowly adapting versus rapidly adapting receptors. **A,** A tendon receptor (Golgi tendon organ) continues to fire action potentials as long as tension is maintained on the tendon. **B,** Most hair receptors fire a short burst of action potentials and are then silent, even if bending of the hair is maintained.

capsulated receptors, but in at least some instances it serves as a mechanical filter, modifying mechanical stimuli before they reach the sensory ending. For example, receptors with lamellated capsules are rapidly adapting, due in large part to these mechanical properties of the capsules. The capsules also have barrier properties (discussed later in this chapter) that may be important in regulating the composition of the fluid surrounding the sensory endings contained within them.

Unencapsulated receptors may be divided into *free nerve endings* and endings with *accessory structures* that do not surround the ending. Free nerve endings, as the name implies, are formed by branching terminations of sensory fibers in the skin, with no obvious specialization around them. Such endings are not restricted to the skin but are found throughout the body. Even though microscopically they look similar to one another, many are known to be nociceptors, others thermoreceptors, and still others may be mechanoreceptors.

### *Cutaneous mechanoreceptors*

In addition to mechanoreceptive free nerve endings, there are five other prominent types of mechanoreceptors found in the skin and adjacent subcutaneous tissue. Two are nonencapsulated endings with accessory structures, and three are encapsulated.

Endings around hairs vary in their degrees of complexity. Those around the base of a cat's whiskers are very elaborate, but those around most ordinary human body hairs are longitudinal neural processes and spiral endings that wrap around the base of the hair (Figure 6-4). Bending the hair is presumed to deform the sensory ending somehow and lead to the production of a generator potential, although the precise molecular events coupling the stimulus at the receptor membrane to the receptor potential are not known for this or for any other mechanoreceptive ending. Most hair receptors are rapidly adapting; they respond well to something brushing across the skin but not to a steady pressure.*

The second type of nonencapsulated receptor is the *Merkel ending,* which is found in both hairy and glabrous skin (see Figure 6-4). The ending is a disc-shaped expansion of the terminal of a sensory fiber, which is inserted into the base of a specialized cell called a Merkel cell. A single fiber branches to innervate several Merkel cells, which tend to occur in groups. Each Merkel cell is situated in the basal layer of the epidermis and contains dense-

*You can easily demonstrate this to yourself; bend a single hair on the back of your hand (or have someone else do it), then hold it in the bent position. You will feel it bending but will almost immediately lose awareness of its new position.

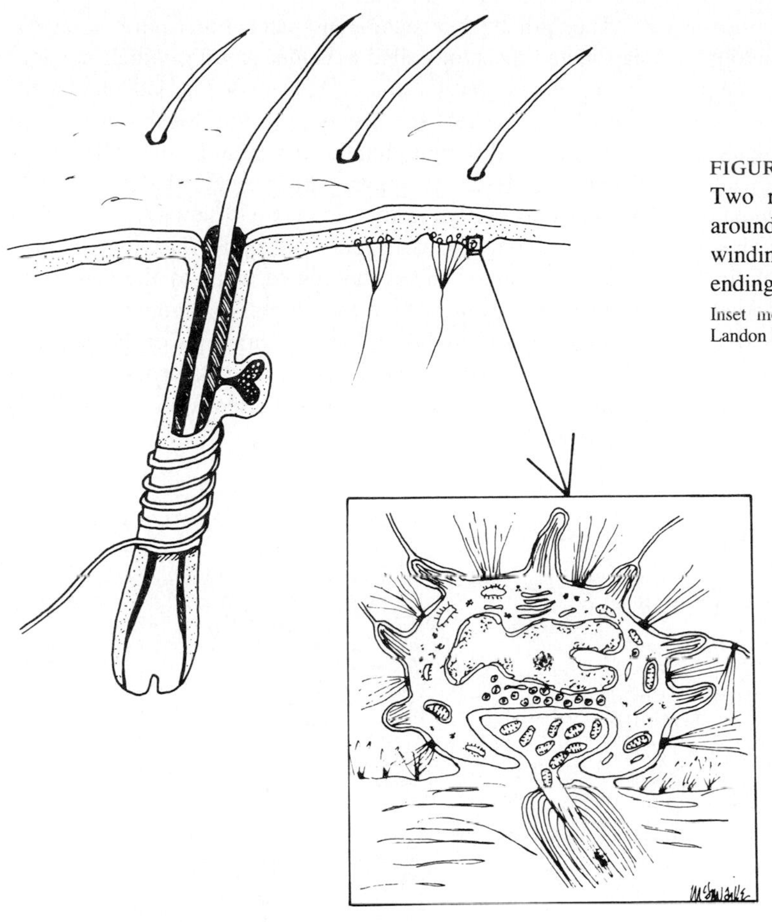

FIGURE 6-4
Two receptor types from hairy skin. Receptor endings wrap around hairs in a wide variety of configurations; a simple helical winding is shown. The inset is an enlarged drawing of a Merkel ending-Merkel cell complex in the basal layer of the epidermis.
Inset modified from Bannister LH: Sensory terminals of peripheral nerves. In Landon DN, editor: The peripheral nerve, London, 1976, Chapman & Hall.

cored vesicles in what looks like a synaptic ending onto the sensory terminal. This apparent synapse led naturally to the hypothesis that the Merkel cell is sensitive to deformation and uses this synapse to pass information about mechanical stimuli along to the nerve ending. However, available evidence suggests that this is not the case and that the nerve ending itself is the mechanoreceptor; the role of the Merkel cell is currently unknown. Recordings from these sensory fibers have shown that Merkel endings are slowly adapting mechanoreceptors.

*Meissner corpuscles* are elongated encapsulated endings in the dermal papillae of hairless skin just beneath the epidermis and are oriented with their long axis perpendicular to the surface of the skin (Figure 6-5). The encapsulation consists of a thin outer capsule and a lamellated stack of epithelial cells within the capsule, each cell oriented perpendicular to the long axis of the capsule. One or more myelinated fibers approach the base of the corpuscle, lose their myelin, and wind back and forth between the stacked cells within the capsule. These are rapidly adapting receptors, and it is assumed that the capsule is important in determining the degree of adaptation. Vertical pressure on a dermal papilla compresses the nerve endings between the stacked capsular cells of a Meissner corpuscle, whereas pressure on a neighboring papilla is not nearly so effective. Meissner corpuscles are quite numerous in the skin of fingertips, and it is thought that they are largely responsible for our ability to perform fine tactile discriminations with our fingertips (Figure 6-6).

*Pacinian corpuscles* are almost as widespread as free nerve endings. They are found subcutaneously over the entire body and in numerous other connective tissue sites. They are wrapped in the ultimate expression of a lamellated capsule and look like an onion in cross section (see Figure 6-5). The capsule consists of many concentric layers of very thin epithelial cells, with fluid spaces between adjacent layers. Pacinian corpuscles are also rapidly adapting, and in this case the role of the capsule is understood. Quickly applied forces are transmitted through the interior of the capsule and reach the ending, but maintained forces are not, as a result of the elastic properties of the capsular lamellae. During maintained pressure, each successive lamella is slightly less deformed than its outer neighbor—imagine indenting the outermost of a series of balloons, one inflated inside another—and the ending itself is not deformed at all. These corpuscles are amazingly sensitive: much like the Merkel endings, they can respond to skin indentations as small as 1 μm.

Because pacinian corpuscles are probably the most rapidly adapting receptors we have, they are poor receptors for pressure but good ones for the rapidly changing mechanical stimulation that we perceive as vibration. That is, a vibratory stimulus causes a steady train of impulses from such an ending, so that in this sense the receptor is "slowly adapting." It is important to understand that slowly adapting receptors, as they are conventionally defined, are simply receptors that respond best to *unchanging* stimuli. Rapidly adapting receptors, on the other hand, respond best to *changing* stimuli, giving a constant output to a stimulus with constant velocity, constant acceleration, or some other temporal property.

The fifth type of cutaneous mechanoreceptor is an encapsulated receptor called a *Ruffini ending,* which is widespread in the dermis and in subcutaneous and other connective tissue sites. It consists of a thin, cigar-shaped capsule traversed longitudinally by strands of collagenous connective tissue. A sensory fiber enters the capsule and branches profusely, so that many small processes are interspersed among the collagenous strands. This is a slowly adapting receptor and is thought to work by the squeezing of sensory terminals between strands of connective tissue when tension is applied to one or both ends of the capsule. Since collagen is not very elastic, the deformation of the endings is maintained as long as the tension is maintained, so adaptation is slow.

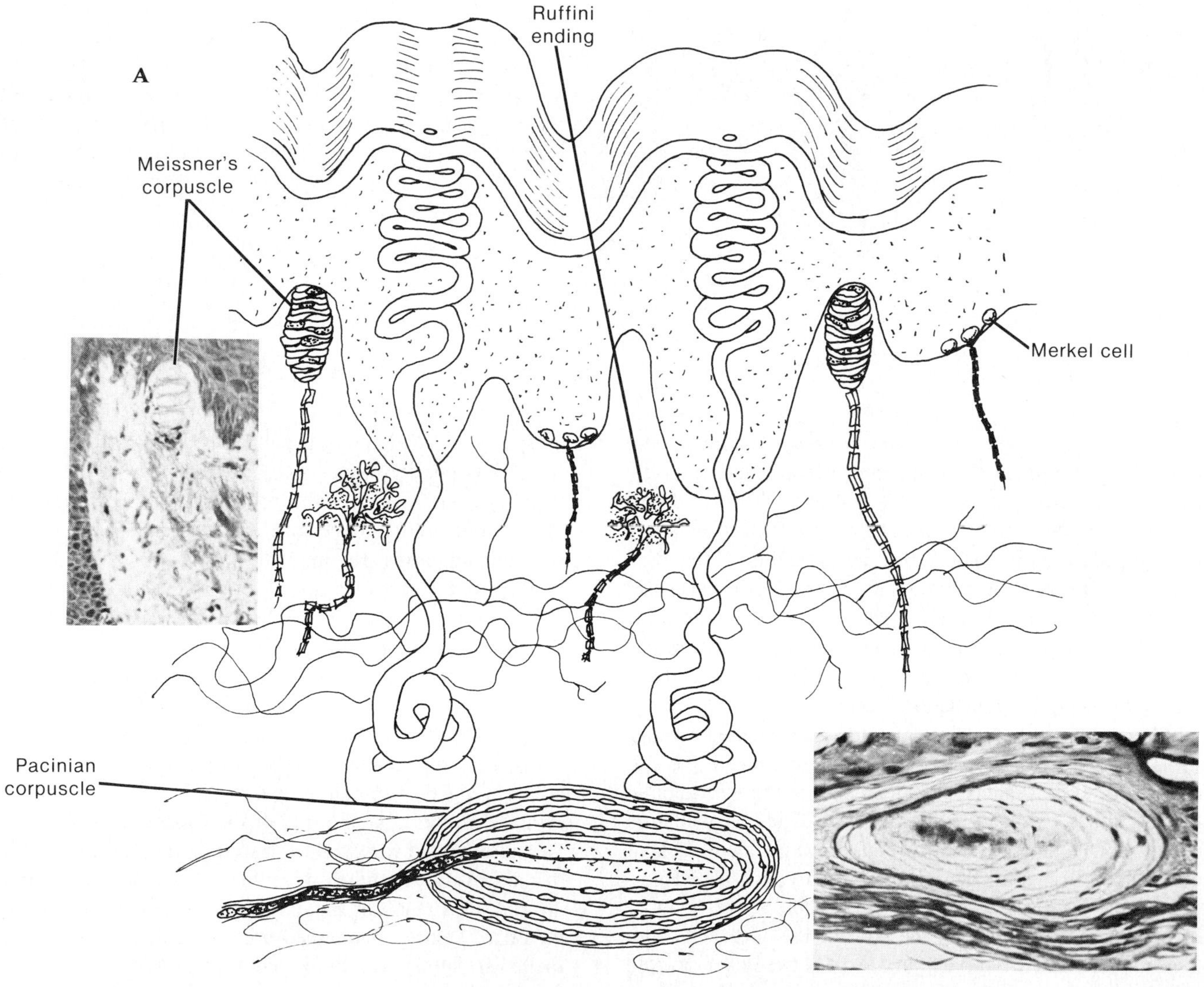


FIGURE 6-5
**A,** Some of the sensory endings found in glabrous skin. The lower inset is a light micrograph of a pacinian corpuscle cut at an oblique angle; the upper inset is a light micrograph of a Meissner corpuscle. Both insets are from monkey skin.
Insets courtesy of Pamela Eller, University of Colorado Health Sciences Center.

### *Other cutaneous receptors*

Thermoreceptors, nociceptors, and some mechanoreceptors are probably all free nerve endings; no pronounced morphological differences are seen among them with presently available techniques. Electrophysiological studies, however, have clearly shown that all exist. Some individual fibers respond selectively to cooling the skin, others to warming it, and still others to stimuli that would be perceived by a conscious animal as touch or as pain. Many of the latter respond not only to damaging mechanical stimuli but also to heat and a variety of chemicals.

### *Patterns of innervation*

The skin is often thought of as a uniform sensory surface varying in hairiness but basically uniform in sensitivity. This is far from true, however; some areas (such as the lips and fingertips) are much more densely innervated than other areas (such as the back). More densely innervated areas can subserve subtler tactile discriminations than can less densely innervated areas because of the close packing of receptors. One way this capability can be measured is in terms of *two-point discrimination,* which refers to the minimum distance by which two stimuli can be separated and still be perceived as two stimuli. This minimum distance is only about 2 mm for the fingertips (see Figure 6-6) but is several centimeters for the back. Corresponding to this two-point discrimination ability is the capacity to localize single stimuli accurately. We can easily detect the movement of a stimulus from one ridge to the next on a fingertip, but we are not nearly so accurate for stimuli delivered to the back of the thigh.

Granted that acuity is better in some areas than in others, many of us still tend to consider the skin a uniform sensory surface, because we think we can detect the occurrence of a stimulus anywhere on it. This too is inaccurate, because receptors are discrete entities whose zones of termination in the skin may not overlap with each other. For example, temperature sensitivity is distributed like polka dots across the skin (more densely in some areas than in others). A fine, cold probe touched to an appropriate spot on the skin elicits a sensation of coolness. The same probe touched to the skin between cold-sensitive spots may elicit only a sensation of touch. Because the skin is more or less densely innervated everywhere, there are probably no places that are insensitive to all stimuli, but a given small location is likely to be most sensitive to a particular *type* of stimulus. In real life, we are usually not stimulated by fine probes, so we are not aware that sensitivity is distributed across the skin in small, selective spots.

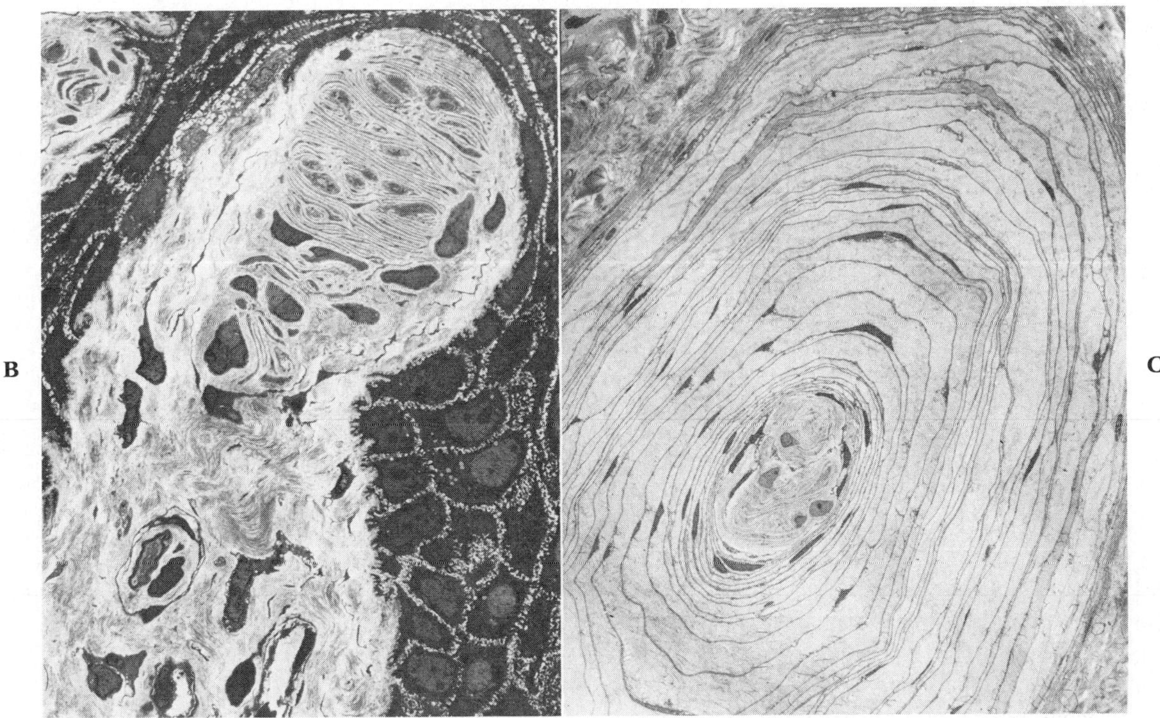


FIGURE 6-5, cont'd
**B** and **C,** Electron micrographs of a Meissner corpuscle and a pacinian corpuscle, respectively. Both are from monkey skin.
Courtesy of Dr. David Moran, University of Colorado Health Sciences Center.

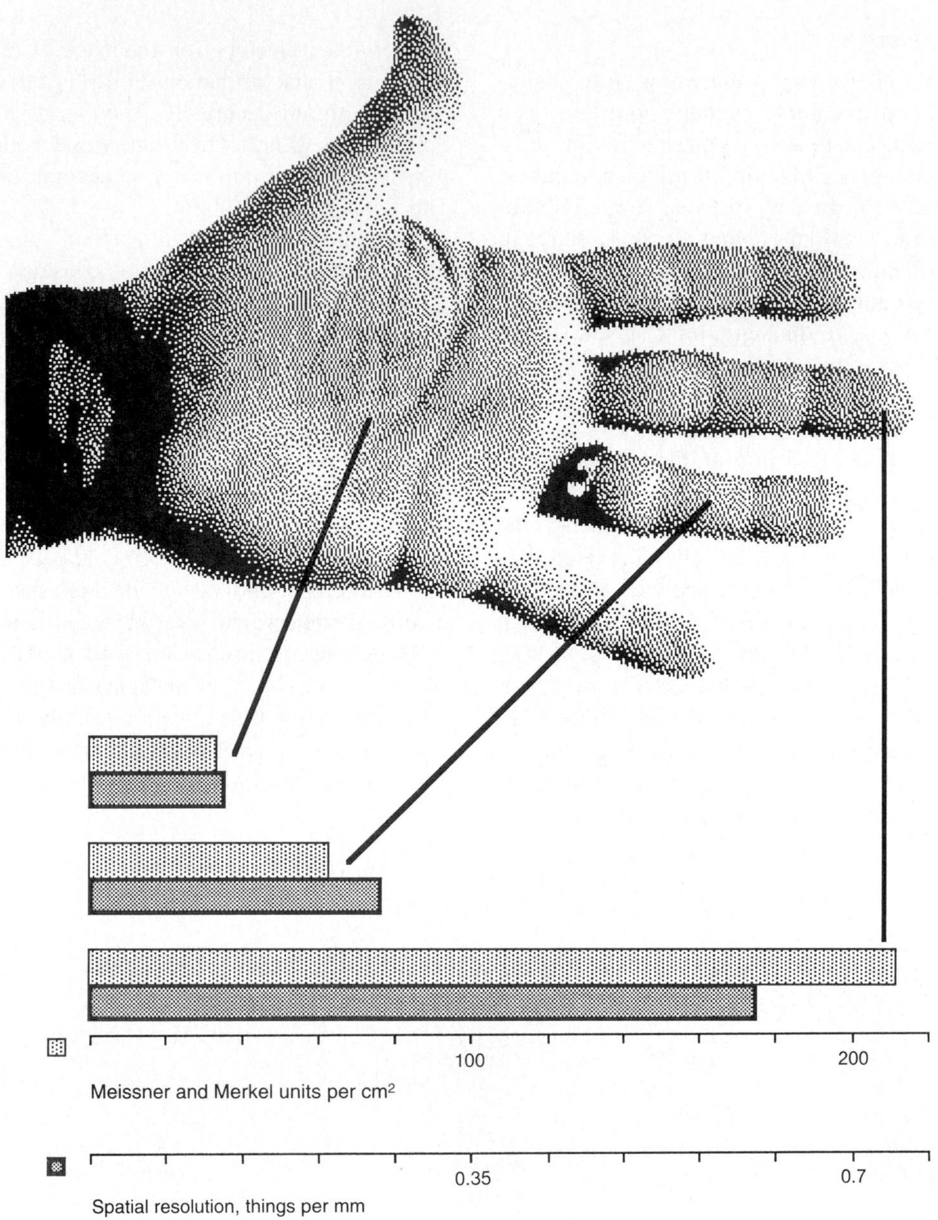


FIGURE 6-6
Correlation of spatial resolution and numbers of cutaneous receptors in different areas of the human hand. Spatial resolution (the reciprocal of the two-point discrimination threshold) was determined in psychophysical experiments, by touching humans with two points and determining the minimum separation needed for them to be recognized as two separate points; this separation is less than 2 mm for fingertips, but more than 8 mm for the palm of the hand. Correspondingly, there are many more Meissner corpuscles and Merkel endings per $cm^2$ in the fingertips than in the palm.
Adapted from an illustration in Vallbo ÅB, Johansson RS: *Human Neurobiol* 3:3, 1984.

## Muscle receptors

Muscle, like other tissues, receives an abundant supply of free nerve endings. The function of these endings is largely unknown, but some are assumed to be involved in muscle pain, while others may be chemoreceptors responsive to changes in extracellular fluid composition during muscle activity.

Muscles are also supplied with two important types of encapsulated receptors: the *muscle spindle,* which is unique to muscle, and the *Golgi tendon organ,* which is similar to a Ruffini ending.

### *Muscle spindles*

Scattered throughout virtually every striated muscle in the body are long, thin, stretch receptors called muscle spindles (Figure 6-7). They are quite simple in principle, consisting of a few small muscle fibers with a capsule surrounding the middle third of the fibers. These fibers are

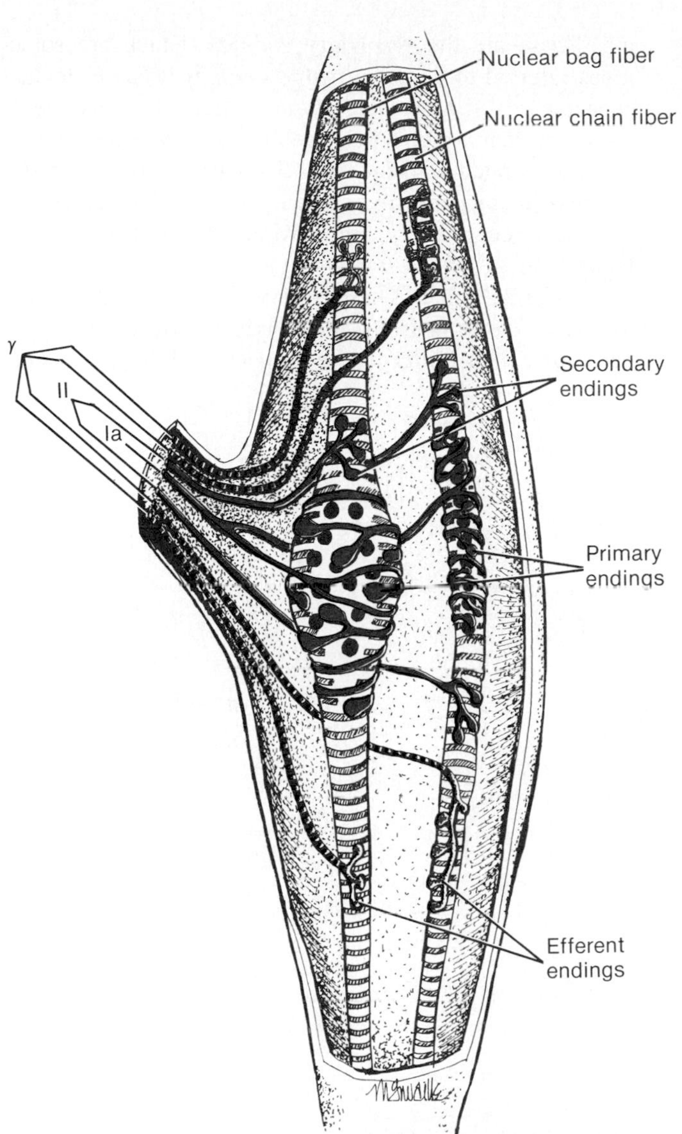


FIGURE 6-7
Simplified diagram of a muscle spindle. A single nuclear bag fiber and a single nuclear chain fiber are shown. A single afferent fiber (group *Ia*) supplies all the intrafusal muscle fibers with primary endings. Several smaller afferents (group *II*) provide secondary endings, mostly to the nuclear chain fibers. Small motor axons (*gamma* motor neurons) of two different types innervate the contractile portions of nuclear bag and nuclear chain fibers. (The Ia-II-gamma terminology is explained later in this chapter.)
Modified from Warwick R, Williams PL, editors: Gray's anatomy, Br. ed 35, Philadelphia, 1975, WB Saunders Co.

called *intrafusal muscle fibers* (from the Latin words *intra,* meaning within, and *fusus,* meaning spindle), in contrast to the ordinary *extrafusal muscle fibers* (from the Latin word *extra,* meaning outside). The ends of the intrafusal fibers are attached to extrafusal fibers, so whenever the muscle is stretched, the intrafusal fibers are also stretched. The central region of each intrafusal fiber has few myofilaments and is noncontractile, but it does have one or more sensory endings applied to it. When the muscle is stretched, the central part of the intrafusal fiber is stretched, and each sensory ending fires impulses.

Numerous specializations occur in this simple basic organization, so that in fact the muscle spindle is one of the most complex receptor organs in the body. Only three of these specializations are described here; their overall effect is to make the muscle spindle adjustable and give it a dual function, part of it being particularly sensitive to the length of the muscle in a static sense and part of it being particularly sensitive to the rate at which this length changes.

1. Intrafusal muscle fibers are of two types. All are multinucleated, and the central, noncontractile region contains the nuclei. In one type of intrafusal fiber, the nuclei are lined up single file; these are called *nuclear chain fibers*. In the other type, the nuclear region is broader, and the nuclei are arranged several abreast; these are called *nuclear bag fibers*. There are typically two or three nuclear bag fibers per spindle and about twice that many chain fibers, but these numbers are variable.

2. There are also two types of sensory endings in the muscle spindle. The first type, called the *primary ending,* is formed by a single very large nerve fiber that enters the capsule and then branches, supplying every intrafusal fiber

in a given spindle (although it innervates* the bag fibers more heavily than the chain fibers). Each branch wraps around the central region of an intrafusal fiber, frequently in a spiral fashion, so these are sometimes called *annulospiral endings*. The second type of ending is formed by a few smaller nerve fibers that branch and primarily innervate nuclear chain fibers on both sides of the primary ending. These are the *secondary endings,* which are sometimes referred to as *flower-spray endings* because of their appearance. Primary endings are selectively sensitive to the onset of muscle stretch but discharge at a slower rate while the stretch is maintained. Secondary endings are less sensitive to the onset of stretch, but their discharge rate does not decline very much while the stretch is maintained.

3. Muscle spindles also receive a motor innervation. The large motor neurons that supply extrafusal muscle fibers are called *alpha motor neurons,* while the smaller

*The word *innervate* means "to supply with nerve endings." The nerve endings can be sensory, as in the case of these stretch-sensitive endings, or motor, as in the endings made by motor neurons on muscle fibers.

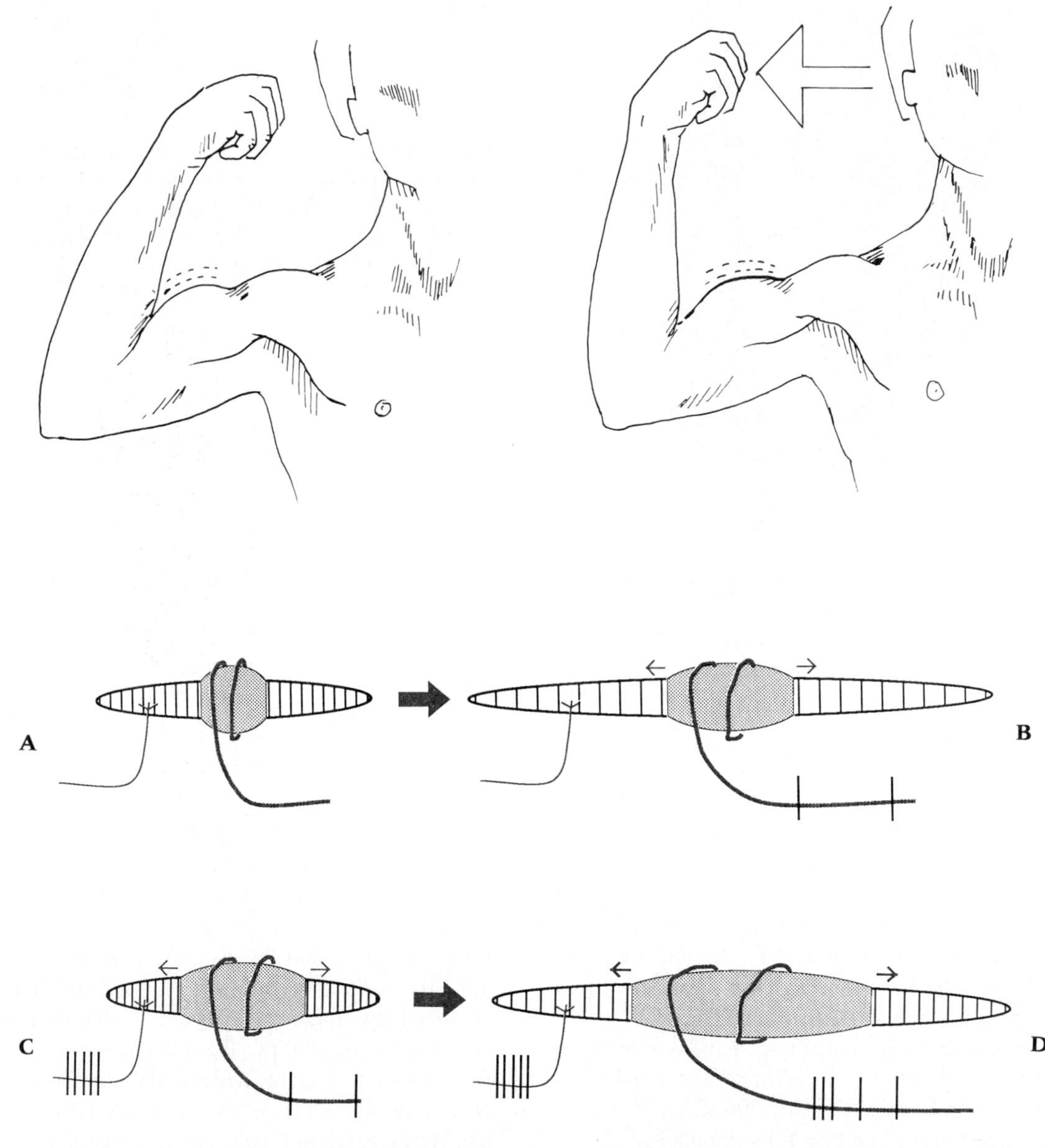


FIGURE 6-8
Mechanism of action of gamma motor neurons. **A,** Muscle spindles in a contracted muscle (in this case the biceps) are unstretched and thus electrically silent. As a result, slight extension of the muscle causes few action potentials **(B).** However, activity of gamma motor neurons "prestretches" the central receptive region of the muscle spindle, causing a few action potentials when the biceps is contracted **(C)** and many more when it is slightly extended **(D).**

ones supplying the contractile portions of intrafusal fibers are called *gamma motor neurons* (or *fusimotor neurons*). Intrafusal fibers are too small and too few to contribute to the strength of a muscle, and firing all the gamma motor neurons to a muscle does not generate significant tension. The function of this motor innervation is discussed in conjunction with motor control systems (Chapter 12), but a simple example can indicate one of the possibilities (Figure 6-8). Consider a muscle spindle in the biceps, and suppose that this muscle is contracted. This will relieve most or all of the tension on the nuclear region of the intrafusal fibers, so the sensory endings will be quite insensitive to muscle stretch that starts from this contracted state. Suppose that, at the same time, the gamma motor neurons to that spindle fire. This will cause the parts of each intrafusal fiber on both sides of the nuclear region to contract. This in turn will generate some tension on the nuclear region and restore its sensitivity. Thus gamma motor neurons can regulate the sensitivity of a muscle spindle so that this sensitivity can be maintained at any given muscle length. Not surprisingly, there are two types of gamma motor neurons, one of which preferentially ends on bag fibers, the other on chain fibers.

This is just one example of feedback control by the nervous system over its sensory pathways. Such control is very common; sometimes it occurs at the level of the receptor (as in this instance), and sometimes it occurs at relay nuclei, but it seems to occur at one or more locations in every sensory pathway.

### *Golgi tendon organs*

Spindle-shaped receptors called Golgi tendon organs are found at the junctions between muscles and tendons. They are similar to Ruffini endings in their basic organization, consisting of interwoven collagen bundles surrounded by a thin capsule (Figure 6-9). A large sensory fiber enters the capsule and branches into fine processes that are inserted among the collagen bundles. It is thought that tension on the capsule along its long axis squeezes these fine processes, and the resulting distortion stimulates them. As in the case of Ruffini endings, these are slowly adapting receptors, since the collagen is nonelastic and the squeezing action is maintained as long as the tension is maintained.

For many years, Golgi tendon organs were studied physiologically by pulling on a tendon while recording from the sensory axon. When they are stimulated in this way, considerable tension must be applied to the tendon before a response is obtained, and so it was thought that these were high-threshold receptors designed to inform the nervous system when muscle tension was reaching dangerous levels. However, the amount of tension actually applied to a tendon organ by such a stimulus is quite small: the muscle acts rather like a rubber band attached to a piece of string, and most of the tension is absorbed by the muscle. However, if tension is generated in a tendon by making its attached muscle contract, the tendon organ is found to be much more sensitive and can actually respond to the contraction of just a few muscle fibers. Thus the Golgi tendon organ very specifically monitors the tension generated by muscle contraction; it is currently considered to play an active role in the process by which the nervous system controls motor activity.

Thus the mode of action of the Golgi tendon organ is quite different from that of the muscle spindle. If a muscle contracts isometrically, tension will be generated across its

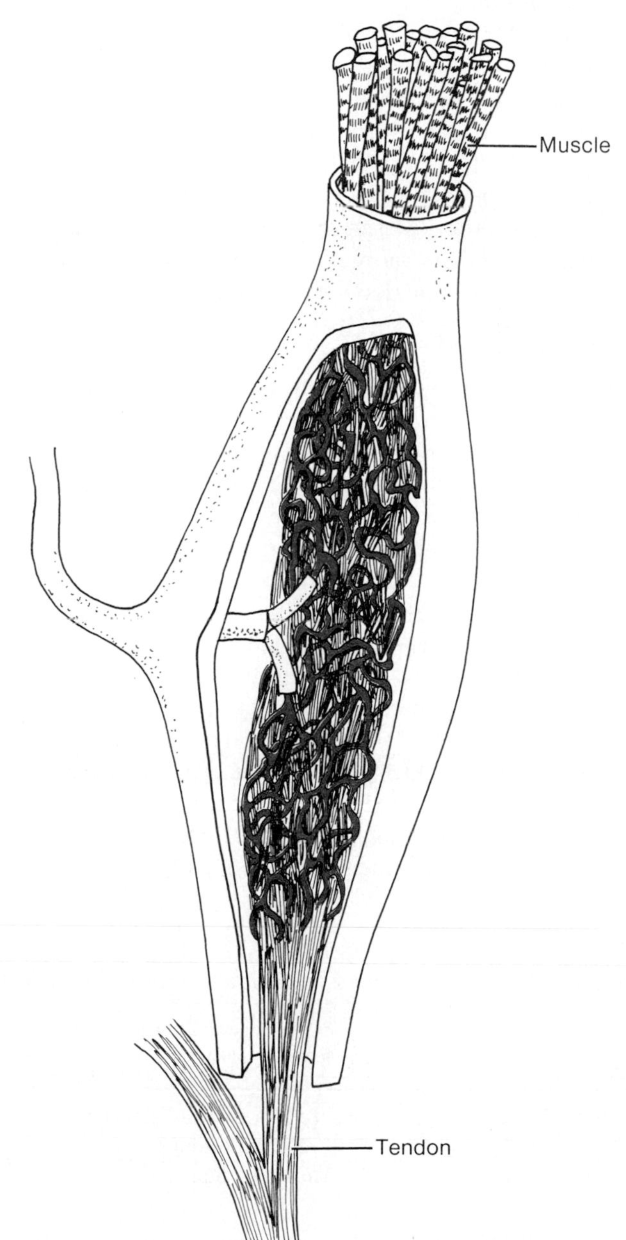


FIGURE 6-9
Golgi tendon organ. A large afferent fiber enters a capsule around part of the myotendinous junction and then breaks up into many branches that interweave with bundles of collagen.

tendons, and the tendon organs will signal this; however, the muscle spindles will signal nothing since muscle length has not changed (assuming that the activity of the gamma motor neurons remains unchanged). On the other hand, a relaxed muscle can be stretched easily, and the muscle spindles will fire; the tendon organs, in contrast, will experience little tension and will remain silent. A muscle, by virtue of these two types of receptors, can simultaneously monitor its own length and tension.

### Other receptors

#### *Joint receptors*

The receptors found in joints and their capsules are similar to some of those found in skin and muscle. In addition to the usual free nerve endings, there are endings equivalent to Golgi tendon organs in the ligaments and Ruffini endings and a few pacinian corpuscles in joint capsules (Table 2). As might be expected from their morphology, a few joint receptors (presumably the pacinian corpuscles) are rapidly adapting, but most are slowly adapting and respond to joint position and movement.

#### *Visceral receptors*

Much less is known about visceral receptors than about the other types discussed in this chapter; they have been studied mostly in terms of their physiology and their reflex effects. They tend to be supplied by thinly myelinated and unmyelinated fibers that terminate as free nerve endings, sometimes with complex branching patterns. Functionally, most of these receptors act at a subconscious level through visceral reflexes. They include (1) mechanoreceptors in the walls of hollow organs (such as the endings in the aortic arch and carotid sinus, which, when stimulated by increased arterial pressure, reflexly cause vasodilation and decreased heart rate), (2) chemoreceptors (such as those of the carotid body, which, when stimulated by changes in blood gases or pH, reflexly cause compensating cardiovascular and respiratory changes), and (3) nociceptors (which can cause severe pain when stimulated, as by distention of an organ or its capsule). In some instances a single visceral receptor may be able to serve as a mechanoreceptor at low discharge frequencies and a nociceptor at higher frequencies.

## PERIPHERAL NERVES

The nerve fibers innervating the receptors described thus far have their cell bodies in dorsal root ganglia adjacent to the spinal cord or, in the case of those serving the head, in various cranial nerve ganglia near the brainstem. The central process of each of these ganglion cells enters the CNS. Each peripheral process joins motor axons emerging from the spinal cord (or brainstem) to form spinal nerves (or cranial nerves). The formal boundary between the central and peripheral nervous systems occurs between the sensory ganglia and the spinal cord/brainstem, at the point where the myelinating cells change from oligodendrocytes to Schwann cells. However, it is more convenient in the present discussion to consider only those portions peripheral to the sensory ganglia (that is, the wrappings and contents of spinal and cranial nerves). Aspects of the sensory ganglia and of the sensory and motor roots of the spinal and cranial nerves are discussed in subsequent chapters.

### Wrappings

Peripheral nerves have three connective tissue coverings, each with a different function. From the outside layer in, these are the *epineurium,* the *perineurium,* and the *endoneurium* (Figure 6-10).

The epineurium is a loose connective tissue sheath surrounding each peripheral nerve. Composed mainly of collagen and fibroblasts, it forms a substantial covering over nerve trunks, then thins to an incomplete layer around smaller branches near their terminations. The abundant longitudinally and spirally arranged collagen fibers of the epineurium are largely responsible for the considerable tensile strength of peripheral nerves. The epineurium is continuous centrally with the dura. Peripherally, it usually

**TABLE 2** *Principal types of somatic receptors found in various tissues**

| | *Free nerve endings with accessory structures* | *Receptors with lamellated capsules* | *Receptors with thin capsules* |
|---|---|---|---|
| Hairy skin | Endings around hairs (R); Merkel endings | Pacinian corpuscles (R) | Ruffini endings |
| Glabrous skin | Merkel endings | Pacinian corpuscles (R)<br>Meissner corpuscles (R) | Ruffini endings |
| Muscle/tendon | | | Muscle spindles; Golgi tendon organs |
| Joints | | Pacinian corpuscles | Ruffini endings; Golgi endings |

*Free nerve endings are not included, since they are ubiquitous. *(R)* indicates that the receptor adapts rapidly to a maintained stimulus.

A

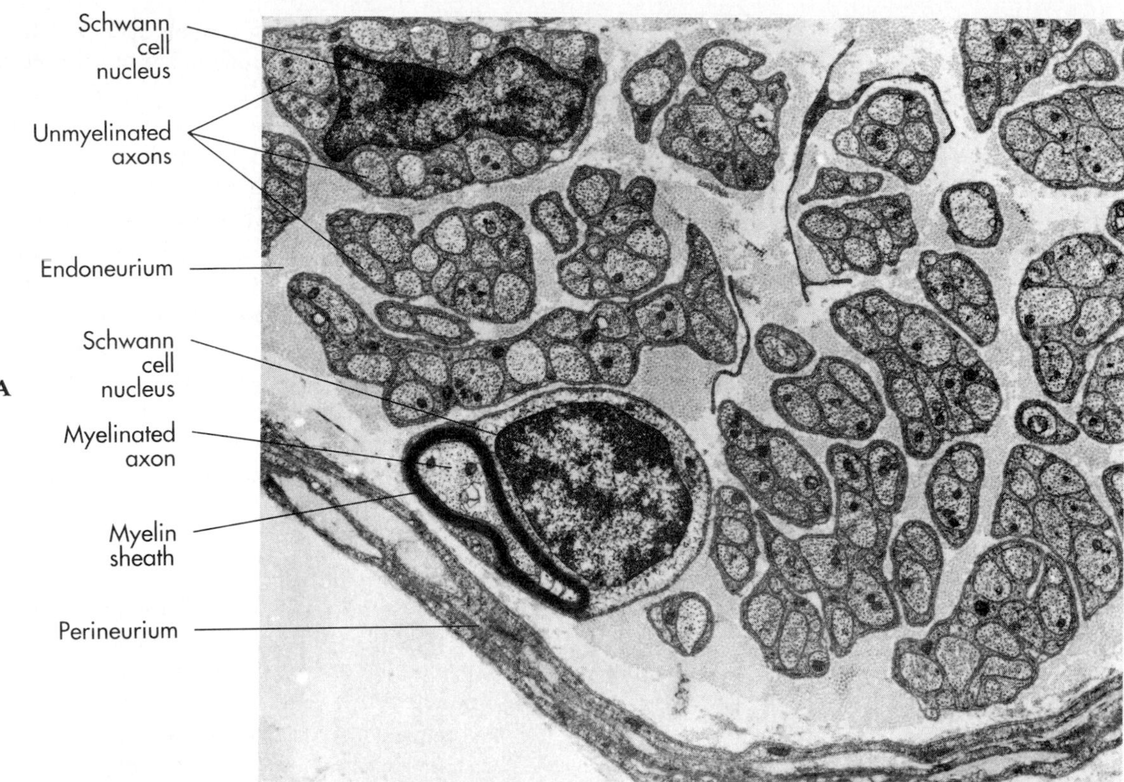


B

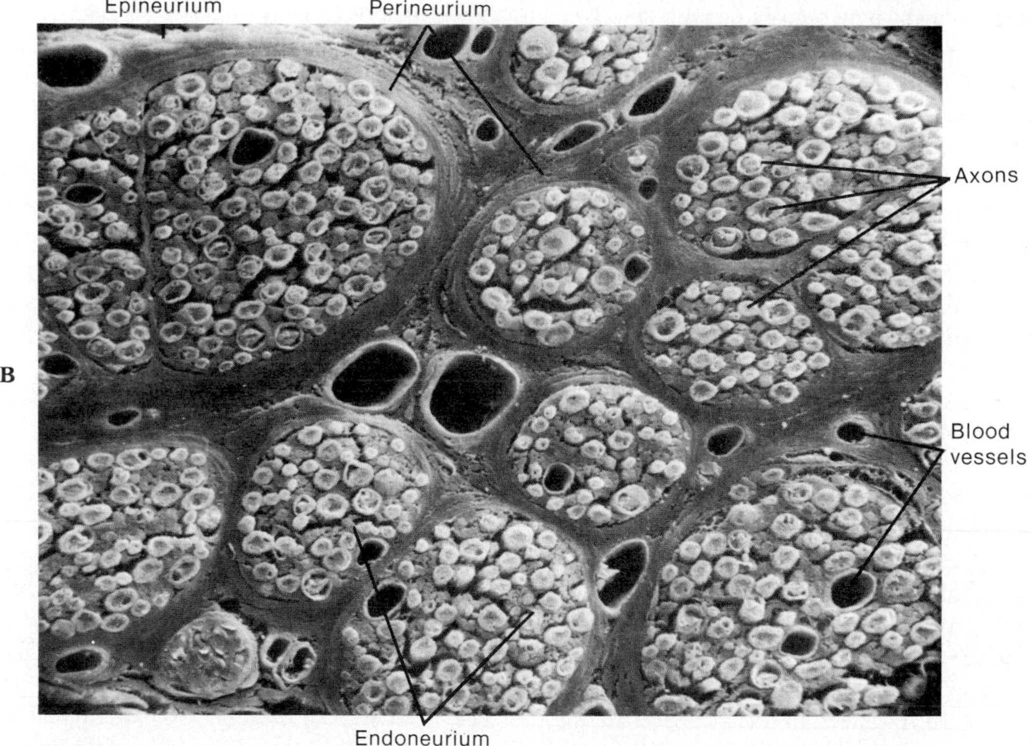


FIGURE 6-10

**A,** Electron micrograph of part of a small, cross-sectioned peripheral nerve of a squirrel monkey. Myelinated and unmyelinated axons, endoneurium and perineurium can be seen, but this nerve was sufficiently small that the epineurium is not evident. (From Moran DT, Rowley, JC III: *Visual Histology,* Philadelphia, 1988, Lea & Febiger. Courtesy of Dr. David Moran, University of Colorado Health Sciences Center.) **B,** Scanning electron micrograph of a freeze-fractured preparation of peripheral nerve.

**B** from Tissues and organs: a text-atlas of scanning electron microscopy by Richard G. Kessel and Randy H. Kardon. W.H. Freeman and Company. Copyright © 1979.

ends near the termination of a nerve fiber, but it may continue as the capsule of Meissner corpuscles and a few other encapsulated endings.

The perineurium, lying within the epineurium, is a layer of thin, concentrically arranged cells with interspersed collagen. Adjacent perineurial cells are connected to one another by tight junctions that effectively isolate the epineurial spaces from the endoneurial spaces around peripheral nerve fibers. In addition, the endothelial cells of capillaries within the perineurium are connected to one another by tight junctions. Thus functional equivalents of the arachnoid barrier and the blood-brain barrier persist in the peripheral nervous system as a *blood-nerve barrier*. The perineurium continues as the capsule of some endings, such as pacinian corpuscles, muscle spindles, and Golgi tendon organs. However, at other places, such as near neuromuscular junctions, the perineurium is open-ended, allowing the endoneurial space around nerve fibers to communicate with the general extracellular space of the body. This may be of clinical importance, since certain toxins and viruses may gain access to the nervous system at these sites.

The endoneurium is the loose connective tissue within the perineurium that continues into nerve fascicles and surrounds individual fibers. In at least some species, these individual endoneurial sheaths are compact enough that they may help to direct the regrowth of nerve fibers after injury.

### Contents

Peripheral nerve fibers come in a wide range of diameters; some are myelinated, others are not. There is some correlation between the size of a fiber and its function, so it has proven useful to subdivide them. Unfortunately, there are two major classification systems, and neither is used universally for all fibers.

The first system is based on conduction velocity. Larger fibers conduct action potentials faster than do smaller fibers. If the compound action potential of a peripheral nerve is recorded at some distance from the site at which the nerve was stimulated electrically, the fast impulses will reach the recording electrode before the slower ones. Conduction velocities (and axonal diameters) are not distributed in a bell-shaped curve but rather in a curve with several peaks. Therefore the remotely recorded compound action potential will have several peaks corresponding to these favored conduction velocities. Three deflections can be easily demonstrated; they are named *A, B,* and *C*. The fibers responsible for the A deflection (the A fibers) are the myelinated sensory and motor fibers. B fibers are myelinated visceral fibers, both preganglionic autonomic fibers and some visceral afferents. C fibers are unmyelinated. The A deflection is complex and was subdivided into $\alpha$, $\beta$, $\gamma$, and $\delta$ peaks ($\alpha$ being the fastest). Although the $\beta$ and $\gamma$ peaks as originally described were probably recording artifacts, the terminology has become established in the literature and is still commonly used. Thus $A\alpha$ fibers are the largest and most rapidly conducting myelinated fibers, and $A\delta$ are the smallest and slowest of the A group.

The second classification system is based on direct microscopic measurement of axonal diameters. In this system myelinated fibers are placed into group *I, II,* or *III* in order of decreasing size. Unmyelinated fibers are group *IV*.

Portions of both systems are commonly used. In general the letter system is used for myelinated efferent fibers and the roman numeral system for myelinated afferents. Unmyelinated fibers are usually referred to as C fibers but may be called group IV. The sizes, conduction velocities, and functional correlates involved in both systems are listed in Table 3 for reference purposes.

The commonly used terminology for efferent fibers is fairly simple. The large axons innervating the extrafusal fibers of skeletal muscle are in the $A\alpha$ category, and the smaller axons innervating intrafusal muscle fibers are in the $A\gamma$ category. The "A" is commonly dropped, and these are simply called $\alpha$ and $\gamma$ motor neurons. Preganglionic autonomic axons are usually called just that but may also be referred to as B fibers.

Myelinated afferents are slightly more complicated. The largest fibers, group I, are found only in muscle nerves; some form the primary endings of muscle spindles and others innervate Golgi tendon organs. To distinguish between them, spindle primary fibers are called *Ia* and tendon organ fibers are called *Ib*. Group II, corresponding to $A\beta$ fibers, is quite diverse and includes the fibers that form the secondary endings of muscle spindles and those that form all the encapsulated receptors of skin and joints. Group III consists of small myelinated afferents that form free nerve endings and includes mechanoreceptors, cold-sensitive thermoreceptors, and some nociceptors. Group III corresponds to $A\delta$, and so these fibers are sometimes referred to as $\delta$ fibers.

## SOME FUNCTIONAL ASPECTS OF THE PERIPHERAL NERVOUS SYSTEM

### Receptors and sensation

Since we have a variety of morphologically distinct types of receptors, it was widely assumed in the past that different types are uniquely responsible for particular sensations. Certainly, the photoreceptor cells of the retina and the hair cells of the cochlea unequivocally form the basis of vision and hearing. This kind of association is true in a very general way for somatic sensation, which has perhaps been shown most elegantly in experiments on human volunteers. Using a technique called *microneurography*, it is possible to insert fine electrodes into human peripheral nerves and stimulate or record from single axons. By recording from single nerve fibers innervating Meissner corpuscles of the fingertip, it has been found that a tiny mechanical indentation of a few micrometers, just enough to cause a single action potential in one nerve fiber, can give

**TABLE 3** *Classification of peripheral nerve fibers*

| *Roman numeral classification* | *Diameter* | *Letter classification* | *Conduction velocity* | *Myelinated* | *Types of structures innervated* |
|---|---|---|---|---|---|
| Ia | 12-20 μm | — | 70-120 m/sec | Yes | Muscle spindle primary endings |
| Ib | 12-20 μm | — | 70-120 m/sec | Yes | Golgi tendon organs |
| — | 12-20 μm | α | 70-120 m/sec | Yes | Efferents to extrafusal muscle fibers |
| II | 6-12 + μm | Aβ* | 30-70 m/sec | Yes | Other encapsulated endings and endings with accessory structures: Meissner corpuscles, Merkel endings, muscle spindle secondary endings, etc. |
| — | 2-10 μm | γ | 10-50 m/sec | Yes | Efferents to intrafusal muscle fibers |
| III | 1-6 μm | Aδ | 5-30 m/sec | Yes | Some nociceptors (sharp pain)<br>Cold receptors<br>Most hair receptors<br>Some visceral receptors |
| — | <3 μm | B | 3-15 m/sec | Yes | Preganglionic autonomic efferents |
| IV | <1.5 μm | C | 0.5-2 m/sec | No | Most nociceptors (dull, aching pain)<br>Some visceral receptors<br>Warmth receptors<br>Few mechanoreceptors<br>Postganglionic autonomic efferents |

*Some afferents in nonmuscle nerves, particularly joint afferents, range up to 17 μm in diameter. Some investigators refer to these larger fibers, in the 12-17 μm range, as Aα and call those in the 6-12 μm range Aβ. Others refer to all nonmuscle afferents larger than 6 μm as Aβ.

rise to perception of the touch. Conversely, stimulation of a fiber electrically, without touching the fingertip, also gives rise to the perception of touch. Since Meissner corpuscles are rapidly adapting, a continuous train of impulses would be expected to signify repeated touches—and subjects do in fact report a sensation of repeated, gentle tapping. In contrast, stimulation of a fiber associated with a slowly adapting Merkel ending gives rise to a sensation of maintained pressure. A train of impulses in the axon from a pacinian corpuscle, which is very rapidly adapting, is interpreted as vibration.

However, thinking of somatic sensation in terms of a unique, one-to-one pairing of specific receptor types and specific sensations is an oversimplification. First, there are counterexamples in which a single receptor type signals different types of stimulation, depending on the location of the receptor. For example, Ruffini endings in the skin are activated by touch, but morphologically similar receptors in joint capsules are activated by changes in limb position. Another example involves free endings. As noted previously, some of these respond best to temperature changes, others to mechanical stimuli, and still others to intense, tissue-damaging stimuli. Second, few situations dealing with mechanical stimuli such as touch and movement involve only one receptor type. The experiments just cited were performed under carefully controlled laboratory conditions, and it seems likely that under ordinary circumstances the overall pattern of activity in an array of receptors is important in determining the resulting sensation. Here again, Ruffini endings provide an instructive example. While touching the skin overlying a Ruffini ending causes its axon to discharge, stimulating the same axon selectively in microneurography experiments causes no sensation at all. Presumably, since any naturally occurring touch stimulates many afferents in addition to the Ruffini ending, the CNS is unable to interpret isolated activity in the latter. Similarly, causing unmyelinated nociceptors to fire in response to chemical irritants produces a sensation of pain; causing the same firing rate with mechanical stimuli (and simultaneously exciting myelinated mechanoreceptor fibers) may produce only a sensation of firm pressure. The central nervous system thus seems to survey all the information coming in from a given area of the body before deciding about the nature of a stimulus.

## Pain

Some free nerve endings have axons classified as group III and others as C fibers. Each of these groups of free nerve endings includes some nociceptors. Corresponding to this, pain is perceived in two different stages. If a painful stimulus is applied abruptly, there is an initial sensation of sharp, pricking, well-localized pain. This is followed by an aching, longer-lasting pain. The initial sharp pain is carried by the more rapidly conducting group III fibers, and since group III is the same as Aδ, it is sometimes referred to as *delta pain*. The aching pain that follows is carried by the more slowly conducting C fibers. This has been verified experimentally on human volunteers, since it is possible to block different classes of nerve fibers selectively. Local anesthetics applied to peripheral nerves block C fibers before myelinated fibers; during the period when only C fibers are blocked, a pinprick is felt only as a sharp, brief pain. Externally applied pressure, however, blocks axons in order of size, so that myelinated fibers can be blocked while C fibers continue to conduct. In this situation, most forms of tactile sensation disappear, and a pinprick is felt only as a dull, aching pain that is even more unpleasant than usual.

The two forms of pain are processed differently within the CNS, so they may be dissociated at sites other than peripheral nerves. This can be of major clinical importance and is discussed further in subsequent chapters.

## Muscle receptors

The identity of the receptors involved in position sense and kinesthesia (conscious awareness of movement) has long been a topic of debate. It was generally assumed in the past that joint receptors are primarily responsible, and that the output of muscle spindles and Golgi tendon organs does not reach consciousness, being utilized in subconscious motor feedback circuits and in reflexes.

This never fit very well with the observation that individuals who have had joint-replacement surgery retain position sense at that joint despite the loss of receptors. This, together with recent experimental work, has led to a reversal in thinking about proprioception; it is currently felt that muscle receptors play a major role, and that joint and cutaneous receptors are of limited importance. If a local anesthetic is injected into the knee joint capsule of a human volunteer or into the skin of the knee, there is no loss of position sense or kinesthesia. However, if tendons of human volunteers are vibrated (through the skin), illusions of movement and altered perceptions of position are experienced at the joints where the muscles of these tendons act. A vibrating stimulus of moderate intensity should be ineffective at activating Golgi tendon organs, but it should activate muscle spindles. In particular, it should excite the primary endings, since these are especially sensitive to changing stimuli. Hence, it is thought that the muscle spindles but not the tendon organs are involved in these illusions and in our sense of limb position and movement. However, the tendon organs may contribute to our sense of the force exerted during a movement.

## Clinical correlations

*Causalgia* sometimes follows injury (such as a partial transection) to a peripheral nerve. The patient has episodes of severe burning pain in the area of distribution of the affected nerve. The pain may be triggered by normally trivial stimuli, such as the mere pressure of clothing, or by emotional states. The exact mechanism of causalgia is not known, but it is usually associated with autonomic disturbances in the affected area and is typically relieved by sympathetic blockade. This has led to the conjecture that efferent sympathetic activity somehow stimulates C fibers at the site of injury, and the subsequent activity is then perceived as pain. A complementary explanation relies on the phenomenon, noted previously, that activity restricted to C fibers (during blockade of the myelinated fibers) causes particularly intense pain. This led some investigators to reason that if myelinated fibers were selectively stimulated in patients with causalgia, then the normal "balance" of activity between large and small fibers would be restored, and the pain would be relieved. Amazingly enough, this works in many patients. Small electrodes placed on the skin over the affected nerve (proximal to the lesion), if adjusted to stimulate only myelinated fibers, can provide dramatic relief from pain. The relief can outlast the electrical stimulus by minutes or even hours.

Most people think that freedom from pain would be a terrific condition. However, pain has a useful function, which is to warn us of damage; its absence is actually a handicap. Some rare individuals are born without the capability to feel pain. They characteristically have many injuries that heal poorly or remain unhealed. They may fracture bones without ever realizing it, have mutilated fingers and toes, or incur serious burns. The deficit may involve only the sensation of pain, but sometimes other forms of sensation are involved as well. The condition takes several different forms. Some patients have a selective loss of C fibers in their peripheral nerves; others have apparently normal nerves, so in these cases the disorder is probably within the CNS.

## ADDITIONAL READINGS


Andres KH, Düring MV: *Morphology of cutaneous receptors.* In Iggo A, editor: *Handbook of sensory physiology.* Vol. II, *Somatosensory system,* New York, 1973, Springer-Verlag.

Bannister LH: *Sensory terminals of peripheral nerves.* In Landon DN, editor: *The peripheral nerve,* London, 1976, Chapman & Hall. *A well-written overview of the anatomy and physiology of somatic, olfactory, and gustatory receptors.*

Burgess PR et al: Signaling of kinesthetic information by peripheral sensory receptors, *Ann Rev Neurosci* 5:171, 1982.

Burkel WE: The histological fine structure of perineurium, *Anat Rec* 158:177, 1967.

Chambers MR et al: The structure and function of the slowly adapting type II mechanoreceptor in hairy skin, *A J Exp Physiol* 57:417, 1972. *The anatomy and physiology of the Ruffini ending of the cat.*

Craske B: Perception of impossible limb position induced by tendon vibration, *Science* 196:71, 1977.

Dow RR, Shinn SL, Ovalle WK, Jr: Ultrastructural study of a blood-muscle spindle barrier after systematic administration of horseradish peroxidase, *Am J Anat* 157:375, 1980.

Dyson C, Brindley GS: Strength-duration curves for the production of cutaneous pain by electrical stimuli, *Clin Sci* 30:237, 1966. *Direct production of both sharp, pricking pain and slow, burning pain by small electrical stimuli.*

Gandevia SC, McCloskey DI: Joint sense, muscle sense, and their combination as position sense, measured at the distal interphalangeal joint of the middle finger, *J Physiol* 260:387, 1976. *Clever experiments taking advantage of an anatomical quirk of the middle finger. This finger can be positioned in such a way that muscles and their receptors are functionally disengaged from its terminal phalanx, so the position sense of the distal interphalangeal joint can be measured both with and without a contribution from muscle receptors.*

Gandevia SC, McCloskey DI, Burke D, Kinaesthetic signals and muscle contraction, *Trends Neurosci* 15:62, 1992. *Our sense of position and movement is more acute during active than during passive movements, providing more evidence for a role of muscle afferents.*

Ghabriel MN, Jennings KH, Allt G: Diffusion barrier properties of the perineurium: an in vivo ionic lanthanum tracer study, *Anat Embryol* 180:237, 1989.

Goodwin GM, McCloskey DI, Matthews PBC: The contribution of muscle afferents to kinaesthesia shown by vibration induced illusions of movement and by the effects of paralysing joint afferents, *Brain* 95:705, 1972. *This paper sparked the recent reinvestigation of the role of muscle spindles in our sense of position and movement. It contains a skeptical review of the earlier literature on this topic as well as several simple but interesting experiments.*

Hallin RG, Torebjörk HE: *Studies on cutaneous A and C fiber afferents, skin nerve blocks and perception.* In Zotterman Y, editor: *Sensory functions of the skin of primates,* Elmsford, NY, 1976, Pergamon Press. *A description of experiments involving recording from the radial nerve; the experimenter notes afferent fiber activity in response to stimulation, and the experimentee reports his sensations, all during selective block of A fibers by pressure or of C fibers by only a local anesthetic.*

Hensel H: *Cutaneous thermoreceptors.* In Iggo A, editor: *Handbook of sensory physiology.* Vol. II, *Somatosensory system,* New York, 1973, Springer-Verlag.

Houk J, Henneman E: Responses of Golgi tendon organs to active contraction of the soleus muscle of the cat, *J Neurophysiol* 30:466, 1967. *Describes experiments demonstrating that tendon organs are really highly sensitive receptors when responding to muscle contraction.*

Hunt CC: Mammalian muscle spindle: peripheral mechanisms, *Physiol Rev* 70:643, 1990.

Iggo A: Sensory receptors in the skin of mammals and their sensory functions, *Rev Neurol* 141:599, 1985.

Iggo A, Muir AR: The structure and function of a slowly adapting touch corpuscle in hairy skin, *J Physiol* 200:763, 1969. *The slowly adapting receptor of this paper is the Merkel ending of the cat.*

Jänig W, Koltzenburg M: On the function of spinal primary afferent fibres supplying colon and urinary bladder, *J Autonom Nerv Sys* 30:S89, 1990. *Single receptors in cats that apparently can signal both normal fullness and painful distention.*

Kenshalo DR, Gallegos ES: Multiple temperature-sensitive spots innervated by single nerve fibers, *Science* 158:1064, 1967.

Kruger L, Perl ER, Sedivic MJ: Fine structure of myelinated mechanical nociceptor endings in cat hairy skin, *J Comp Neurol* 198:137, 1981.

Landau W, Bishop GH: Pain from dermal, periosteal, and fascial endings and from inflammation: electrophysiological study employing differential nerve block, *Arch Neurol Psychiatr* 69:490, 1953. *The volunteers in this case were the authors themselves who, with admirable fortitude, studied the effects of pressure blocks and local anesthetics on the pain caused by needles, bee stings, and other methods.*

Low FN: *The perineurium and connective tissue of peripheral nerve.* In Landon DN, editor: *The peripheral nerve,* London, 1976, Chapman & Hall.

Macefield G, Gandevia SC, Burke D: Conduction velocities of muscle and cutaneous afferents in the upper and lower limbs of human subjects, *Brain* 112:1519, 1989. *Evidence that human muscle afferents may not conduct as rapidly as those of cats and other experimental animals, and that they may be no faster than large-diameter cutaneous afferents.*

Matthews PBC: *Mammalian muscle receptors and their central actions,* London, 1973, Edward Arnold.

Matthews PBC: Where does Sherrington's "muscular sense" originate? Muscles, joints, corollary discharges? *Ann Rev Neurosci* 5:189, 1982.

McCloskey DI et al: Sensory effects of pulling or vibrating exposed tendons in man, *Brain* 106:21, 1983. *Heroic experiments in which one of the investigators had the tendon of his own extensor hallucis longus transected and then pulled on.*

Meyer GA, Fields HL: Causalgia treated by selective large fibre stimulation of peripheral nerve, *Brain* 95:163, 1972.

Ochoa J, Torebjörk E: Sensations evoked by intraneural microstimulation of single mechanoreceptor units innervating the human hand, *J Physiol* 342:633, 1983.

Pease DC, Quilliam TA: Electron microscopy of the Pacinian corpuscle, *J Biophys Biochem Cytol* 3:331, 1957.

Sato J, Perl ER: Adrenergic excitation of cutaneous pain receptors induced by peripheral nerve injury, *Sci* 251:1608, 1991.

*Recent evidence indicating that partial nerve injury may make the sensory terminalis of C fibers sensitive to sympathetic stimulation, thus leading or contributing to causalgia.*

Schoultz TW, Swett JE: The fine structure of the Golgi tendon organ, *J Neurocytol* 1:1, 1972.

Shanthaveerappa TR, Bourne GH: Perineural epithelium: a new concept of its role in the integrity of the peripheral nervous system, *Science* 154:1464, 1966.

Sinclair D: *Mechanisms of cutaneous sensation,* New York, 1981, Oxford University Press.

Thrush DC: Congenital insensitivity to pain: a clinical genetic and neurophysiological study of four children from the same family, *Brain* 96:369, 1973.

Vallbo ÅB, Johansson RS: Properties of cutaneous mechanoreceptors in the human hand related to touch sensation, *Hum Neurobiol* 3:3, 1984. *Good review of the properties of skin receptors, as determined by recording from individual sensory axons of human volunteers.*

Vallbo ÅB et al: Somatosensory, proprioceptive, and sympathetic activity in human peripheral nerves, *Physiol Rev* 59:919, 1979.

Van Hees J, Gybels J: C nociceptor activity in human nerve during painful and nonpainful skin stimulation, *J Neurol Neurosurg Psych* 44:600, 1981. *Direct demonstration that a given level of activity in the axon of a nociceptor can be interpreted as pain in some situations but not in others.*

Widdicombe JG: *Enteroceptors.* In Hubbard JI, editor: *The peripheral nervous system,* New York, 1974, Plenum Press.

Winkelmann RK, Lambert EH, Hayles AB: Congenital absence of pain, *Arch Derm* 85:325, 1962.

# CHAPTER 7

# Spinal Cord

The spinal cord is the traditional starting point for a detailed consideration of the central nervous system (CNS). It is a uniformly organized part of the CNS and also one of the simplest (in a relative sense), but many principles of cord function apply to other levels of the nervous system. It is, at the same time, extraordinarily important in the day-to-day activities we tend not to think about. In it reside all the motor neurons supplying the muscles we use to move our bodies around, as well as most autonomic efferents. It also receives all the sensory input from the body and part of the head and performs the initial processing operations on most of this input.

## GROSS ANATOMY

An adult human spinal cord appears surprisingly small on first inspection, being only about 42 to 45 cm long and about 1 cm in diameter at its widest point. It weighs about 35 g, so one could be mailed for just two stamps. It is anatomically segmented—not obviously like an earthworm but in terms of the nerve roots attached to it (Figure 7-1). A continuous series of dorsal (=posterior) rootlets enters the cord in a shallow longitudinal groove (the *posterolateral sulcus*) on its posterolateral surface, and a continuous series of ventral (=anterior) rootlets leaves from the poorly defined *anterolateral sulcus*. The dorsal and ventral rootlets from discrete sections of the cord coalesce to form *dorsal* and *ventral roots,* which in turn join to form *spinal nerves*. Each dorsal root bears a *dorsal root ganglion* just proximal to the junction between dorsal and ventral roots; it contains the cell bodies of the primary sensory neurons whose processes travel through that particular spinal nerve. A portion of the cord that gives rise to a spinal nerve constitutes a *segment*. There are 31 segments in the human spinal cord: 8 *cervical,* 12 *thoracic,* 5 *lumbar,* 5 *sacral,* and 1 *coccygeal*.

The spinal cord itself, stripped of its dorsal and ventral rootlets, gives no obvious sign of segmentation. Rather, it is a continuous column with two enlargements, which ends caudally in the pointed *conus medullaris* (Figure 7-2). The two enlargements occur in those regions of the cord that supply the upper and lower extremities and therefore contain increased numbers of motor neurons and interneurons. The limits of the enlargements are not distinct, but the *cervical enlargement* (which supplies the upper extremities) is conventionally considered to extend from the fifth cervical to the first thoracic segment (C5 to T1), inclusive. The *lumbar* (or *lumbosacral*) *enlargement* (which supplies the lower extremities) extends from the second lumbar to the third sacral segment (L2 to S3).

The spinal cord approaches its adult length long before the vertebral canal does. Until the third month of fetal life, both grow at about the same rate, and the cord fills the canal. Thereafter the body and the vertebral column grow faster than the spinal cord does, so that at the time of birth the spinal cord ends at the third lumbar vertebra. A small additional amount of differential growth in the vertebral column occurs subsequent to this, and in the adult the cord ends at about the level of the disk between the first and second lumbar vertebrae. However, the spinal nerves still exit through the same intervertebral foramina as they did early in development, and each dorsal root ganglion remains at the level of the appropriate foramen. Proceeding from cervical to sacral levels the dorsal and ventral roots become progressively longer, since they have longer and longer distances to travel before reaching their sites of exit from the vertebral canal (Figure 7-2). The *lumbar cistern,* from the end of the spinal cord at vertebral level L1 to L2 to the end of the dural sheath at vertebral level S2, is filled with this collection of dorsal and ventral roots, collectively referred to as the *cauda equina* (Latin for horse's tail) (Figure 7-3).

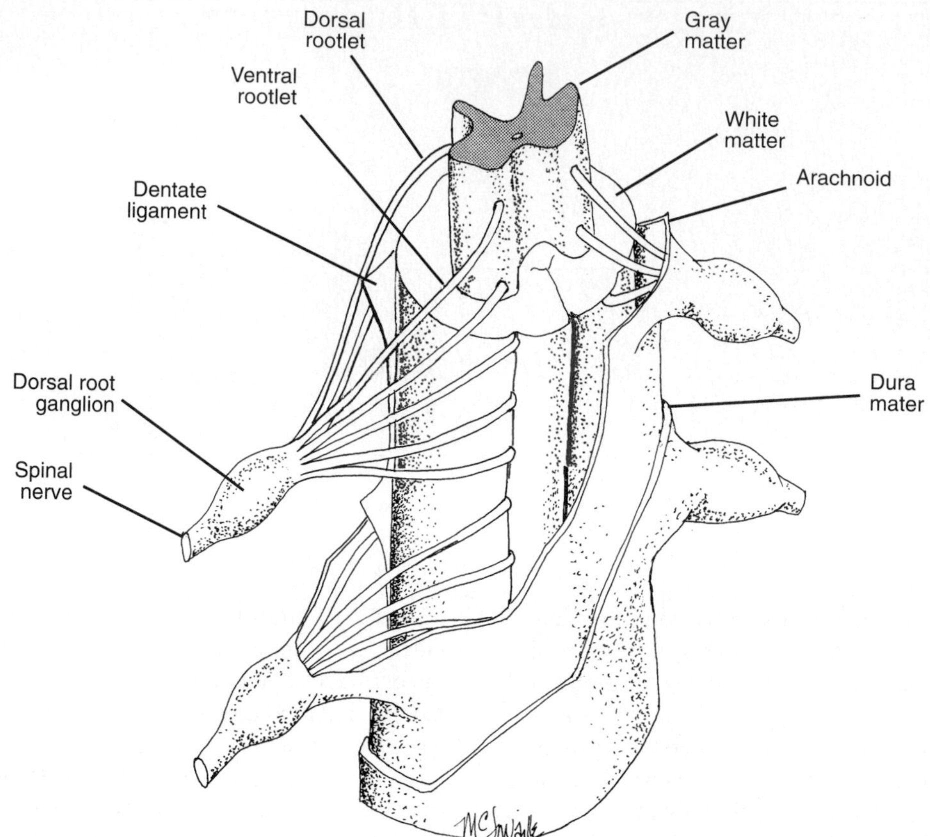


FIGURE 7-1
Portion of the spinal cord, showing its relationship to meninges and spinal nerves. The portion in color, giving rise to a single spinal nerve, represents a single segment.

Each of the first seven cervical nerves leaves the vertebral canal *above* the corresponding vertebra; for instance, the first cervical nerve leaves between the occiput and the first cervical vertebra (the atlas), the second leaves between the first and second cervical vertebrae (the atlas and the axis), and so on. However, because there are only seven cervical vertebrae, the eighth cervical nerve leaves between the seventh cervical and first thoracic vertebrae, and each of the subsequent nerves leaves *below* the corresponding vertebra.

The meningeal coverings of the spinal cord were described in Chapter 3 (see Figures 3-13 and 7-1). The cord is suspended within an arachnoid-lined dural tube by the dentate ligaments, which are extensions of the pia mater. In addition, the caudal end of the cord is anchored to the end of the dural tube by the *filum terminale,* an extension of the pial covering of the conus medullaris. The filum terminale then acquires a dural outer layer and in turn is anchored to the coccyx.

## INTERNAL STRUCTURE

In cross section the spinal cord consists of a roughly H-shaped area of gray matter that floats like a butterfly in a surround of white matter. The gray matter can be divided into *horns* and the white matter into *funiculi* (from the Latin *funiculus* meaning string) (Figure 7-4). Keep in mind that the spinal cord is, to a great extent, a longitudinally organized structure, even though it is most conveniently studied in cross section. For example, the posterior gray horns are continuous cell columns rather than a series of discrete nuclei, and at any given level the posterior horn cells interact with cells from many other levels.

In addition to the posterolateral and anterolateral sulci, several other longitudinal grooves indent the cross-sectional outline of the cord (Figure 7-4). The deep *anterior median fissure* extends almost to the center of the cord; at the apex of this fissure, only a thin zone of white matter (the *anterior white commissure*) and a thin zone of gray matter separate the central canal from the subarachnoid

A

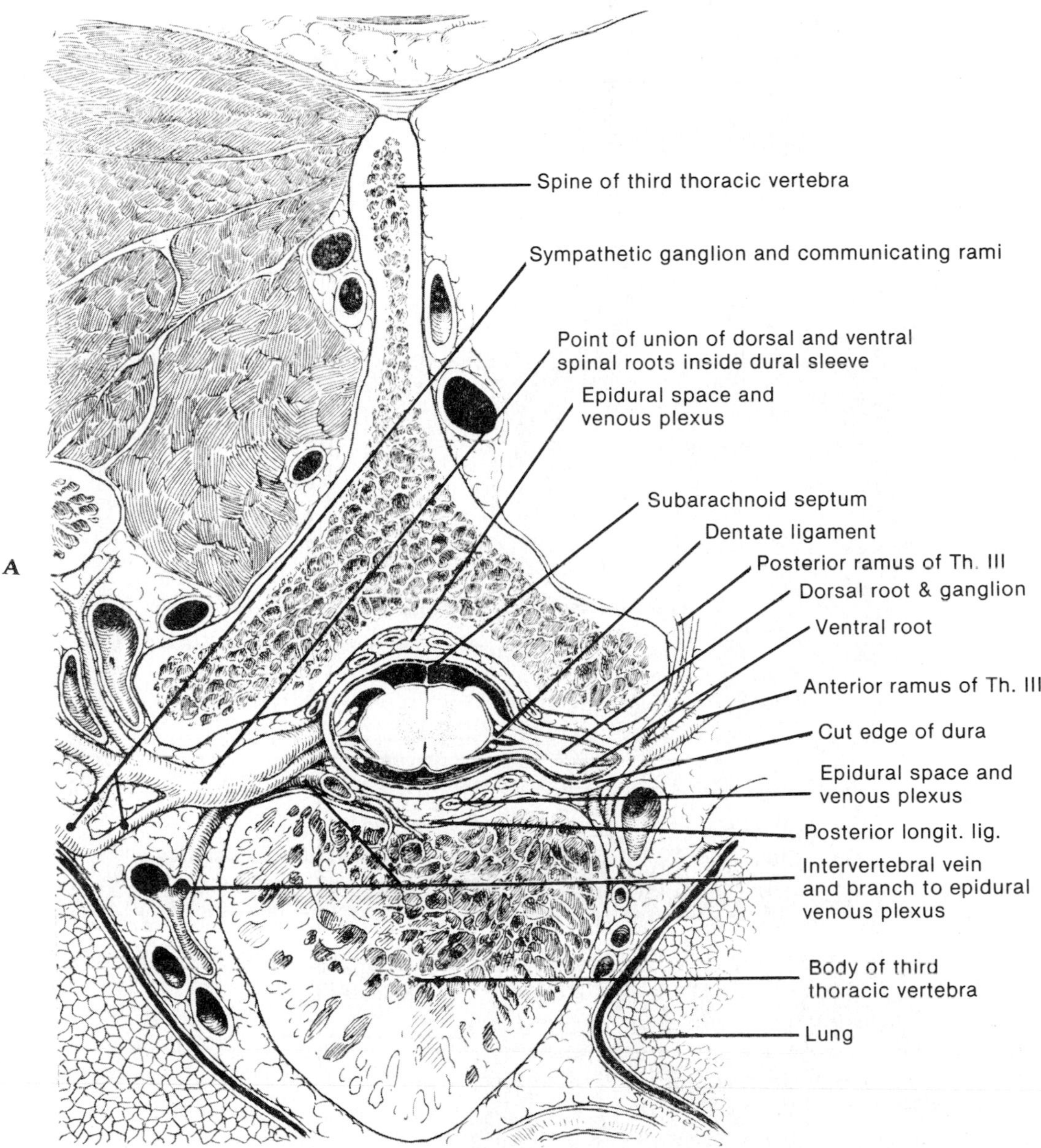


FIGURE 7-2
Relationships between spinal cord, vertebrae, and vertebral column. **A,** Section through the third thoracic vertebra and the spinal cord at that level.

From Mettler FA: Neuroanatomy, ed 2, St. Louis, 1948, The CV Mosby Co.

*Continued.*

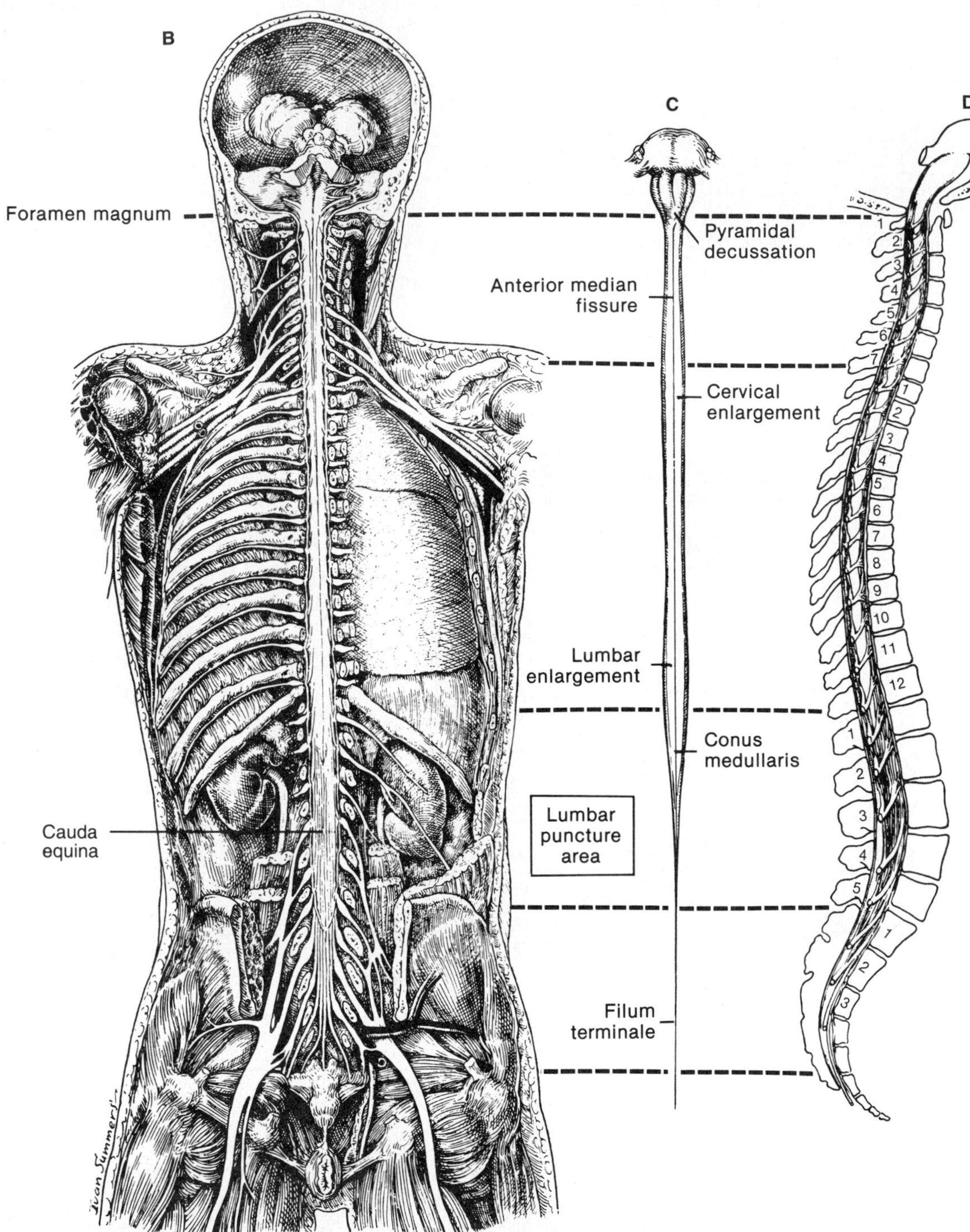


FIGURE 7-2, cont'd
**B,** Posterior surface of a spinal cord within a vertebral canal dissected from the back. **C,** How the anterior surface of the same spinal cord would look after removal of dura, arachnoid, and spinal nerves. **D,** Spinal cord exposed from the lateral direction, showing the way in which the cord ends at about the L1-L2 level and spinal nerves travel progressively longer distances in the cauda equina to reach their exits from the vertebral canal.

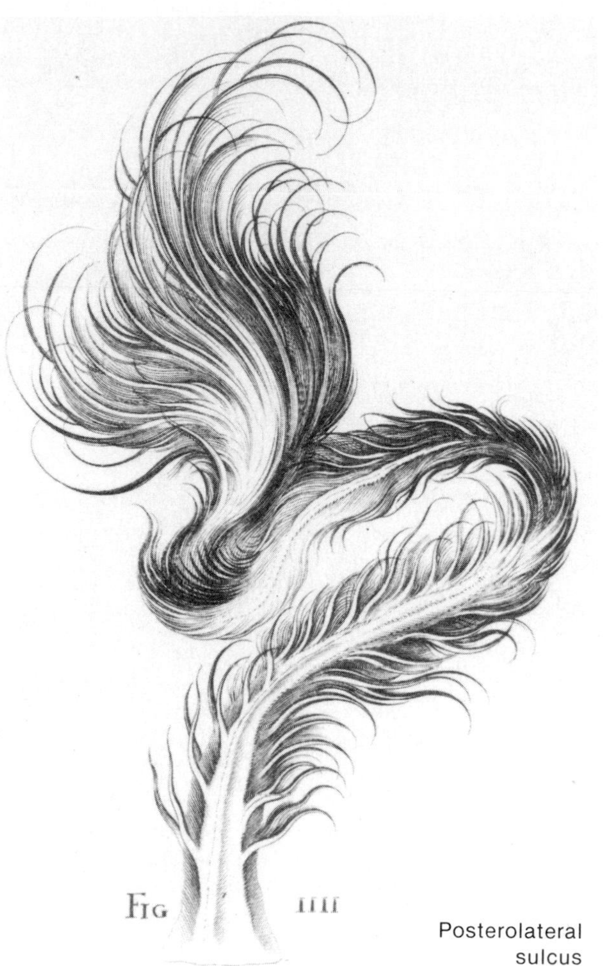


FIGURE 7-3
A depiction of the cauda equina from *Historia Anatomica Humani Corporis* by Andreas Laurentius (Frankfurt, 1600, Becker), who was apparently the first to name and illustrate this structure. The dissection from which this illustration was made was "obtained by immersion in water, suggesting a horse's tail." My thanks to Dr. Francis Schiller, University of California, San Fransisco for calling attention to this illustration *(Neurol* 38:161, 1988).

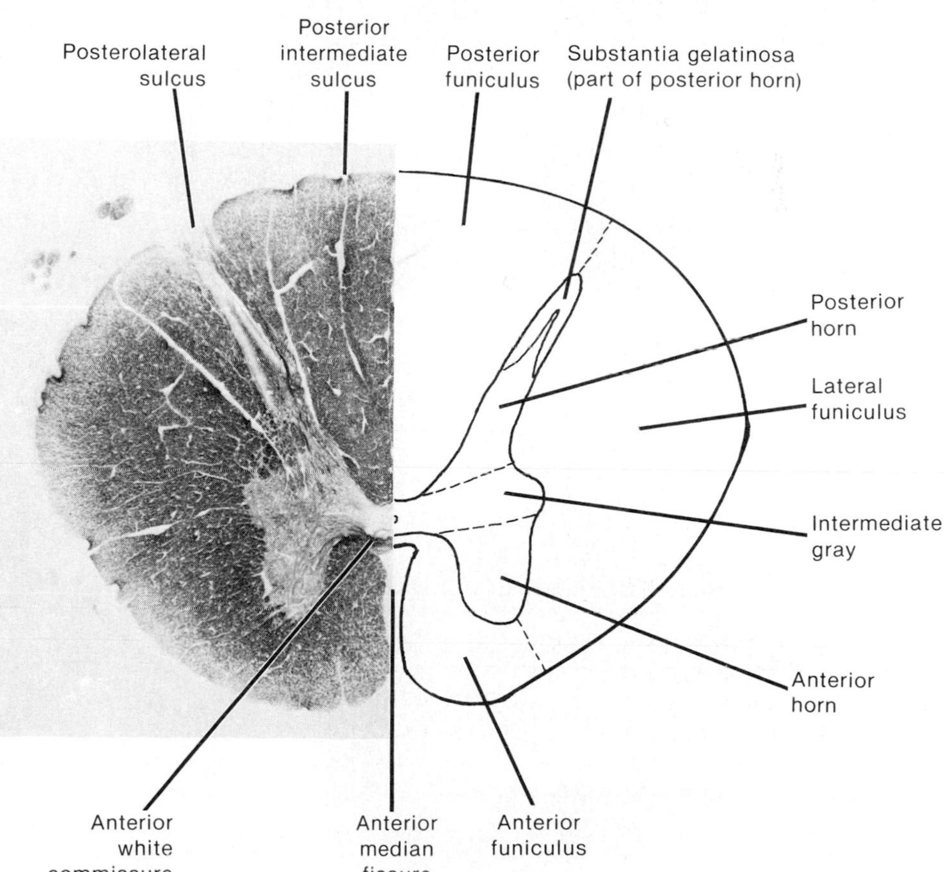


FIGURE 7-4
General cross-sectional anatomy of the spinal cord, represented in this case by the second cervical segment.

A

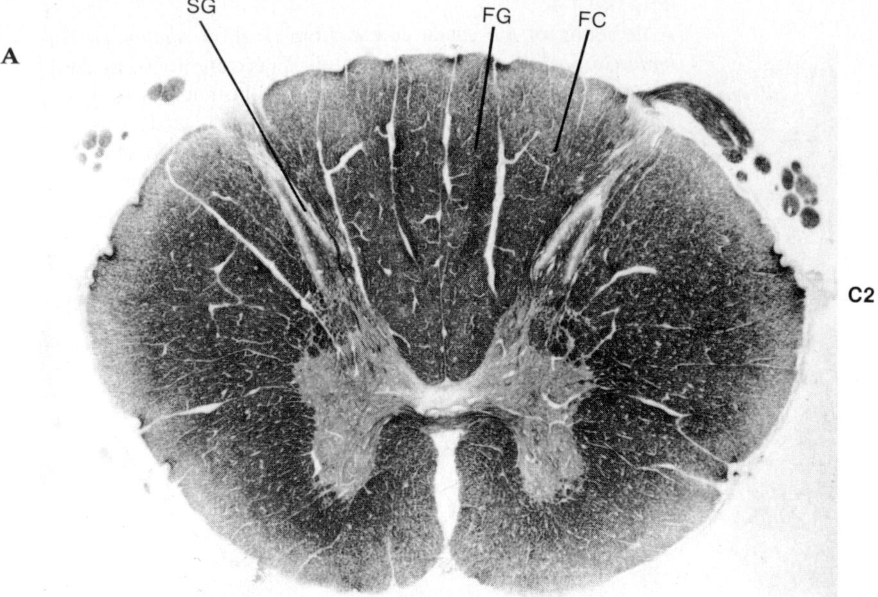


B

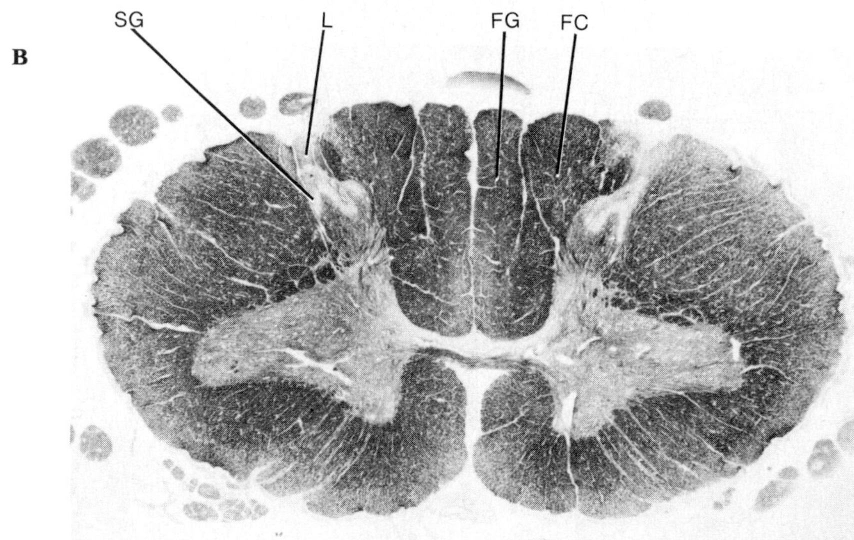


FIGURE 7-5
Cross sections of the spinal cord at various levels; note the large lateral extensions of the anterior horns in C8 and L2. Scale mark is 5 mm for all sections. *C,* Clarke's nucleus; *FC,* fasciculus cuneatus; *FG,* fasciculus gracilis; *IL,* intermediolateral cell column; *L,* Lissauer's tract; *SG,* substantia gelatinosa. *Continued.*

C

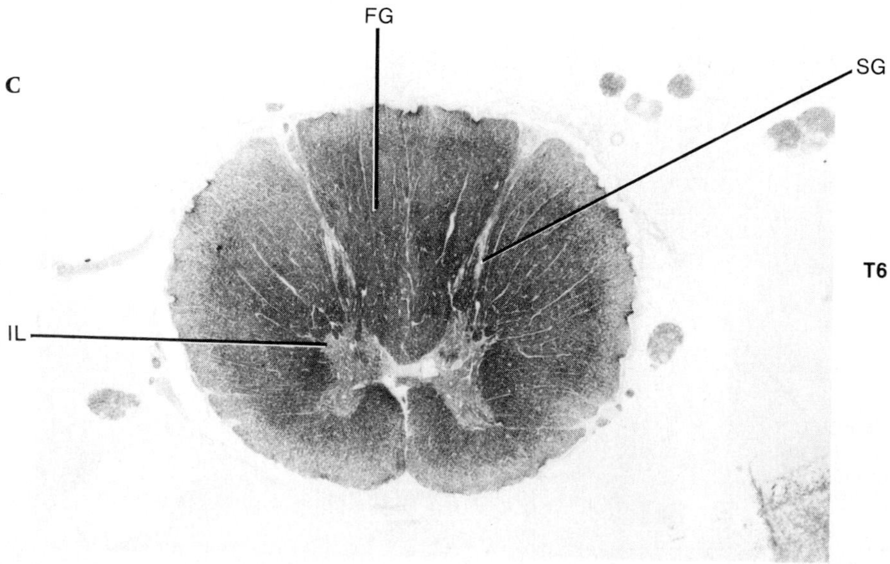

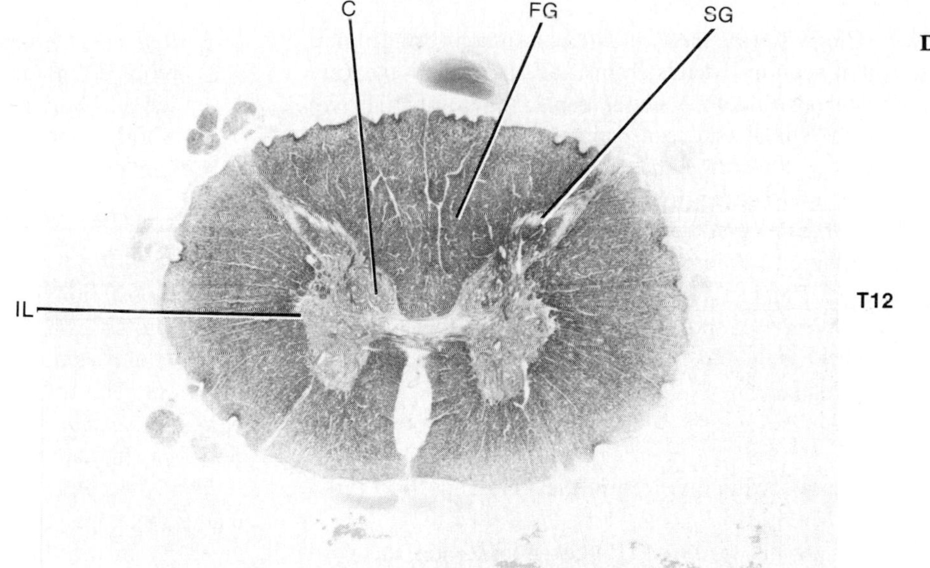


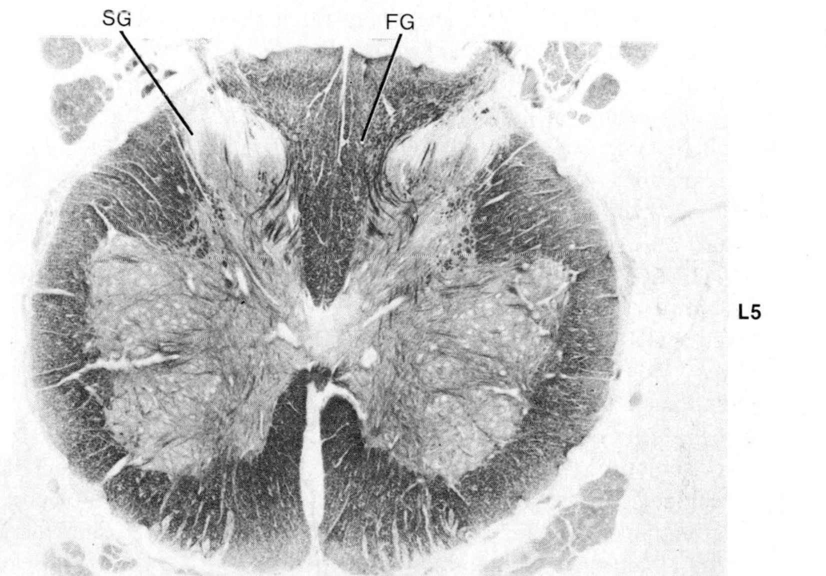


FIGURE 7-5, cont'd
Cross sections of the spinal cord at various levels; note the large lateral extensions of the anterior horns in C8 and L2. Scale mark is 5 mm for all sections. *C*, Clarke's nucleus; *FC*, fasciculus cuneatus; *FG*, fasciculus gracilis; *IL*, intermediolateral cell column; *L*, Lissauer's tract; *SG*, substantia gelatinosa.

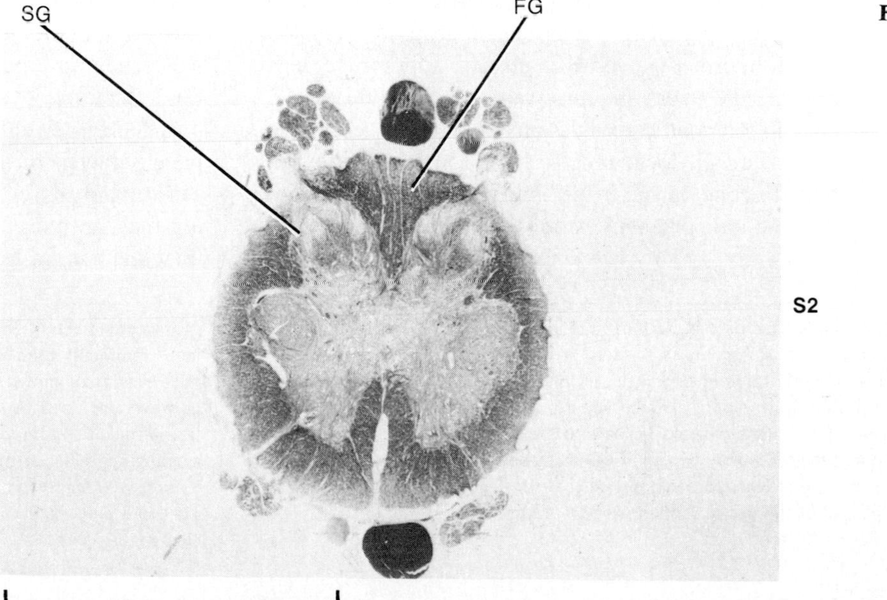

space. The *posterior median sulcus* is much less distinct, but a glial septum extends from it all the way to the gray matter surrounding the central canal. Therefore the two sides of the spinal cord can communicate with each other through only a narrow band of neural tissue. Since the fibers of many ascending pathways cross the midline in the spinal cord, this small area where crossing occurs can become important clinically in diseases affecting the center of the cord. Finally, at cervical and upper thoracic levels, a *posterior intermediate sulcus* is found. Another glial septum projects from this sulcus, partially subdividing each posterior funiculus.

## GENERAL ORGANIZATION

The spinal cord is involved in the following three types of activity.

1. *Sensory processing.* Afferent fibers enter the cord via the dorsal roots* and then end primarily on the ipsilateral side of the CNS. They may reach their site of termination either by ascending directly and uncrossed to relay nuclei in the medulla or by synapsing on neurons in the ipsilateral gray matter of the spinal cord. The relay cells in the spinal gray matter or the medulla then project their axons through defined sensory pathways to more rostral structures. In subsequent discussions of these sensory pathways, it may sometimes sound as if a particular primary afferent synapses on only one relay cell and sends its information into one and only one pathway. However, it is important to realize that each primary afferent fiber gives rise to many branches and feeds into more than one ascending sensory pathway as well as into local reflex circuits. It is estimated, for example, that a single Ia afferent from a muscle spindle may give rise to 500 or more branches within the spinal cord.
2. *Motor outflow.* The motor neurons that innervate skeletal muscle are located in the anterior horns, and many preganglionic autonomic neurons are located in the intermediate gray matter of appropriate segments. The axons of these motor neurons leave the cord in the ventral roots. Activity in these neurons is modulated by local reflex circuits and by pathways that descend through the spinal white matter from the cerebral cortex and from various brainstem structures.
3. *Reflexes.* Certain specified afferent inputs cause stereotyped motor outputs, as in the familiar knee jerk reflex. Many of these involve neural circuitry that is wholly contained within the spinal cord; several examples are discussed in this chapter.

*The Bell-Magendie law, a long-standing neuroanatomical tenet, states that the dorsal root comprises solely primary afferent fibers and the ventral root solely efferent fibers of various sorts. However, it now appears that a significant number of the ventral root fibers of the cat are finely myelinated or unmyelinated primary afferents. Preliminary findings indicate that the same may be true for humans and that the ventral root afferents may be at least partially responsible for the persistence or the return of pain after the dorsal roots have been sectioned.

## SPINAL GRAY MATTER

### Posterior horn

The posterior horn consists mainly of interneurons whose processes remain within the spinal cord and of tract cells whose axons collect into long ascending sensory pathways. This area of gray matter contains two prominent parts, the *substantia gelatinosa* and the *body* of the posterior horn, that are present at all spinal levels.

The substantia gelatinosa is a distinctive region of gray matter that caps the posterior horn at all spinal levels (Figure 7-5). In myelin-stained preparations this region looks pale compared with the rest of the gray matter, since it deals mostly with finely myelinated and unmyelinated sensory fibers that carry pain and temperature information. Between the substantia gelatinosa and the surface of the cord is a relatively pale-staining area of white matter called *Lissauer's tract.** This tract stains more lightly than the rest of the white matter, because it contains the finely myelinated and unmyelinated fibers with which the substantia gelatinosa deals.

The body of the posterior horn consists mainly of interneurons and tract cells that transmit many types of somatic and visceral sensory information. In this respect it functionally overlaps parts of the intermediate gray matter.

### Anterior horn

The anterior horn contains the cell bodies of the large motor neurons that supply skeletal muscle (Figure 7-6). These alpha motor neurons, also referred to as *lower motor neurons,* are the only means by which the nervous system can exercise control over body movements, whether voluntary or involuntary; a number of different pathways and parts of the nervous system can influence these lower motor neurons, but they alone can effect muscle contraction. Destruction of the lower motor neurons supplying a muscle or interruption of their axons therefore causes complete paralysis of that muscle. Lower motor neuron lesions cause paralysis of a type called *flaccid paralysis,* indicating that the muscle is limp and uncontracted. Reflex contractions can no longer be elicited, and the muscle slowly

*Lissauer's tract is an unusual case in which an eponym is becoming more commonly used rather than fading away. For many years Lissauer's tract was also known by the descriptive term *dorsolateral fasciculus.* However, as described elsewhere in this chapter, the dorsal part of the lateral funiculus is now known to contain some distinctively important ascending and descending pathways. As a result, many now refer to the latter area of spinal white matter as the *dorsolateral fasciculus* or *funiculus.* To avoid ambiguity, Lissauer's tract is probably best referred to by its eponymous name.

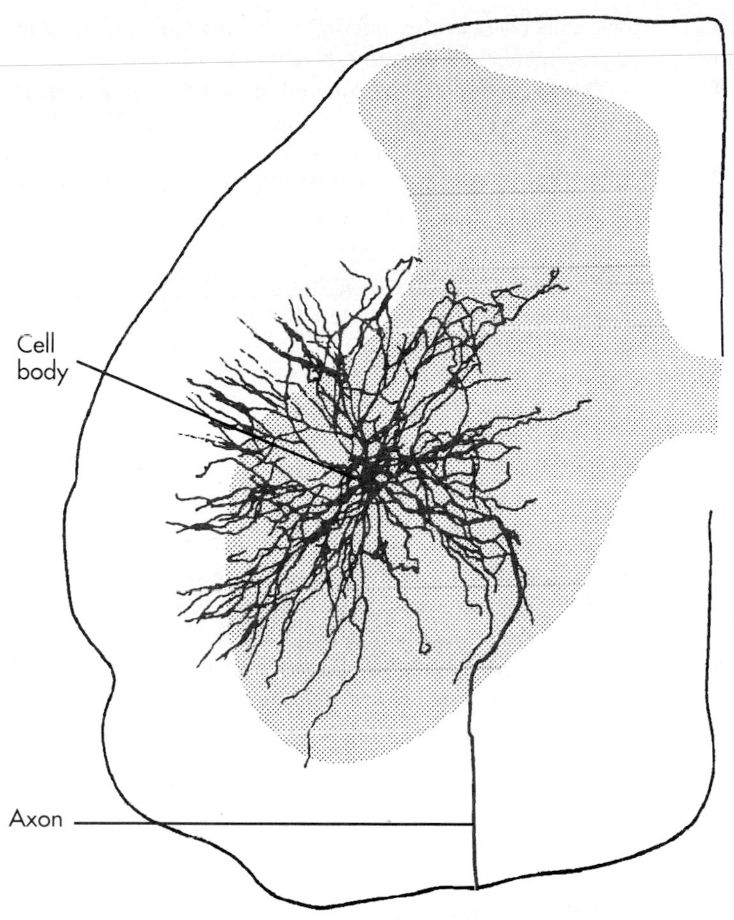


FIGURE 7-6
A single motor neuron from the lumbar spinal cord of an adult cat. A marker substance (horseradish peroxidase) was injected from the intracellular tip of a microelectrode, and the neuron was subsequently reconstructed from a series of sections. The extent and complexity of the dendritic trees of real neurons are obviously different from those of the "cartoon" neurons in most of the diagrams in this book. Modified from Ulfhake B et al: *J Comp Neurol* 278:69, 1988.

atrophies (for reasons that are not completely understood). This occurs, for example, in poliomyelitis, a viral disease that attacks the motor neurons of the anterior horn, and in injuries in which ventral roots are damaged.

Alpha motor neurons occur in groups, separated from one another by areas of interneurons; the groups that innervate axial muscles are medial to those that innervate limb muscles. In the cervical and lumbar enlargements, which contain the limb motor neurons, the anterior horns are enlarged laterally (see Figure 7-5). Smaller gamma motor neurons are interspersed with alpha motor neurons in all such groups. They innervate the intrafusal muscle fibers of muscle spindles, and so they are also referred to as *fusimotor neurons*.

Two columns of motor neurons in the anterior horn of the cervical cord are recognized as separate entities. The *spinal accessory nucleus* extends from the caudal medulla to about C5. The axons of these motor neurons emerge from the lateral surface of the spinal cord just posterior to the dentate ligament as a separate series of rootlets that form the accessory nerve (see Figure 2-15). The *phrenic nucleus,* containing the motor neurons that innervate the diaphragm, is located in the medial portion of the anterior horn in segments C3 to C5. This makes injuries to the upper cervical spinal cord a matter of grave concern, since destruction of the descending pathways that control the phrenic nucleus and other respiratory motor neurons renders a patient unable to breathe.

### Intermediate gray matter

The gray matter that is intermediate to the anterior and posterior horns has some characteristics of both and also contains the spinal preganglionic autonomic neurons. In addition, at some levels it includes a distinctive region called *Clarke's nucleus*.

From T1 through L2 or L3, the preganglionic sympathetic neurons for the entire body lie in a column of cells, the *intermediolateral cell column,* which forms a pointy lateral horn on the spinal gray matter (see Figure 7-5). Their axons leave through the ventral roots. Cells in a corresponding location in segments S2 to S4 form the *sacral parasympathetic nucleus* but do not form a distinct lateral horn. Their axons leave through the ventral roots and synapse on the postganglionic parasympathetic neurons for the pelvic viscera.

Clarke's nucleus (or *nucleus dorsalis*) is a rounded collection of large cells located on the medial surface of the base of the posterior horn from about T1 to L2 or L3. It is particularly prominent at lower thoracic levels (see Figure 7-5). This is an important relay nucleus for the transmission of information to the cerebellum and also plays a role in forwarding proprioceptive information from the leg to the thalamus. Because of its prominent role in sensory processing, it is considered by many to be part of the posterior horn.

The remainder of the intermediate gray matter is a collection of various tract cells, sensory interneurons, and interneurons that synapse on motor neurons.

### Rexed's laminae

In 1952 Rexed devised a system for subdividing the gray matter of the cat's spinal cord into layers, or laminae. The same system has since been applied to the cords of other mammals, including humans (Figure 7-7). *Lamina I* (also called the *marginal zone*) is a thin layer of gray matter that covers the substantia gelatinosa, *lamina II* is the substantia gelatinosa, and *laminae III through VI* are the body of the posterior horn; *lamina VII* roughly corresponds to the intermediate gray matter but also includes Clarke's nucleus and large extensions into the anterior horn; *lamina VIII* comprises some of the interneuronal zones of the anterior horn, while *lamina IX* is the clusters of motor neurons embedded in the anterior horn; *lamina X* is the zone of gray matter surrounding the central canal.

This terminology has proved useful for experimental anatomists and physiologists, since the histological differences between the laminae correspond to functional differences (Table 4). For example, the functional dichotomy between large- and small-diameter peripheral nerve fibers is maintained to a great extent in the patterns of termination of these fibers in the spinal gray: there are prominent (though not exclusive) terminations of pain and temperature afferents in laminae I and II, tactile afferents from cutaneous nerves in lamina III, and Ia muscle spindle afferents in laminae VI, VII, and IX.

## REFLEXES

A reflex is an involuntary, stereotyped response to a sensory input. All reflex pathways therefore must involve at least a receptor structure and associated afferent neuron (with its cell body in a dorsal root ganglion or some other sensory ganglion) and an efferent neuron (with its cell body within the CNS). With the exception of the *stretch reflex,* all reflexes involve one or more interneurons as well.

Reflexes range from the very simple ones described in

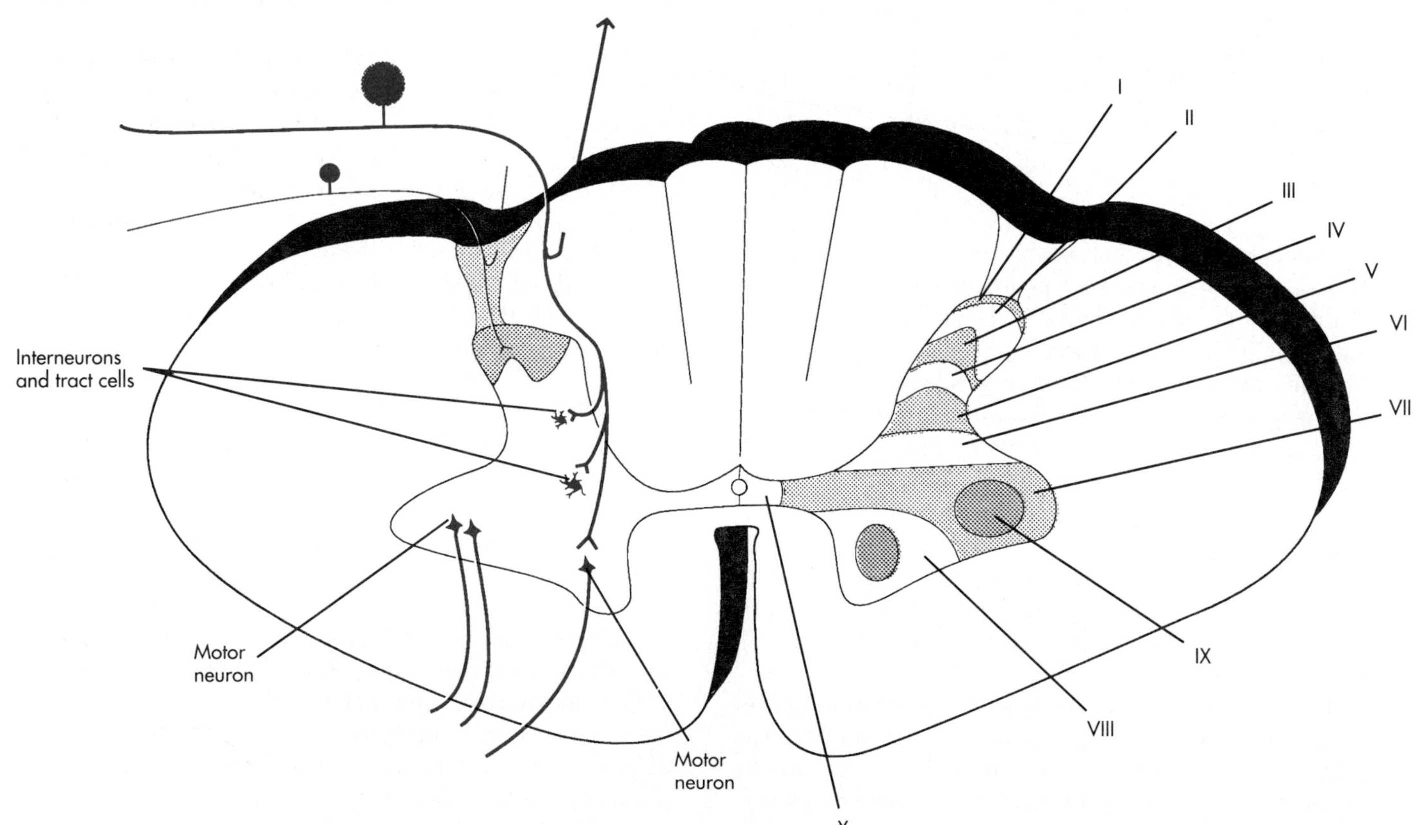


FIGURE 7-7
Laminae of Rexed are indicated on the right, and the general kinds of cells and connections in these different areas are indicated on the left. Notice that large diameter, heavily myelinated afferents enter medially through the posterior funiculus, whereas small diameter afferents enter laterally near the substantia gelatinosa. This corresponds to the way in which tactile and proprioceptive information is processed, relative to pain and temperature information.

**TABLE 4** *Important subdivisions of spinal cord gray matter*

| *Nucleus* | *Levels* | *Lamina* | *Function* |
|---|---|---|---|
| Marginal zone | all | I | Some spinothalamic tract cells |
| Substantia gelatinosa | all | II | Modulate pain and temperature |
| Body of posterior horn | all | III-VI | Sensory processing |
| Clarke's nucleus | T1-L2/L3 | VII | Posterior spinocerebellar tract cells |
| Intermediolateral column | T1-L2/L3 | VII | Preganglionic sympathetics |
| Sacral parasympathetic nucleus | S2-S4 | VII | Preganglionic parasympathetics → pelvic viscera |
| Accessory nucleus | Medulla-C5 | IX | Motor neurons → trapezius and sternocleidomastoid |
| Phrenic nucleus | C3-C5 | IX | Motor neurons → diaphragm |

this chapter (which serve as a useful introduction to neural integration and are the basis for common clinical tests) to neural subroutines so complex that calling them "reflexes" seems an oversimplification. For example, a cat with its spinal cord transected at thoracic levels can, under certain conditions, perform coordinated walking movements with its hind limbs. If its hind feet are placed on a moving treadmill, the gait changes in a predictable fashion with the speed of the treadmill, from alternating stepping movements at low speeds to galloping movements (in which both legs move together in phase) at higher speeds.

## Stretch reflex

All skeletal muscles have a tendency, more pronounced in some than others, to contract in response to being stretched. The reflex arc responsible for this contraction is the simplest possible, since it involves only two neurons and a single intervening synapse. It is therefore sometimes referred to as the *monosynaptic reflex* or the *myotatic reflex* (from the Greek words *mys* meaning muscle and *tasis* meaning stretch). The afferent limb of the arc is a Ia afferent with its associated muscle spindle primary ending. Central processes of the Ia afferent make synapses within the spinal cord directly on the alpha motor neurons that innervate the muscle containing the stimulated spindle (Figure 7-8).

The stretch reflex is commonly used for clinical testing purposes. Tapping the patellar tendon, as in the familiar *knee jerk reflex,* stretches the quadriceps slightly. Ia endings in quadriceps muscle spindles are excited and in turn excite quadriceps alpha motor neurons; these cause the quadriceps to contract, completing the reflex. Similarly,

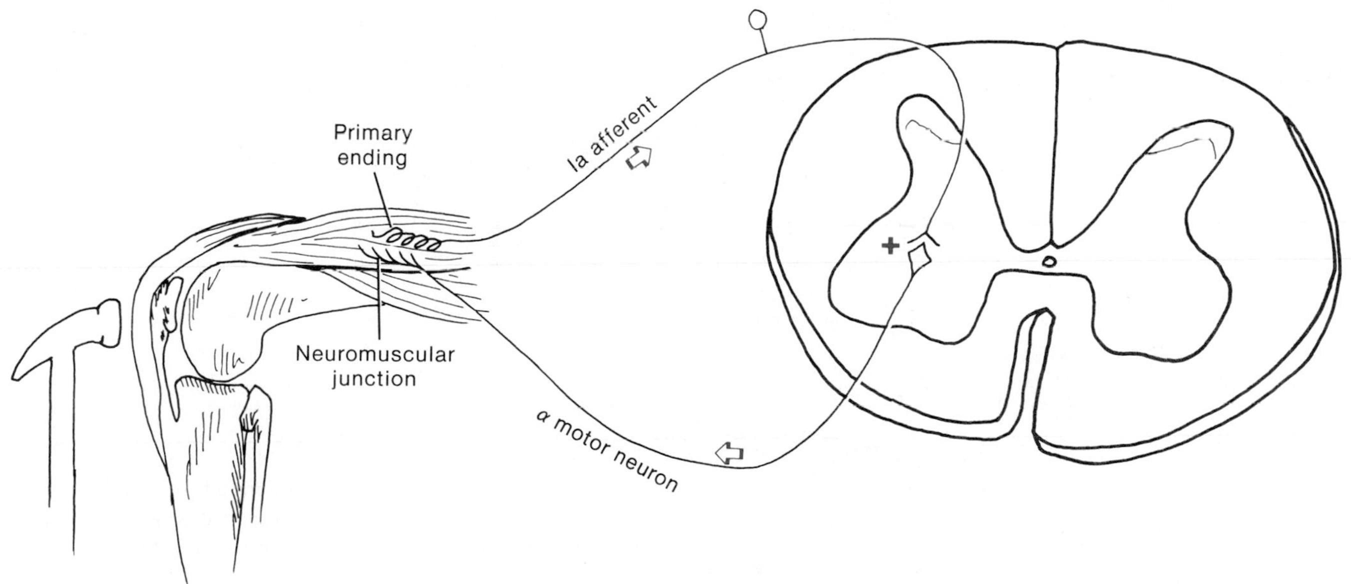


FIGURE 7-8
Stretch reflex. Striking the patellar tendon activates muscle spindle primary endings, which then monosynaptically excite alpha motor neurons that innervate the stretched muscle.

tapping the Achilles tendon stretches the gastrocnemius slightly, thereby causing a reflex contraction. Since stretch reflexes are usually elicited by tapping a tendon, they are often referred to as *deep tendon reflexes* (sometimes abbreviated as DTRs). One should remember that even though the reflex is studied in this manner, the responsible receptors are actually in the muscles attached to the tapped tendons.

Stretch reflexes are thought to be important for the constant automatic corrections we perform during movements and postures (although other reflexes may in fact be even more important for this function). As an example, when we stand still and upright, we actually sway to and fro a bit. Each time we sway in one direction, some muscles are stretched and the resulting reflex contraction helps return us toward the desired position.

There must, however, be more to the stretch reflex system, or we would be unable to sit. Sitting should stretch the quadriceps much as tapping the patellar tendon does; reflex contraction of the quadriceps would then be expected to make us stand up again. The answer to this apparent dilemma lies in the gamma motor neurons. During the act of sitting, the gamma motor neurons to quadriceps muscle spindles decrease their firing rate. This decreases the excitability of the quadriceps spindles just enough that they do not respond to the stretch imposed by sitting. The activities of the alpha and gamma motor neuron populations are coordinated generally during movements; this is discussed in more detail in Chapter 12.

### Autogenic inhibition

Stimulation of a Ib fiber, from a Golgi tendon organ, has an effect opposite to that of stimulating a Ia fiber: the alpha motor neurons that innervate the muscle connected to that tendon organ are inhibited. This effect is termed *autogenic inhibition* and involves an inhibitory interneuron between the afferent and efferent fibers (Figure 7-9).

The normal role of this reflex arc is unclear at present. It is frequently stated that it is protective in nature, preventing muscles from developing excess tension. However, in view of the great sensitivity of tendon organs to actively generated tension, it is clear that the reflex should be activated long before hazardous levels are reached. Therefore it seems likely that autogenic inhibition plays an as-yet-unknown role in ordinary motor activities.

Clinically this reflex may be manifested in a phenome-

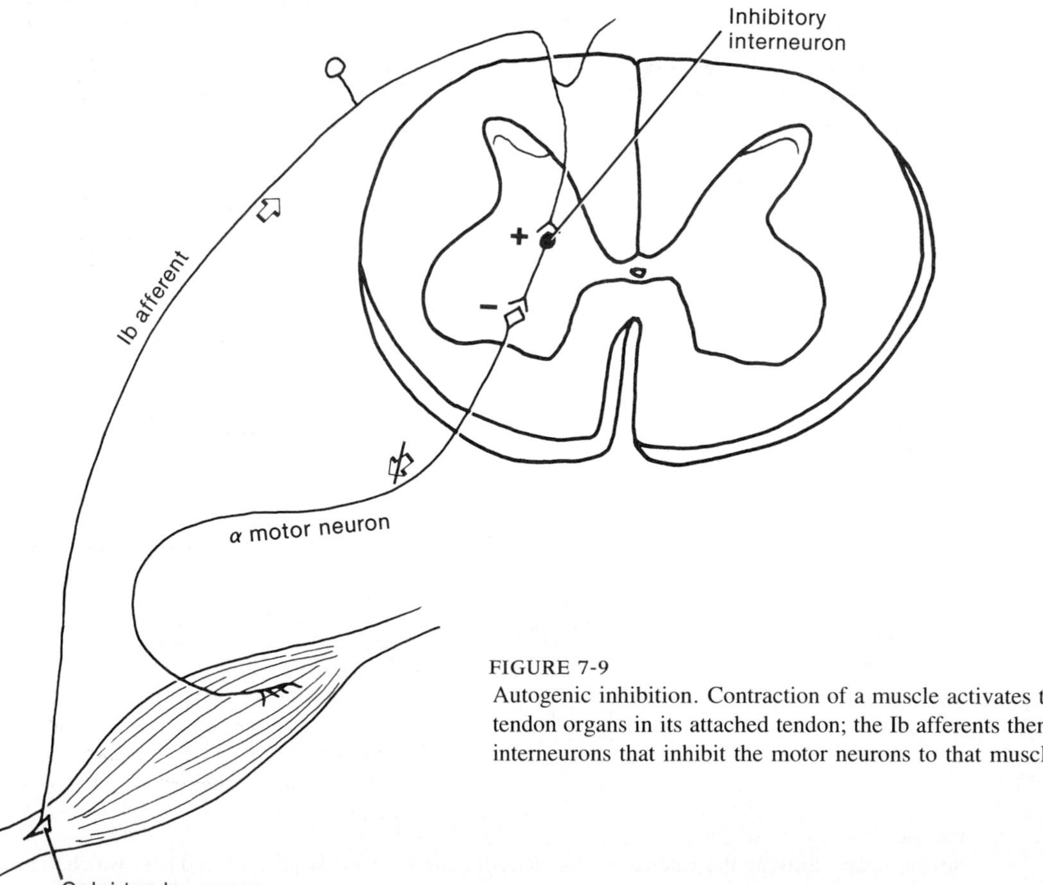


FIGURE 7-9
Autogenic inhibition. Contraction of a muscle activates the Golgi tendon organs in its attached tendon; the Ib afferents then activate interneurons that inhibit the motor neurons to that muscle.

non called the *clasp-knife response*. In certain pathological conditions following damage to descending motor pathways, the resistance of muscles to manipulation is greatly increased. Thus one would have considerable difficulty flexing the leg of an individual with such a condition. If sufficient force is applied, however, the leg slowly flexes until at some point all resistance suddenly disappears and the leg collapses in flexion like a clasp knife snapping shut. This collapse of resistance is commonly attributed to autogenic inhibition initiated by Golgi tendon organs, although other receptors may also be involved.

## Flexor reflex

Whereas stretch reflexes and autogenic inhibition are initiated by muscle or tendon receptors and primarily involve the muscle stretched or tensed, the *flexor reflex* is initiated by cutaneous receptors and involves a whole limb. A familiar example is withdrawal from a painful stimulus; after accidentally touching something painfully hot, we automatically remove the offended hand from that vicinity by flexing the arm to which it is attached.

The flexor reflex pathways in the spinal cord are normally held in a somewhat inhibited state by descending influences from the brainstem, so that only noxious stimuli result in a strong reflex. If these descending influences are removed, either surgically in experimental animals or as a result of certain pathological conditions, reflex flexion can result from harmless tactile stimulation. This indicates that most or all cutaneous receptors feed into the pathway, but ordinarily only nociceptors have a powerful enough influence to cause a reflex withdrawal.

Since the flexor reflex involves an entire limb, its pathway must spread over several spinal segments to include the motor neurons innervating all the various flexor muscles of that limb. This spreading occurs in two ways. First, all primary afferent fibers bifurcate on entering the spinal

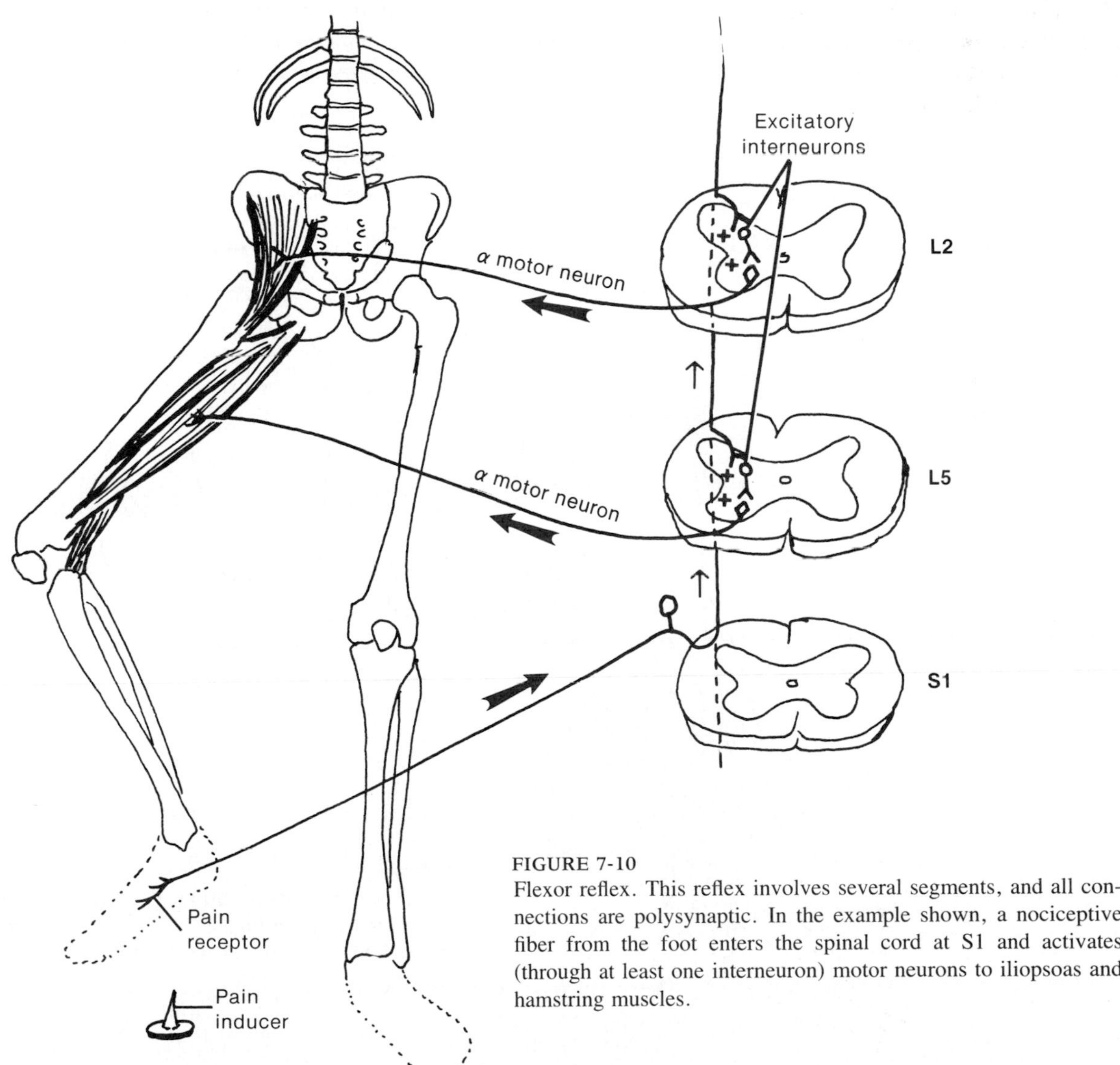


FIGURE 7-10
Flexor reflex. This reflex involves several segments, and all connections are polysynaptic. In the example shown, a nociceptive fiber from the foot enters the spinal cord at S1 and activates (through at least one interneuron) motor neurons to iliopsoas and hamstring muscles.

cord, and their processes then extend one or more segments in both rostral and caudal directions. Second, the flexor pathway includes at least one interneuron, which itself may have processes extending over several segments (Figure 7-10).

Although this reflex is usually called the flexor reflex, the term "withdrawal reflex" is also used and is perhaps more appropriate. The reflex is not an all-or-none phenomenon for a given limb but rather shows different patterns depending on which portion of the limb is stimulated (the pattern being appropriate to withdraw the stimulated area). It would be imprudent to flex a lower extremity when a painful stimulus was applied to the anterior surface of the thigh, since this would drive the thigh into the stimulus. In such a situation, it would make much more sense to activate the extensors, which is in fact what happens. Modification of the reflex response so that it reflects the area being stimulated is called *local sign*.

### Reciprocal and crossed effects

So far, we have given a simplified description of reflex circuits, including only the most direct and dominant motor effects. However, these reflexes also include weaker influences on other muscles of the same limb and even of contralateral limbs.

It would clearly be easier to shorten a stretched muscle if the motor neurons to its synergists were excited and those to its antagonists inhibited. This actually does occur and is a general principle in all reflexes; reflex activity in a given muscle produces similar activity in its ipsilateral synergists and the opposite activity in its ipsilateral antagonists (Figure 7-11). Thus the standard tap on the patellar tendon causes not only excitation of quadriceps motor neurons but also inhibition (through an interneuron) of motor neurons to the hamstring muscles. If one extensor muscle of the thigh were selectively stretched, its motor neurons would be monosynaptically excited, as would those of all the other thigh extensors. After stimulation of a Golgi tendon organ the pattern is just the reverse. If tension is applied to the patellar tendon, the quadriceps is inhibited and the hamstring muscles are excited, both actions occurring through interneurons. Finally, the flexor reflex is accompanied by inhibition of the extensors of that limb.

The crossed effects in reflex actions are most easily un-

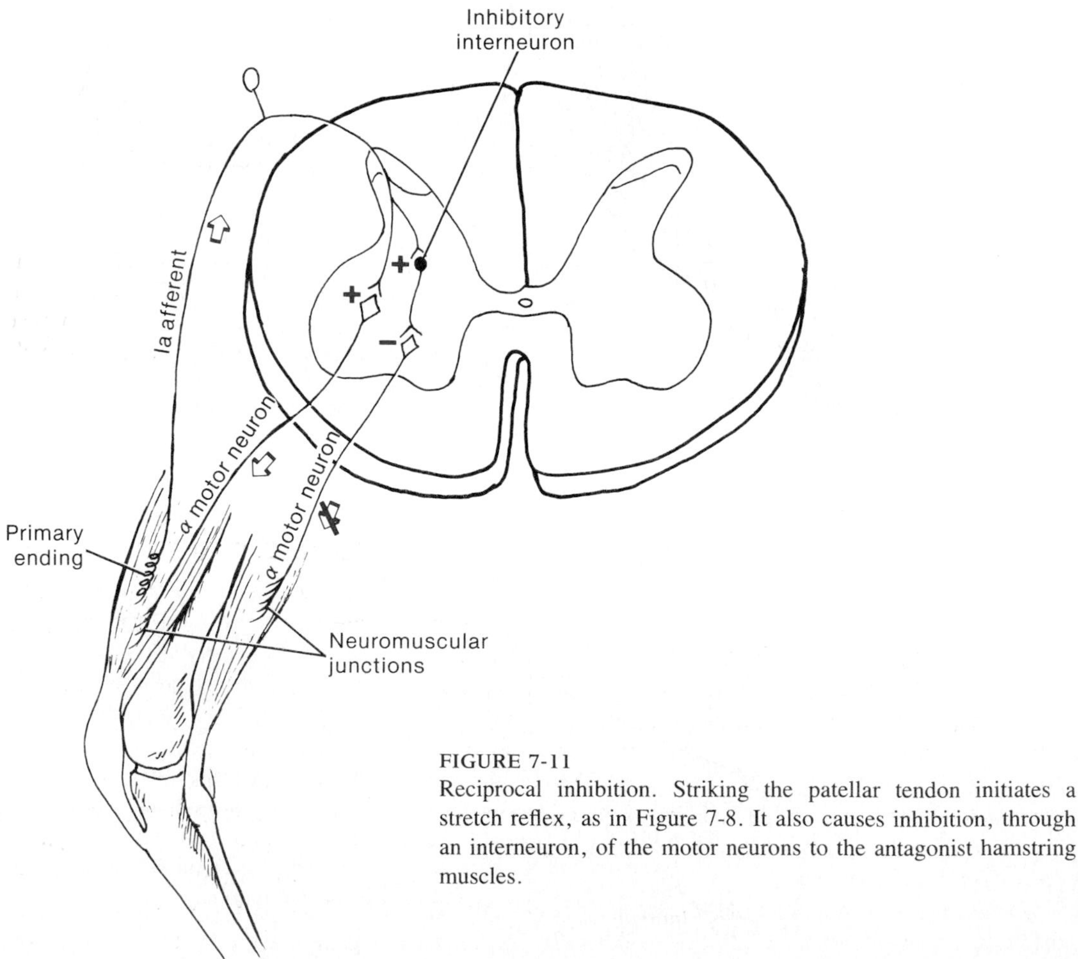


FIGURE 7-11
Reciprocal inhibition. Striking the patellar tendon initiates a stretch reflex, as in Figure 7-8. It also causes inhibition, through an interneuron, of the motor neurons to the antagonist hamstring muscles.

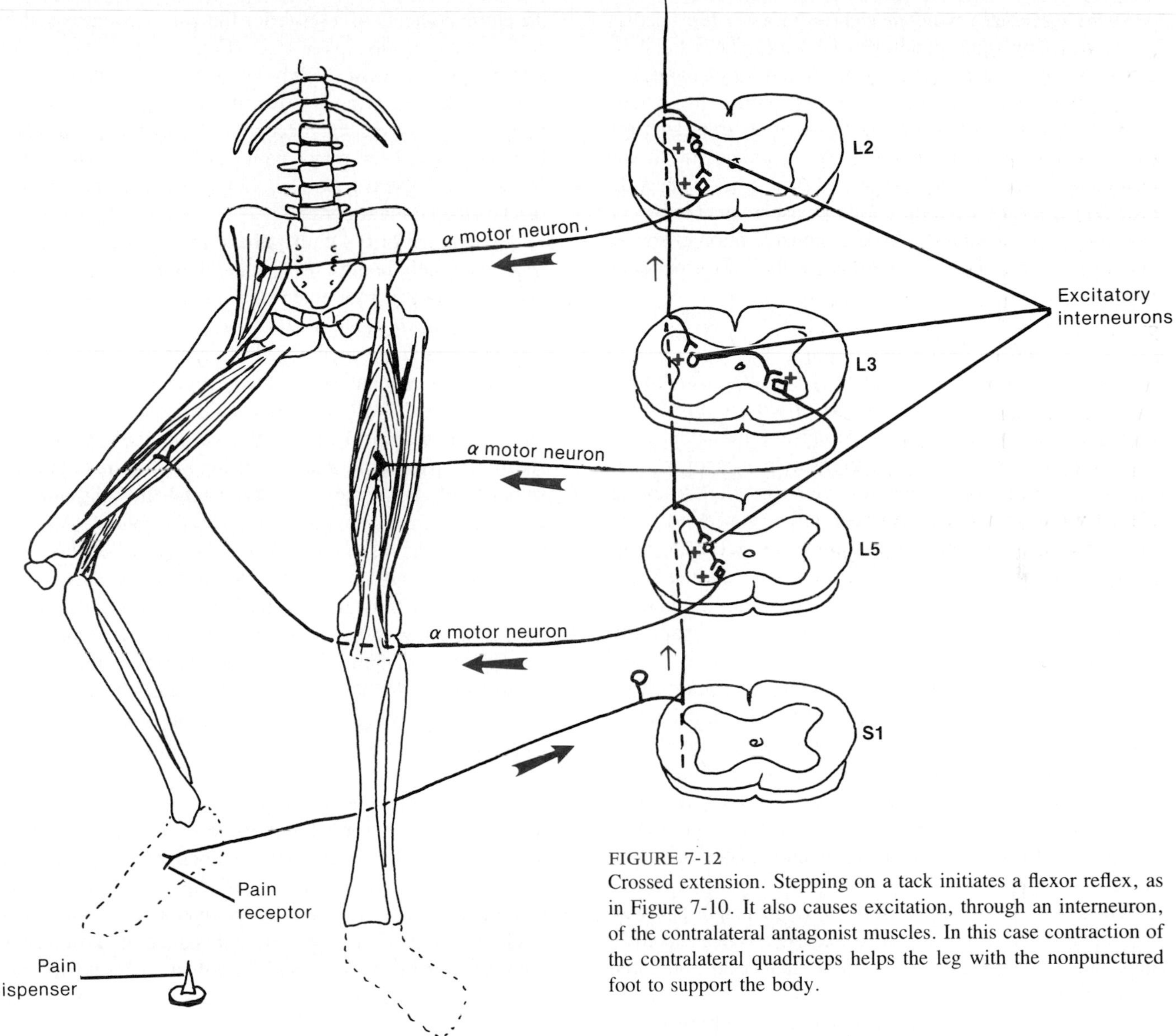


FIGURE 7-12
Crossed extension. Stepping on a tack initiates a flexor reflex, as in Figure 7-10. It also causes excitation, through an interneuron, of the contralateral antagonist muscles. In this case contraction of the contralateral quadriceps helps the leg with the nonpunctured foot to support the body.

derstood with reference to the flexor reflex (Figure 7-12). If the only effect of stepping on a tack with the right foot were withdrawal of the right leg, the maladaptive behavior of falling over and possibly landing on the tack might follow. This is avoided by a simultaneous and opposite pattern of activity in the contralateral limb; as the right leg flexes and withdraws, the left leg extends and is thus better able to support the body. Similar observations have been made after stimulation of muscle spindles and Golgi tendon organs, although the effects on contralateral antagonists are not pronounced.

These crossed effects may be the basic building blocks for more complex subroutines, such as those for the coordinated stepping movements referred to earlier.

## SPINAL WHITE MATTER

The nerve fibers in the white matter of the spinal cord are of three general types:

1. Long ascending fibers projecting to the thalamus, the cerebellum, or various brainstem nuclei
2. Long descending fibers projecting from the cerebral cortex or from various brainstem nuclei to the spinal gray matter
3. Shorter *propriospinal* fibers interconnecting various spinal cord levels, such as the fibers responsible for the coordination of flexor reflexes.

Fibers having similar connections tend to travel together, forming the various tracts of the spinal cord. Propriospinal fibers mostly remain in a thin shell surrounding the gray matter called the *propriospinal tract* or *fasciculus proprius* (the Latin word *fasciculus* means little bundle); descending tracts are found primarily in the lateral and anterior funiculi; ascending tracts are found in all funiculi.

A great many ascending and descending tracts have been described, largely on the basis of their origins and terminations; the function of some is unknown. In this chapter we describe the largest and best-known tracts descending from the cerebral cortex or ascending to the cerebellum or the thalamus. We defer consideration of several other tracts until the structures where they arise or terminate are discussed.

## Ascending pathways

As mentioned previously, there is a tendency to think of individual primary afferents as performing a single function (for example, either participating in a particular reflex arc or transmitting information to a single ascending tract). Single fibers are drawn that way in textbooks for convenience and clarity, but in fact each primary afferent probably participates in one or more reflex arcs and also in one or more ascending tracts. In a similar way, there is a tendency to think of particular sensory functions as uniquely associated with particular tracts (for example, pain with one tract and touch with another), so that damage to an ascending tract should result in total loss of some sensory function. This is not actually the case, and most kinds of sensory information reach the thalamus and the cerebellum by more than one route. Why this is so and the consequences in an intact nervous system are not understood, but one result is that the loss of a single tract can often be compensated for, to a surprising extent, by the remaining tracts.

The following section describes the principal pathways by which somatic sensory information reaches the thalamus and the cerebellum. Information that reaches the thalamus is relayed to the cerebral cortex and perceived consciously. Information that reaches the cerebellum is used in the regulation of motor patterns; we are not consciously aware of cerebellar activity.

### *Pathways to the thalamus and cortex*

There are two traditionally important routes for somatic sensory information to reach the thalamus (the *posterior column-medial lemniscus* pathway and the *spinothalamic tract*), and several more recently discovered routes that may also be of considerable importance. Two generalizations may be made about ascending somatosensory pathways of the spinal cord:

1. Most somatosensory information travels in more than one pathway.
2. Tracts in the posterior half of the cord ascend uncrossed (that is, ipsilateral to the dorsal roots whose information they carry), whereas those in the anterior half of the cord cross the midline as they form.

*Posterior columns.* The term "posterior column" refers to the entire contents of a posterior funiculus, exclusive of its share of the propriospinal tract (Figure 7-13). The posterior columns consist mainly of ascending collaterals of large myelinated primary afferents carrying impulses from various kinds of mechanoreceptors.* This has traditionally been considered the major pathway by which information from low-threshold cutaneous, joint, and muscle receptors reaches the cerebral cortex.

A large majority of the fibers in a posterior column have their cell bodies in ipsilateral dorsal root ganglia. Where the dorsal root enters the spinal cord, it segregates itself into *medial* and *lateral divisions*. The medial division contains large myelinated afferents, whereas the lateral division contains small, finely myelinated or unmyelinated afferents. Fibers of the medial division enter the posterior column. Most of them give off numbers of collaterals to the spinal gray matter and finally terminate at some spinal level, but some reach the caudal medulla and synapse there. Caudal to T6, each posterior column is an undivided bundle called the *fasciculus gracilis* (the Latin word *gracilis* means slender). Rostral to T6, fibers may leave the fasciculus gracilis, but few if any are added. Afferents entering rostral to T6 accumulate in a second bundle, roughly triangular in shape and lateral to the fasciculus gracilis, called the *fasciculus cuneatus* (the Latin word *cuneus* means wedge). A glial partition (the *posterior intermediate septum*) extends inward to partially separate the two.

At each successive spinal level, fibers entering the posterior columns add on laterally to those already present. A lamination results, with layers of fibers from sacral levels most medial and layers from cervical levels most lateral (see Figure 7-13). This sort of arrangement, in which particular portions of the body are represented in particular regions of a pathway or nucleus, is called *somatotopic* organization and is characteristic of most sensory and motor pathways.

Those posterior column fibers that reach the brainstem synapse in the *nucleus gracilis* or the *nucleus cuneatus* (the *posterior column nuclei*) in the caudal medulla. Second-order fibers arising in these nuclei cross the midline and form the *medial lemniscus* (the Latin word *lemniscus* means ribbon), a flattened bundle of fibers that proceeds rostrally through the brainstem and terminates in the thalamus. Third-order fibers arising in the thalamus (specifically in the *ventral posterolateral nucleus* of the thalamus, or *VPL*) ascend through the internal capsule to synapse mainly in the cortex of the postcentral gyrus, the primary somatosensory cortex.

When the primary afferents of the posterior columns

*Significant numbers of unmyelinated fibers have recently been noted in the posterior columns, but at this point little is known of their significance. Some are branches of primary visceral afferents.

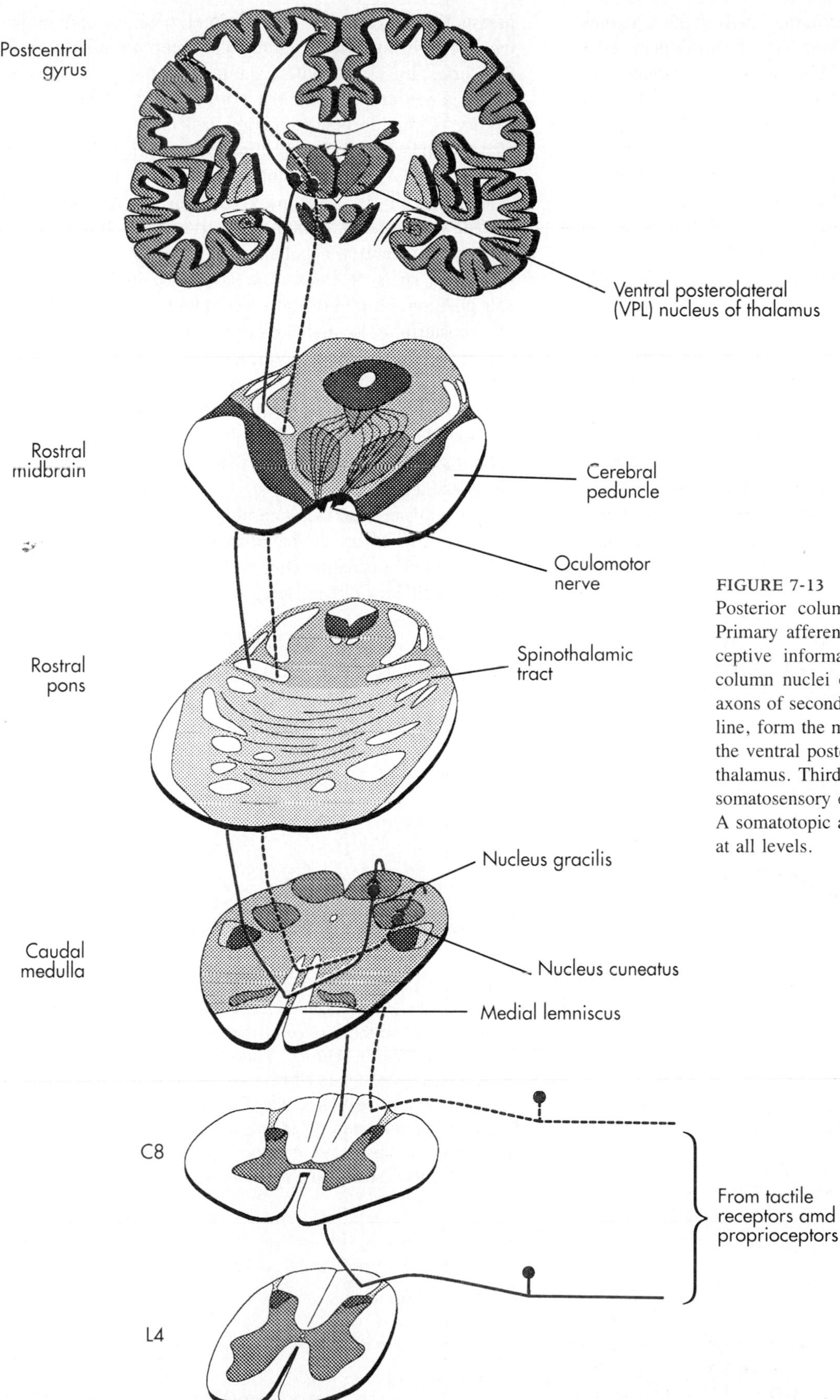


FIGURE 7-13
Posterior column-medial lemniscus pathway. Primary afferents carrying tactile and proprioceptive information synapse in the posterior column nuclei of the ipsilateral medulla. The axons of second order cells then cross the midline, form the medial lemniscus, and ascend to the ventral posterolateral (VPL) nucleus of the thalamus. Third order fibers then project to the somatosensory cortex of the postcentral gyrus. A somatotopic arrangement of fibers is present at all levels.

terminate in the posterior column nuclei, they maintain their somatotopic organization. Fibers from sacral levels terminate in the most medial portions of the nucleus gracilis, and fibers from cervical levels terminate in the most lateral portions of the nucleus cuneatus. A somatotopic arrangement is found throughout the rest of this pathway, so that information from sacral segments travels through a particular part of the medial lemniscus, projects to a particular portion of the VPL, and proceeds to a particular region of the postcentral gyrus. This does not mean that the sacral-to-cervical sequence remains along a medial-to-lateral line throughout the pathway, but rather that sacral information remains segregated from cervical information at all points along the way to somatosensory cortex. You may find it easier to keep track of the somatotopic arrangement of the pathway at different levels if you envision it as an actual map of the body (a *homunculus,* from the Latin word meaning little person), with sacral and lumbar levels corresponding to the legs, thoracic to the trunk, and cervical to the arms and neck. Viewed in this way, the homunculus is lying down with its feet toward the midline, up to the level of the posterior column nuclei. Its subsequent gyrations are described in the next chapter.

As might be expected from the types of afferents contained in the posterior columns, this pathway carries information relevant to the conscious appreciation of touch, pressure, and vibration and of joint position and movement. Since input from cutaneous receptors also reaches the cortex by other routes, damage to the posterior columns causes impairment, but not abolition, of tactile sensibility. Complex discrimination tasks are more severely affected than is simple detection of stimuli. (For this reason, whereas posterior column function is commonly tested clinically by touching a vibrating tuning fork to the surface of the body, a more effective test is having a patient try to identify a pattern drawn on the skin.) Other functions, such as *kinesthesia* (sense of body movement and position), are classically considered to be totally lost after posterior column destruction.* The result is a distinctive type of *ataxia* (incoordination of muscular activity); the brain is unable to direct motor activity properly without sensory feedback as to the current position of parts of the body. This ataxia is particularly pronounced when the patient's eyes are closed, so that visual compensation is not possible.

*Spinothalamic tract.* Collaterals of some touch- and pressure-sensitive fibers in the posterior columns, as well as collaterals of mechanoreceptive, thermoreceptive, and nociceptive fibers of the lateral division of the dorsal root,

*Although, as discussed later in this chapter, severe kinesthetic deficits imply additional damage to nearby structures.

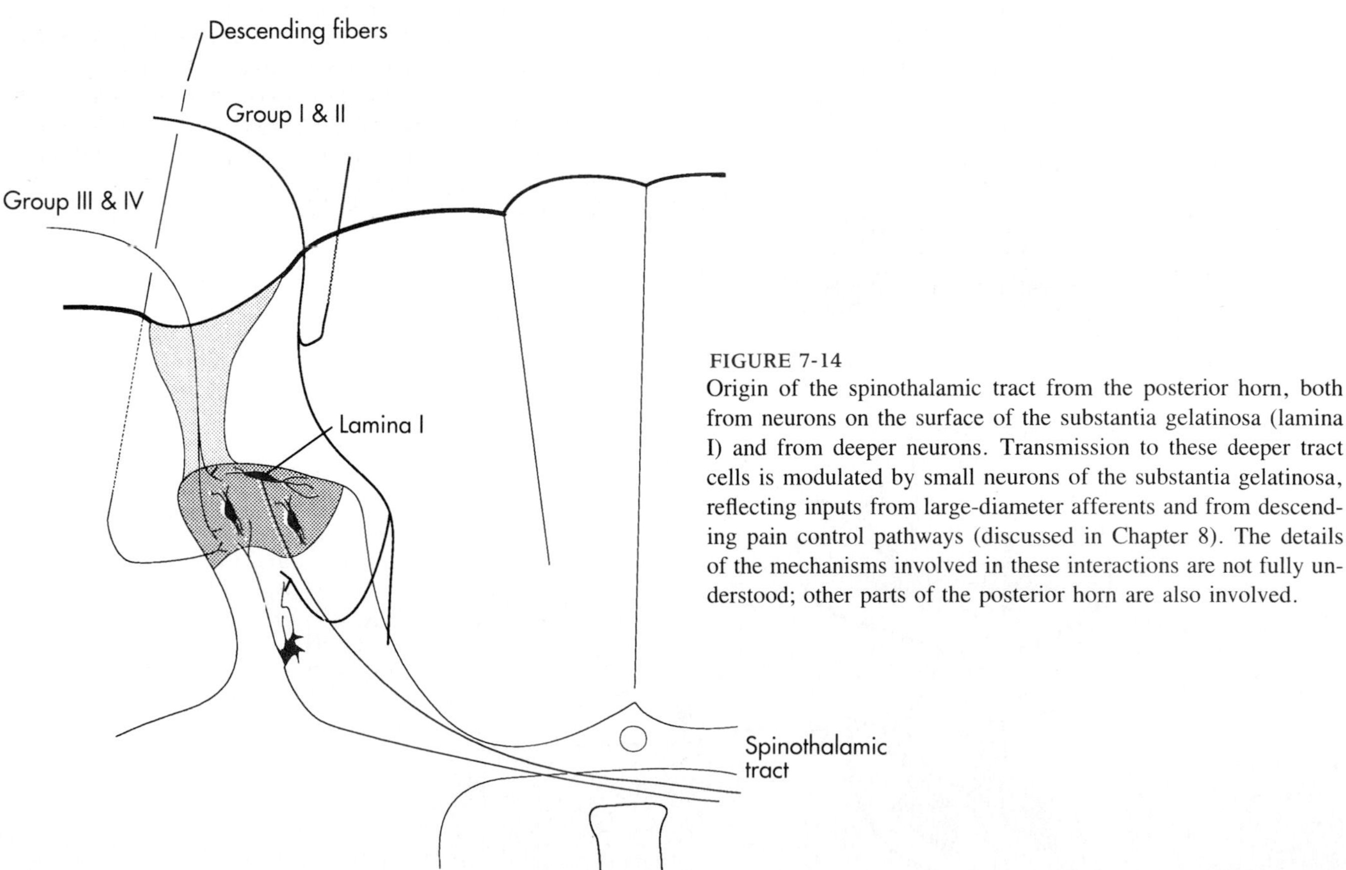


FIGURE 7-14
Origin of the spinothalamic tract from the posterior horn, both from neurons on the surface of the substantia gelatinosa (lamina I) and from deeper neurons. Transmission to these deeper tract cells is modulated by small neurons of the substantia gelatinosa, reflecting inputs from large-diameter afferents and from descending pain control pathways (discussed in Chapter 8). The details of the mechanisms involved in these interactions are not fully understood; other parts of the posterior horn are also involved.

enter the posterior horn and synapse in or near the substantia gelatinosa (Figure 7-14). Although these afferents end in the substantia gelatinosa, the latter cells do not give rise to the spinothalamic tract. Rather, the same afferents make additional synapses on dendrites of neurons whose cell bodies are located deeper in the posterior horn or on the surface of the substantia gelatinosa (Figures 7-14 and 7-15). These second-order cells of the pain and temperature pathway then send their axons across the midline with a slight rostral inclination to form the *spinothalamic tract** (Figures 7-16 and 7-17). This is one alternate pathway by which mechanoreceptive input reaches the thalamus and cerebral cortex, but more importantly it is the primary pathway for pain and temperature information. The tract occupies most of the anterior half of the lateral funiculus. New fibers join the spinothalamic tract at its ventromedial edge, so that this tract, like the posterior columns, is somatotopically organized. Fibers from the most caudal segments occupy its most dorsolateral portion, and those from more rostral segments occupy more ventromedial portions.

The spinothalamic tract was traditionally subdivided into the lateral and anterior spinothalamic tracts, the former subserving pain and temperature sensation and the latter some aspects of tactile sensation. It now appears, however, that all these types of fibers are intermingled to a great extent, and the whole complex is now referred to as a single spinothalamic tract. On the other hand, the spinothalamic pathway can be subdivided on the basis of the origin, destination, and probable function of the fibers. One subset of spinothalamic fibers arises from laminae I and V and projects directly to its own part of the VPL and adjoining nuclei of the thalamus in the same somatotopic fashion as the medial lemniscus. This has been called the *neospinothalamic tract;* some investigators feel that it has a special role in the appreciation of sharp, pricking, well-localized pain (related to that mediated by Aδ fibers). A second subset, arising mainly from the intermediate gray and parts of the anterior horn (laminae VI to VIII), projects to different parts of the thalamus (the intralaminar and other nuclei) without a somatotopic arrangement.

*Information about pain and temperature, much as in the case of tactile and proprioceptive information, travels in multiple parallel pathways. "Spinothalamic tract" is used here as a convenient umbrella term for this collection of tracts (described briefly in the next text paragraph), all of which deal with pain and temperature but some of which do not even reach the thalamus. A commonly used alternate term for this group of tracts, one that avoids the ambiguity of calling all of them spinothalamic, is the *anterolateral pathway*.

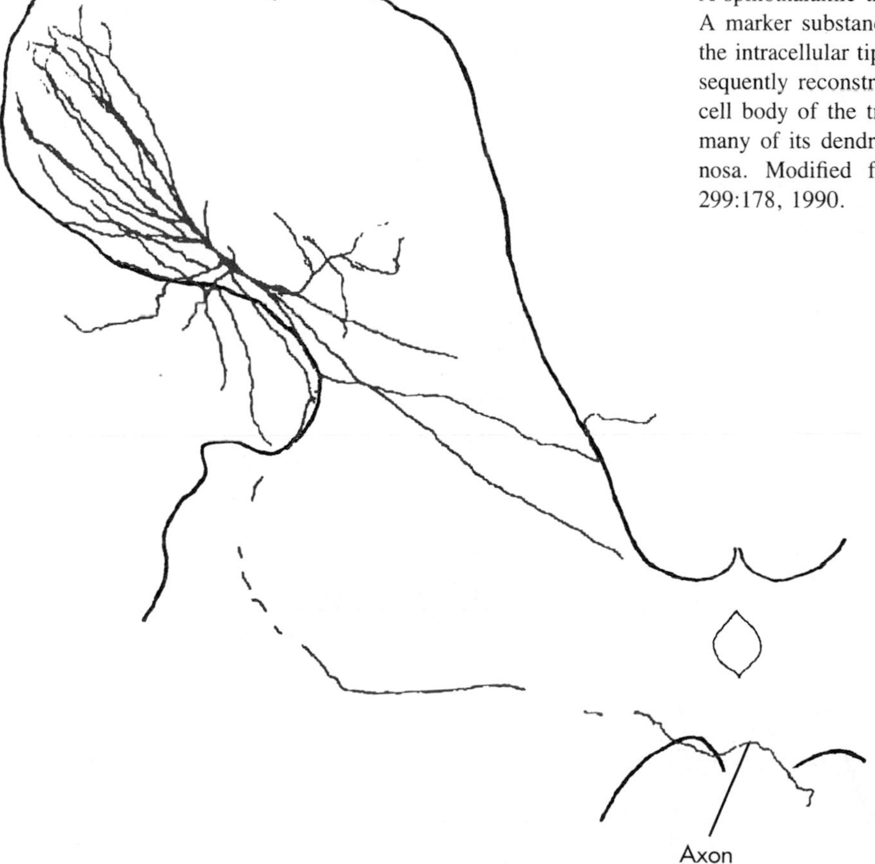


FIGURE 7-15
A spinothalamic tract neuron from the spinal cord of a monkey. A marker substance (horseradish peroxidase) was injected from the intracellular tip of a microelectrode, and the neuron was subsequently reconstructed from a series of sections. Although the cell body of the tract cell is located deep in the posterior horn, many of its dendrites extend upwards into the substantia gelatinosa. Modified from Westlund KN et al.: *J Comp Neurol* 299:178, 1990.

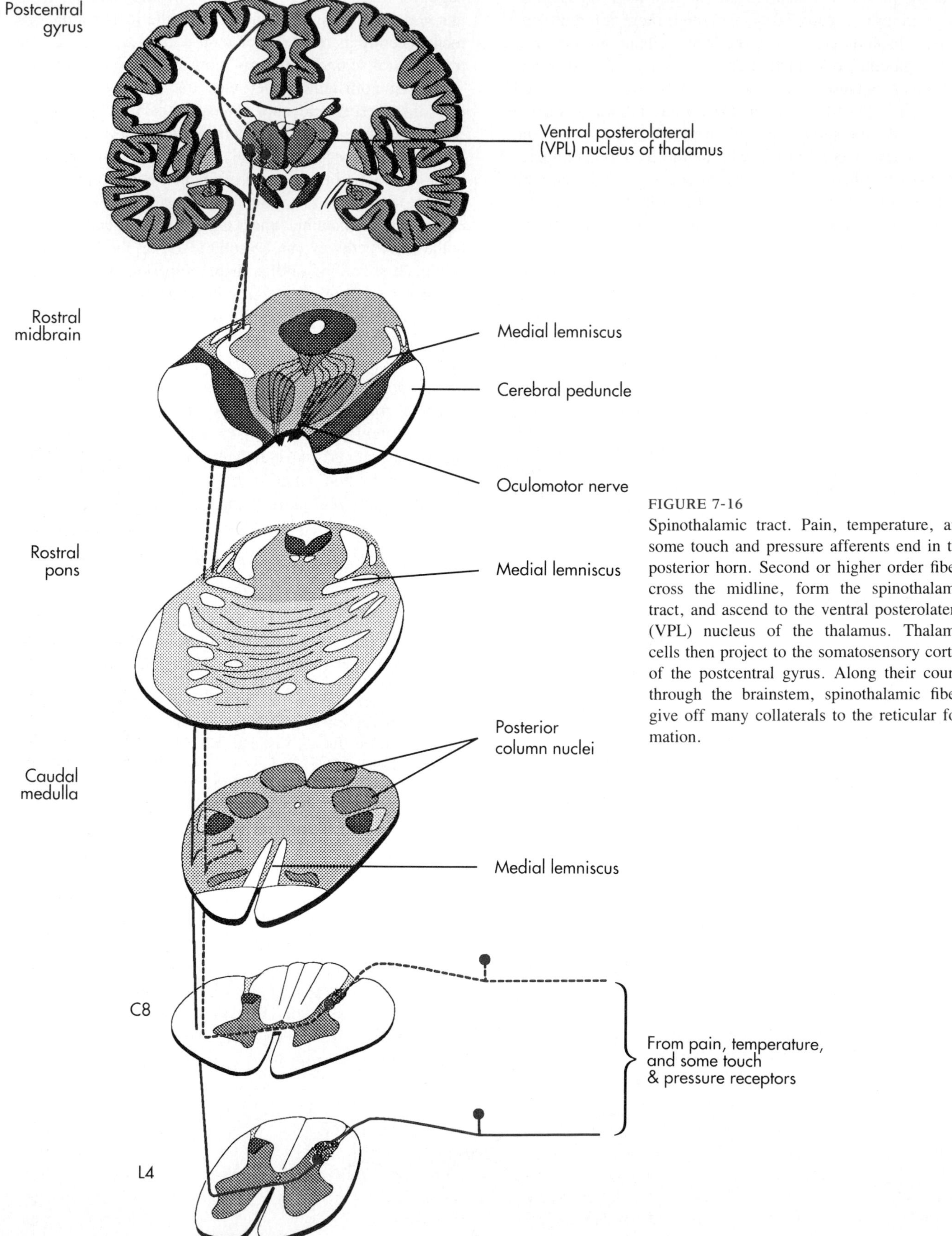


FIGURE 7-16
Spinothalamic tract. Pain, temperature, and some touch and pressure afferents end in the posterior horn. Second or higher order fibers cross the midline, form the spinothalamic tract, and ascend to the ventral posterolateral (VPL) nucleus of the thalamus. Thalamic cells then project to the somatosensory cortex of the postcentral gyrus. Along their course through the brainstem, spinothalamic fibers give off many collaterals to the reticular formation.

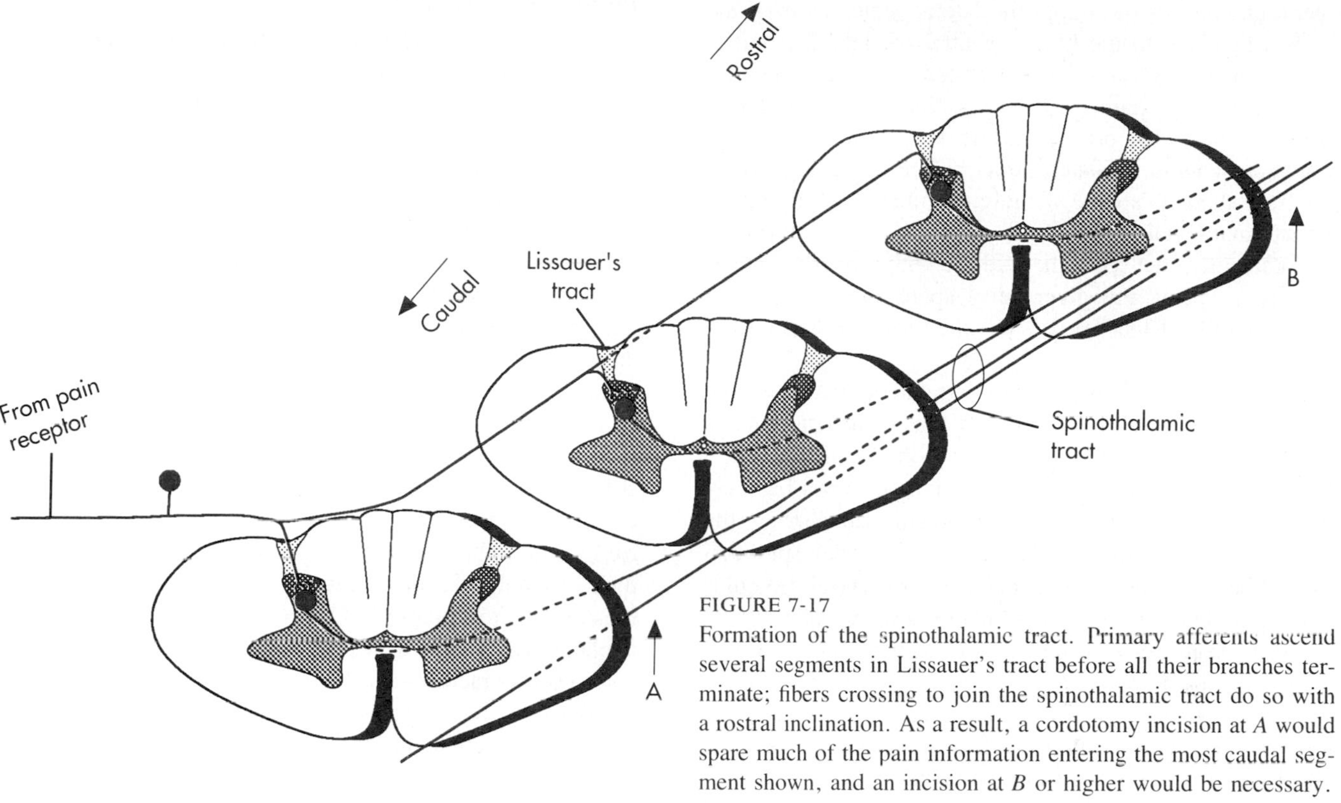


FIGURE 7-17
Formation of the spinothalamic tract. Primary afferents ascend several segments in Lissauer's tract before all their branches terminate; fibers crossing to join the spinothalamic tract do so with a rostral inclination. As a result, a cordotomy incision at *A* would spare much of the pain information entering the most caudal segment shown, and an incision at *B* or higher would be necessary.

Many of the latter projections are indirect, following a polysynaptic course through the reticular formation, which makes up much of the core of the brainstem (Chapter 8), and so they are more properly called *spinoreticular fibers*. Those that do pass directly to the intralaminar nuclei have been called the *paleospinothalamic tract*. There is some evidence that these, together with the spinoreticular fibers, have a special role in the sensation of dull, aching, poorly localized pain related to that mediated by C fibers. Finally, a collection of *spinomesencephalic* fibers, also arising mainly from laminae I and V, probably plays an important role in pain control (discussed in Chapter 8). All these neospinothalamic, paleospinothalamic, spinomesencephalic, and spinoreticular fibers are intermingled or adjacent to one another in the spinal cord, but the neospinothalamic component pursues a separate course in the brainstem, as discussed in the next chapter.

The role of the substantia gelatinosa in the transmission of pain information is incompletely understood at the present time. Anatomically it consists of large numbers of small cells among which finely myelinated and unmyelinated cutaneous afferents terminate (muscle and visceral afferents apparently bypass the substantia gelatinosa). Very few of these small cells give rise to long ascending axons; rather, they interact with tract cells and interneurons that also receive input from pain and temperature afferents (see Figure 7-14). The substantia gelatinosa is therefore strategically organized to regulate the access of pain and temperature information to the spinothalamic tract. The notion of the dependence of the perception of pain on the balance of activity in large and small afferents was referred to briefly in Chapter 6. The substantia gelatinosa is apparently one site at which these activities are compared and the transmission of pain information is modulated.

Although the spinothalamic tract carries some tactile and pressure information, a great deal also travels in the posterior column system, so destruction of the spinothalamic tract causes no significant tactile deficit. There are, however, several types of sensation (in addition to pain and temperature) subserved more or less predominantly by the spinothalamic tract. These are itch (and probably tickle) sensations, pressure sensations from bladder and bowel, and sexual sensations. However, with the exception of itch (and possibly tickle), this information is carried bilaterally, so unilateral damage generally results in little dysfunction. This may be considered a particularly elegant example of the providence of nature.

The spinothalamic tract is, however, the principal pathway for somatic pain sensations, and its destruction produces contralateral analgesia. An operation to destroy the tract (called a *cordotomy* or *chordotomy*) is sometimes performed on patients suffering from intractable pain. This operation consists of cutting the lateral funiculus from the dentate ligament to the line of ventral rootlets. The cut is usually made several segments rostral to the highest dermatomal level of pain, for two reasons (see Figure 7-17). First, collaterals of primary afferents may ascend one or more segments in Lissauer's tract before synapsing, so input from these is spared if the cut is made at the highest dermatomal level of pain. Second, the axons that form the spinothalamic tract cross the midline with a rostral inclination, so a cut at any given level spares fibers that arise contralaterally at that level, since they join the tract rostral to the cut.

Cordotomy provides prompt contralateral analgesia, but surprisingly the analgesia is usually not permanent. After a varying interval (generally several months), the patient's pain frequently returns. The reason is not known but may be the increasing efficacy of a few uncrossed fibers in the contralateral spinothalamic tract, of additional spinothalamic fibers located more dorsally in the lateral funiculus or of a limited number of pain fibers in other pathways.

*Other somatosensory pathways.* In recent years additional routes for the transmission of tactile and proprioceptive (and to a lesser extent, pain) information have been described. One such route consists of nonprimary afferents, fibers with their cell bodies in the posterior horn, that nevertheless project to the posterior column nuclei. Some of these travel within the posterior columns, but others travel in the posterior part of the lateral funiculus. The latter route seems to be particularly important for conveying proprioceptive information from the leg to the nucleus gracilis.

Another alternate route is the *spinocervical tract*. Primary afferents conveying information from hair receptors, some other tactile receptors, and some nociceptors synapse on tract cells in the body of the posterior horn (mainly laminae III and IV). These tract cells send their axons ipsilaterally through the posterior part of the lateral funiculus as the spinocervical tract. The spinocervical tract then terminates in the small *lateral cervical nucleus,* which is embedded in the lateral funiculus of the first two cervical segments. The axons of neurons in the lateral cervical nucleus then cross the midline, join the medial lemniscus as it forms in the caudal medulla, and ascend to the VPL.

The size and importance of these alternate pathways in the lateral funiculus are not known for humans, although both are known to exist in monkeys. They are mentioned here because evidence is slowly accumulating that they are important complements to the posterior column system. In monkeys, for example, combining a lesion of the posterior part of the lateral funiculus with a lesion of the ipsilateral posterior column results in a much more severe and long-lasting deficit than does damage to the posterior column alone.

### *Pathways to the cerebellum*

*Posterior spinocerebellar tract.* Collaterals of posterior column fibers conveying tactile, pressure, and proprioceptive information (mainly the latter, from muscle spindles and Golgi tendon organs) synapse on neurons of Clarke's nucleus. These then send their axons into the lateral funiculus of the same side, forming the *posterior spinocerebellar tract* (Figure 7-18). This tract, a curved band of fibers extending from the dorsal root entry zone to the dentate ligament, lies at the surface of the spinal cord. Fibers in the tract project ipsilaterally to the vermis of the cerebellum through the *inferior cerebellar peduncle*. Collaterals of some of these fibers end in the nucleus gracilis, providing an important route by which nonprimary afferents transmit proprioceptive information from the leg to the posterior column-medial lemniscus system. Since Clarke's nucleus does not exist caudal to L2 or L3, neither does the posterior spinocerebellar tract. However, afferents from segments caudal to L2 or L3 ascend to that level in the fasciculus gracilis to synapse in Clarke's nucleus. This probably explains why Clarke's nucleus is so large at upper lumbar and lower thoracic levels (Figure 7-5), since at these levels it has a large backlog of afferent input to process.

The posterior spinocerebellar tract is principally concerned with the ipsilateral leg. Most spinocerebellar-type afferents that enter in cervical and upper thoracic segments (for example, those representing the arm) do not project to Clarke's nucleus. Rather, they travel in the fasciculus cuneatus to a nucleus in the medulla analogous to Clarke's nucleus called the *lateral* (or *external*) *cuneate nucleus* because it is located just lateral to the nucleus cuneatus (Figure 8-6). Axons of these cells form the *cuneocerebellar tract,* which also projects ipsilaterally to the vermis of the cerebellum through the inferior cerebellar peduncle.

*Anterior spinocerebellar tract.* Cells in the body of the lumbosacral posterior horn, together with cells on the lateral surface of the anterior horn (called spinal border cells), give rise to the *anterior spinocerebellar tract*. Although this tract is also concerned primarily with the leg, it differs from the posterior spinocerebellar tract in three important respects. First, inputs to these tract cells are more complex; they come not only from group I muscle afferents (mainly Golgi tendon organs) but also from a wide variety of cutaneous receptors, from spinal interneurons, and from fibers of descending tracts. Second, the tract is crossed at the level of the spinal cord, in contrast to the posterior spinocerebellar tract, which ascends uncrossed to an ipsilateral termination in the cerebellum. Finally, the anterior spinocerebellar tract takes a roundabout route to the cerebellum (Figure 7-18). It ascends as far as the rostral pons, then turns caudally and enters the cerebellum via the *superior cerebellar peduncle*. There, most of its fibers recross the midline before ending in the vermis of the anterior

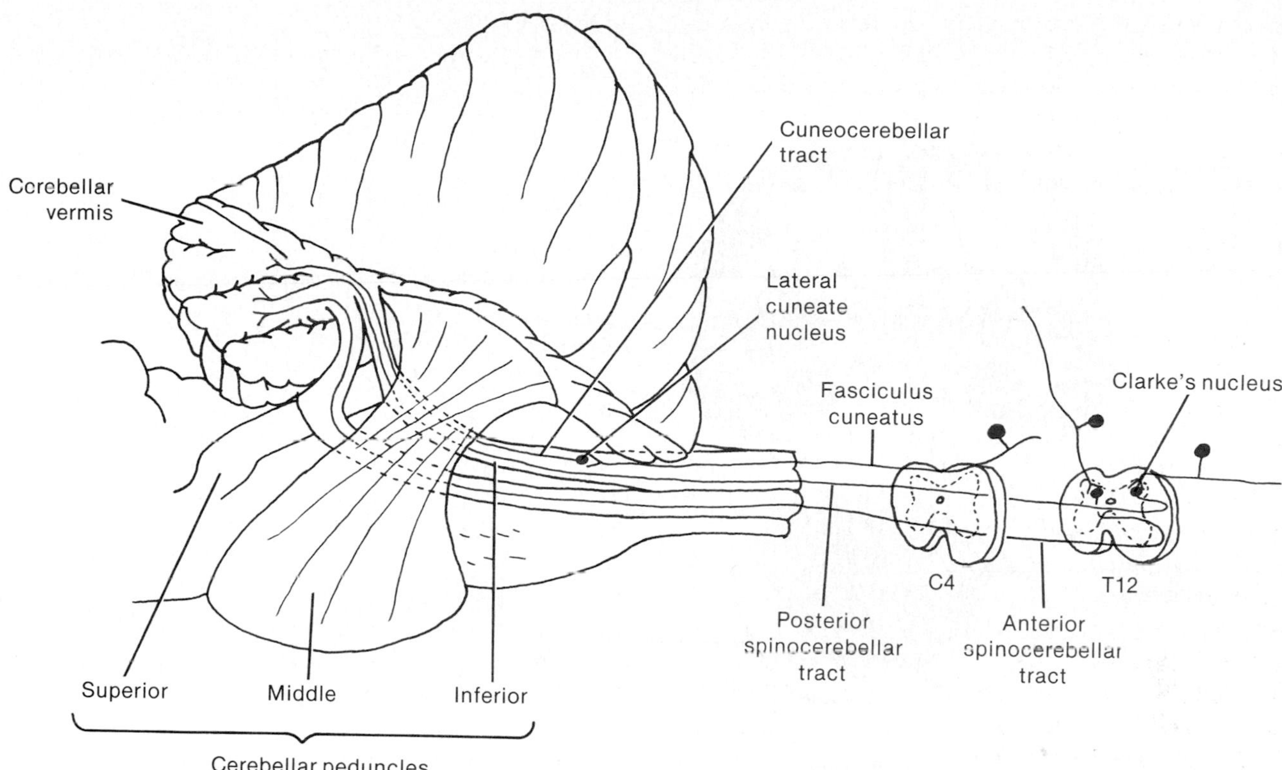


FIGURE 7-18
Spinocerebellar and cuneocerebellar tracts. Mechanoreceptive afferents from the lower extremity synapse in Clarke's nucleus, whose cells give rise to the ipsilateral posterior spinocerebellar tract, which enters the inferior cerebellar peduncle and ends ipsilaterally in the vermis of the anterior lobe. Similar afferents also end on other cells of the spinal gray matter, whose axons form the contralateral anterior spinocerebellar tract; this tract ascends to the pons, loops over the superior cerebellar peduncle, and recrosses in the vermis of the anterior lobe. Mechanoreceptive afferents from the upper extremity ascend to the medulla in the fasciculus cuneatus and end in the lateral cuneate nucleus (analogous to Clarke's nucleus); these cells give rise to the cuneocerebellar tract, which enters the inferior cerebellar peduncle and ends ipsilaterally in the vermis of the anterior lobe. The rostral spinocerebellar tract is not shown in this diagram.
Modified from Nieuwenhuys R et al: *The human central nervous system,* New York, 1978, Springer-Verlag.

lobe, so they too ultimately end in the cerebellum on the side ipsilateral to their origin.

A presumed forelimb equivalent of the anterior spinocerebellar tract, called the *rostral spinocerebellar tract,* originates from the posterior horn of lower cervical segments. Little is known of its properties, and it is mentioned here mainly for reasons of symmetry.

Clinically detectable deficits that can be attributed with confidence to damage to the spinocerebellar tracts are rare, partially because the spinocerebellar tracts are rarely if ever affected in isolation. Even in the family of inherited diseases referred to as the spinocerebellar atrophies, other areas of the cord are always affected as well. For example, the most common type of spinocerebellar atrophy is Friedreich's ataxia. This disorder is characterized by loss of coordination, which is consistent with cerebellar damage, but also by other impairments not consistent with cerebellar damage, such as disturbed tactile sensation and proprioception and loss of reflexes. Correspondingly widespread damage is found in and around the spinal cord, affecting not only the posterior spinocerebellar tracts but also the posterior columns and some dorsal root fibers. If the spinocerebellar tracts were selectively affected, one would not expect any sensory changes at all, since the cerebellum and its connections have nothing directly to do with sensation.

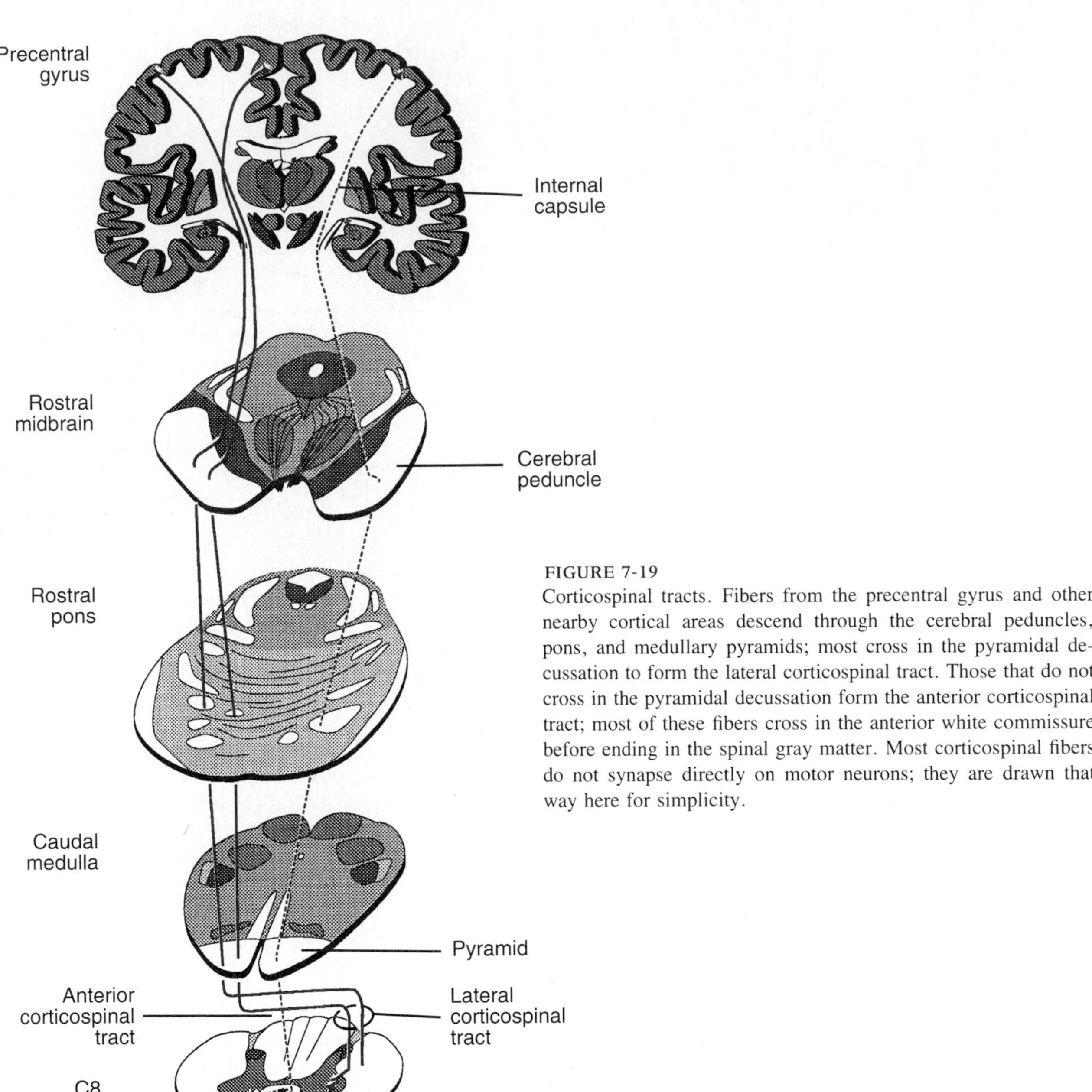


FIGURE 7-19
Corticospinal tracts. Fibers from the precentral gyrus and other nearby cortical areas descend through the cerebral peduncles, pons, and medullary pyramids; most cross in the pyramidal decussation to form the lateral corticospinal tract. Those that do not cross in the pyramidal decussation form the anterior corticospinal tract; most of these fibers cross in the anterior white commissure before ending in the spinal gray matter. Most corticospinal fibers do not synapse directly on motor neurons; they are drawn that way here for simplicity.

## Descending pathways

The alpha and gamma motor neurons of the anterior horn are regulated in a variety of ways by supraspinal centers. Some of these centers are located in the brainstem and are discussed in later chapters. The major descending outflow is from the cerebral cortex, particularly the precentral gyrus. This *corticospinal* system is dealt with at length in Chapter 12, but a few basic concepts are introduced here.

### *Corticospinal tract*

The *lateral corticospinal tract* (Figure 7-19) is a large, crossed, descending tract that contains the approximately 85% of fibers from the contralateral pyramid that cross in the pyramidal decussation. It is also known as the *pyramidal tract* and occupies the posterior portion of the lateral funiculus medial to the posterior spinocerebellar tract. Its fibers originate in the cerebral cortex (in the precentral gyrus and nearby areas); descend through the cerebral peduncle, basal pons, and medullary pyramid; decussate; and end in the anterior horn or intermediate gray matter. They terminate on the motor neurons of the anterior horn or, more often, on smaller interneurons that in turn synapse on these motor neurons. Lateral corticospinal fibers are arranged somatotopically, with those destined for more caudal cord levels located more laterally.

The difference between fibers of the pyramidal tract and the motor axons of the ventral root should be clearly understood. Alpha motor neurons (and the ventral root fibers these neurons give rise to) contact striated muscle directly and are called *lower motor neurons*. They are also sometimes called the "final common pathway" of the motor system, since, as noted earlier, they are the only means by which the nervous system can exercise control over body movements. Interruption of the lower motor neurons supplying a muscle causes flaccid paralysis and, eventually, atrophy of the muscle.

Neurons with axons that descend from the cerebral cortex or brainstem and end on lower motor neurons, either directly or by way of an interneuron, are called *upper motor neurons*.* An upper motor neuron lesion caused by corticospinal damage—often referred to clinically as a pyramidal lesion, although there are problems with this designation (see Chapter 12)—has very different effects from those of a lower motor neuron lesion. Characteristically,

*Some use this term in a more restricted sense to refer only to corticospinal neurons.

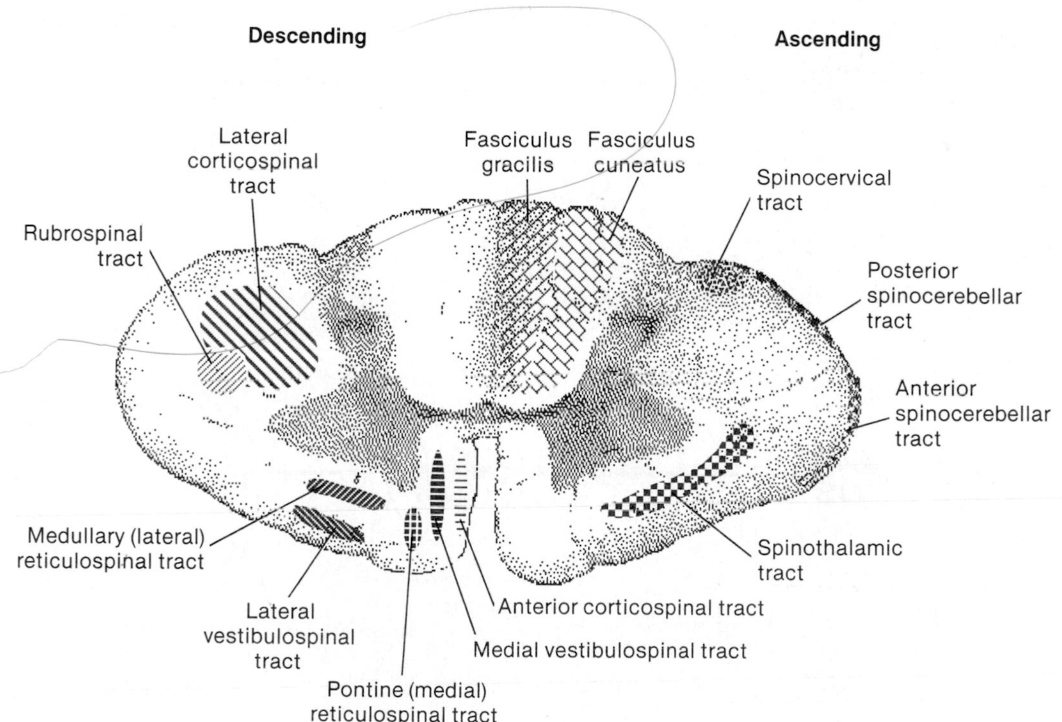


FIGURE 7-20
Summary diagram of the principal tracts present in the lower cervical spinal cord. Descending pathways are indicated on the left, ascending pathways on the right. Not all of these tracts were mentioned in this chapter. The medullary (lateral) reticulospinal and pontine (medial) reticulospinal tracts are discussed in Chapter 8; the lateral vestibulospinal and medial vestibulospinal tracts are discussed in Chapter 9; and the rubrospinal tract is discussed in Chapter 12.

the muscles involved show hyperactive reflexes. Their resting tension is increased (that is, they are *hypertonic*), and there is paralysis or weakness *(paresis)*, particularly of fine voluntary movements. This complex of symptoms is referred to as *spastic paralysis*. A number of pathological reflexes are associated with upper motor neuron lesions. The best known is *Babinski's sign*—dorsiflexion of the big toe and fanning of the others in response to firmly stroking the sole of the foot. (Note that Babinski's sign is either present or not present; it is not "positive" or "negative.")

The 15% or so of the fibers in each pyramid that do not cross in the pyramidal decussation continue into the anterior funiculus (located adjacent to the anterior median fissure) as the *anterior corticospinal tract* (Figures 7-19 and 7-20). These fibers also terminate on motor neurons or interneurons of the anterior horn or intermediate gray matter, mainly in cervical and thoracic segments. Many of them cross in the anterior white commissure before synapsing, but some do not. Strictly speaking, the term "pyramidal tract" refers to the combination of lateral and anterior corticospinal tracts.

## AUTONOMIC NERVOUS SYSTEM

The goings on of our cardiac and smooth muscles and our glands proceed, for the most part, without conscious supervision—indeed, in spite of attempts at conscious supervision. For instance, we automatically digest our food, regulate our heartbeat, sweat when appropriate, and divert blood to active muscles. Because of the relative automaticity of such functions, the afferents and efferents that innervate these organs are referred to as the *autonomic nervous system*.*

The autonomic nervous system has three subdivisions: the *sympathetic, parasympathetic,* and *enteric nervous systems*. Although less well known than the other two, the enteric nervous system perhaps best exemplifies the concept of automatic, self-regulating function. It consists of two interconnected plexuses (the *myenteric plexus* [of Auerbach] and the *submucous plexus* [of Meissner]), in-

*The autonomic nervous system as originally defined consists only of visceral efferents. However, most now use the term to refer to afferents as well.

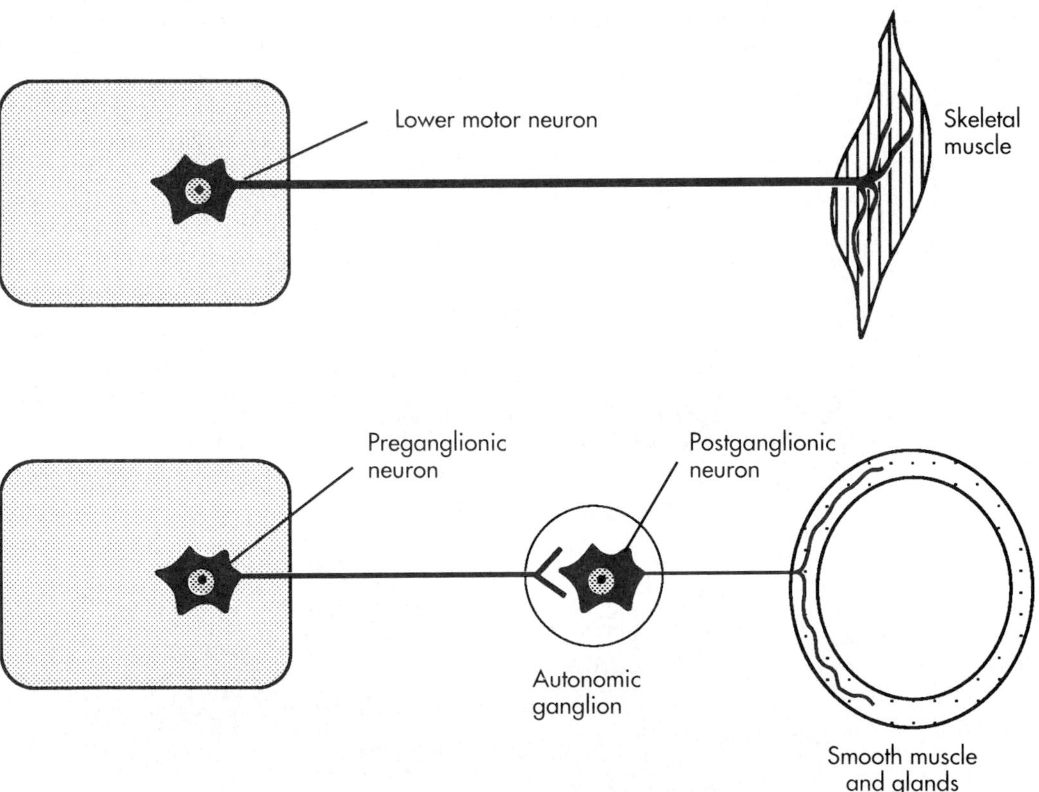


FIGURE 7-21
Schematic diagram of one major difference between somatic and autonomic efferents. The axons of lower motor neurons leave the spinal cord through ventral roots (or leave the brainstem through cranial nerves) and reach skeletal muscle directly. The autonomic system, in contrast, uses a two-neuron path. The axons of preganglionic neurons leave through ventral roots or cranial nerves and end on postganglionic neurons in autonomic ganglia outside the CNS. Axons of postganglionic neurons then innervate smooth muscles and glands.

cluding sensory neurons, interneurons, and visceral motor neurons, in the walls of the alimentary canal; all of these neurons and their processes lie entirely outside the CNS. The plexuses are quite extensive. It has been estimated that they contain $10^8$ neurons, a number comparable to the number of neurons in the entire spinal cord. The enteric nervous system accounts for the observation that near-normal coordinated gut motility persists even in the total absence of connections between the gut and the CNS. The normally present sympathetic and parasympathetic connections between the gut and the CNS allow for modulation of this motility.

The sympathetic and parasympathetic divisions of the autonomic nervous system, on the other hand, have a more familiar organization. Similar to the somatic portions of the nervous system considered thus far, there are visceral sensory fibers, ascending visceral sensory pathways, visceral reflex arcs, and descending pathways that control the activity of visceral motor neurons. One fundamental difference is that sympathetic and parasympathetic efferents originating in the central nervous system do not reach their targets directly; rather, a two-neuron chain is involved (Figure 7-21). The first neuron, referred to as a *preganglionic neuron,* has its cell body in the CNS. Its axon terminates in a peripheral ganglion on the second neuron, termed a *postganglionic neuron*. Preganglionic fibers are thinly myelinated (group B), whereas postganglionic fibers are unmyelinated. Sympathetic ganglia are located near the CNS; parasympathetic ganglia are located near the organs they innervate (Figure 7-22). The sympathetic and parasympathetic nervous systems also differ in the neurotransmitter used by their postganglionic neurons (see Figure 7-22). The preganglionic neurons of both systems liberate acetylcholine onto the postganglionic neurons. Postganglionic parasympathetic neurons also release acetylcholine onto their targets. Most postganglionic sympathetic neurons, in contrast, release norepinephrine (a prominent exception is the sympathetic innervation of sweat glands, which is cholinergic). Other differences between the sympathetic and parasympathetic systems are reviewed briefly in the following sections.

### Parasympathetic nervous system

Preganglionic parasympathetic fibers originate from neurons in two widely separated parts of the CNS, the brainstem and the sacral spinal cord (Figure 7-23). They travel in sacral spinal nerves or in certain cranial nerves (III, VII, IX, and most important, X, as discussed further in Chapter 9) to ganglia in or near their targets. Postganglionic neurons in these peripheral parasympathetic ganglia then innervate the target organ. Relative to the case in sympathetic ganglia, there is little divergence in parasym-

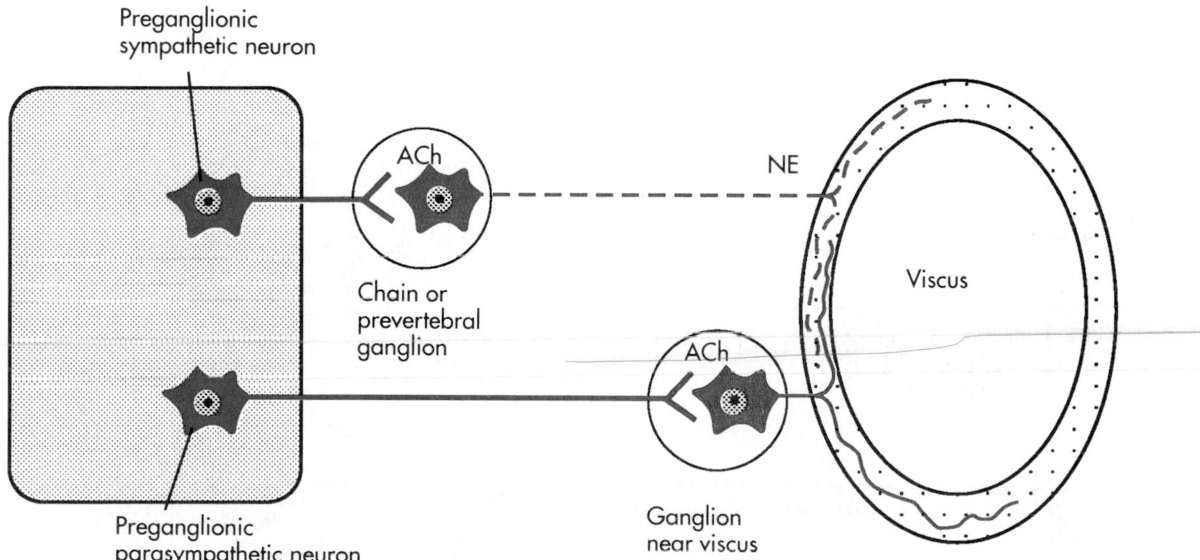


FIGURE 7-22
Major differences between the sympathetic and parasympathetic systems. The axons of preganglionic sympathetic neurons end in ganglia near the spinal cord, whereas those of preganglionic parasympathetic neurons travel a longer distance and reach ganglia near the innervated organ. The preganglionic neurons of both systems use acetylcholine *(ACh)* as their neurotransmitter, but at the synapses of postganglionic neurons the parasympathetic system uses acetylcholine and the sympathetic system typically uses norepinephrine *(NE)*.

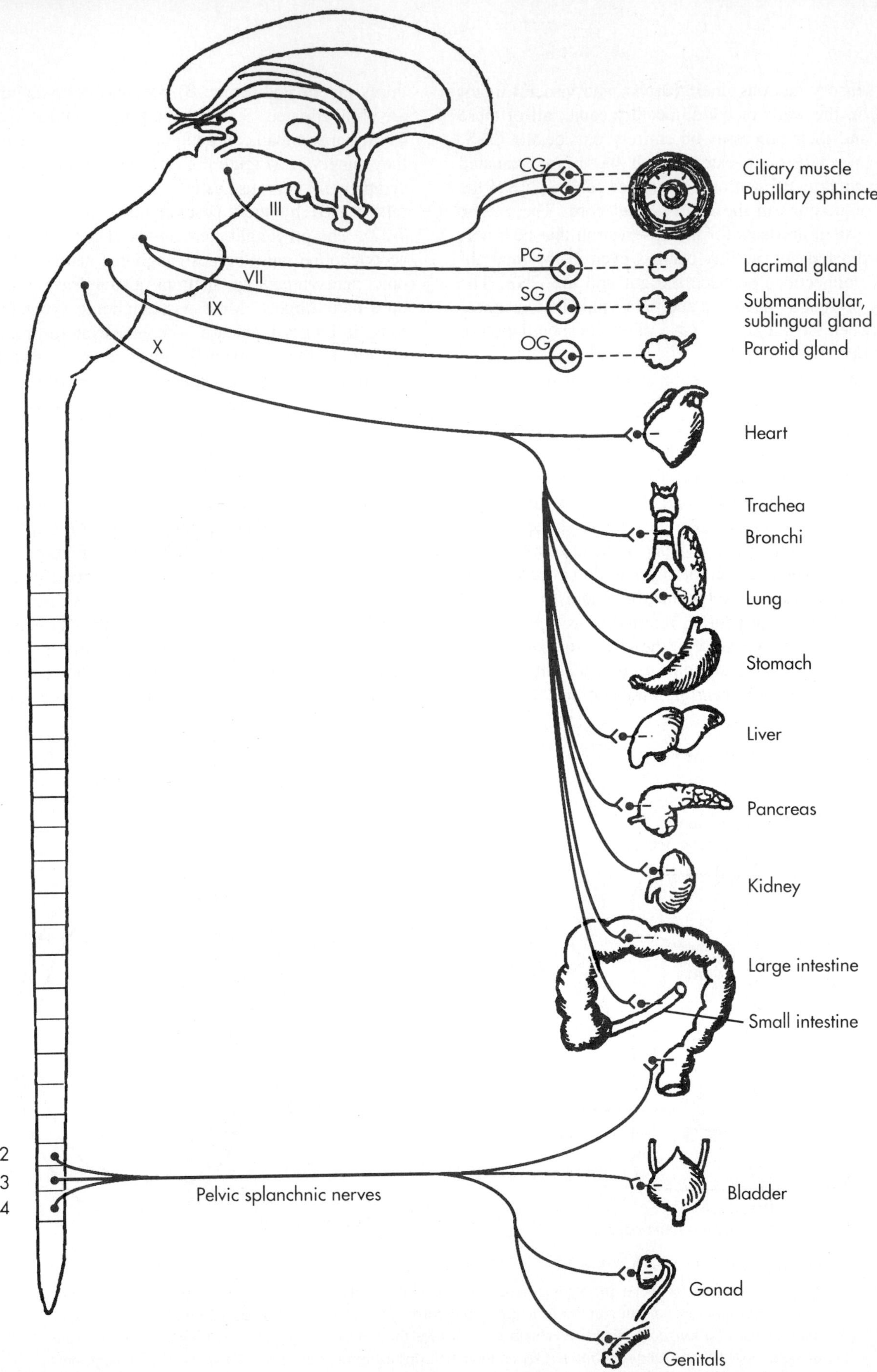


FIGURE 7-23
Origin and distribution of parasympathetic efferents. Although the cranial nerves have distinct and separate parasympathetic contents, there is substantial overlap in the contents of ventral roots S2 to S4. Abbreviations: CG, ciliary ganglion; OG, otic ganglion; PG, pterygopalatine ganglion; SG, submandibular ganglion. (Adapted from Mettler FA: *Neuroanatomy*, ed. 2, St. Louis, 1948, The C.V. Mosby Co.)

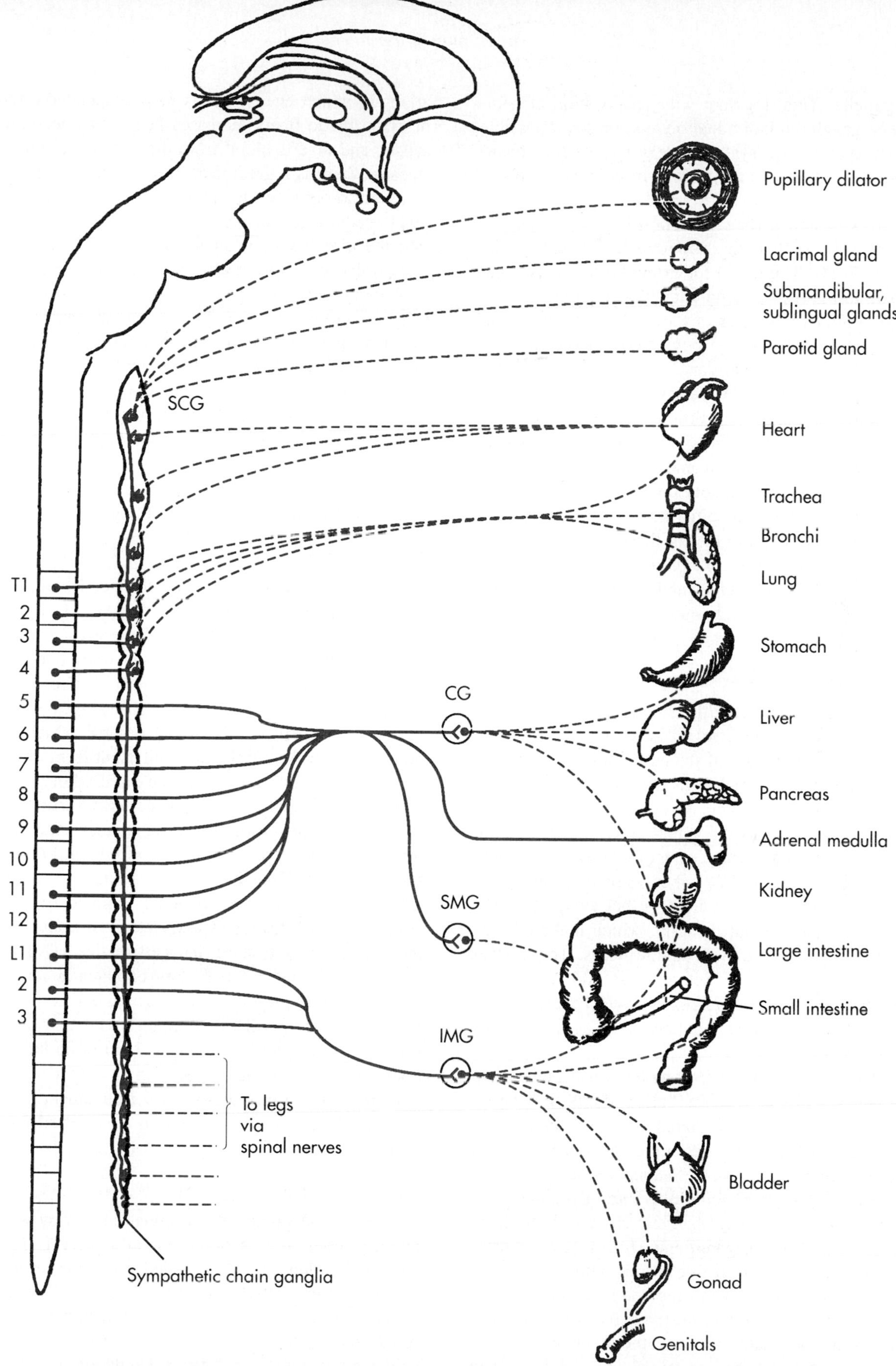


FIGURE 7-24

Origin and distribution of sympathetic efferents. Postganglionic neurons that live in sympathetic chain ganglia and project to the body wall and upper extremity are omitted from the diagram to avoid excessive complexity; their axons travel in spinal nerves in a way analogous to that indicated for the lower extremity supply. Abbreviations: CG, celiac ganglion; IMG, inferior mesenteric ganglion, SCG, superior cervical ganglion; SMG, superior mesenteric ganglion. (Adapted from Mettler FA: *Neuroanatomy*, ed. 2, St. Louis, 1948, The C.V. Mosby Co.)

pathetic ganglia. This, together with the location of parasympathetic ganglia in individual organs, makes it possible for the parasympathetic system to exert restricted, localized control. Sympathetic activation, in contrast, tends to be more widespread.

The parasympathetic (or *craniosacral*) outflow goes almost exclusively to thoracic, abdominal, and pelvic viscera (Figure 7-23). There are, for example, no parasympathetic fibers to the limbs. (One clinically important exception is the pupillary sphincter of the eyeball; the parasympathetic fibers included in the oculomotor nerve serve as the efferent limb of the pupillary light reflex [Figure 11-14].) In a general sense, the parasympathetic system enhances energy storage. Activation of parasympathetic nerves causes decreased cardiac output and blood pressure, increased peristalsis in the gut and salivation, as well as pupillary constriction and bladder contraction. Visceral afferents traveling with sacral spinal nerves and with cranial nerves IX and X are appropriate for these functions, carrying information about things like blood pressure and chemistry and fullness of the bladder and gastrointestinal tract. Cranial nerves VII, IX, and X also carry information from taste buds, obviously relevant to energy intake.

### Sympathetic nervous system

Preganglionic sympathetic fibers originate from neurons in the thoracic and upper two or three lumbar segments (Figure 7-24). This division of the autonomic nervous system therefore is also referred to as the *thoracolumbar outflow*. The preganglionic fibers travel in spinal nerves to ganglia relatively close to the spinal cord. Some of these ganglia form an interconnected *sympathetic chain* adjacent to the spinal cord (Figure 7-2), whereas others, referred to as *prevertebral ganglia,* are a little farther away. The major exception is the adrenal medulla, which is directly innervated by preganglionic sympathetic fibers. The adrenal medulla develops from the neural crest and, similar to postganglionic sympathetic neurons, its cells secrete norepinephrine; it can therefore be thought of as a displaced sympathetic ganglion.

Sympathetic fibers are more widely distributed than parasympathetic fibers, reaching all parts of the body. Preganglionic fibers exit the spinal cord in thoracic and lumbar nerves and then travel from the spinal nerves to the sympathetic chain via *white communicating rami,* so called because the preganglionic fibers are myelinated and hence white. Some end in sympathetic chain ganglia, from which unmyelinated postganglionic fibers rejoin spinal nerves via *gray communicating rami*. Others continue through the chain without synapsing and reach prevertebral ganglia. Postganglionic fibers destined for the head, thorax, and limbs originate in sympathetic chain ganglia, whereas those destined for abdominal and pelvic viscera originate in prevertebral ganglia.

Generally, the sympathetic system prepares us for situations in which energy needs to be expended. Activation of sympathetic fibers increases heart rate, decreases peristalsis, and diverts blood from the gut to skeletal muscles. Because there is a great deal of divergence in sympathetic ganglia and because sympathetic stimulation causes the adrenal medulla to secrete norepinephrine and epinephrine into the circulation, sympathetic activation tends to produce widespread and relatively long-lasting effects.

Although in some instances, such as effects on gut motility and heart rate, the sympathetic and parasympathetic systems have opposite effects, in other instances one or the other is unopposed or both act cooperatively. For example, sweat glands and limb vasculature receive only sympathetic innervation, but the parasympathetic system is the dominant influence in control of the pupil and the bladder. The two systems cooperate in male sexual function; erection is mediated primarily by parasympathetic fibers and ejaculation is mediated by sympathetic fibers.

### Referred pain

Visceral afferent fibers, with their cell bodies in T1 to L2 or L3 dorsal root ganglia, accompany sympathetic efferents in spinal nerves. Some of these carry information that subserves visceral reflexes and does not reach consciousness, such as data about vascular tone. Others, unlike parasympathetic nerves, carry messages about distortion or inflammation of visceral organs, which are interpreted as pain. Visceral pain is different from somatic pain in that it is poorly localized to the diseased organ and commonly is *referred* to an area of the body surface. The area to which the pain is referred corresponds to the dermatome innervated by the spinal segment to which the visceral afferents project. Thus the heart is supplied by visceral afferents that enter the cord in upper thoracic segments, and coronary artery disease is associated with pain referred to the left side of the chest and part of the left arm (angina pectoris). The most satisfactory explanation available for referred pain at present is that visceral and somatic pain fibers at a given level of the spinal cord converge on the same spinothalamic tract cells, and our brain interprets spinothalamic tract impulses as pain in the somatic region. The functional utility of such an arrangement is not clear, but knowledge of typical patterns of referred pain is important clinically.

## VASCULAR SUPPLY OF THE SPINAL CORD

The arterial supply of the spinal cord is by way of vertebral arteries and of branches, ultimately from the thoracic and abdominal aorta, called *radicular arteries*. Each vertebral artery gives rise to a *posterior spinal artery,* which proceeds along the line of attachment of the dorsal roots, and to an *anterior spinal artery*. The two anterior spinal arteries fuse to form a single midline vessel that courses along the anterior median fissure of the spinal cord (Figures 5-1 and 7-25). The posterior spinal arteries and

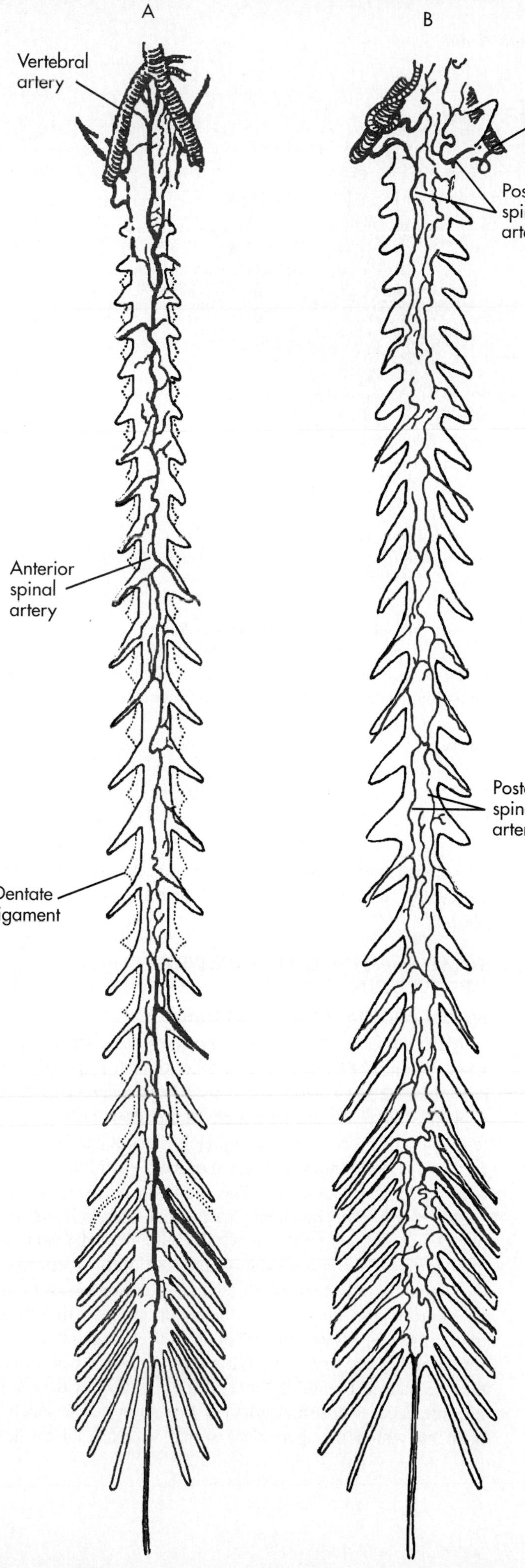


FIGURE 7-25

Arterial supply of the spinal cord. *A,* The anterior surface of the spinal cord, showing the midline anterior spinal artery and the series of radicular arteries that supply blood to it below upper cervical levels. The pattern of these radicular arteries is variable from one individual to another; in this example there are two large radicular arteries helping to supply caudal levels of the cord, although in most individuals there is only one. *B,* The posterior surface of the same spinal cord, demonstrating the plexiform arterial network that is conventionally referred to as paired posterior spinal arteries. (Redrawn from Mettler FA: *Neuroanatomy,* ed. 2, St. Louis, 1948, The C.V. Mosby Co.)

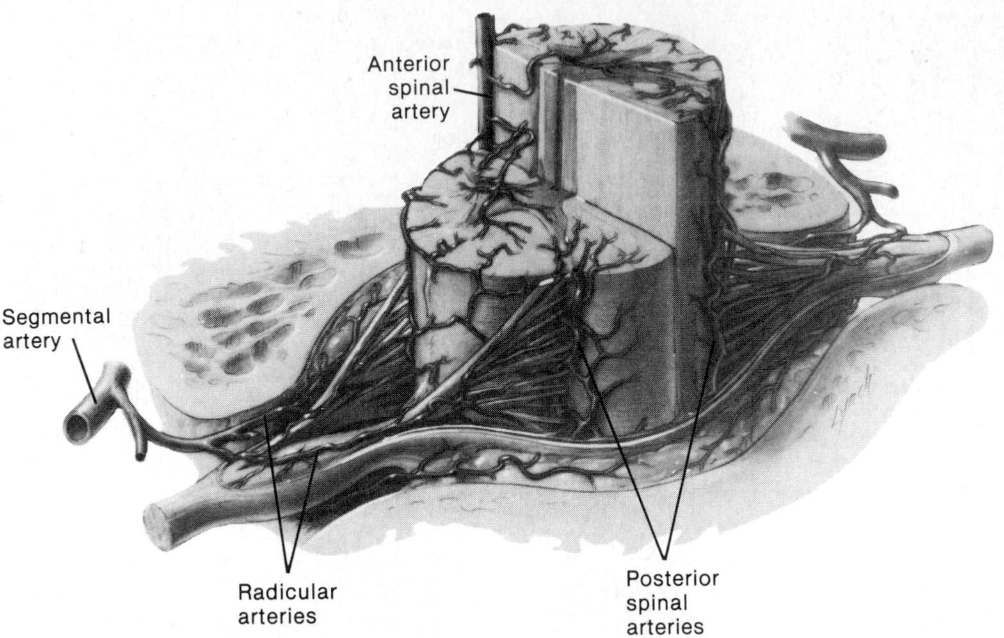


FIGURE 7-26
Arterial supply of the spinal cord. The anterior spinal artery, through hundreds of branches that pass either circumferentially or through the anterior median fissure, supplies the anterior two thirds of the cord. The posterior spinal arteries, really a paired arteriolar plexus, supply the posterior third of the cord. Both anterior and posterior spinal arteries receive contributions along their course from radicular arteries.
From Toole JF: *Cerebrovascular disorders,* ed 4, New York, 1990, Raven Press.

the midline anterior spinal artery supply upper cervical levels with blood from the vertebral arteries. Below this, all three spinal arteries form a more or less continuous series of anastomoses with radicular arteries for the length of the cord. The spinal arteries are rather small; beginning with lower cervical segments, the spinal cord depends on these radicular arteries for its survival. One particular radicular artery, present at spinal cord level T12 to L2 in most individuals, is called the *great radicular artery* (or *artery of Adamkiewicz*) and may provide the entire arterial supply for the caudal two thirds of the spinal cord.

The very long anterior spinal artery, which is usually a continuous vessel for the length of the spinal cord, gives rise to a series of hundreds of central and circumferential branches that supply the anterior two thirds of the spinal cord, including the base of the posterior horn and a variable portion of the lateral corticospinal tract (Figure 7-26). The posterior spinal arteries, which are really more of a plexiform network of small arteries, supply the posterior columns, substantia gelatinosa, dorsal root entry zone, and a variable portion of the lateral corticospinal tract.

Venous drainage is by a series of six irregular, plexiform channels: one each along the anterior and posterior midlines and one along the line of attachment of the dorsal and ventral roots of each side. These are drained by *radicular veins,* which in turn empty into the *epidural venous plexus.*

## SOME FUNCTIONAL ASPECTS OF THE SPINAL CORD

### Spinal cord lesions and spinal shock

If the spinal cord of a cat is transected at a midcervical level, you might expect, among other things, a spastic (upper motor neuron) paralysis of its whole body. This does happen eventually, but first there is a period, lasting for a few days, of more or less completely flaccid paralysis and areflexia. Deep tendon reflexes then begin to return and finally become hyperactive. The areflexic period is called *spinal shock.* The mechanism of spinal shock is incompletely understood, but the whole sequence of events is thought to be a consequence of interruption of fibers from the brainstem and cerebrum descending to spinal cord motor neurons and interneurons. In addition to corticospinal tracts, there are a number of other descending influences, some facilitatory and some inhibitory. Spinal shock would thus be caused by sudden loss of a collection of descending influences whose net effect is facilitatory. The mechanism by which this period of spinal shock resolves into spasticity is not fully understood. It may be the result, at least in part, of the formation of new synaptic connections. The degeneration of the endings of descending fibers would leave vacant synaptic sites at various places on motor neurons and interneurons, adjacent to intact reflex connections. Multiplication of these reflex connections to fill up the vacated sites would be expected to increase the sensitivity and intensity of reflexes. Other mechanisms, such as increased sensitivity to the transmitter substances released at remaining synapses, may also be involved.

Spinal shock occurs in humans as well, even in cases of contusion of the spinal cord, in which total or near-total recovery can be expected. It may last for weeks or even months in cases of complete transection. A complicating factor in spinal shock is the complete loss of bladder function (and loss of a sensation of distention) that accompanies it. Early catheterization is called for to minimize bladder distention and consequent damage. With proper care, even in cases of complete cord transection, a state of automatic or reflex emptying of the bladder develops.

Partial lesions of the spinal cord are (fortunately) much more common than complete transections. Complete transection of one side of the cord (hemisection), although rare, results in an instructional complex of symptoms called the *Brown-Séquard syndrome*. After a period of spinal shock (particularly prominent in those areas subserved by the damaged portion of the cord), a spastic paralysis develops below the lesion and ipsilateral to it because of interruption of the lateral corticospinal tract. Tactile, vibratory, and position senses are disturbed ipsilaterally below the lesion because of interruption of the posterior column. There is loss of pain and temperature sensation *contralateral* to the lesion, beginning one or two segments caudal to the lesion, as a result of interruption of the spinothalamic tract. This is one of many examples of *crossed findings* (that is, some symptoms referable to one side of the head or body and others to the other side), which may seem strange and inexplicable unless one understands the anatomical sites at which different pathways cross the midline.

*Syringomyelia* (the Greek word *syrinx* means tube) is a disease of the central part of the spinal cord in which a tubelike enlargement of the central canal develops, typically at lower cervical or upper thoracic levels. As the syrinx enlarges, surrounding neural tissue is destroyed. The first damage is to fibers crossing through the limited available area around the central canal (Figure 7-4). The next area damaged is usually the anterior horn. The result is a distinctive combination of loss of pain and temperature sensation bilaterally over the arms and shoulders (as a result of the damage to crossing fibers) and weakness and atrophy of the muscles of the hands (as a result of anterior horn damage). Of course, if the syrinx occurred at a different spinal level, the symptoms would be referred to a correspondingly different part of the body.

### *Posterior columns*

The posterior columns provide a particularly instructive example of the notion that sensory information travels in multiple pathways, so that damage to a single pathway seldom causes total loss of a function. Classical views of the posterior columns as the pathway responsible for fine tactile discrimination and kinesthesia (sense of position and movement) were based mostly on clinical observations. However, selective lesions of the posterior columns are rare. For example, any process impinging on the posterior columns, such as a tumor, would probably also affect the adjacent posterior horns and dorsal roots, as well as the ascending pathways in the posterior part of the lateral funiculus. Tabes dorsalis, a disease process seen in the late stages of neurosyphilis, was traditionally regarded as typifying posterior column damage. Tabetic patients show all the symptoms one would expect if the classical view were correct: their two-point discrimination and vibratory sense are impaired; their sense of movement and position is impaired, and they have great difficulty walking unless they can watch their limbs; and if they try to stand erect with their eyes closed and their feet together, they tend to sway and fall *(Romberg's sign)*. Consistent with this, there is pronounced degeneration in the posterior columns. However, there is also degeneration of dorsal root fibers, particularly the heavily myelinated fibers of the medial division, so mechanoreceptive input to all spinal pathways is affected to some extent.

If the posterior columns of a monkey are selectively transected surgically, there is severe impairment initially. The animal has great difficulty coordinating the affected limbs and tends to neglect and not use them. Over a period of months a remarkable recovery ensues, particularly if the animal is encouraged to use those limbs. After this recovery process, movement and coordination appear nearly normal, tactile threshold is normal, and two-point discrimination and position sense are only slightly impaired. What remains permanently impaired is the ability to use somatosensory information for more complex tasks, for example, judging the shape of an object pressed against the skin *(stereognosis)* or the direction or speed of a stimulus moving across the skin.

The acute and chronic effects of posterior column damage leave little doubt that the posterior columns are ordinarily involved in a major way in kinesthesia and tactile sensation. On the other hand, the degree of recovery that occurs also leaves little doubt that much of this information reaches the thalamus by additional routes. One of these additional routes is undoubtedly the ascending fibers in the posterior part of the lateral funiculus, bound for the posterior column nuclei or the lateral cervical nucleus. These fibers lie near the surface of the cord and can be transected without damaging the lateral corticospinal tract. Such a lesion by itself has no particular effects, but when added to a posterior column lesion, it makes the effects of the latter much more severe and prolonged.

## ADDITIONAL READINGS


Applebaum ML et al: Organization and receptive fields of primate spinothalamic tract neurons, *J Neurophysiol* 38:572, 1975.

Appenzeller O: *The autonomic nervous system: an introduction to basic and clinical concepts,* ed. 4, Amsterdam, 1990, Elsevier.

Barson AJ: The vertebral level of termination of the spinal cord during normal and abnormal development, *J Anat* 106:489, 1970.

Basbaum AI: Conduction of the effects of noxious stimulation by short-fiber multisynaptic systems of the spinal cord in the rat, *Exp Neurol* 40:699, 1973. *A series of experiments showing that rats can learn to avoid painful stimuli even after hemisection of both sides of the spinal cord, which should transect the long ascending fibers of both sides.*

Batzdorf U, editor: *Syringomyelia: current concepts in diagnosis and treatment,* Baltimore, 1991, Williams & Wilkins.

Besson JM, Chaouch A: Peripheral and spinal mechanisms of nociception, *Physiol Rev* 67:67, 1987.

Brown AG: The spinocervical tract, *Prog Neurobiol* 17:59, 1981.

Bryan RN, Coulter JD, Willis WD: Cells of origin of the spinocervical tract in the monkey, *Exp Neurol* 42:574, 1974.

Calne DB, Pallis CA: Vibratory sense: a critical review, *Brain* 89:723, 1966. *Interesting reading, with a review of old clinical observations.*

Cervero F, Iggo A: The substantia gelatinosa of the spinal cord: a critical review, *Brain* 103:717, 1980.

Cervero F, Morrison JFB, editors: *Visceral sensation,* vol. 67, *Prog Brain Res,* Amsterdam, 1986, Elsevier.

Cervero F, Sharkey KA: More than just gut feelings about visceral sensation, *Trends Neurosci* 8:188, 1985. *A brief review of a neglected topic—the pathways and mechanisms used by visceral afferents.*

Chung K, Coggeshall RE: Unmyelinated primary afferent fibers in dorsal funiculi of cat sacral spinal cord, *J Comp Neurol* 238:365, 1985.

Coggeshall RE: Law of separation of function of the spinal roots, *Physiol Rev* 60:716, 1980.

Collins WF, Nulsen FE, Randt CT: Relation of peripheral nerve fiber size and sensation in man, *Arch Neurol* 3:381, 1960. *Post cordotomy abolition of the painful consequences of controlled electrical stimulation of the sural nerve.*

Creed RS et al: *Reflex activity of the spinal cord,* reprinted with annotations by D.P.C. Lloyd, New York, 1972, Oxford University Press.

Crock HV, Yoshizawa H: *The blood supply of the vertebral column and spinal cord in man,* New York, 1977, Springer-Verlag.

Davidoff RA: The dorsal columns, *Neurol* 39:1377, 1989. *A good recent review of the complications lurking in this seemingly simple pathway.*

deGroat WC et al: Mechanisms underlying the recovery of urinary bladder function following spinal cord injury, *J Autonom Nerv Sys* 30:S71, 1990.

Dennis SG, Melzack R: Pain-signalling systems in the dorsal and ventral spinal cord, *Pain* 4:97, 1977.

Furness JB, Costa M: *The enteric nervous system,* Edinburgh, 1987, Churchill Livingstone.

Gillilan LA: The arterial blood supply of the human spinal cord, *J Comp Neurol* 110:75, 1958.

Gillilan LA: Veins of the spinal cord, *Neurol* 20:860, 1970.

Glees P, Soler J: Fibre content of the posterior column and synaptic connections of nucleus gracilis, *Z Zellforsch* 36:381, 1951. *Documents the fact that, at least in the cat, only about 25% of the fibers that enter the posterior columns actually reach the posterior column nuclei; the rest end within the spinal cord.*

Grillner A: *Locomotion in the spinal cat.* In Stein RB et al, editors: *Control of posture and locomotion: advances in behavioral biology,* vol. 7, New York, 1973, Plenum Press. *Walking with the hind limbs by cats whose spinal cords had been transected at low thoracic levels.*

Ha H: Cervicothalamic tract in the rhesus monkey, *Exp Neurol* 33:205, 1971.

Hosobuchi Y: The majority of unmyelinated afferent axons in human ventral roots probably conduct pain, Pain 8:167, 1980.

Jenny A, Smith J, Decker J: Motor organization of the spinal accessory nerve in the monkey, *Brain Res* 441:352, 1988.

Keswani NH, Hollinshead WH: Localization of the phrenic nucleus in the spinal cord of man, *Anat Rec* 125:683, 1956.

Kuhn RA: Functional capacity of the isolated human spinal cord, *Brain* 73:1, 1950. *A careful study of the course of events after complete transection of the spinal cord, particularly spinal shock and its gradual fading.*

Kuo DC, DeGroat WC: Primary afferent projections of the major splanchnic nerve to the spinal cord and gracile nucleus of the cat, *J Comp Neurol* 231:421, 1985.

Liddell EGT, Sherrington C: Reflexes in response to stretch (myotatic reflexes), *Proc R Soc Lond,* series B, 96:212, 1924.

Matthews PBC: The 1989 James A.F. Stevenson memorial lecture. The knee jerk: still an enigma, *Can J Physiol Pharmacol* 68:347, 1990.

Melzack R, Wall PD: Pain mechanisms: a new theory, *Science* 150:971, 1965. *A seminal paper, in which the modulating effect of the substantia gelatinosa on pain transmission was proposed in a scheme called the "gate control theory" of pain. While apparently wrong in some of its details, the gate control theory has nevertheless been very influential on pain research since 1965.*

Mense S: Structure-function relationships in identified afferent neurones, *Anat Embryol* 181:1, 1990. *A review of recent elegant demonstrations of how single primary afferents with known functions end in precisely defined patterns in the spinal cord.*

Miller S, van der Meché FGA: Coordinated stepping of all four limbs in the high spinal cat, *Brain Res* 109:395, 1976.

Morin F: A new spinal pathway for cutaneous impulses, *Am J Physiol* 183:245, 1955. *The original physiological description of the spinocervical tract.*

Nathan PW, Smith MC: The location of descending fibres to sympathetic preganglionic vasomotor and sudomotor neurons in man, *J Neurol Neurosurg Psychiatry* 50:1253, 1987.

Nathan PW, Smith MC, Cook AW: Sensory effects in man of lesions of the posterior columns and of some other afferent pathways, *Brain* 109:1003, 1986. *"The total evidence from all the relevant cases shows that the major pathway subserving every kind of mechanoreception is in the posterior third of the cord."*

Nathan PW, Smith MC, Deacon P: The corticospinal tracts in man. Course and location of fibres at different segmental levels, *Brain* 113:303, 1990.

Norrsell U: Behavioral studies of the somatosensory system, *Physiol Rev* 60:327, 1980.

Nudo RJ, Masterton RB: Descending pathways to the spinal cord: A comparative study of 22 mammals, *J Comp Neurol* 277:53, 1988.

Oscarsson O: *Functional organization of spinocerebellar paths.* In Iggo A, editor: *Handbook of sensory physiology,* vol. II: Somatosensory system, New York, 1973, Springer-Verlag.

Perl ER: Effects of muscle stretch on excitability of contralateral motoneurones, *J Physiol* 145:193, 1959.

Petras JM: Spinocerebellar tract neurons in the rhesus monkey, *Brain Res* 130:146, 1977.

Rexed B: The cytoarchitectonic organization of the spinal cord in the cat, *J Comp Neurol* 96:415, 1952.

Rodríguez-Baera A et al: Anterior spinal arteries. Origin and distribution in man, *Acta Anatom* 136:217, 1989.

Rustioni A, Hayes NL, O'Neill SO: Dorsal column nuclei and ascending afferents in macaques, *Brain* 102:95, 1979. *An account of the nonprimary afferents ascending to nuclei gracilis and cuneatus in the posterior columns and the posterior part of the lateral funiculus.*

Rymer WZ, Houk JC, Craggo PE: Mechanisms of the clasp-knife reflex studied in an animal model, *Exp Brain Res* 37:93, 1979. *Physiological experiments suggesting that Golgi tendon organs cannot entirely account for the clasp-knife reflex and that group III and IV muscle afferents may be involved.*

Shealy CN, Mortimer JT, Hagfors NR: Dorsal column electroanalgesia, *J Neurosurg* 32:560, 1970. *Another example of treating pain by shifting the balance of activity toward large-fiber afferent systems, this time by stimulating the posterior columns.*

Siekert RG, Dale AJD: *Vascular disease of the spinal cord.* In Goldensohn ES, Appel SH, editors: *Scientific approaches to clinical neurology,* Philadelphia, 1977, Lea & Febiger.

Smith MC, Deacon P: Topographical anatomy of the posterior columns of the spinal cord in man: the long ascending fibers, *Brain* 107:671, 1984.

Snyder R: The organization of the dorsal root entry zone in cats and monkeys, *J Comp Neurol* 174:47, 1977.

Truex RC et al: The lateral cervical nucleus of cat, dog and man, *J Comp Neurol* 139:93, 1970.

Uddenberg N: Functional organization of long second-order afferents in the dorsal funiculus, *Exp Brain Res* 4:377, 1968. *Physiological description of the minority of fibers in the posterior column that are not primary afferents.*

Vierck CJ Jr: Alterations of spatio-tactile discrimination after lesions of primate spinal cord, *Brain Res* 58:69, 1973. *Some speculations on how primates compensate for loss of a posterior column, plus experiments to show the much greater deficits caused by damage to both a posterior column and the posterior part of the ipsilateral lateral funiculus.*

Vierck CJ Jr, Luck MM: Loss and recovery of reactivity to noxious stimuli in monkeys with primary spinothalamic cordotomies, followed by secondary and tertiary lesions of other cord sectors, *Brain* 102:233, 1979.

Wall PD, Noordenbos W: Sensory functions which remain in man after complete transection of dorsal columns, *Brain* 100:641, 1977. *A description of the surprising sensory capabilities left in two unfortunate patients after transection of all but one anterior quadrant of the cord. "We conclude that patients with dorsal column lesions do not lose one or more of the classical primary modalities of sensation but lose an ability to carry out tasks where they must simultaneously analyse spatial and temporal characteristics of the stimulus."*

Weaver TA, Walker AE: Topical arrangement within the spinothalamic tract of the monkey, *Arch Neurol Psychiatry* 46:877, 1941.

White JC, Sweet WH: *Pain and the neurosurgeon: a forty year experience,* Springfield, Ill, 1969, Charles C Thomas.

Willis WD, Coggeshall RE: *Sensory mechanisms of the spinal cord,* ed 2 New York, 1991, Plenum Press. *A well-written, thoroughly documented review of the literature.*

Willis WD, Kenshalo DR Jr, Leonard RB: The cells of origin of the primate spinothalamic tract, *J Comp Neurol* 188:543, 1979.

Yaksh TL: *Spinal afferent processing,* New York, 1986, Plenum Press.

CHAPTER

# 8

# Brainstem

The spinal cord continues rostrally into the brainstem (Figure 8-1), which performs spinal cord-like functions for the head. It contains the lower motor neurons for the muscles of the head and does the initial processing of general afferent information concerning the head. However, the brainstem does much more than this, and its activities may be divided (not very cleanly) into three general types: *conduit functions, cranial nerve functions,* and *integrative functions*.

The need for conduit functions is apparent, since the only way for ascending tracts to reach the thalamus or cerebellum (or for descending tracts to reach the spinal cord) is through the brainstem. Many of these tracts, however, are not straight-through affairs, and identifiable relay nuclei in the brainstem are frequently involved.

The cranial nerves contain not only the head's equivalent of spinal nerve fibers but also those involved in the special senses of olfaction, sight, hearing, equilibrium, and gustation, or taste (Table 5). The olfactory and optic nerves project directly to the telencephalon and diencephalon, respectively, but the others project to or emerge from the brainstem. Thus a wide assortment of sensory and motor nuclei related to cranial nerve function can be found at various brainstem levels.

A number of integrative functions are organized at the level of the brainstem, such as complex motor patterns, aspects of respiratory and cardiovascular activity, and even some regulation of the level of consciousness itself. Much of this is accomplished by the *reticular formation,* which forms the central core of the brainstem.

It is clear that these three general types of activity are far from mutually exclusive. For example, ascending pathways to the thalamus arise not only in the spinal cord, but also from cranial nerve nuclei; the latter therefore have a hybrid conduit and cranial nerve function. However, this parcellation does provide a useful framework on which to organize a treatment of the brainstem. It is difficult to learn about this portion of the nervous system all at once, so it is presented here in two parts. This chapter describes the overall anatomy of the brainstem and presents a series of sections showing the locations of some prominent nuclei and of major ascending and descending tracts. The next chapter describes the central connections of cranial nerves III to XII; at the end of that chapter is a similar series of sections, labeled in more detail, with summary descriptions of the contents of various tracts and nuclei (Figures 9-41 to 9-49).

## GROSS ANATOMY

### Medulla

The medulla is vaguely scoop shaped. The "handle" corresponds to the *caudal* or *closed* portion containing a central canal continuous with that of the spinal cord. The open portion of the scoop corresponds to the *rostral* or *open medulla,* in which the central canal expands as the fourth ventricle. The apex of the V-shaped caudal fourth ventricle, where it narrows into the central canal, is called the *obex* (Figures 8-2 and 8-3).

The longitudinal grooves of the surface of the spinal cord continue into the medulla. They divide the surface of the caudal, and part of the rostral, medulla into a series of columns that completely encircle it (Figure 8-2). The anterior median fissure is briefly interrupted by the pyramidal decussation at the junction between spinal cord and brainstem but then continues rostrally to the edge of the pons, separating the two pyramids (Figures 8-2 and 8-3). Proceeding around in a posterior direction, the anterolateral sulcus marks the other side of the pyramid. The rootlets of the hypoglossal nerve (XII) emerge from this sulcus, mainly in the rostral medulla. The rootlets of the glosso-

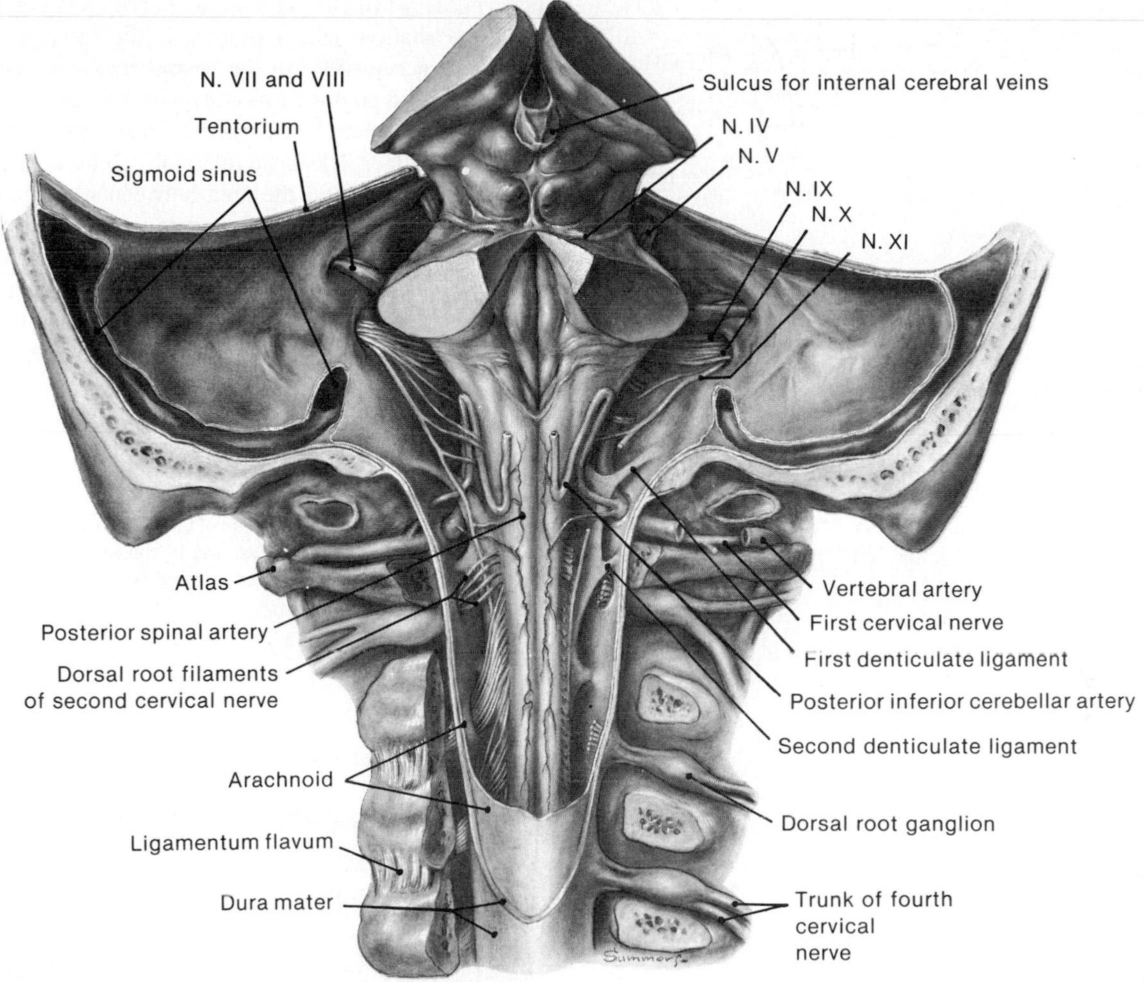


FIGURE 8-1

Posterior aspect of the brainstem and upper spinal cord. The cerebellum and cerebral hemispheres have been removed.

From Mettler FA: *Neuroanatomy*, ed. 2, St. Louis, 1948, The CV Mosby Co.

**TABLE 5** *Highly simplified overview of cranial nerve functions**

| *Cranial nerve* | *Main sensory function* | *Main motor function* |
|---|---|---|
| I. Olfactory | Smell | — |
| II. Optic | Sight | — |
| III. Oculomotor | — | Eye movements, pupil and lens function |
| IV. Trochlear | — | Eye movements |
| V. Trigeminal | Facial sensation | Chewing |
| VI. Abducens | — | Eye movements |
| VII. Facial | Taste | Facial expression |
| VIII. Vestibulocochlear | Hearing, equilibrium | — |
| IX. Glossopharyngeal | Taste | Swallowing |
| X. Vagus | Thoracic and abdominal viscera | Speech, swallowing; thoracic and abdominal viscera |
| XI. Accessory | — | Head and shoulder movements |
| XII. Hypoglossal | — | Tongue movements |

*For more details see Table 6 (p. 180) and Chapter 9.

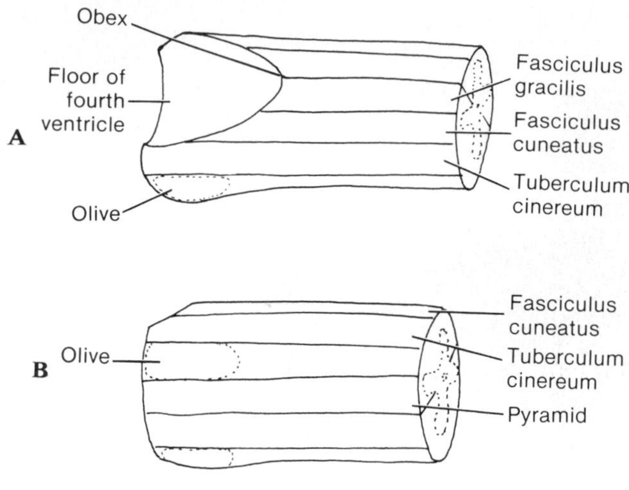


FIGURE 8-2
Surface features of the medulla. **A,** Seen from above and to the left. **B,** Seen from below and to the left.

pharyngeal nerve (IX) and vagus nerve (X)* emerge from the same shallow lateral groove as the spinal part of the accessory nerve (XI). In the rostral medulla, the column between the hypoglossal rootlets and the vagal and glossopharyngeal rootlets is enlarged to form an oval swelling called the *olive*. The posterolateral sulcus also continues into the medulla, and the area between it and the line of rootlets of IX and X is referred to as the *tuberculum cinereum*. Beneath the tuberculum cinereum is the *spinal tract of the trigeminal nerve,* which, as explained in the next chapter, is the head's equivalent of Lissauer's tract. Finally, the posterior columns continue into the medulla.

*The most caudal vagal filaments join the accessory nerve briefly while passing through the jugular foramen, and so are often considered separately as the *cranial part of the accessory nerve*. However, in most other aspects of their origin, course, and termination they resemble vagal fibers (see Chapter 9). Hence there is a growing tendency to include these caudal filaments as part of the vagus, and to consider the fibers emerging from the lateral surface of the upper cervical cord as the definitive accessory nerve.

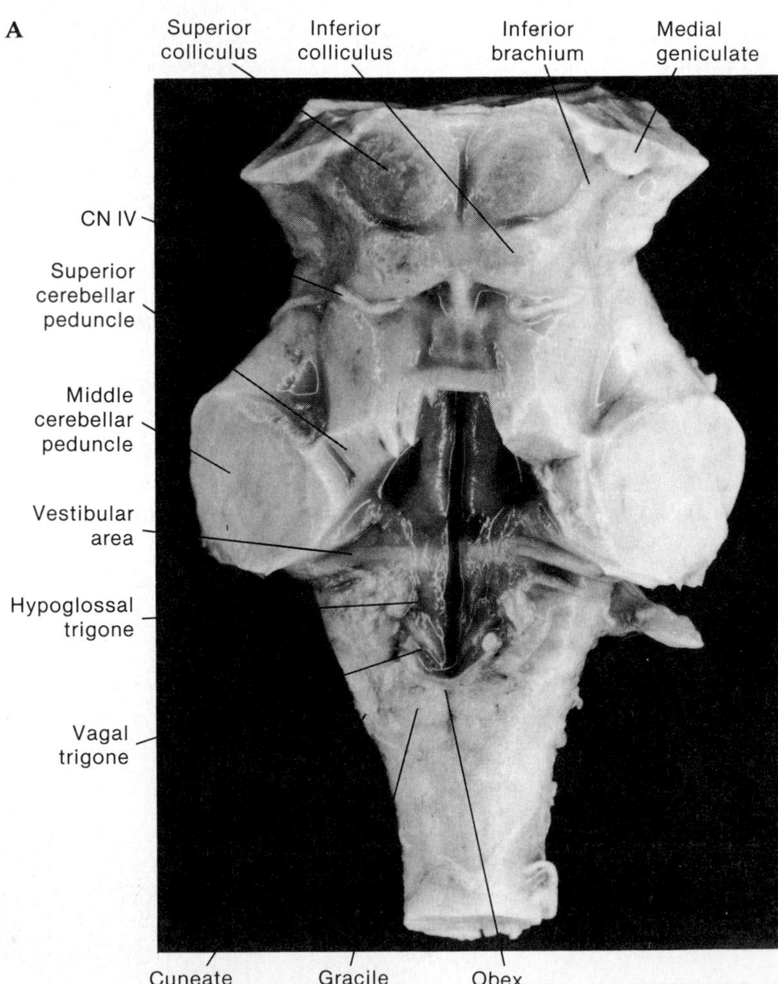


FIGURE 8-3
Posterior **(A)**, anterior **(B)**, and lateral **(C)** aspects of the brainstem, after the cerebellum and cerebrum were removed. Actual length is 6 cm.

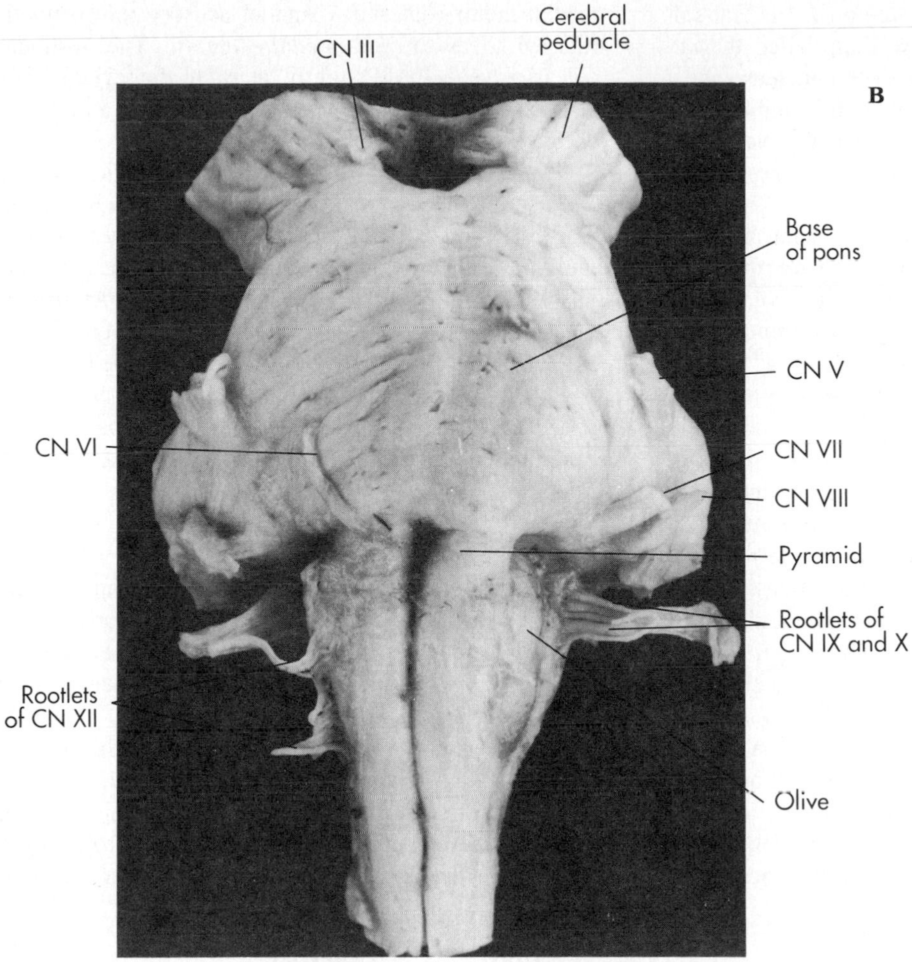

B
CN III
Cerebral peduncle
Base of pons
CN V
CN VI
CN VII
CN VIII
Pyramid
Rootlets of CN IX and X
Rootlets of CN XII
Olive

FIGURE 8-3, cont'd.
For legend see opposite page.

C
Rootlets of CN XI
Tuberculum cinereum
CN IX & X
CN VIII
CN VII
Middle cerebellar peduncle
Lateral lemniscus
Inferior colliculus
Superior colliculus
Inferior brachium
CN IV
Cerebral peduncle
CN V
Base of pons
CN XII
Pyramid
Olive
CN VI

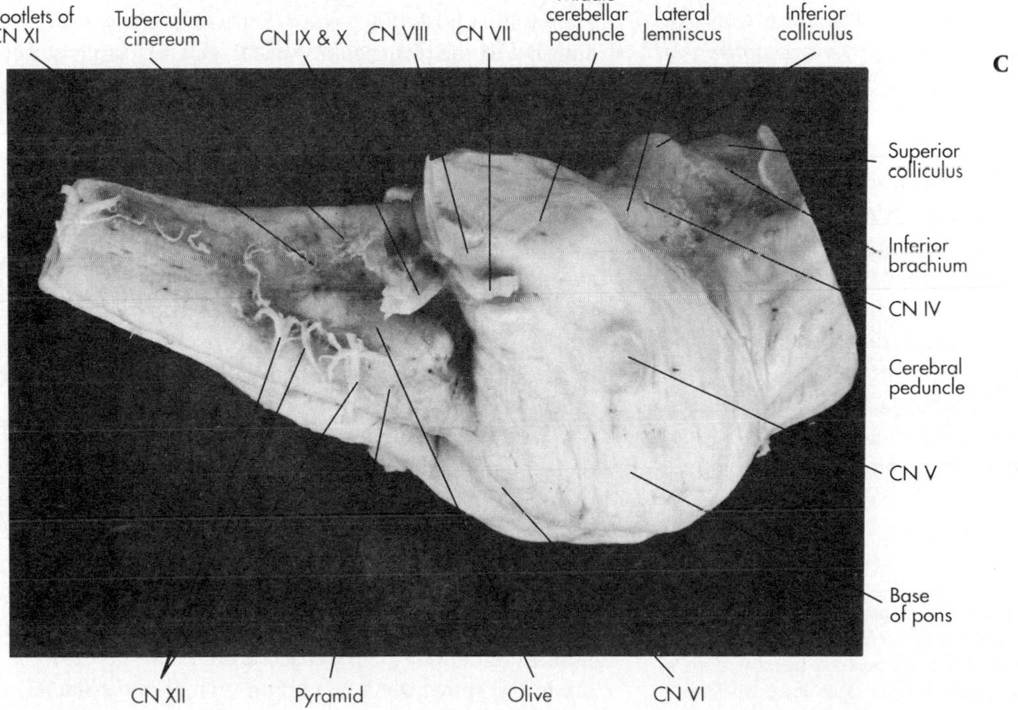

The fasciculus cuneatus, adjacent to the posterolateral sulcus, extends rostrally to a small swelling called the *cuneate tubercle,* which marks the site of the nucleus cuneatus. The fasciculus gracilis, adjacent to the midline, extends rostrally to a similar small swelling called the *gracile tubercle* (or *clava*), which marks the site of the nucleus gracilis.

If the cerebellum is removed (as it has been in Figure 8-3), one can peer down on the floor of the fourth ventricle. Here, too, various grooves and elevations signify the presence of underlying nuclei. The sulcus limitans can sometimes be followed rostrally along the floor of the ventricle into the pons. As in the embryonic spinal cord, it is a line of separation between motor nuclei (now medial to it) and sensory nuclei (now lateral to it; see Figure 1-11). The portion of the medulla and pons immediately beneath the floor of the ventricle, lateral to the sulcus limitans, is mostly occupied by vestibular nuclei and is referred to as the *vestibular area*. The area medial to the sulcus limitans overlies a series of motor nuclei, three of which make visible elevations. In the medulla, the hypoglossal nucleus and the dorsal motor nucleus of the vagus make small triangular swellings, appropriately called the *hypoglossal* and *vagal trigones*. Farther rostrally, in the pons, is another elevation called the *facial colliculus*. This elevation is not caused by an underlying motor nucleus of the facial nerve but instead is the location of the abducens nucleus; fibers destined for the facial nerve loop over it at this location on their way out of the brainstem.

### Pons

The pons is dominated by the massive, transversely oriented structure on its ventral surface from which it derives its name (Figures 8-3 and 8-4). Pons is the Latin word for bridge, and this portion of it (called the *ventral portion of the pons,* or *basal pons*) looks like a bridge interconnecting the two cerebellar hemispheres. Actually, though, it does not interconnect them. Rather, many of the fibers descending in a cerebral peduncle synapse in scattered nuclei of the ipsilateral half of the basal pons. These nuclei in turn project their fibers across the midline, after which they funnel into the middle cerebellar peduncle *(brachium pontis*)* and finally enter the cerebellum.

The trigeminal nerve (V) enters the brainstem at the midpons, and three others enter (or leave) along the groove between the basal pons and the medulla (Figure 8-3). The abducens nerve (VI) is the smallest and most medially located of these three, exiting where the pyramid emerges from the basal pons. The facial nerve (VII) is farther lateral and consists of two parts: a larger and more medial motor root and a smaller sensory root (sometimes referred to as the *intermediate nerve*). The vestibulocochlear nerve (VIII) is slightly lateral to the facial nerve and also has two parts: a vestibular division and a more lateral cochlear division.

The superior cerebellar peduncle *(brachium conjunctivum)* forms much of the roof of the fourth ventricle in the pons. It emerges from the cerebellum, moves toward the midline and the brainstem, and enters the latter near the junction between the pons and midbrain. At this same junction, the trochlear nerve (IV) emerges from the dorsal surface of the brainstem. The superior cerebellar peduncle is covered in the rostral pons by a flattened band of fibers called the *lateral lemniscus,* which forms part of the ascending auditory system and terminates in the inferior colliculus.

### Midbrain

The midbrain is characterized by four bumps (the paired superior and inferior colliculi) on its posterior surface and by the large cerebral peduncles on its anterior surface. The oculomotor nerve (III) emerges from the interpeduncular fossa between the peduncles.

The broad low ridge extending rostrally from the inferior colliculus is the *brachium of the inferior colliculus* (usually shortened to *inferior brachium*). This is a continuation of the ascending auditory pathway, projecting from the inferior colliculus to the thalamic relay nucleus for hearing (the *medial geniculate nucleus*).

## INTERNAL STRUCTURE

At any given brainstem level rostral to the obex, three general areas can be identified in cross section. These are (1) the area posterior to the ventricular space, (2) the area anterior to the ventricular space, and (3) large structures "appended" to the anterior surface of the brainstem. (In the caudal medulla the central canal is surrounded by structures, including some that will be anterior to the ventricular space at more rostral levels).

The only place where the portion posterior to the ventricular space contains a substantial amount of neural tissue is the midbrain. Here this region is called the *tectum* (Latin for roof) and consists of the superior and inferior colliculi. In the pons and rostral medulla, the fourth ventricle is covered posteriorly by the superior and inferior medullary vela (and, of course, the cerebellum).

The area anterior to the ventricular space is called the *tegmentum* (Latin for covering) as a general term. The tegmentum contains most of the structures to be described in this and the next chapter: the reticular formation, cranial nerve nuclei and tracts, ascending pathways from the spinal cord, and some descending pathways.

The structures appended to the anterior surface of the brainstem contain fibers descending from the cerebral cortex to the spinal cord, to certain cranial nerve nuclei, or to

*Brachium is the Latin word for arm and is used neuroanatomically to refer to some prominent bands of white matter extending from or to an area of gray matter. In this case the brachium pontis—literally "the arm of the pons"—extends dorsally from the pons to reach the cerebellum.

pontine nuclei, which in turn project to the cerebellum. These appended structures are the large fiber bundles of the cerebral peduncles, the basal pons, and the pyramids of the medulla.

Although the brainstem is derived embryologically from a serial array of vesicles, in the adult it no longer possesses an organization quite so neat (Figure 8-4). For example, the basal pons usually extends rostrally to a point ventral to the tectum of the midbrain; the pineal gland and part of the thalamus extend caudally to a point dorsal to the tectum of the midbrain. Since the most instructive way to study the brainstem is to consider a series of parallel sections through it (all perpendicular to its long axis), I have ignored minor inconveniences like the intrusion of the basal pons under the midbrain and have used, for the purposes of the following discussion, reference transverse planes that subdivide the brainstem into six parts: caudal and rostral medulla, caudal and rostral pons, and caudal and rostral midbrain.

The following discussion points out major brainstem structures at these levels and the locations of tracts that begin or end in the spinal cord. The next chapter deals with the cranial nerves and their tracts and nuclei. Finally, as noted previously, the material of both chapters is integrated in a series of extensively labeled sections at the end of Chapter 9 (Figures 9-41 to 9-49).

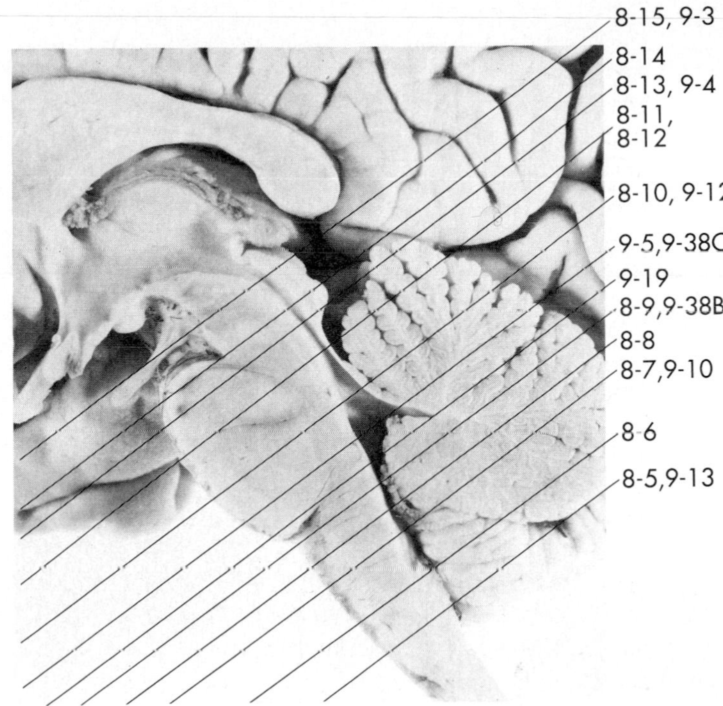


FIGURE 8-4
Planes of sections seen in Figures 8-5 to 8-15 and in some figures in Chapter 9.

## Caudal medulla

The caudal (closed) medulla extends from the caudal edge of the pyramidal decussation (where the medulla becomes continuous with the spinal cord) to the obex, which marks the caudal end of the fourth ventricle.

The caudal medulla (Figures 8-5 and 8-6) looks somewhat like the spinal cord. Part of the anterior horn is still present caudally (Figure 8-5), as are structures similar to Lissauer's tract and part of the posterior horn. The latter two are actually the *spinal tract* and *spinal nucleus of the trigeminal nerve*. These are the head's equivalent of Lissauer's tract and the substantia gelatinosa (that is, they deal with pain, temperature, and some tactile information).

The fasciculi gracilis and cuneatus continue into the caudal medulla but are gradually replaced by the posterior column nuclei (nucleus gracilis and nucleus cuneatus). The nucleus cuneatus begins and ends a bit rostral to the nucleus gracilis, so even in Figure 8-6 part of the fasciculus cuneatus is still present. Postsynaptic fibers leave these two nuclei in a ventral direction and arch across the midline to form the contralateral medial lemniscus, a vertically oriented band of fibers (Figure 8-6). These decussating fibers are part of the collection of *internal arcuate fibers* and are sometimes called the *sensory decussation*. Throughout the medulla, the medial lemniscus is organized so that fibers representing cervical segments are most posterior (that is, as though the homunculus were standing upright).

Adjacent to the nucleus cuneatus and embedded in the fasciculus cuneatus is the *lateral* (or *external*) *cuneate nucleus* (Figure 8-6). This is the forelimb equivalent of Clarke's nucleus, and the axons of these cells join the posterior spinocerebellar tract in the inferior cerebellar peduncle at a slightly more rostral level.

The spinothalamic tract is one of several that are not so compact or heavily myelinated as the medial lemniscus and therefore cannot be distinguished clearly in myelin-stained sections. However, this tract maintains more or less the same location (the ventrolateral portion of the tegmentum) during its passage through the brainstem, at least until it reaches the rostral midbrain.

The prominent pyramids and their decussation are located most anteriorly in the caudal medulla. Each pyramid consists of corticospinal fibers that originated in ipsilateral cerebral cortex and are (mostly) bound for the contralateral anterior horn.

Most of the area traversed by internal arcuate fibers in Figure 8-6 is *reticular formation*. A casual observer, looking at this region in photographs like these, will not see much. This is, to a first approximation, what distinguishes the reticular formation from the rest of the brainstem; the posterior column nuclei, for example, *look* like nuclei, whereas the reticular formation just looks like the uniform neural tissue filling the gaps between identifiable structures throughout the brainstem tegmentum. In fact, though, the

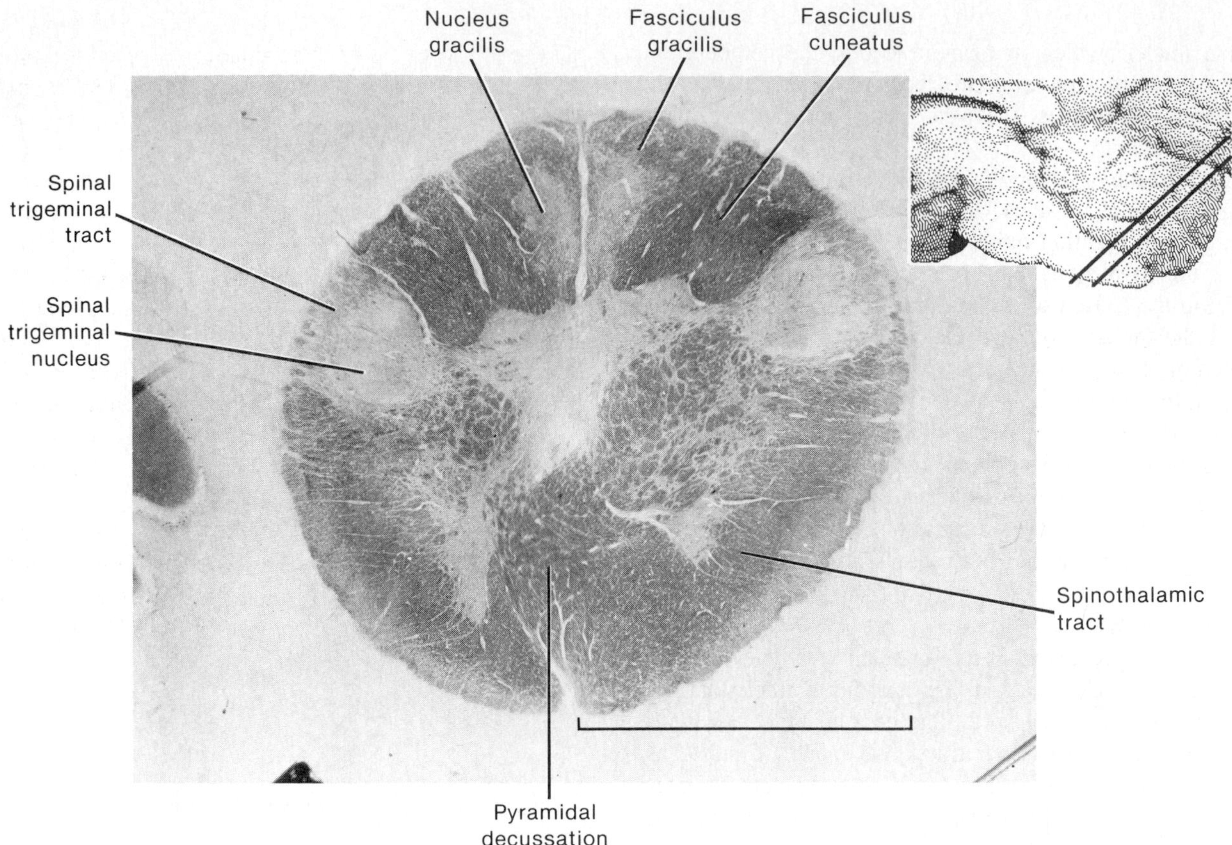


FIGURE 8-5
Caudal medulla, at the level of the pyramidal decussation. Scale mark = 5 mm.

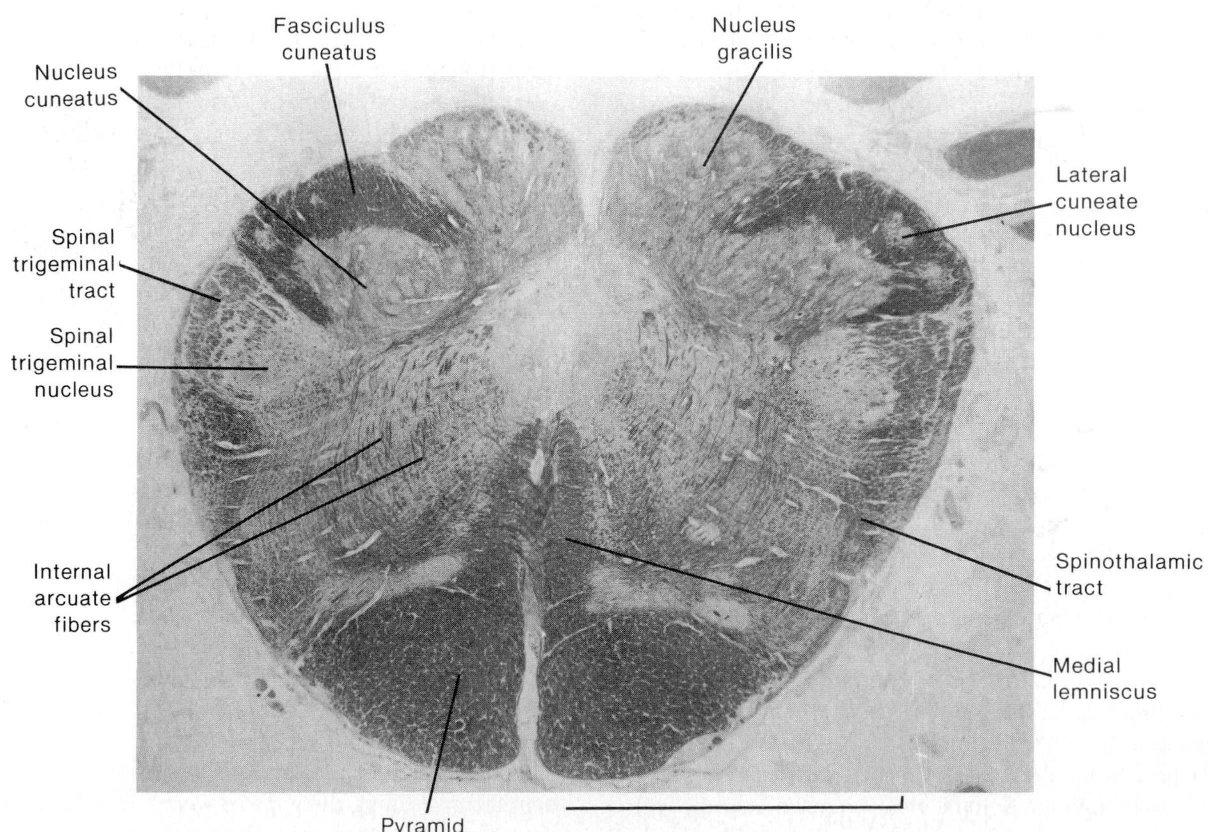


FIGURE 8-6
Caudal medulla just caudal to the obex. Scale mark = 5 mm.

reticular formation is organized—but on a microscopic level, as discussed briefly later in this chapter.

## Rostral medulla

The rostral (open) medulla, as defined here, extends from the obex to the rostral wall of the lateral recess, where the inferior cerebellar peduncle turns posteriorly to enter the cerebellum. The rostral medulla (Figures 8-7 and 8-8) no longer looks much like the spinal cord, partly because the walls of the embryonic neural tube have been pushed outward to form the floor of the fourth ventricle (see Figure 1-11).

The caudal boundary (the obex) is approximately coincident with the caudal edge of the *inferior olivary nucleus,* a prominent structure that is responsible for the surface swelling called the olive (Figure 8-3). The inferior cerebellar peduncle is located dorsolaterally at these levels and grows progressively larger as it continues rostrally (compare Figures 8-7 and 8-8). Fibers can be seen leaving the medially facing mouth (or *hilus*) of the inferior olivary nucleus, arching across the midline, and joining the contralateral inferior cerebellar peduncle. These too are internal arcuate fibers. More and more are added at progressively more rostral levels of the medulla, increasing the size of the peduncle.

Medial to the inferior olivary nucleus is the medial lemniscus, which still has the shape of a flattened band with a dorsal-ventral axis. Anterior to the medial lemniscus is the pyramid. Fascicles of the hypoglossal (XII) nerve (Figures 8-3 and 8-7) emerge lateral to the pyramid in the groove between it and the inferior olivary nucleus. Posterior to the medial lemniscus, near the floor of the fourth ventricle, is a small but distinctive bundle of fibers that can be followed all the way to the midbrain. This is the *medial longitudinal fasciculus (MLF),* which is involved in vestibular functions and eye movements.

The spinothalamic tract remains in the ventrolateral portion of the tegmentum, just above the inferior olivary nucleus, as does the anterior spinocerebellar tract. The posterior spinocerebellar tract moves posteriorly and joins the inferior cerebellar peduncle.

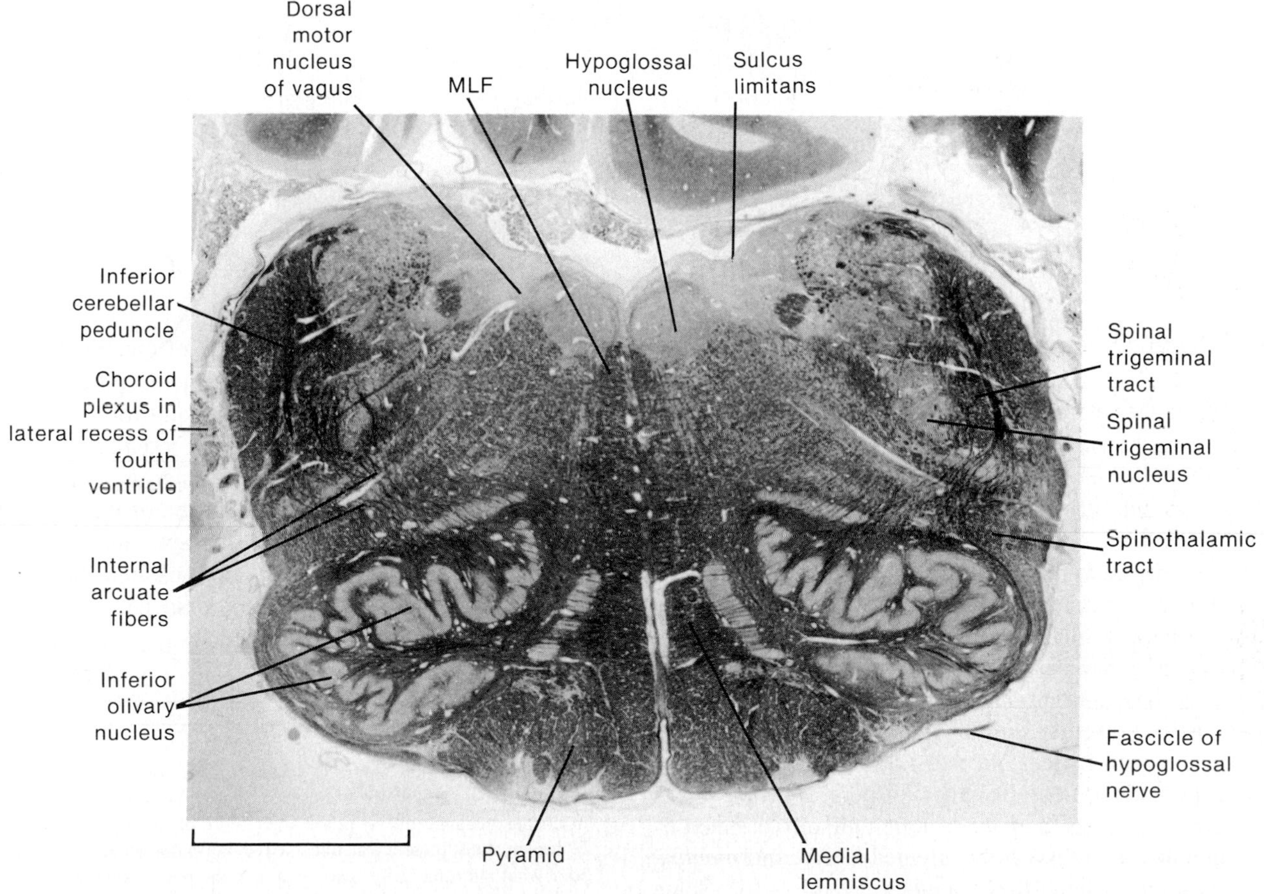


FIGURE 8-7
Rostral medulla just rostral to the obex. Scale mark = 4 mm.

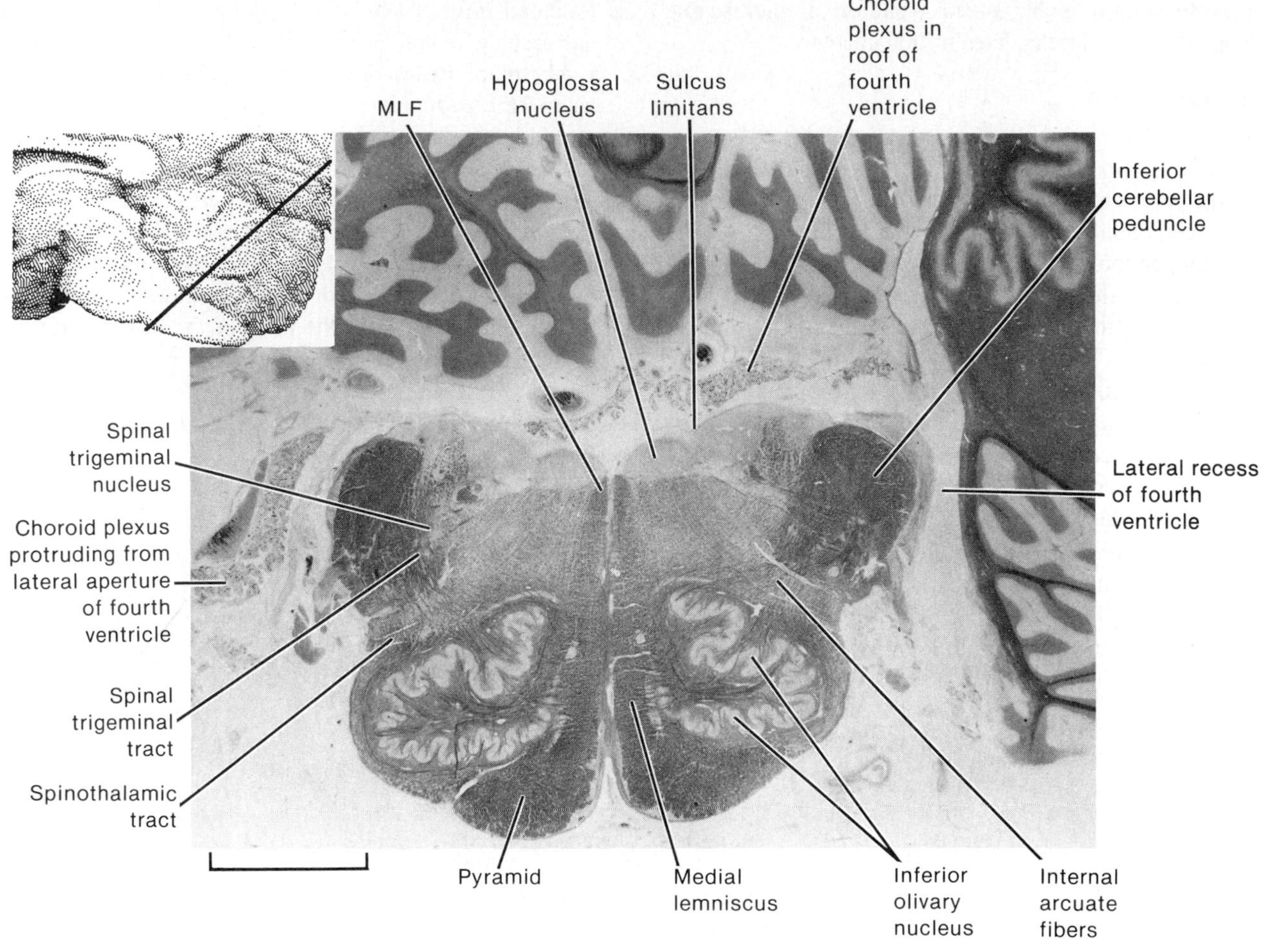


FIGURE 8-8
Rostral medulla near the pontomedullary junction. Scale mark = 5 mm.

## Caudal pons

The caudal pons, as defined here, extends from the rostral wall of the lateral recess of the fourth ventricle to the point of attachment of the trigeminal nerve. In the caudal pons the inferior olivary nucleus ends, and the inferior cerebellar peduncle bends posteriorly and enters the cerebellum (Figure 8-9). The MLF is in the same relative position as it was previously, adjacent to the midline and the floor of the fourth ventricle.

As the inferior olivary nucleus ends, the medial lemniscus assumes a more oval shape, as though it had previously been held upright against the midline. Now the homunculus is allowed to slump down slowly into a horizontal position, with its feet directed laterally (Figure 8-10).

The pyramidal tract becomes dispersed in the basal pons, which contains bundles of longitudinally oriented fibers, bundles of transversely oriented fibers, and *pontine nuclei* scattered among these bundles (Figure 8-10). Some of the longitudinally oriented fibers are those of the pyramidal tract. Most of the others are *corticopontine fibers;* these fibers originate in many areas of the cerebral cortex and terminate in ipsilateral pontine nuclei. Fibers arising in the pontine nuclei cross the midline and form the massive middle cerebellar peduncle (brachium pontis).

The spinothalamic tract and the anterior spinocerebellar tract remain in the ventrolateral portion of the tegmentum. Spinoreticular fibers related to the spinothalamic system terminate medial to the direct spinothalamic fibers in the reticular formation throughout the brainstem, as do collaterals of direct spinothalamic fibers.*

*All direct spinothalamic fibers in humans (that is, those projecting directly to the thalamus from the spinal cord) follow the classic spinothalamic pathway through the brainstem. That is, both neospinothalamic and paleospinothalamic fibers, in the strict sense of the term, travel together. However, the spinoreticular fibers leave the spinothalamic tract and travel somewhat more medially, particularly in the pons. Some authors include the polysynaptic spinoreticulothalamic pathway in the term "paleospinothalamic," so the reader may encounter descriptions of a medial paleospinothalamic tract, as opposed to a more laterally situated neospinothalamic tract.

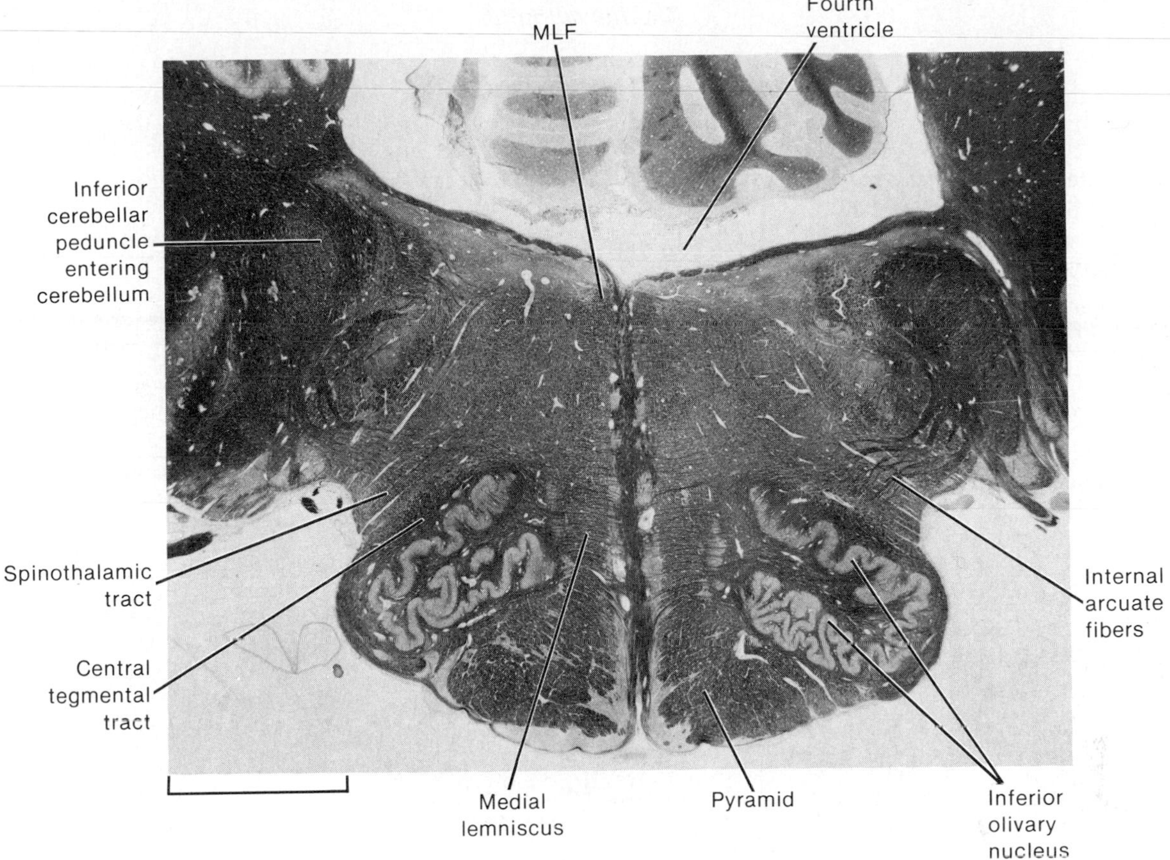


FIGURE 8-9
Caudal pons in the transition region from medulla to pons. Plane of section indicated in the inset in Figure 8-10. Scale mark = 5 mm.

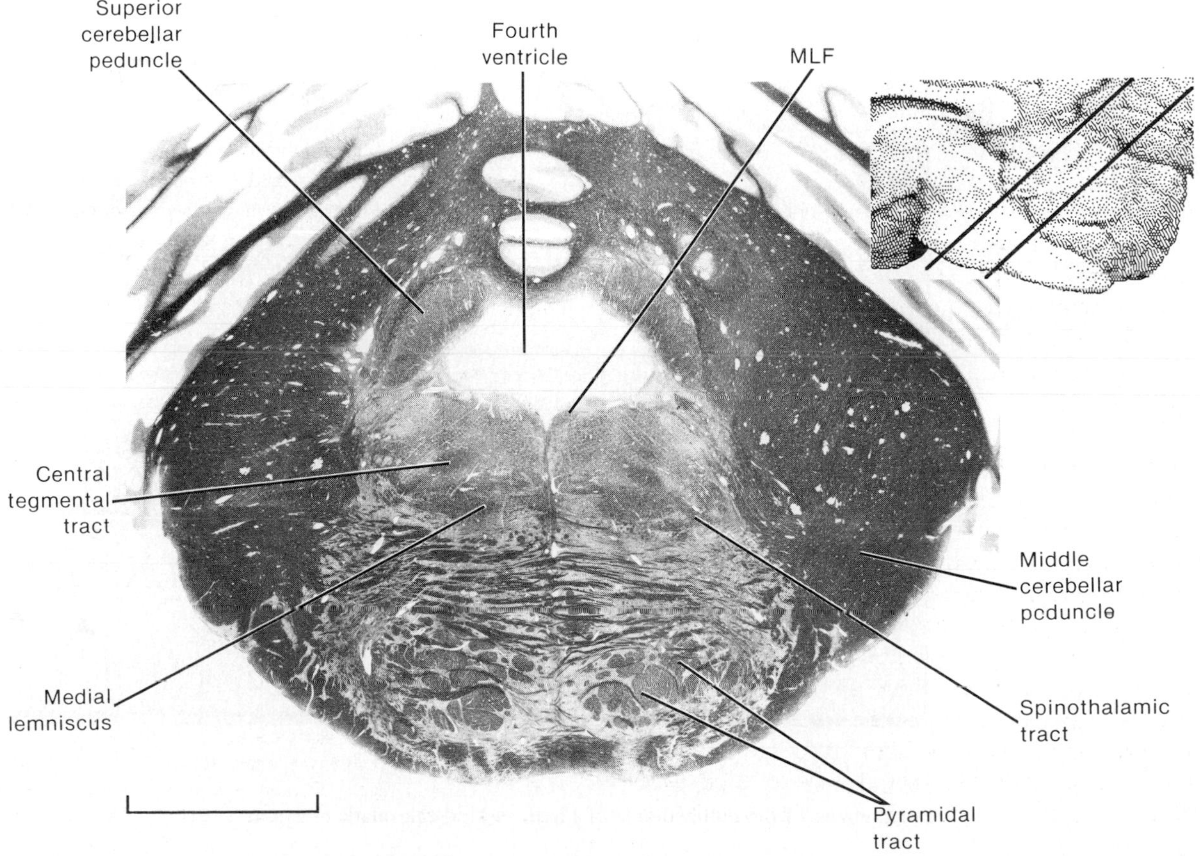


FIGURE 8-10
Midpons near the level of entry of the trigeminal nerve. Scale mark = 8 mm.

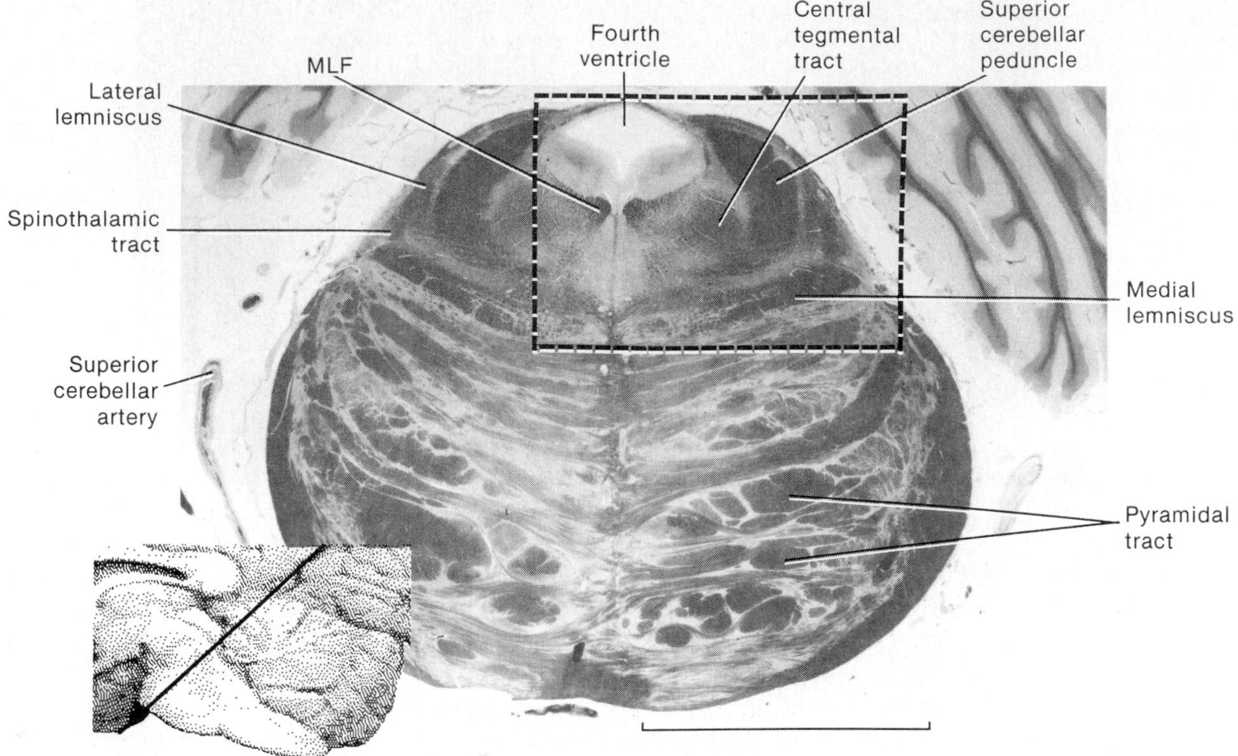


FIGURE 8-11
Rostral pons near the pons-midbrain junction. Scale mark = 1 cm.

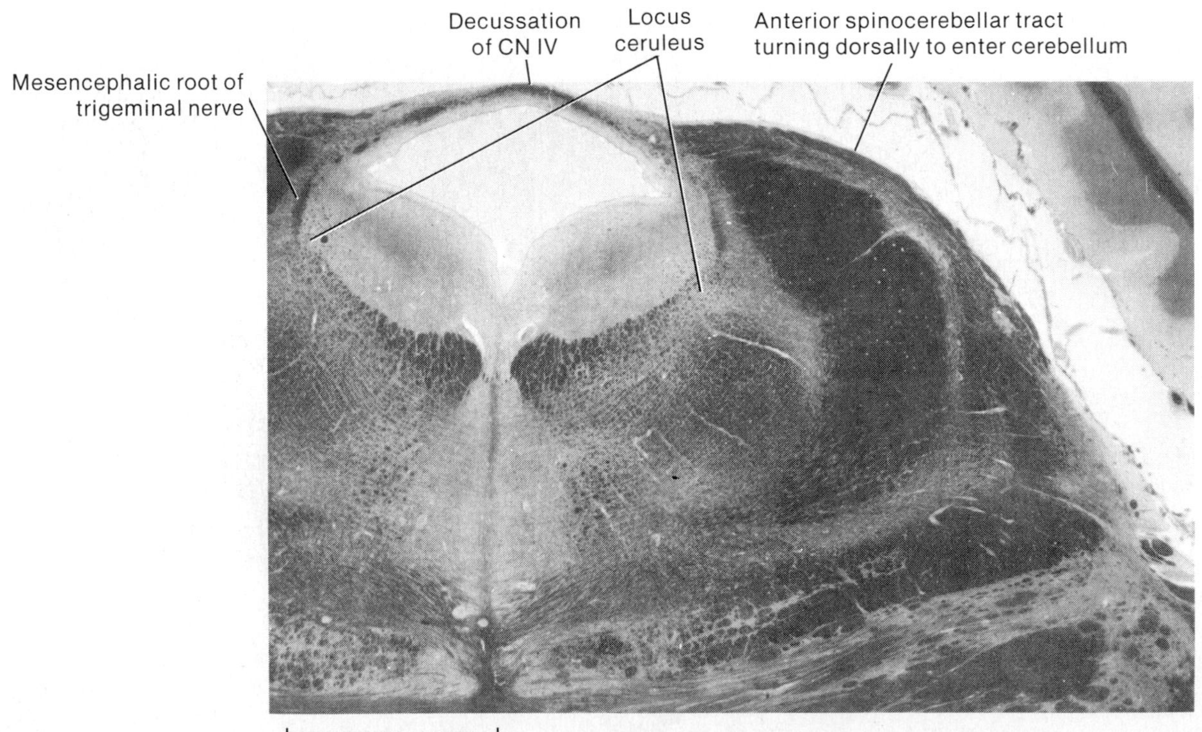


FIGURE 8-12
Enlargement of the outlined area of Figure 8-11. Scale mark = 2 mm.

## Rostral pons

The rostral pons extends from the attachment point of the trigeminal nerve (V) to the beginning of the cerebral aqueduct, which is about at the point of emergence of the trochlear nerve (IV). The MLF is visible throughout the rostral pons, as is the basal pons (Figure 8-11). The fourth ventricle narrows as the cerebral aqueduct is approached, and the superior cerebellar peduncle (brachium conjunctivum) becomes apparent in the wall of the ventricle. This is the major outflow from the cerebellum, projecting to the thalamus and to other structures.

The medial lemniscus gradually takes on a more flattened profile, now with a medial-lateral axis, and assumes a transverse orientation at the junction between the basal pons and the pontine tegmentum. As in the caudal pons, the homunculus is arranged so that its feet are most lateral. As the medial lemniscus moves laterally, it approaches the spinothalamic tract; from here through the midbrain, the two are adjacent.

The anterior spinocerebellar tract moves posteriorly onto the surface of the superior cerebellar peduncle (Figure 8-12). From here it turns caudally and enters the cerebellum, traveling "backwards" along the peduncle.

Near the floor of the fourth ventricle is a collection of pigmented cells that contain neuromelanin and appear blue-black in unstained brain tissue (Figure 8-12). This is the *locus ceruleus* (Latin for blue spot), a long thin nucleus that has been the subject of much research and interest in recent years. Cells of the locus ceruleus contain the neurotransmitter norepinephrine and innervate virtually the entire CNS, from the spinal cord to cerebral cortex.

Some of these cells send their axons to one particular site, such as the hypothalamus or the hippocampal formation. Others have widely branched axons, and a single neuron of the locus ceruleus can have synaptic terminals in the diencephalon, spinal cord, and cerebral cortex. (Prior to the discovery of the latter connection, it had been thought that no fibers arising caudal to the diencephalon reached the cerebral cortex; several counterexamples are now known.) The function of the locus ceruleus is not known with certainty, but it has been surmised from the widespread connections of this nucleus that it has some sort of overall biasing effect on the central nervous system. Consistent with this notion is the finding that the discharge rate of locus ceruleus neurons increases as an animal's state of arousal increases, decreases with drowsiness, and is nearly abolished in sleep.

The locus ceruleus and the axons leaving it constitute one example of a chemically coded neural pathway, in the sense that these neurons use norepinephrine as their neuro-

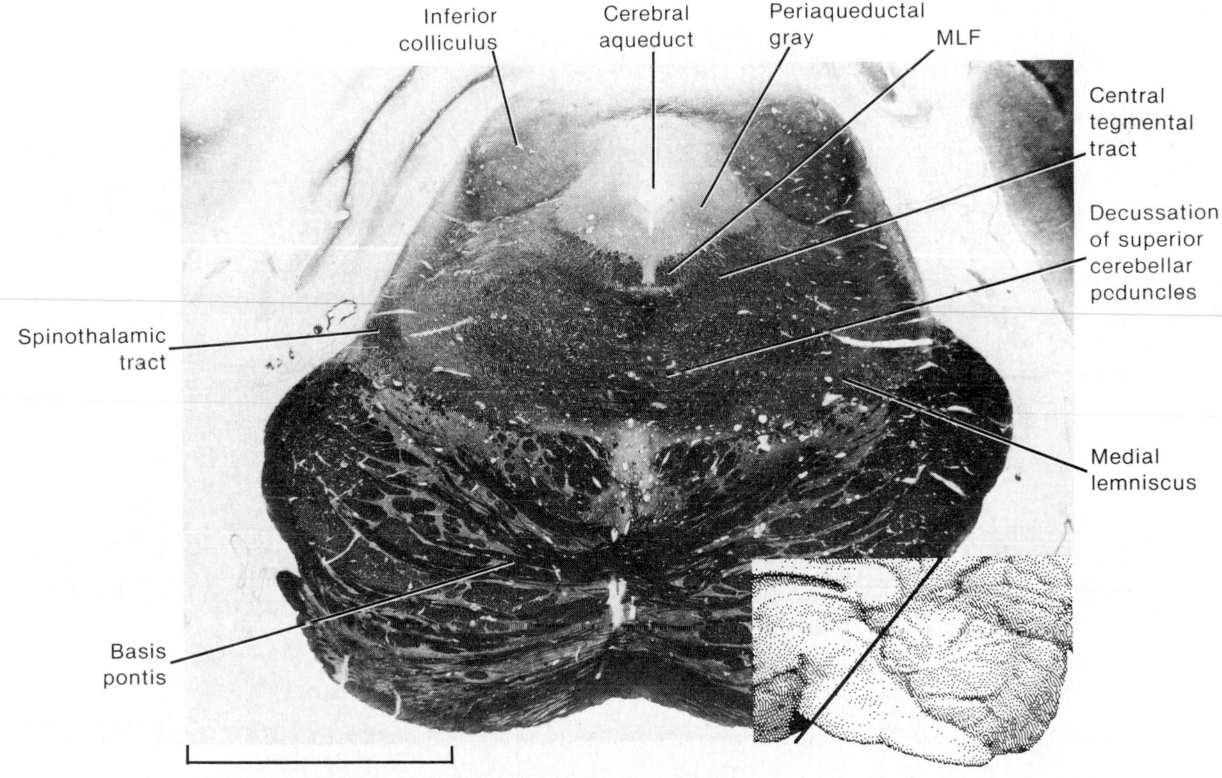


FIGURE 8-13
Caudal midbrain at the level of the inferior colliculus. Scale mark = 1 cm.

transmitter. Knowledge about other neurotransmitters and neuromodulators* and about other chemically coded pathways has accumulated rapidly in recent years. The number of known or strongly suspected neurotransmitters and neuromodulators currently stands at about 50; there are undoubtedly dozens more to be found. Some of these chemically coded neuronal systems correspond to previously known neuroanatomical pathways, whereas others do not. One reason that they have generated so much interest is that dysfunction of specific chemically coded systems is likely to correspond to particular kinds of neurological diseases; better understanding of such systems may therefore lead to improved pharmacologic treatment. Additional examples are cited later in this chapter and elsewhere, particularly in Chapter 17.

*A neurotransmitter is a substance that causes brief potential changes in postsynaptic neurons by means of short-lived permeability increases. Other substances released at synapses can cause much longer-lasting changes in postsynaptic neurons, modulating their response to conventional neurotransmitters. Such substances, which include some biogenic amines and small peptides, are therefore called neuromodulators.

## Caudal midbrain

The caudal midbrain is essentially the part that contains the inferior colliculi. It extends from the point of emergence of the trochlear nerve to the *intercollicular groove*. The fourth ventricle has narrowed into the cerebral aqueduct (Figure 8-13), the superior cerebellar peduncles sink deeper into the midbrain tegmentum and begin to decussate, and the MLF continues on its usual course. The basal pons protrudes rostrally under the caudal midbrain tegmentum. The inferior colliculus is (literally) a prominent nuclear mass. Ventromedial to it, encircling the aqueduct, is a particularly pale-staining region of gray matter called, appropriately enough, the *periaqueductal gray*.

The medial lemniscus is still a flattened band of fibers, now curving a bit dorsally, and the spinothalamic tract is dorsal to it at the surface of the brainstem. At slightly more rostral levels (Figure 8-14), the spinothalamic fibers are arranged in a band just beneath the brachium of the inferior colliculus. Damage here would be expected to abolish pain and temperature sensations over the entire contralateral half of the body. This was done for a time in a surgical procedure called *mesencephalic tractotomy,* in the hope of relieving intractable pain. However, because of unexpected and undesirable side effects (discussed later), the operation is seldom performed.

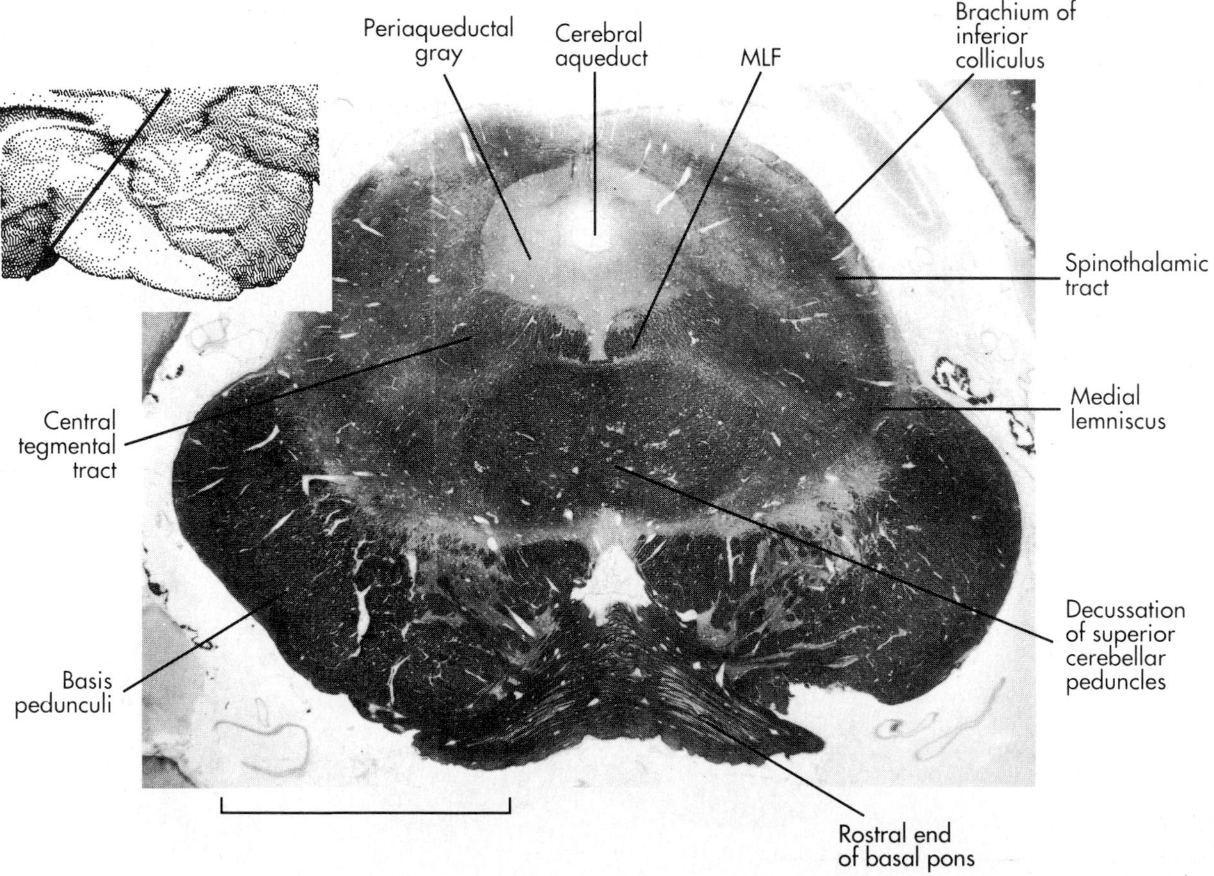


FIGURE 8-14
Mid-midbrain at the level of the intercollicular groove. Scale mark = 1 cm.

## Rostral midbrain

The rostral midbrain contains the superior colliculi. It extends from the intercollicular groove to the *posterior commissure*. Figure 8-15 shows a section through the rostral midbrain. At this level the MLF is ending, decussation of the superior cerebellar peduncles is complete, and in their place the large *red nucleus* becomes visible on each side. Some fibers from the contralateral half of the cerebellum end here, but most continue on to the thalamus. Anterior to the red nucleus is the *substantia nigra* (pale in myelin-stained preparations but dark in unstained or cell-stained preparations). The pigmented cells characteristic of the dorsal part of the substantia nigra provide another example of a chemically coded system. These neurons use dopamine for their neurotransmitter, ending profusely on neurons of the putamen and caudate nucleus. As discussed in Chapter 13, malfunction of this system results in Parkinson's disease.

Ventral to the substantia nigra is a massive bundle of fibers commonly referred to as the cerebral peduncle.* This bundle consists principally of descending corticopontine and corticospinal fibers. The oculomotor nerve (III) emerges into the space between the cerebral peduncles (the interpeduncular fossa). Several parts of the diencephalon (the pineal gland and some thalamic nuclei) hang back over and alongside the rostral midbrain.

*Strictly speaking, the term *cerebral peduncle* refers to all of the midbrain anterior to the superior colliculus, and the term *basis pedunculi* (or *crus cerebri*) refers to the massive fiber bundle in the anterior part of the peduncle. However, in common usage, *basis pedunculi* and *cerebral peduncle* are becoming more or less interchangeable, both referring to the fiber bundle.

At rostral midbrain levels, the medial lemniscus and the spinothalamic tract form a continuous curved band of fibers. Spinomesencephalic fibers (sometimes referred to as the *spinotectal tract*) that have accompanied the spinothalamic tract through the brainstem terminate in the periaqueductal gray, adjacent regions of the reticular formation and certain portions of the superior colliculus.

# RETICULAR FORMATION

## Nature

The reticular formation is an apparently (but not actually) diffusely organized area that forms the central core of the brainstem (Figure 8-16). It has been likened to a hot dog surrounded by a bun of discrete tracts and nuclei.† The reason it appears to be diffusely organized is twofold.

1. Its pattern of connectivity is characterized by a great deal of convergence and divergence, so that a single cell may respond to several different sensory modalities or to stimuli applied practically anywhere on the body.

†Earnest, Michael: Personal communication, 1974.

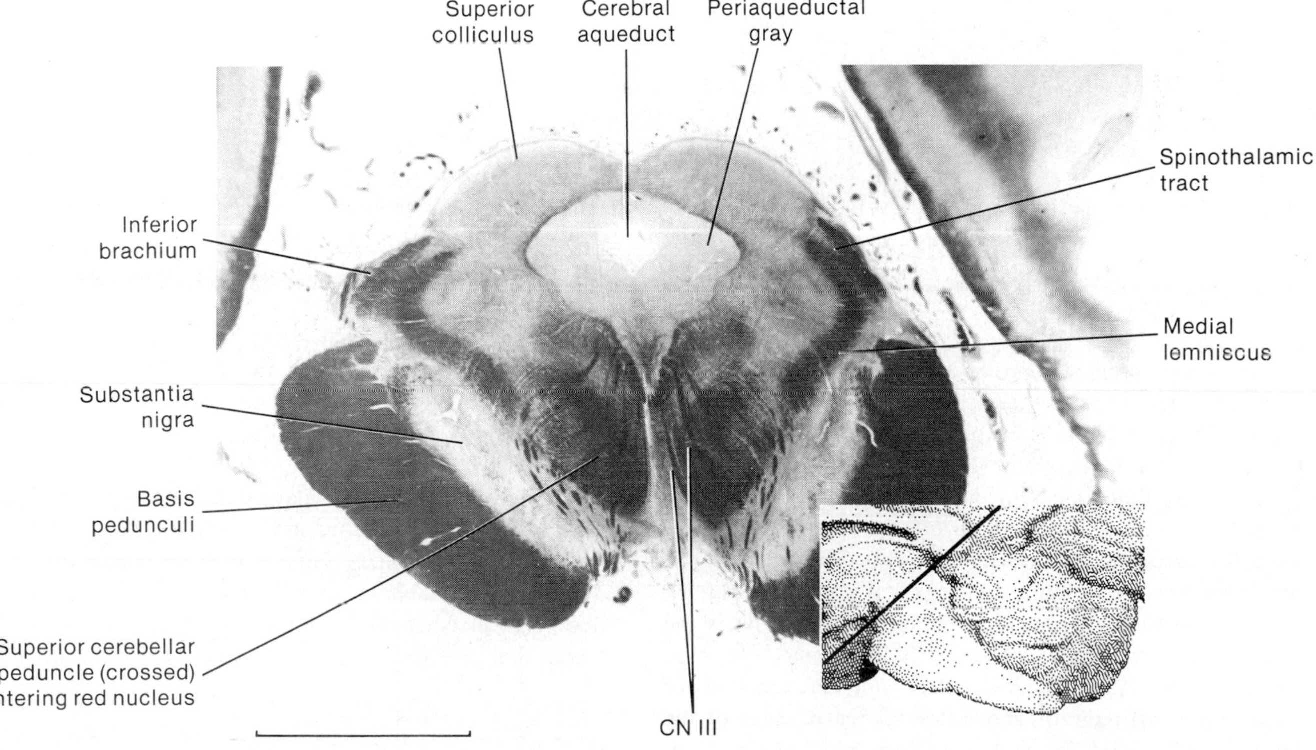


FIGURE 8-15
Rostral midbrain at the level of the superior colliculus. Scale mark = 1 cm.

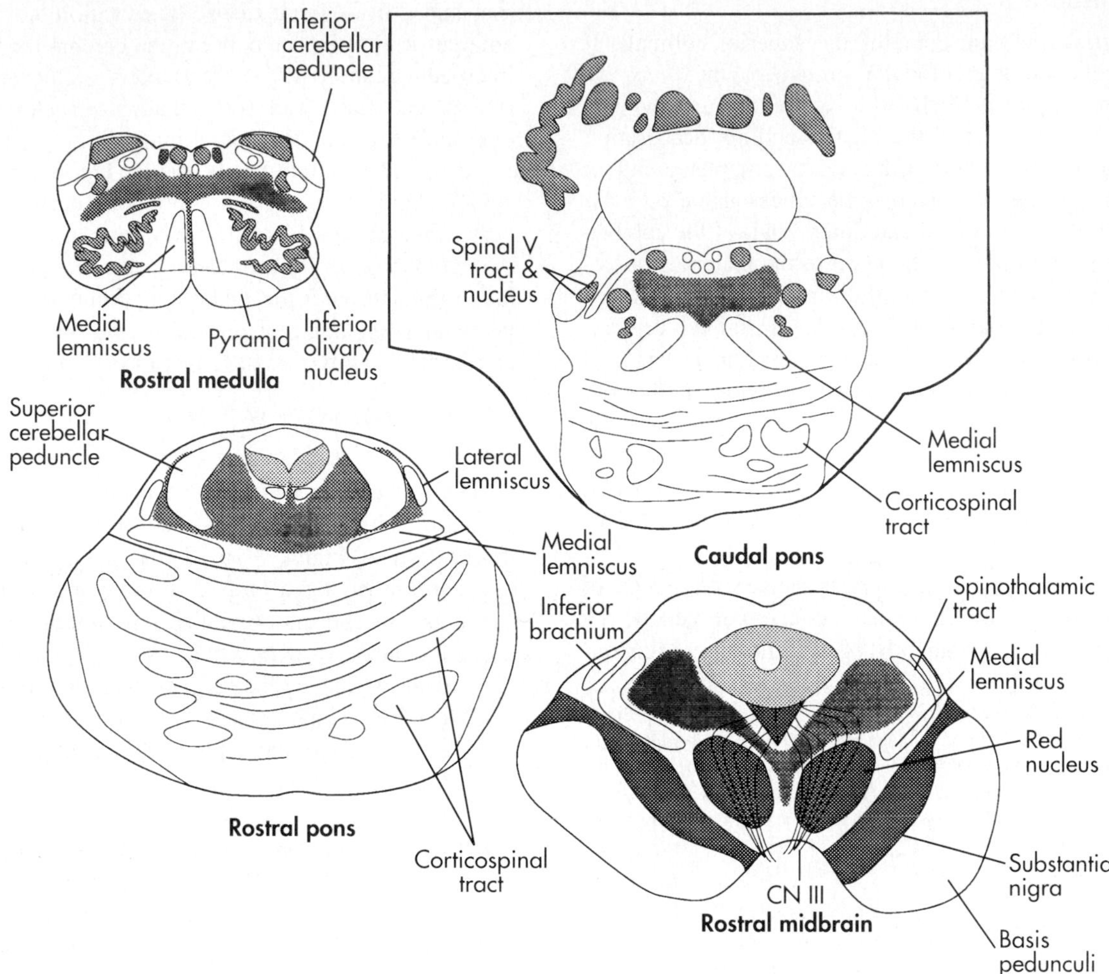


FIGURE 8-16
Approximate extent of the reticular formation at four different brainstem levels, indicated by color stippling.

2. Although it is involved in several quite separate functions, the areas involved in these functions overlap considerably, almost as though several nuclei had been scrambled together and dispersed along the brainstem, while their constituent cells retained their original connections.

At most levels of the brainstem, the reticular formation can be divided into three longitudinal zones arranged in a medial to lateral sequence. The *raphe nuclei* (from the Greek word *rhaphe* meaning seam, referring to the midline seam of the brainstem) are thin plates of cells in and immediately adjacent to the sagittal plane. Like the cells of the locus ceruleus, raphe neurons have exceedingly far flung connections; in this case, however, serotonin is the neurotransmitter (see Chapter 17). The *medial zone,* alongside the midline raphe nuclei, contains a mixture of large and small neurons and is the source of most of the long ascending and descending projections from the reticular formation. Some of the neurons in the medial zone of the rostral medullary reticular formation are so large that this area is referred to as the *gigantocellular reticular nucleus*. Finally, the *lateral zone,* which is particularly prominent in the rostral medulla and caudal pons, is primarily concerned with cranial nerve reflexes and visceral functions. These reticular zones have been further subdivided into a series of nuclei based on histology, connections, and function, although such nuclei cannot be distinguished easily in conventionally prepared sections such as those shown in Figures 9-41 to 9-49.

Many reticular neurons have extensive and complex axonal projections. Some innervate multiple levels of the spinal cord, while others send numerous collaterals to the brainstem and diencephalon (but generally not directly to the cerebral cortex*). A few may even have bifurcating axons that give rise to both ascending and descending con-

*Groups of monoamine-containing cells (see Chapter 17), like those of the locus ceruleus, are an exception. Certain of these cell groups are considered to be part of the reticular formation.

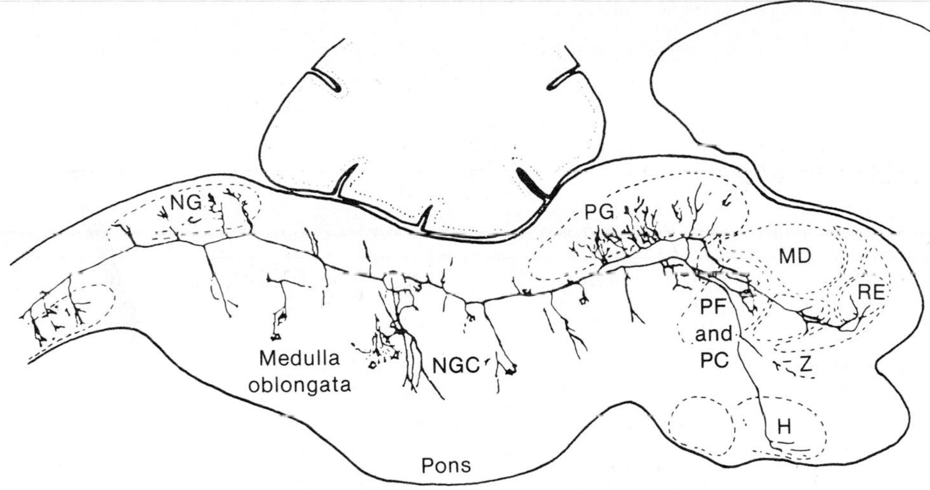


FIGURE 8-17
Drawing of a Golgi-stained parasagittal section from the brain of a young rat. The single stained cell in the pontine reticular formation has an axon that bifurcates and ends in wide areas of the CNS. If one cell has projections this extensive, imagine the complexity of the reticular formation as a whole. *H,* Hypothalamus; *MD, PC, PF,* and *RE,* thalamic nuclei (dorsomedial, paracentral, parafascicular, and reuniens); *NG,* nucleus gracilis; *NGC,* part of the pontine reticular formation (gigantocellular nucleus); *PG,* periaqueductal gray; *Z,* zona incerta (part of the diencephalon).

From Scheibel ME, Scheibel AB: Structural substrates for integrative patterns in the brain stem reticular core. In Jasper HH, et al, editors: *Reticular formation of the brain,* Boston, 1958, Little, Brown & Co.

nections (Figure 8-17). Reticular neurons also have large fields of dendrites, sometimes spreading out in a plane perpendicular to the long axis of the brainstem, that allow them to receive synaptic inputs from ascending sensory pathways, descending cortical axons, and a variety of other sources. A look at the processes of a single reticular cell in a single plane (Figure 8-17) should demonstrate why the reticular formation has been a tremendously difficult area of the brain to study; still, some progress has been made.

## Functions and connections

The reticular formation is involved in four general types of function: motor control, sensory control, visceral control, and control of consciousness.

### *Motor control*

Motor control has several different aspects.

1. Certain reticular regions are closely related to the cerebellum and its motor control functions. A fairly discrete collection of cells in the medullary reticular formation called the *lateral reticular nucleus* can often be resolved adjacent to the spinothalamic tract in conventionally prepared brainstem sections. It extends rostrally to midolivary levels and caudally into the caudal medulla, receiving direct spinoreticular fibers and collaterals of spinothalamic fibers and projecting to the cerebellum. It also receives input from the red nucleus, so it is more than a straightforward somatosensory relay to the cerebellum. Collections of reticular neurons near the medullary midline, collectively called the *paramedian reticular nucleus,* also project to the cerebellum. Afferents to the paramedian nucleus arise in the cerebellum and in other locations, including the cerebral cortex. Finally, the *reticular tegmental nucleus,* located between the medial lemnisci in the rostral pons, receives inputs from the cerebral cortex and other sites and projects to the cerebellum.
2. There are two *reticulospinal tracts* arising from the medial zone of the pontine and the rostral medullary reticular formation. Fibers from the pons descend with the ipsilateral MLF and travel through the ventral funiculus in the spinal cord (Figure 8-18). Those from the medulla descend bilaterally in the ventral part of the lateral funiculus.

The reticulospinal tracts are a major alternate route (to the pyramidal tract) by which spinal motor neurons are controlled. These reticular neurons receive projections from many areas, including the basal ganglia, red nucleus, and substantia nigra. Input from widespread areas of the cerebral cortex, particularly the somatosensory and motor cortex, seems to be especially important. Most of these descending fibers travel to their reticular terminations in the *central tegmental tract* (Figures 8-9 to 8-15). This is a complex tract containing afferents to, and efferents from, the reticular formation and descend-

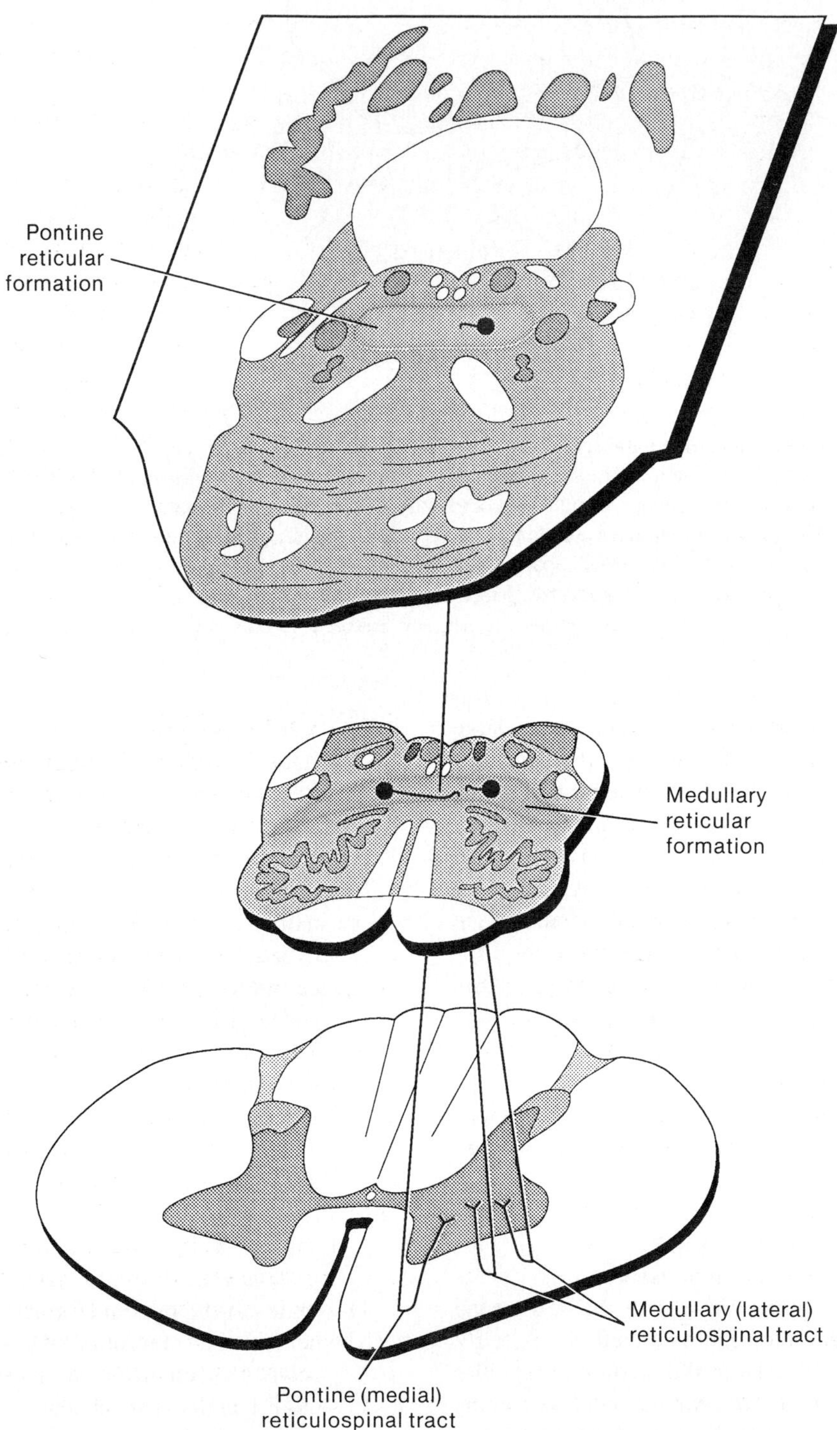


FIGURE 8-18
Medullary and pontine reticulospinal tracts.

ing projections from the red nucleus to the inferior olivary nucleus.

3. The reticulospinal tracts also carry descending motor commands generated within the reticular formation itself. Just as the spinal cord contains the basic neural machinery for simple (and some not-so-simple) reflexes, so the reticular formation contains the neural machinery for considerably more complex patterns of movement. A cat whose brainstem has been surgically separated from its diencephalon can, after a recovery period, walk and run spontaneously, properly right itself if tipped over, and assume a variety of complex postures. There have been cases of human infants born without cerebral hemispheres who were nevertheless capable of apparently normal yawning, stretching, suckling, and orienting behavior. It is assumed that their reticular formations formed the basis for these activities.

### *Sensory control*

Reticular neurons exert some control over activity in spinal reflex arcs and also over the access of sensory information to ascending pathways. Tonic inhibition of flexor reflexes originates in the reticular formation, with the result that only noxious stimuli can normally evoke such a reflex. In addition, stimulation of certain regions of the medullary reticular formation causes inhibition of some sensory interneurons and tract cells in the spinal cord. This seems to be important in the regulation of pain perception, as discussed a little later in this chapter.

### *Visceral control*

A great deal of visceral information reaches the reticular formation, which programs appropriate responses to environmental changes and projects to the autonomic nuclei of the brainstem and spinal cord. Centers controlling inspiration, expiration, and the normal rhythm of breathing have been identified physiologically in the medulla and pons. Other centers controlling heart rate and blood pressure have been identified in the medullary reticular formation.

The hypothalamus also gives rise to numerous fibers concerned with autonomic regulation. Many of those involved in sympathetic control traverse the brainstem near the spinothalamic tract and reach mainly the ipsilateral (but to some extent the contralateral) intermediolateral cell column of the spinal cord. The numbers and types of synapses in the pathway are not completely understood, but at least some of the fibers reach the spinal cord directly from the hypothalamus. Interruption of the descending sympathetic pathway causes ipsilateral *Horner's syndrome,* which refers to a combination of miosis (small pupil), ptosis (drooping eyelid), and enophthalmos (recession of the eyeball; this is more apparent than real). Horner's syndrome may be accompanied by flushing and lack of sweating in ipsilateral skin of the face and part of the body.

### *Control of consciousness*

Ascending projections from the reticular formation terminate in the thalamus, subthalamus, hypothalamus, and basal ganglia. The functions of most of these are poorly understood, but those to the thalamus seem to be particularly important. They terminate (as do the paleospinothalamic fibers) in the intralaminar nuclei, which in turn project to widespread areas of the cortex. Activity in this pathway is essential for the maintenance of a normal state of consciousness, and bilateral damage to these fibers as they traverse or originate in the midbrain reticular formation results in prolonged coma. This is an astounding notion: a normal, intact cerebrum is incapable of functioning in a conscious manner by itself; sustaining input from the brainstem reticular formation is required. The portion of the reticular formation that provides this input is known as the *ascending reticular activating system* (ARAS). It is important to understand that the ARAS is defined by physiological criteria; it is not synonymous with the anatomically defined reticular formation but rather is a portion of it. Modulation of the ARAS has a basic role in the sleep-wakefulness cycle, as discussed later in this book.

## VASCULAR SUPPLY

The brainstem depends chiefly on the vertebral-basilar system for its blood supply (Figures 8-19 and 8-20). The caudal medulla has a supply much like that of the spinal cord. Anterior and lateral portions are supplied by the anterior spinal artery and/or small branches of the vertebral artery. Posterior portions are supplied by the posterior spinal artery and/or small branches of the posterior inferior cerebellar artery (PICA). The rostral medulla receives a varying supply. Anterior and medial structures, such as the pyramid and the medial lemniscus, depend on some combination of vertebral branches and the anterior spinal artery. Lateral and posterior structures, such as the spinothalamic tract and the inferior cerebellar peduncle, depend on the PICA and, to a lesser extent, on the posterior spinal artery.

Most of the pons is supplied by unnamed *paramedian* and *circumferential* branches of the basilar artery. The anterior inferior cerebellar artery (AICA) and the superior cerebellar artery contribute branches to the middle and superior cerebellar peduncles and to dorsal and lateral portions of the pontine tegmentum.

The supply of the midbrain is chiefly from the posterior cerebral artery, with some contribution from the superior cerebellar artery caudally. In addition, the anterior choroidal artery and the posterior communicating artery may send branches to the cerebral peduncle.

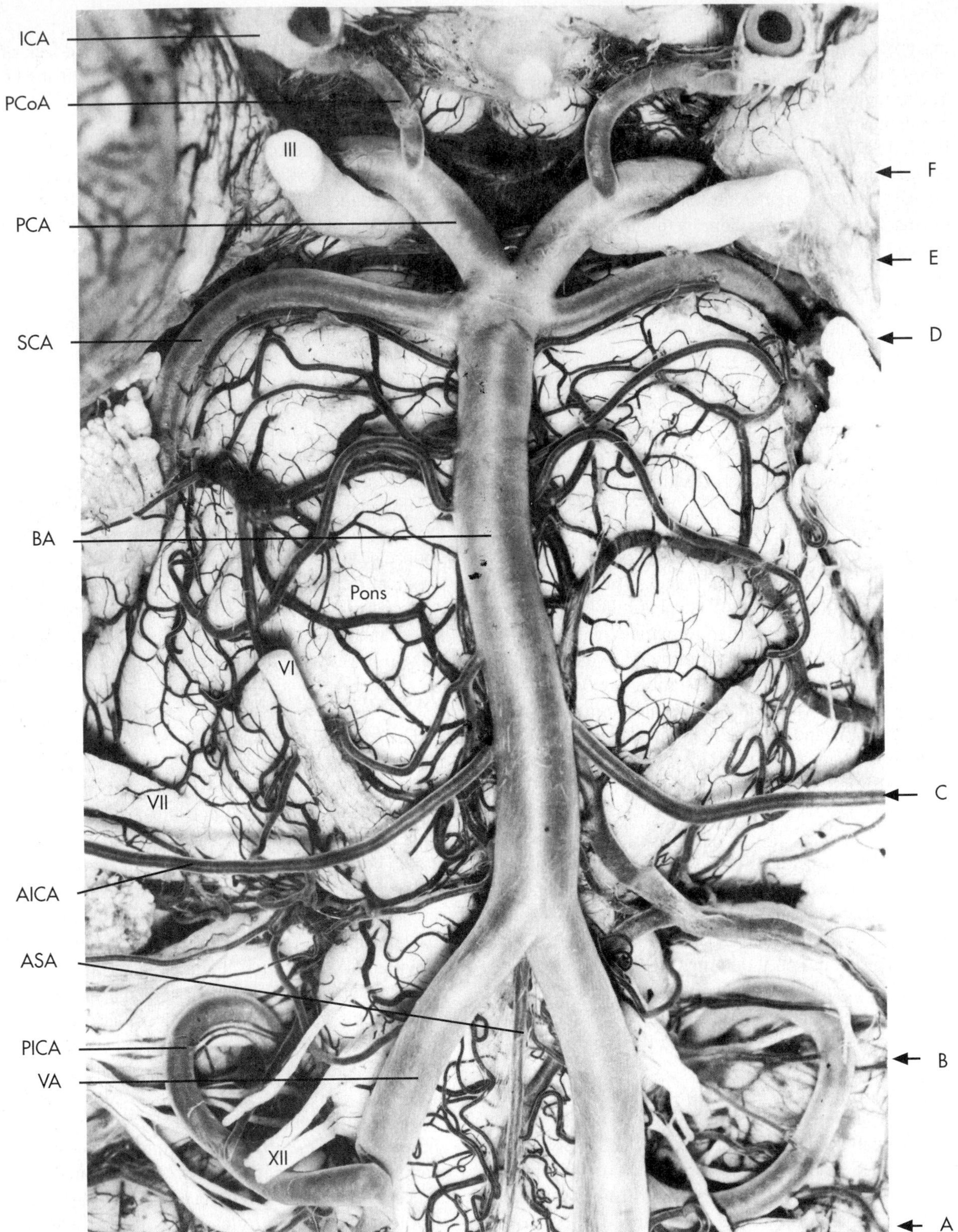


FIGURE 8–19
The anterior surface of a human brainstem, after its arteries had been injected with a mixture of gelatin and Indian ink. Arteries of the vertebral-basilar systems can be seen clearly, overlying the various divisions of the brainstem. By considering where different vessels and branches leave the vertebral-basilar system, one can imagine the vascular supply of each brainstem level; the arrows on the right indicate the levels for which vascular territories are charted in Figure 8–20. *AICA*, Anterior inferior cerebellar artery; *ASA*, Anterior spinal artery; *BA*, Basilar artery; *ICA*, Internal cartoid artery; *PCA*, Posterior cerebal artery; *PCoA*, Posterior communicating artery; *PICA*, Posterior inferior cerebellar artery; *SCA*, Superior cerebellar artery; *VA*, Vertebral artery.

From Duvernoy HM: *Human Brainstem Vessels*, New York, 1978, Springer-Verlag, Inc. Courtesy of Dr. H.M. Duvernoy, Faculte de Medecine, Universite de Franche-Comte.

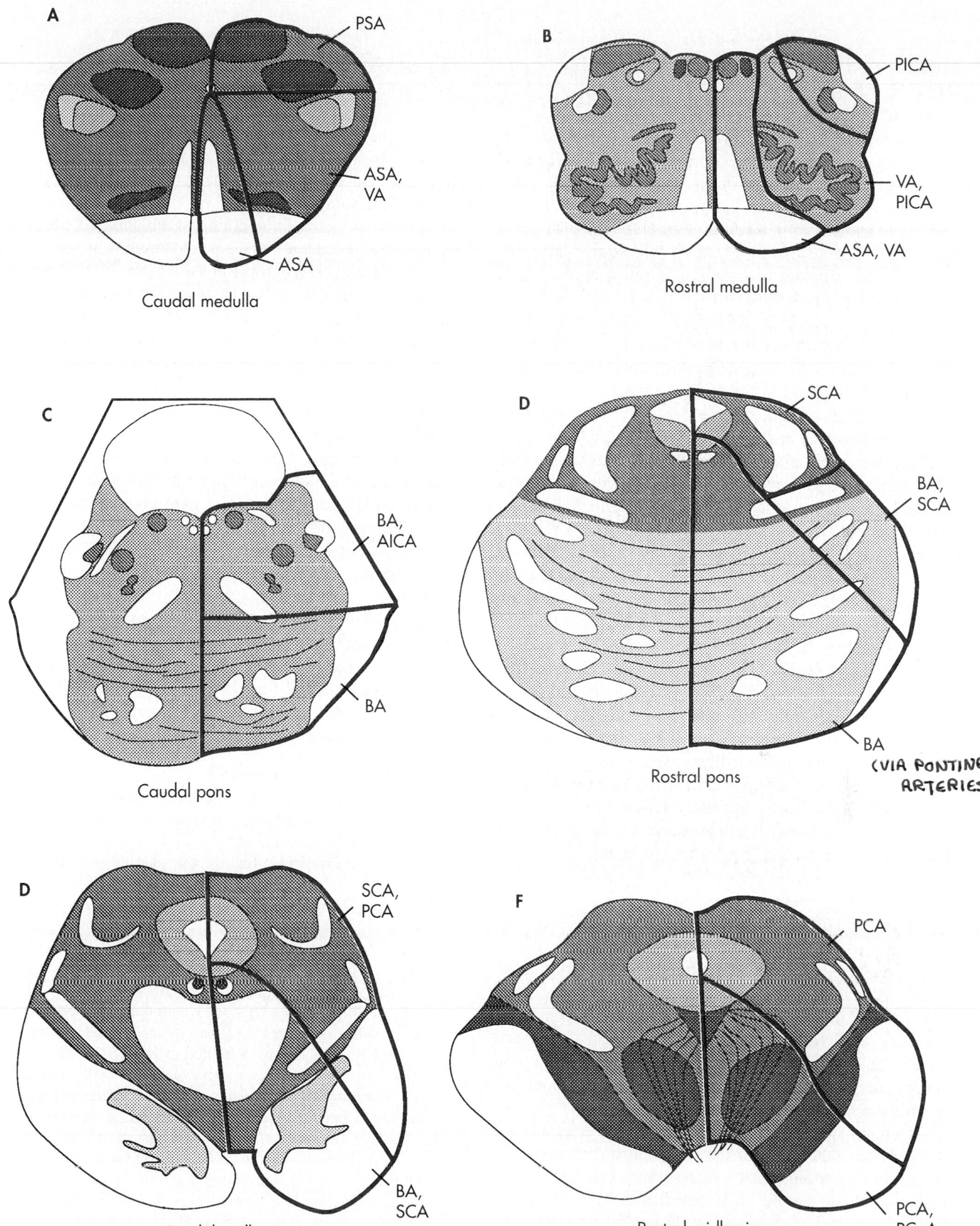


FIGURE 8-20
Approximate arterial supply of various brainstem levels; corresponding levels of an intact brainstem are indicated in Figure 8-19. While there is variability from one individual to another, different vertebral-basilar branches, or combinations of these branches, typically supply wedge-shaped areas at each brainstem level. The zones of damage in brainstem strokes frequently correspond to these wedge-shaped areas. *PSA*, posterior spinal artery; other abbreviations as in Figure 8-19.

## SOME FUNCTIONAL ASPECTS OF THE BRAINSTEM

### Pain pathways

As noted in Chapter 7, a cordotomy is sometimes performed for the surgical relief of intractable pain. When the pain involves an entire side of the body, the spinothalamic tract has occasionally been sectioned in the medulla (an operation known as a *medullary tractotomy*). This is a rather more serious operation than a cordotomy, partly because of the difficulty of obtaining surgical access to the medulla and partly because of the risk to vital structures located in the medulla. Therefore, attempts have been made in the past to cut the spinothalamic tract in other, less risky sites in the brainstem. A mesencephalic tractotomy, cutting the tract in the midbrain where it is near the surface of the brainstem (Figure 8-14), seems feasible on anatomical grounds and has been attempted in several instances. However, although medullary tractotomies abolish contralateral pain over the whole body (much as a high cervical cordotomy would), a mesencephalic tractotomy often had a less favorable outcome. In a large percentage of the latter cases, the patients developed a new form of pain shortly after the operation. A pinprick, or sometimes just a light touch, on the contralateral side of the body would cause an excruciating, deep, burning pain that was frequently felt to be worse than the original problem. The operation therefore is no longer performed. What was the cause of this unfortunate outcome? A medullary tractotomy, like a cordotomy, interrupts both spinothalamic and spinoreticular fibers, but mesencephalic tractotomy interrupts only the spinothalamic fibers, since the spinoreticular fibers have by this time moved medially and terminated in the reticular formation. Apparently activity in this spinoreticulothalamic pathway, in the absence of direct spinothalamic activity, somehow causes the *dysesthesia*.

### Endorphins and enkephalins

Opium and its derivatives, especially morphine, have long been used for pain control. The mechanism of their action has been a topic of great interest; if this mechanism could be understood, it might then be possible to design new pain-killing drugs that would not cause tolerance and addiction to develop. Over the past 20 years, pharmacological and anatomical-physiological studies have converged to produce extremely exciting data about this mechanism.

Electrical stimulation (through implanted electrodes) of the periaqueductal gray of the midbrain of rats causes an analgesia so profound that major surgery can then be performed without the aid of an anesthetic. This electrically induced analgesia is blocked by drugs that antagonize the action of morphine. Similar stimulation of the periaqueductal gray of humans can abolish intractable pain, an effect also blocked by opiate antagonists. This seemed to imply that morphine mimics a pain-killing substance that is produced by the brain and released by stimulation of the periaqueductal gray. Two closely related pentapeptides called *enkephalins* (from the Greek words meaning "in the head"), having powerful opiate properties, have been isolated from mammalian brains and are found in high concentration in the periaqueductal gray and in the posterior horn of the spinal cord.

One way in which midbrain stimulation (or morphine administration) depresses pain transmission is via a pathway that travels through the posterior part of the lateral funiculus, terminates in the ipsilateral posterior horn, and inhibits the interneurons and the tract cells of the spinothalamic tract. However, the direct projections from the periaqueductal gray to the spinal cord are relatively sparse. For the most part this pain-control pathway involves a synapse in the medulla, either in one of the raphe nuclei *(nucleus raphe magnus)* or in adjacent areas of the medullary reticular formation. This pathway can be activated by stressful or painful stimuli, which appears to provide a partial explanation for the suppression of pain experienced by people in emergency situations. The classic example of this is soldiers wounded in battle who nevertheless continue to function and are not nearly as distressed as one would expect.

Endogenous sustances with opiate activity (collectively called *endorphins*), of which the enkephalins are one example, are widespread in the nervous system and participate in many neural functions in addition to pain control. Conversely, not all aspects of pain control are accounted for by the enkephalin system.

## ADDITIONAL READINGS


Amaral DG, Sinnamon HM: The locus coeruleus: neurobiology of a central noradrenergic nucleus, *Prog Neurobiol* 9:147, 1977. *An extensive review.*

Basbaum AI, Fields HL: Endogenous pain control mechanisms: review and hypothesis, *Ann Neurol* 4:451, 1978.

Basbaum AI, Fields HL: Endogenous pain control systems: brainstem spinal pathways and endorphin circuitry, *Ann Rev Neurosci* 7:309, 1984. *An updating of the 1978 review by the same authors, with new details.*

Basbaum AI, Ralston DD, Ralston HJ III: Bulbospinal projections in the primate: a light and electron microscopic study of a pain-modulating system, *J Comp Neurol* 250:311, 1986.

Beecher HR: Pain in men wounded in battle, *Ann Surg* 123:96, 1946. *A fascinating paper showing that wounds we would expect to be terribly painful may not be, depending in part on the circumstances surrounding the incurrence of the injury.*

Bonica JJ et al: *Biochemistry and modulation of nociception and pain.* In Bonica JJ, editor: *The management of pain,* ed 2, Philadelphia, 1990, Lea and Febiger.

Bradford HF: *Chemical neurobiology: an introduction to neurochemistry,* New York, 1986, W.H. Freeman & Co.

Cohen MI: Neurogenesis of respiratory rhythm in the mammal, *Physiol Rev* 59:1105, 1979.

Drake CG, McKenzie KG: Mesencephalic tractotomy for pain, *J Neurosurg* 10:457, 1953.

Engberg I, Lundberg A, Ryall RW: Reticulospinal inhibition of transmission in reflex pathways, *J Physiol* 194:201, 1968.

Foote SL, Bloom FE, Aston-Jones G: Nucleus locus ceruleus: new evidence of anatomical and physiological specificity, *Physiol Rev* 63:844, 1983.

Hobson JA, Brazier MAB, editors: *The reticular formation revisited: specifying function for a nonspecific system,* International Brain Res. Organization monograph series, vol. 6, New York, 1980, Raven Press.

Hosobuchi Y, Adams JE, Linchitz R: Pain relief by electrical stimulation of the central gray matter in humans and its reversal by naloxone, *Science* 197:183, 1977. *Evidence that the analgesia caused by stimulation of the periaqueductal gray has properties in common with morphine analgesia.*

Hughes J: Isolation of an endogenous compound from the brain with pharmacological properties similar to morphine, *Brain Res* 88:295, 1975.

Jacobs BL: Single-unit activity of locus ceruleus neurons in behaving animals, *Prog Neurobiol* 27:183, 1986.

Kneisley LW, Biber MP, La Vail JH: A study of the origin of brain stem projections to monkey spinal cord using the retrograde transport method, *Exp Neurol* 60:116, 1978.

Kuhar MJ, Pert CB, Snyder SH: Regional distribution of opiate receptor binding in monkey and human brain, *Nature* 245:447, 1973.

Loewy AD, Araujo JC, Kerr FWL: Pupillodilator pathways in the brain stem of the cat: anatomical and electrophysiological identification of a central autonomic pathway, *Brain Res* 60:65, 1973.

Luiten PGM et al: The course of paraventricular hypothalamic efferents to autonomic structures in medulla and spinal cord, *Brain Res* 329:374, 1985.

Mayer DJ, Price DD, Rafii A: Antagonism of acupuncture analgesia in man by the narcotic antagonist naloxone, *Brain Res* 121:368, 1977. *A provocative paper providing initial evidence that acupuncture works by somehow causing the release of enkephalins.*

Mehler WR: Some neurological species differences—*a posteriori, Ann NY Acad Sci* 167:424, 1969. *Tracing ascending tracts through the brainstem in a phylogenetic series of mammals from opossums to people.*

Mitani A et al: Descending projections from the gigantocellular tegmental field in the cat: cells of origin and their brainstem and spinal cord trajectories, *J Comp Neurol* 268:546, 1988.

Nygren L-G, Olson L: A new major projection from locus coeruleus: the main source of noradrenergic nerve terminals in the ventral and dorsal columns of the spinal cord, *Brain Res* 132:85, 1977.

Olszewski J, Baxter D: *Cytoarchitecture of the human brainstem,* Philadelphia, 1954, JB Lippincott Co.

Peterson BW: *The reticulospinal system and its role in the control of movement.* In Barnes CD, editor: *Brainstem control of spinal cord function,* Orlando, Fla., 1984, Academic Press.

Reynolds DV: Surgery in the rat during electrical analgesia induced by focal brain stimulation, *Science* 164:444, 1969.

Riley HA: *An atlas of the basal ganglia, brain stem and spinal cord,* New York, 1960, Hafner.

Saper CB et al: Direct hypothalamo-autonomic connections, *Brain Res* 117:305, 1976.

Steriade M, McCarley RW: *Brainstem control of wakefulness and sleep,* New York, 1990, Plenum Press. *A recent, extensive review of the structure, connections, and electrophysiology of the reticular formation.*

Willis WD, Haber LH, Martin RF: Inhibition of spinothalamic tract cells and interneurons by brain stem stimulation in the monkey, *J Neurophysiol* 40:968, 1977.

CHAPTER

# 9

# *Cranial Nerves*

The caudal medulla looks somewhat similar to the spinal cord, but this similarity seems to disappear at more rostral levels of the brainstem. One of the complicating factors is the arrangement of the tracts and nuclei associated with cranial nerves III to XII. These tracts and nuclei appear discouragingly intricate on first inspection, but there is a common way of systematizing the cranial nerves so that their central connections make sense. This is in terms of the *functional components* contained within each nerve.

Spinal nerves contain sensory and motor fibers. Some of each kind are related to visceral structures and some to somatic structures. A given spinal nerve fiber can therefore be placed in one of the following four categories, each of which is prefixed by the word "general":

1. *General somatic afferent (GSA)* fibers are related to receptors for pain, temperature, and mechanical stimuli in somatic structures such as skin, muscles, and joints.
2. *General visceral afferent (GVA)* fibers are related to receptors in visceral structures such as the walls of the digestive tract.
3. *General visceral efferent (GVE)* fibers are preganglionic autonomic fibers.
4. *General somatic efferent (GSE)* fibers innervate skeletal muscle (that is, they are the axons of alpha and gamma motor neurons).

By and large the cell bodies on which spinal afferents synapse and the cell bodies of spinal efferent fibers are located in portions of the spinal gray matter predictable from its embryological development (Figure 9-1, *A*). The sulcus limitans separates the alar plate (which develops into the posterior horn) from the basal plate (which develops into the anterior horn). Within both the alar and the basal plate, cells concerned with visceral function tend to be located nearer the sulcus limitans. This is shown most clearly in the adult by the location of the cell bodies of GVE fibers in the intermediolateral cell column. Thus for each of the four spinal functional components there is a corresponding column of cells in the spinal gray matter. The GSA and GSE columns extend the length of the cord; the GVA and GVE columns are found at spinal levels T1 to L2 or L3 and S2 to S4.

All four of the spinal functional components are found in various cranial nerves, where they subserve the same functions for the head. Three additional components are also found among the cranial nerves; these new components are prefixed by the word "special":

1. *Special somatic afferent (SSA)* fibers are related to the special senses of sight, hearing, and equilibrium.
2. *Special visceral afferent (SVA)* fibers are related to the special senses of smell and taste.
3. *Special visceral efferent (SVE)* fibers innervate certain striated muscles with a special embryological origin, referred to as the branchiomeric muscles. Structures that develop into the gill arches (or branchial arches) in fish develop instead into various structures in and near the head and neck in humans. Branchiomeric muscles (notably the muscles of the larynx, pharynx, and face) are associated with these branchial arch structures. Functionally and histologically, branchiomeric muscles are identical to ordinary skeletal muscle. However, since they tend to be concentrated around the mouth at the junction between visceral and somatic areas, the motor fibers that innervate them are conventionally called SVE fibers. The classification is sometimes confusing (particularly since the sensory fibers to these muscles are called GSA fibers), but it is a tradition of long standing. The important point is that the motor

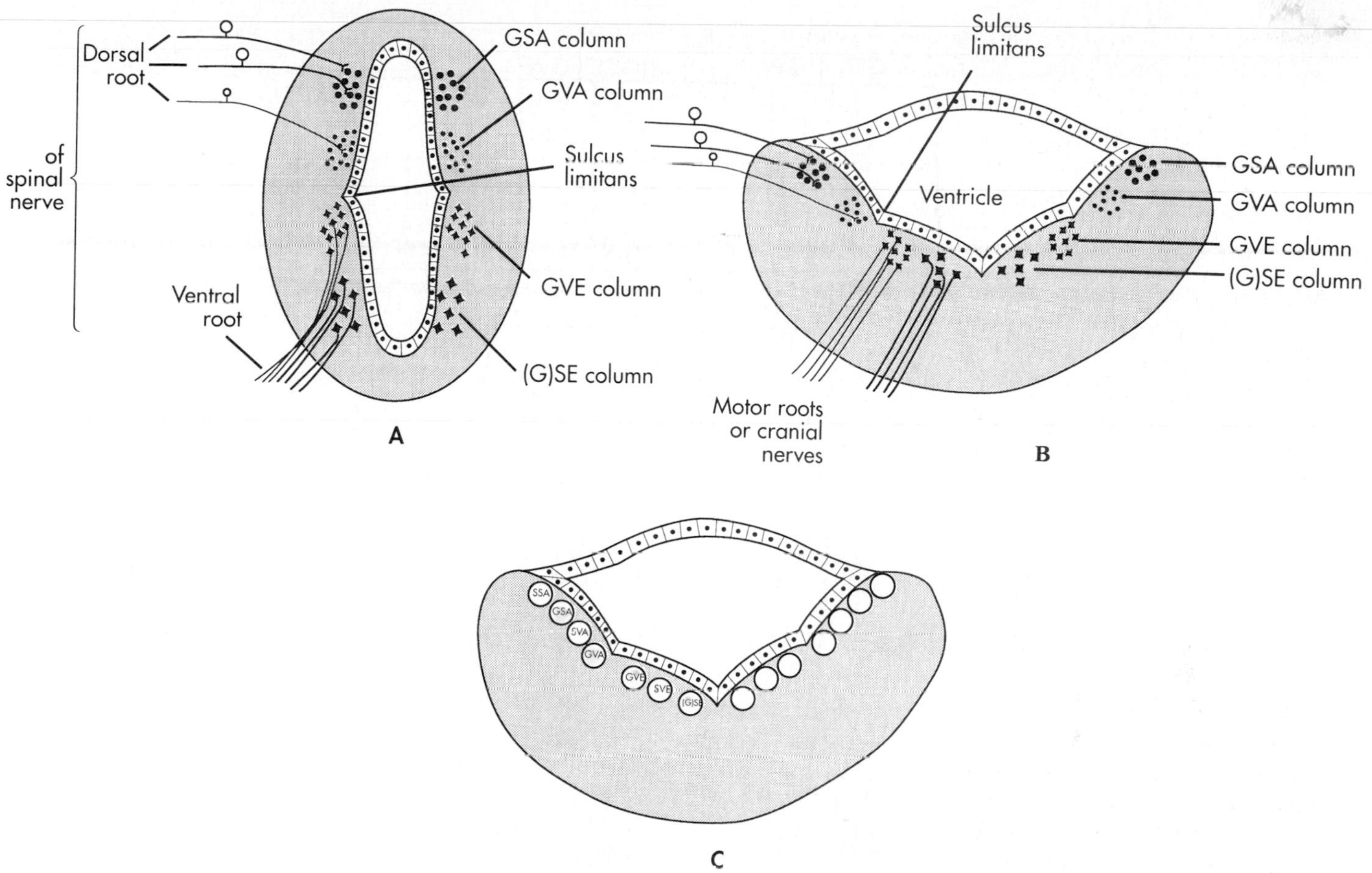


FIGURE 9-1
Arrangement of cranial nerve nuclei in the brainstem. **A,** Arrangement of the general afferent and efferent cell columns in the embryonic spinal cord. **B,** Movement of these columns to the floor of the fourth ventricle in the embryonic rhombencephalon. **C,** Further subdivision of these cell columns, showing the "ideal" locations of the cranial nerve nuclei, corresponding to the seven functional components.

neurons for branchiomeric muscles have a distinctive location in the brainstem, different from that of ordinary somatic motor neurons.

There are no special somatic efferent fibers, so GSE fibers are often referred to simply as *somatic efferent (SE)* fibers.

As in the case of the spinal cord, the locations of the cell bodies where cranial nerve afferents terminate or cranial nerve efferents originate can be predicted (to some extent) from the embryology of the brainstem. The walls of the neural tube spread apart in the medulla and pons to form the floor of the fourth ventricle (see Figure 1-11). The sulcus limitans runs longitudinally along the floor of the adult ventricle, still separating sensory alar plate derivatives (now lateral) from motor basal plate derivatives (now medial) (Figure 9-1, *B*). As in the case of the spinal cord, cells concerned with visceral function tend to be located nearer the sulcus limitans.

Ideally the cell columns subserving the special components of the cranial nerves would be located adjacent to those for the corresponding general components, as indicated in Figure 9-1, *C*. The actual arrangement in the adult brainstem is not quite so simple as in this idealized diagram, for two principal reasons. First, the cell columns of the brainstem are not continuous as are those of the spinal cord; rather, they are interrupted and form a series of nuclei so that all components may not be present in a given transverse plane (Figures 9-2, *A* and 9-10). Second, in a few instances, portions of a cell column migrate away from their expected locations (Figure 9-2, *B* ). For example, most SVE neurons are located in the ventrolateral part of the tegmentum rather than in the floor of the ventricle adjacent to other efferent neurons. The actual locations of cranial nerve nuclei in the rostral medulla are shown in Figure 9-2, *B;* also indicated are the types of functional components in each of the cranial nerves of the brainstem. However, this is only meant to be a convenient summary, and not all cranial nerves project to or originate from the rostral medulla.

It can be seen from Figure 9-2, *B* that no cranial nerve

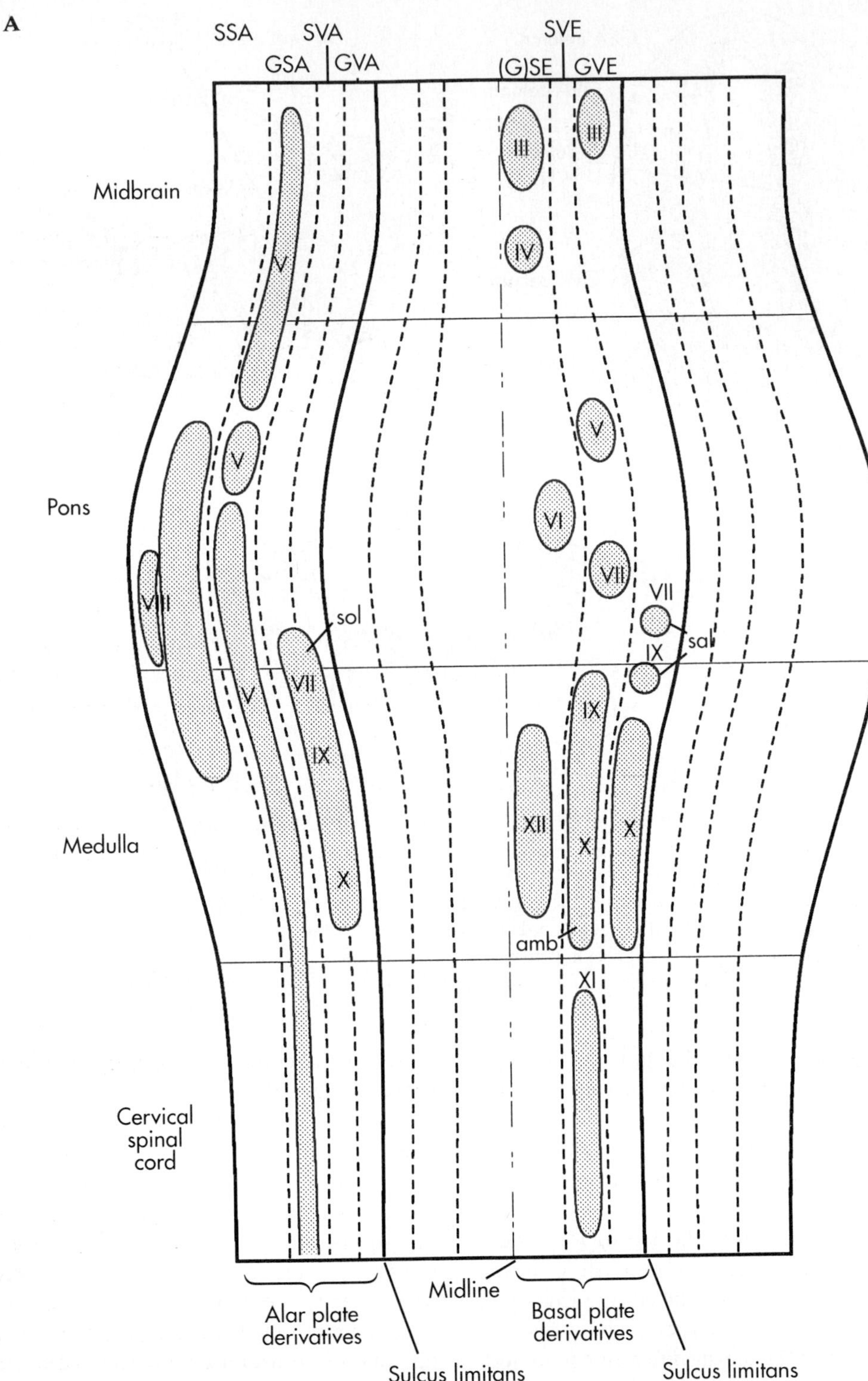


FIGURE 9-2
**A,** The longitudinal arrangement of functional types of cranial nerve nuclei in the brainstem, indicating their derivation from cell columns. Abbreviations: amb, nucleus ambiguus; sal, superior and inferior salivatory nuclei; sol, nucleus of the solitary tract. (Adapted from Nieuwenhuys R et al: *The human central nervous system: a synopsis and atlas,* ed. 3, New York, 1988, Springer-Verlag.) **B,** Drawing of an actual section through the rostral medulla of an adult brain. On the left the nuclei corresponding to the seven functional components are indicated. On the right the cranial nerves containing each of these components are indicated; cranial nerves I and II are not included nor are some minor components such as the few GSA fibers in cranial nerve VII. Not all the nerves listed actually emerge at this brainstem level; they are included here for summary purposes.

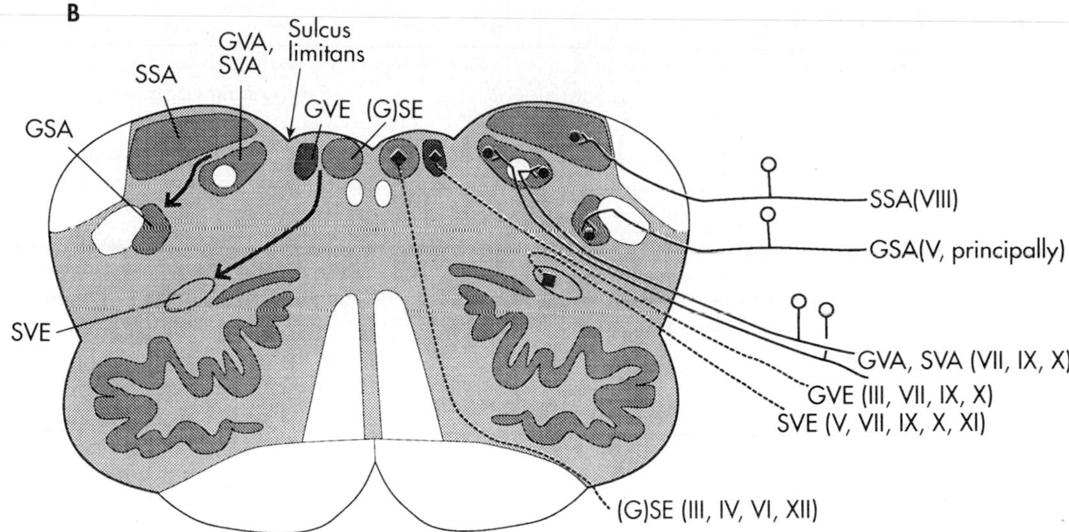


FIGURE 9-2, cont'd
For legend see opposite page.

contains all seven functional components. If the components of all the nerves are tabulated (as in Table 6), it becomes apparent that there are three types of cranial nerves. Some nerves (III, IV, VI, and XII) contain GSE fibers and little or nothing else, so they may be referred to as *somatic efferent nerves*. Others (I, II, and VIII) contain special sensory fibers (SSA or SVA) and nothing else. The remaining nerves (V, VII, IX, X, and XI) are somewhat more complex and tend to contain several components; all innervate branchial arch musculature (that is, they contain SVE fibers), so they are called *branchiomeric nerves*.

Presenting the cranial nerves requires dealing with a considerable amount of material; the remainder of this chapter is divided into three more or less distinct sections discussing the somatic efferent nerves, the branchiomeric nerves, and a particular special sensory nerve, the eighth nerve. Since cranial nerves I and II are not attached to the brainstem but rather are directly related to the forebrain, they are considered separately in later chapters. At the end of this chapter, as mentioned previously, is a series of brainstem sections with labels and summary descriptions indicating the locations and contents of important brainstem structures (see Figures 9-41 to 9-49).

## SOMATIC EFFERENT NERVES (III, IV, VI, AND XII)

The somatic efferent nerves are the simplest of the cranial nerves, since each contains only one functional component (GSE fibers), except for cranial nerve III, which has a small but important complement of GVE fibers.* The nuclei of origin of all these nerves are located adjacent to the midline near the aqueduct or the floor of the fourth ventricle, as would be expected from their embryological origins.

### Oculomotor nerve (III)

Cranial nerve III supplies the levator palpebrae superioris and all the internal and external muscles of the ipsilateral eye except the lateral rectus, superior oblique, and dilator pupillae. The fibers originate in the wedge-shaped *oculomotor nucleus,* which is located at the ventral edge of the periaqueductal gray in the rostral midbrain (Figure 9-3). They then proceed ventrally and arch through the midbrain tegmentum in several separate bundles that join to form the nerve just as they emerge into the interpeduncular fossa (see Figure 8-15).

The oculomotor nucleus actually consists of a series of longitudinal cell columns, or subnuclei. The column supplying the levator palpebrae superioris is located in the midline and innervates this muscle on both sides. The column supplying the superior rectus projects to the contralateral eye. The columns supplying the medial rectus, inferior oblique, and inferior rectus all project to the ipsilateral eye. Finally, a column including preganglionic parasympathetic (GVE) neurons, which straddles the midline and is known by the tenacious eponym *Edinger-Westphal nucleus,* projects to the ipsilateral ciliary ganglion. The ciliary ganglion in turn innervates the sphincter pupillae and the ciliary muscle.

The partly crossed-partly uncrossed nature of the oculo-

*The course of proprioceptive fibers (for example, from stretch receptors) from extraocular muscles and muscles of the tongue has long been a matter of contention. The hypoglossal nerve almost certainly contains lingual proprioceptive fibers for part or all of its course. Those from the extraocular muscles travel in cranial nerves III, IV, and VI within the orbit, then join the ophthalmic division of the trigeminal nerve for the rest of their course to the brainstem. Eye muscle proprioceptors may play a role in depth perception or its development, but the function of lingual proprioceptors is largely unknown.

**TABLE 6** *Contents of the cranial nerves*

| *Nerve* | *Functional component* | *Origin or termination within CNS* | *Peripheral sensory or motor ending* |
|---|---|---|---|
| I (olfactory) | SVA | Olfactory bulb | Originates in olfactory epithelium |
| II (optic) | SSA | Lateral geniculate nucleus and superior colliculus | Originates in ganglion cells of retina |
| III (oculomotor) | (G)SE | Oculomotor nucleus | Superior, inferior, and medial recti; inferior oblique; levator palpebrae superioris |
| | GVE | Edinger-Westphal nucleus (part of oculomotor nucleus) | Sphincter pupillae, ciliary muscle* |
| IV (trochlear) | (G)SE | Trochlear nucleus | Superior oblique |
| V (trigeminal) | GSA | Spinal and main sensory nuclei | Skin and deep tissues of head; dura mater |
| | | Mesencephalic nucleus | Muscle spindles and other mechanoreceptors |
| | SVE | Trigeminal motor nucleus | Muscles of mastication, tensor tympani, and a few others |
| VI (abducens) | (G)SE | Abducens nucleus | Lateral rectus |
| VII (facial) | GSA | Spinal trigeminal nucleus | Outer ear |
| | SVA | Solitary nucleus | Taste buds of palate and anterior ⅔ of tongue |
| | GVA | Solitary nucleus | Some mucous membranes of nasopharynx |
| | GVE | Superior salivatory nucleus | Submandibular, sublingual salivary glands; lacrimal gland* |
| | SVE | Facial motor nucleus | Muscles of facial expression; stapedius |
| VIII (vestibulocochlear) | SSA | Cochlear and vestibular nuclei | Organ of Corti; cristae of semicircular canals; maculae of utricle and saccule |
| IX (glossopharyngeal) | GSA | Spinal trigeminal nucleus | Outer ear |
| | SVA | Solitary nucleus | Taste buds of posterior third of tongue |
| | GVA | Solitary and spinal trigeminal nuclei | Carotid body and sinus; mucous membranes of nasal and oral pharynx and middle ear |
| | GVE | Inferior salivatory nucleus | Parotid gland* |
| | SVE | Nucleus ambiguus | Pharynx (stylopharyngeus) |
| X (vagus) | GSA | Spinal trigeminal nucleus | Outer ear |
| | SVA | Solitary nucleus | Taste buds of epiglottis |
| | GVA | Solitary and spinal trigeminal nuclei | Thoracic and abdominal viscera; mucous membranes of larynx and laryngeal pharynx |
| | GVE | Dorsal motor nucleus, nucleus ambiguus | Thoracic and abdominal viscera* |
| | SVE | Nucleus ambiguus | Larynx and pharynx† |
| XI (accessory) | SVE | Accessory nucleus (cervical cord) | Sternocleidomastoid; trapezius |
| XII (hypoglossal) | (G)SE | Hypoglossal nucleus | Muscles of tongue |

*Final destination after synapse in a parasympathetic ganglion.

†Axons of the most caudal of these neurons innervate laryngeal muscles and are often referred to separately as the cranial root of XI.

motor nerve is a curious fact but one of limited clinical significance. This is because the oculomotor nuclei of the two sides are so close to one another that a central lesion in this vicinity is likely to damage both nuclei. On the other hand, once a given oculomotor nerve emerges from the brainstem, it supplies only ipsilateral muscles, so a lesion of the third nerve affects only one eye. Therefore the dissociated finding of paralysis of the superior rectus on one side and of other extraocular muscles on the opposite side is rarely encountered (although there are occasional cases of unilateral nuclear damage in which these deficits are found).

Damage to one oculomotor nerve causes a series of deficits. The eye ipsilateral to the lesion deviates laterally, since the medial rectus is now paralyzed and the lateral rectus is unopposed. This is called *lateral strabismus,* indicating that the eyes are misaligned because one of them deviates away from the midline. As a result, the patient complains of *diplopia* (double vision) and is unable to move the affected eye vertically or medially. The ipsilateral levator palpebrae superioris is paralyzed, so *ptosis* occurs. In addition, the sphincter pupillae and ciliary muscle are nonfunctional. The pupil on the affected side is dilated *(mydriasis)* as a result of the now unopposed dilator pupil-

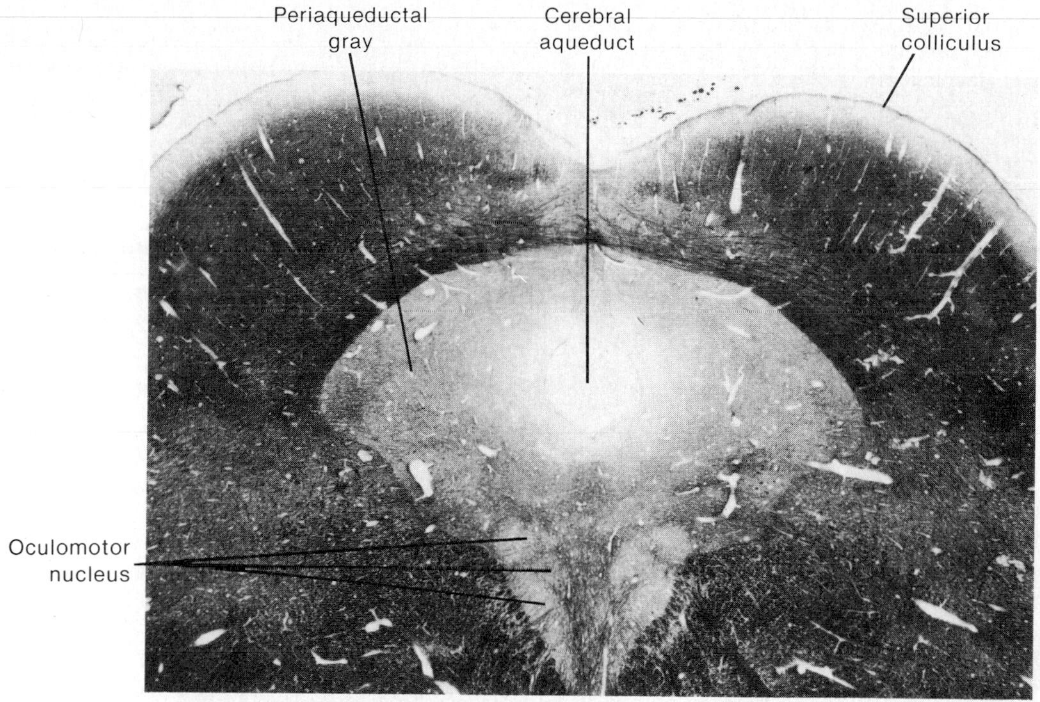


FIGURE 9-3
Section through the rostral midbrain showing the oculomotor nucleus. This figure is an enlargement of part of a section similar to that shown in Figure 8-15. The oculomotor nucleus is actually a tight cluster of subnuclei, each of which innervates a different muscle.

lae and does not constrict in response to light*; the lens cannot be focused on near objects.

Along the course of the oculomotor nerve from brainstem to orbit, the GVE fibers from the Edinger-Westphal nucleus travel in a superficial location and are therefore especially susceptible to external pressures. A dilated pupil, unresponsive to light, may be the first clinically detectable sign of something pressing on the third nerve.

Since ptosis and pupils of unequal size accompany Horner's syndrome, one might think this syndrome could be confused with third nerve damage. However, in Horner's syndrome the ptosis is on the same side as a nonfunctional dilator pupillae, hence on the same side as the *smaller* pupil. On the other hand, the ptosis following third nerve damage is on the same side as a nonfunctional sphincter pupillae, hence on the same side as the *larger* pupil. Also, the ptosis following third nerve damage is more pronounced and is usually accompanied, of course, by defective eye movements and lateral strabismus.

## Trochlear nerve (IV)

Cranial nerve IV supplies the superior oblique muscle. Its cell bodies of origin are located in the contralateral *trochlear nucleus*. This is a small nucleus (since it has only one small muscle to supply) located at the level of the inferior colliculus, where it indents the medial longitudinal fasciculus (MLF) (Figure 9-4). Fibers leaving the nucleus turn caudally in the periaqueductal gray, then arch dorsally to decussate and leave the brainstem at the pons-midbrain junction. The trochlear nerve is thus unique in two respects: it is the only cranial nerve attached to the dorsal aspect of the brainstem and the only one to originate entirely from a contralateral nucleus.*

Damage to the trochlear nerve results in much less drastic and noticeable deficits than does damage to either the oculomotor or the abducens nerve. The superior oblique muscle helps to move the eye downward and laterally, so attempted movement in these directions (typically in reading or in descending stairs) may cause diplopia.

*Both pupils normally constrict when light is shone into either eye. This is the pupillary light reflex, which is discussed further in Chapter 11.

*This probably reflects an adaptation to maintain certain relationships between head movements and eye movements. The details are beyond the scope of this book, but consider the following example. Tilting your head toward your left shoulder evokes a reflex counterrotation of your eyes. The principal muscles that need to contract in this counterrotation are the left superior oblique and superior rectus, and the right inferior oblique and inferior rectus. Since fibers to the superior oblique and superior rectus cross before leaving the brainstem, all the lower motor neurons needed for this counterrotation are located on the right side of the brainstem.

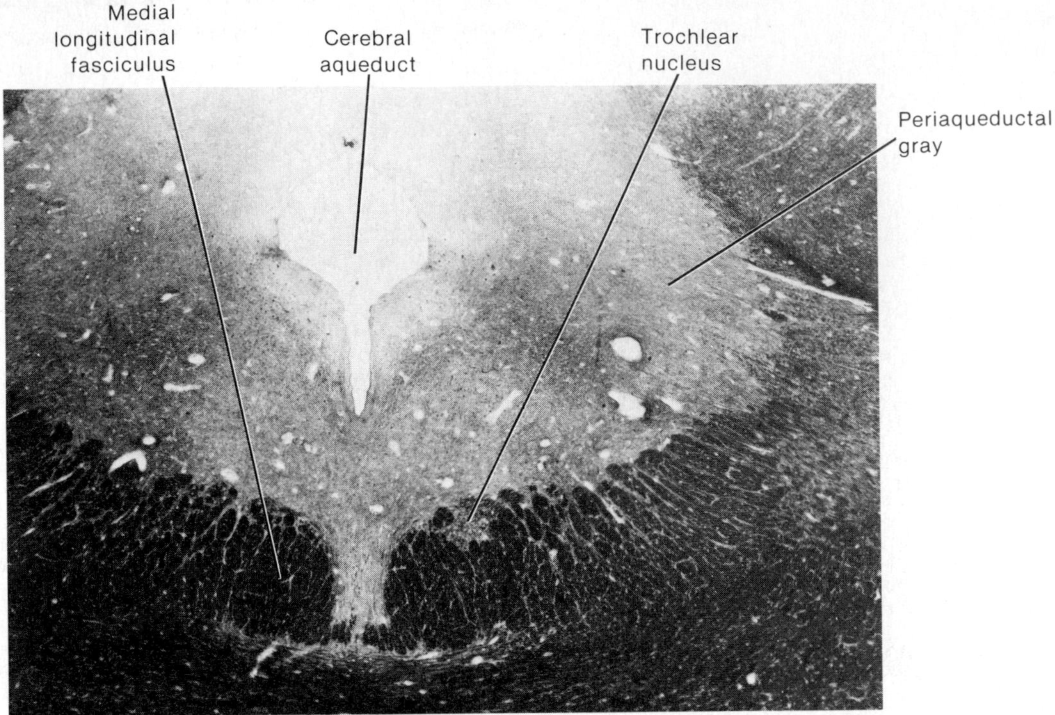


FIGURE 9-4
Section through the caudal midbrain showing the trochlear nucleus. This figure is an enlargement of part of a section similar to that shown in Figure 8-13.

## Abducens nerve (VI)

Cranial nerve VI supplies the lateral rectus muscle. The fibers originate from the ipsilateral *abducens nucleus,* which is located in the caudal pons beneath the floor of the fourth ventricle (Figure 9-5). Medial to this nucleus are two bundles of fibers. The more medial of the two is the MLF. Between the MLF and the abducens nucleus are motor fibers of the facial nerve, which take an unusual course in leaving the brainstem. They originate in the facial nucleus (Figures 9-5, *B* and 9-19), which is located in the ventrolateral part of the pontine tegmentum at about the same level as the abducens nucleus. The facial fibers project dorsomedially, wrap around the abducens nucleus, and turn back ventrally to exit from the brainstem (Figure 9-6). The place where these fibers wrap around the abducens nucleus is called the *internal genu of the facial nerve.* The abducens nucleus, together with the internal genu, is responsible for the facial colliculus in the floor of the fourth ventricle (see Figure 8-3).

### *Lateral gaze*

Damage to the abducens nerve causes a *medial strabismus* (that is, the affected eye deviates medially) as a result of the action of the now-unopposed medial rectus muscle. The individual may be able to move the affected eye to the midline (but not past it) by relaxing its medial rectus muscle (Figure 9-7, *A*). Damage to the abducens nucleus causes the same deficit but with a significant addition. In this case, not only can the individual not move the ipsilateral eye laterally, but it is also impossible to move the contralateral eye medially when trying to look toward the side of the lesion (Figure 9-7, *B*). This is called *lateral gaze paralysis* and occurs because the abducens nucleus contains not only lateral rectus motor neurons but also an approximately equal number of *internuclear neurons*. The axons of these internuclear neurons project through the MLF to the motor neurons controlling the contralateral medial rectus muscle (Figure 9-8).

The function of the MLF in lateral gaze may be understood by considering that both eyes normally work together. For example, when we look to one side, one lateral rectus muscle contracts, and the contralateral medial rectus muscle also contracts. The pathway that interconnects the abducens, trochlear, and oculomotor nuclei to make these sorts of movements possible is the MLF. Vertical movements and the higher centers that direct coordinated eye movements are discussed in a later chapter, but for purely horizontal movements the crucial interconnecting fibers are those that arise from the internuclear neurons in the abducens nucleus (Figure 9-8). These cells send their axons across the midline at the level of the abducens nucleus to join the contralateral MLF. These axons then ascend to the

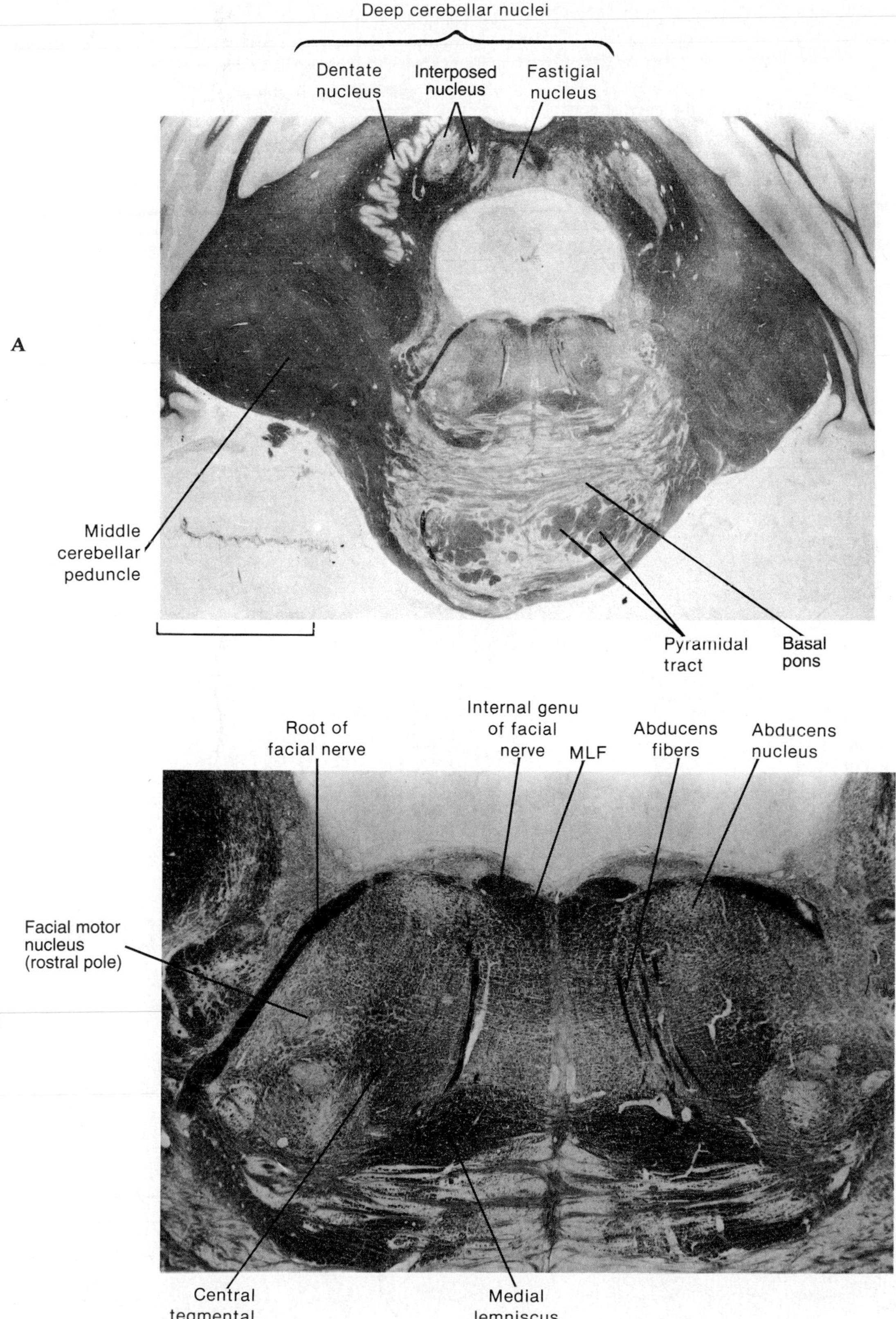


FIGURE 9-5
Section through the caudal pons showing the abducens nucleus and fibers of the facial nerve cut at different points along their course. **A,** Scale mark = 1 cm. **B,** Enlargement of a portion of **A.**

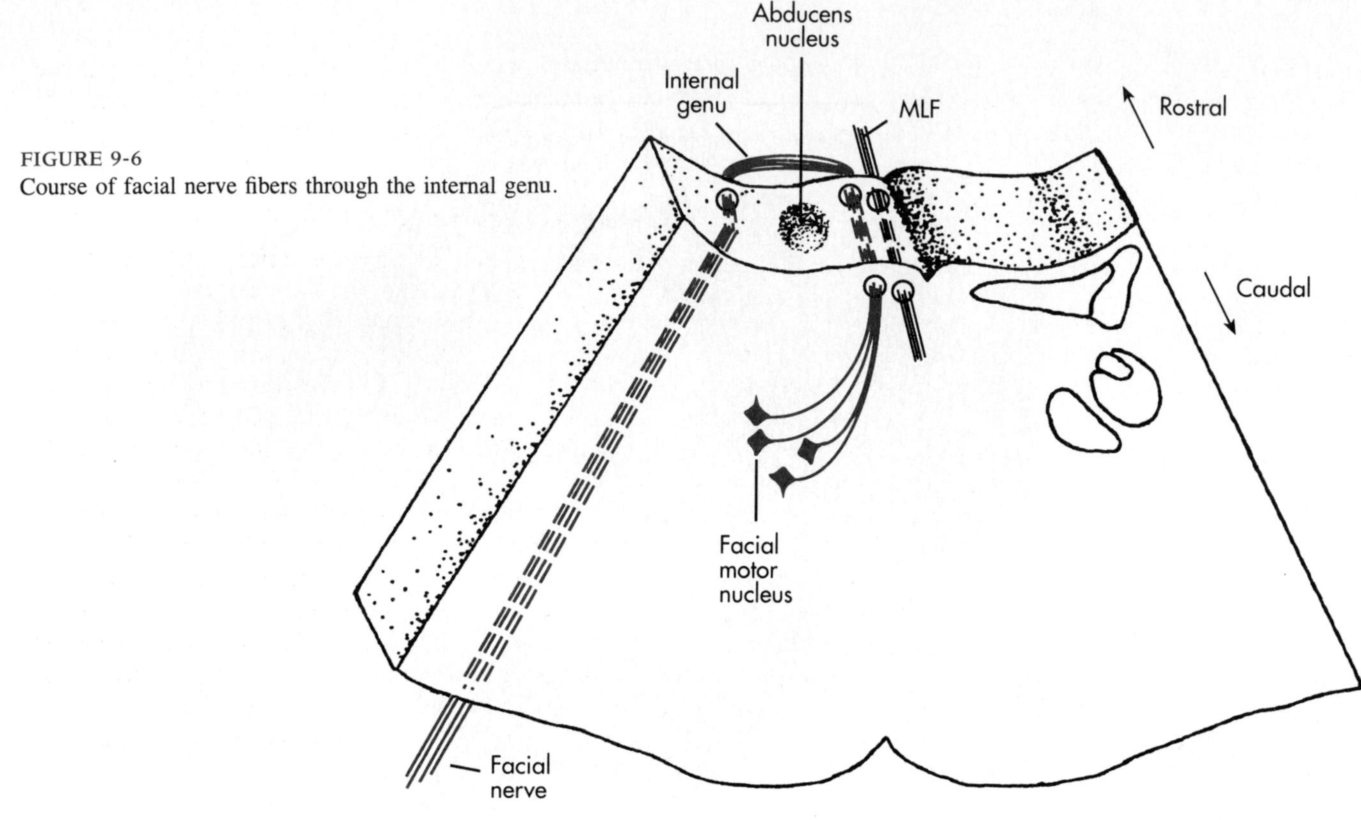


FIGURE 9-6
Course of facial nerve fibers through the internal genu.

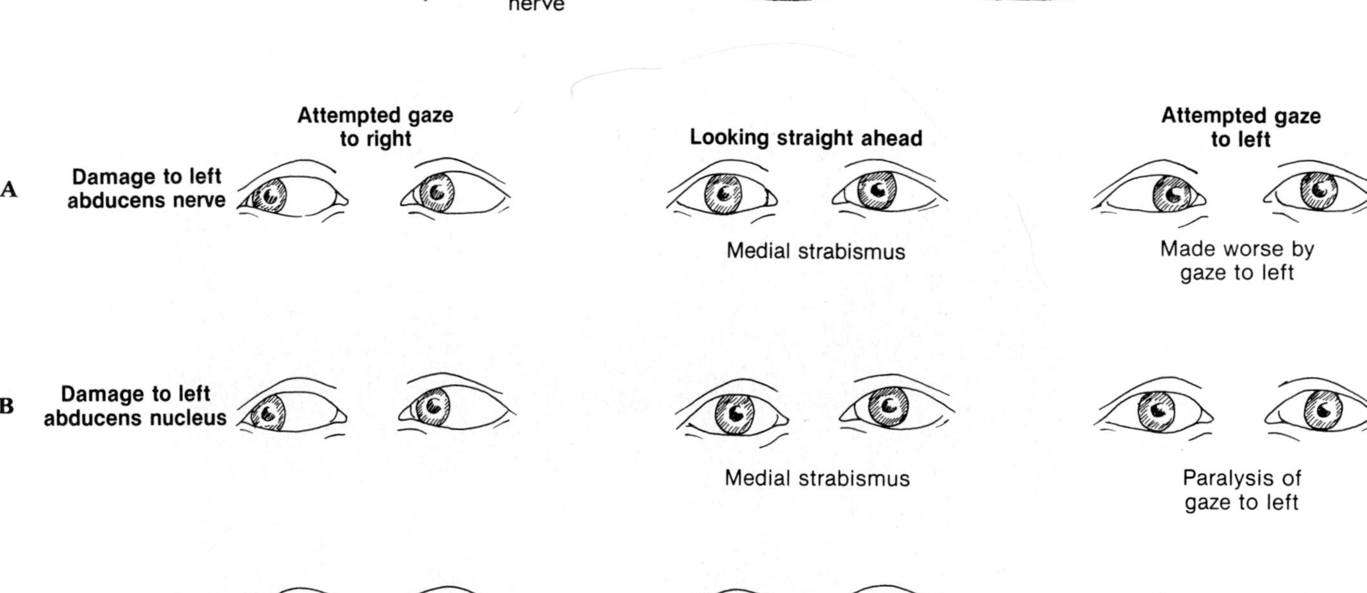


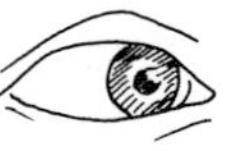
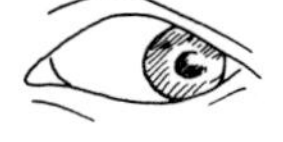

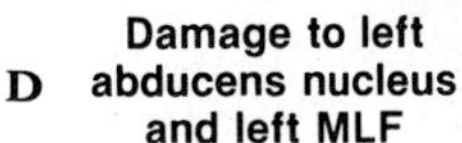

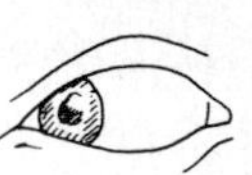
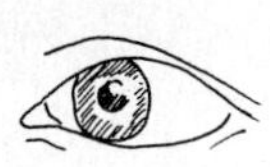
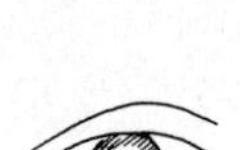
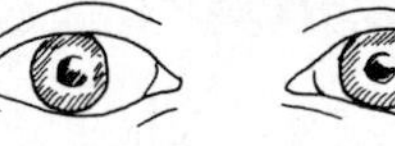
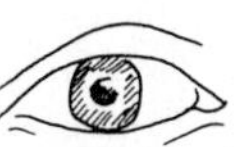
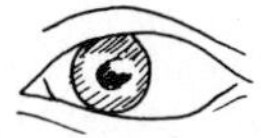


FIGURE 9-7
Deficits of horizontal gaze following damage to the abducens/MLF system as indicated in Figure 9-8. **A,** Abducens palsy. **B,** Lateral gaze paralysis. **C,** Internuclear ophthalmoplegia. **D,** A "one-and-a-half" (combination of **B** and **C**).

oculomotor nucleus, where they make excitatory synapses on medial rectus motor neurons. Simultaneous firing of abducens motor neurons and internuclear neurons thus results in coordinated lateral gaze.

Damage to one MLF removes this excitatory influence from medial rectus motor neurons, so the eye ipsilateral to the lesion fails to move medially past the midline during attempted horizontal gaze (Figures 9-7, *C,* and 9-8). Since both abducens nuclei are intact, full lateral movements of both eyes are still possible. This condition has the ponderous name *internuclear ophthalmoplegia** (often abbreviated as INO).

Another eye movement disorder, clinically called a *one-and-a-half,* is rarely seen but is nevertheless instructive. It is caused by damage in the vicinity of the abducens nucleus and is characterized by the patient's inability to move either eye toward the side of the lesion in lateral gaze, or to move the eye on the side of the lesion in gaze toward the opposite side (Figure 9-7, *D*). Thus of the two directions of horizontal gaze (right and left), the patient has only half of one intact. This is caused by destruction of one abducens nucleus plus destruction of fibers from the contralateral internuclear neurons as they join the MLF on the side of the lesion (Figure 9-8).

*Literally, "paralysis of the eye caused by damage between the nuclei."

## Hypoglossal nerve (XII)

Cranial nerve XII supplies the intrinsic and most extrinsic muscles of the tongue. The fibers originate in the ipsilateral *hypoglossal nucleus,* which extends from the caudal medulla to the rostral part of the rostral medulla (Figures 9-9 and 9-10). This nucleus is situated adjacent to the midline just beneath the floor of the fourth ventricle and forms an elevation there called the hypoglossal trigone or triangle (Figure 8-3). Hypoglossal axons proceed ventrally and emerge as a series of rootlets in the groove between the pyramid and the olive (Figures 8-3, 8-7, and 9-10).

Damage to the hypoglossal nerve causes weakness of one side of the tongue and, since this would be a lower motor neuron lesion, atrophy of that side of the tongue as well. This weakness is most easily demonstrated by asking the patient to protrude his or her tongue; the tongue deviates *toward* the side of the lesion (that is, toward the weak

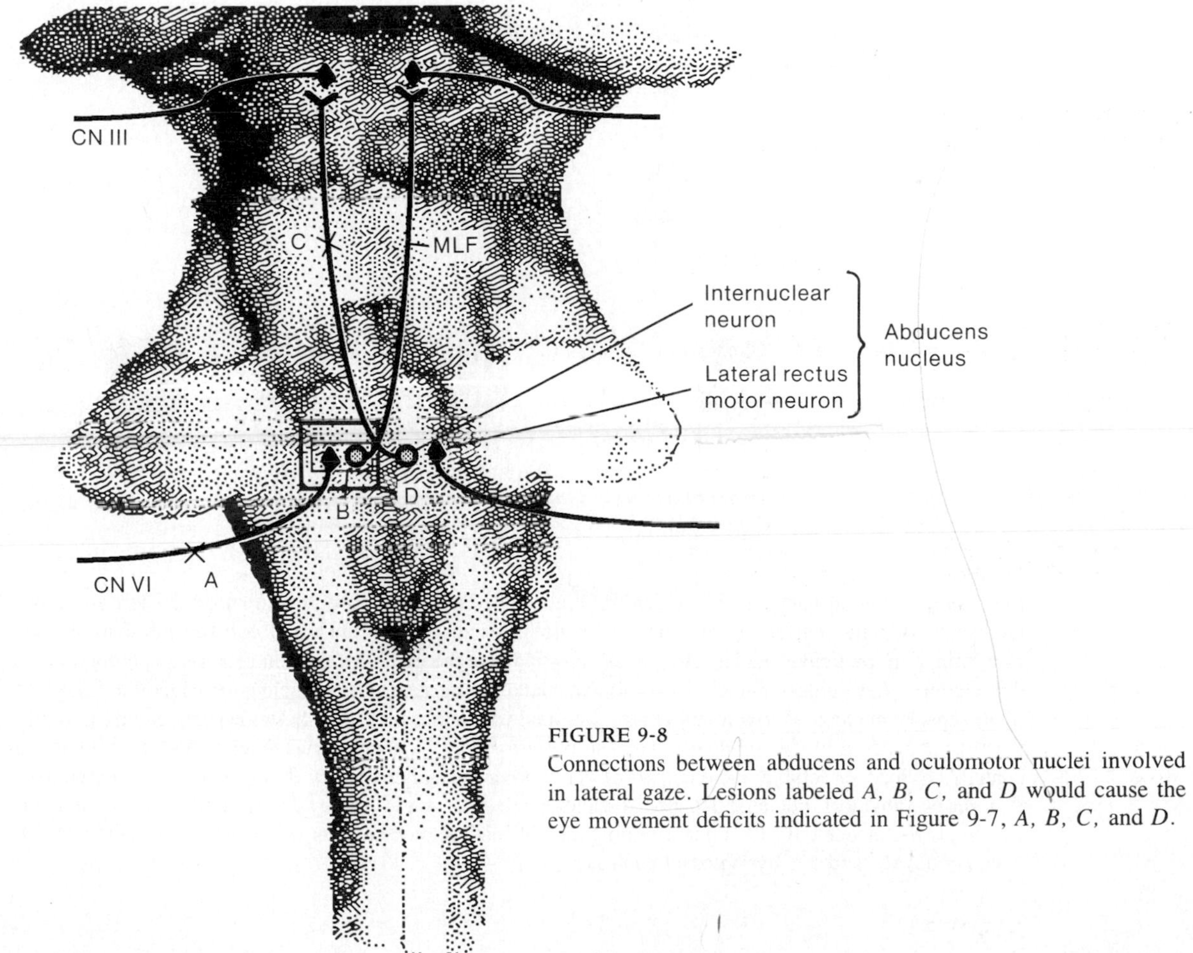


FIGURE 9-8
Connections between abducens and oculomotor nuclei involved in lateral gaze. Lesions labeled *A, B, C,* and *D* would cause the eye movement deficits indicated in Figure 9-7, *A, B, C,* and *D.*

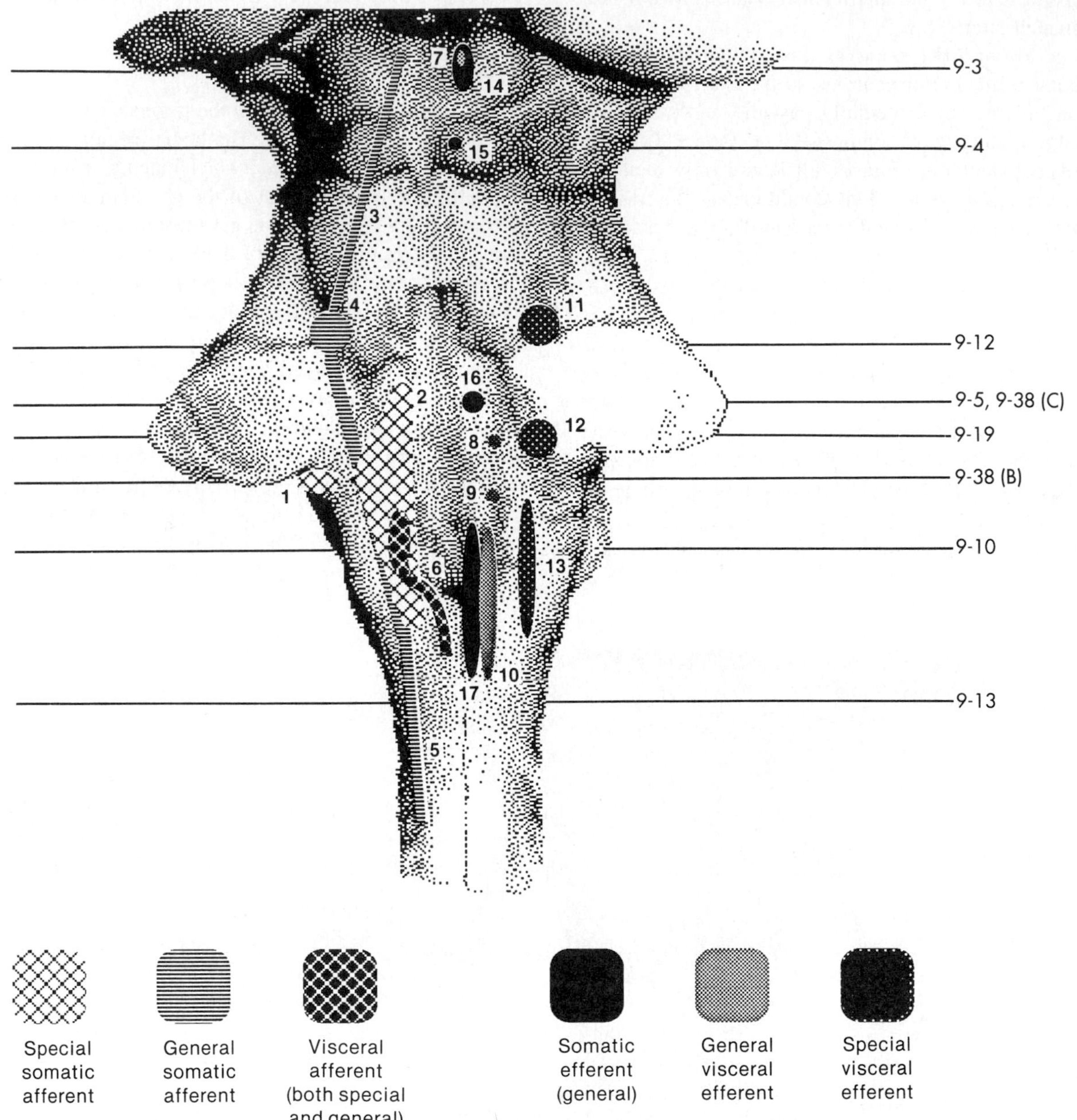


FIGURE 9-9
Locations of cranial nerve nuclei within the brainstem. Sensory nuclei are shown on the left and motor nuclei on the right. Different hatchings and stipplings indicate the functional components that originate or terminate in particular nuclei. Horizontal lines indicate the planes of section of various photographs in this chapter. *1,* Cochlear nuclei; *2,* vestibular nuclei; *3,* mesencephalic nucleus of trigeminal nerve; *4,* main sensory nucleus of trigeminal nerve; *5,* spinal trigeminal nucleus (shown here as ending abruptly, whereas actually it blends gradually with the posterior horn of upper cervical segments); *6,* solitary nucleus; *7,* Edinger-Westphal nucleus (part of oculomotor nuclear complex); *8,* superior salivatory nucleus; *9,* inferior salivatory nucleus; *10,* dorsal motor nucleus of vagus nerve; *11,* trigeminal motor nucleus; *12,* facial motor nucleus; *13,* nucleus ambiguus; *14,* oculomotor nucleus; *15,* trochlear nucleus; *16,* abducens nucleus; and *17,* hypoglossal nucleus.

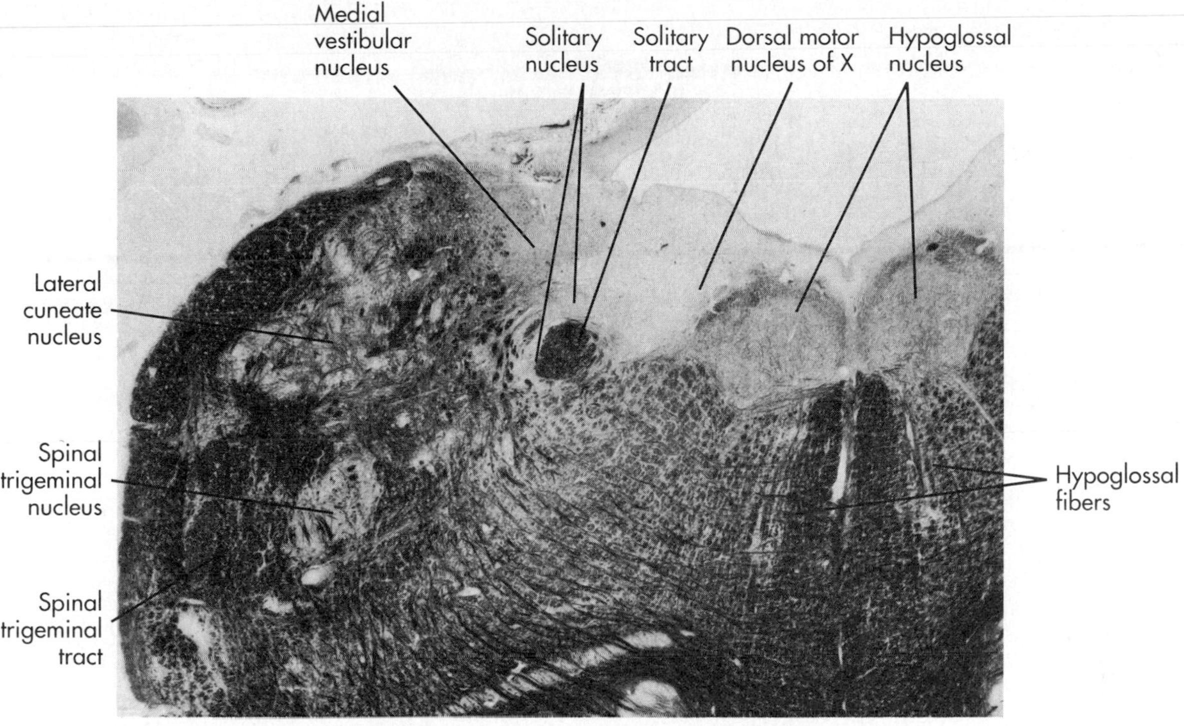


FIGURE 9-10
Section through the rostral medulla showing the hypoglossal nucleus and other cranial nerve nuclei. This figure is an enlargement of part of a section similar to that shown in Figure 8-7.

side). Bilateral hypoglossal lesions may cause difficulties in both speaking and eating.

## BRANCHIOMERIC NERVES (V, VII, IX, X, AND XI)

The branchiomeric nerves all innervate striated muscle of branchial arch origin (that is, they all contain SVE fibers). With the possible exception of cranial nerve XI, they all contain other components as well. In spite of this, each has one function with which it tends to be associated: the trigeminal nerve (V) is the major general sensory nerve for the head; the facial nerve (VII) is the motor nerve for facial expression; the glossopharyngeal nerve (IX) is the most important conveyor of taste and pharyngeal sensations; the vagus nerve (X) carries the parasympathetic outflow to the thoracic and abdominal viscera; and the accessory nerve (XI) is the motor nerve for the sternocleidomastoid and trapezius muscles.

### Trigeminal nerve (V)

With respect to somatic sensory innervation, cranial nerve V and its connections are to the head what the dorsal roots and spinal cord are to the body. That is, the trigeminal system is ultimately responsible for the transmission of tactile, proprioceptive, and pain and temperature information from the head to the cerebral cortex, cerebellum, and reticular formation. The primary afferent fibers are distributed peripherally in the three divisions of the trigeminal nerve (the *ophthalmic* [$V_1$], *maxillary* [$V_2$], and *mandibular* [$V_3$] divisions), in the pattern shown in Figure 9-11.

#### *Trigeminal motor nucleus*

There is also one motor nucleus, a special visceral efferent (SVE) nucleus, associated with the trigeminal nerve. This nucleus is called the *trigeminal motor nucleus*. It innervates the muscles of the first branchial arch, which consist mainly of the muscles of mastication. They also include the tensor tympani (discussed later) and several other small muscles. The nucleus is located in the midpons at the level of attachment of the trigeminal nerve to the brainstem (Figure 9-12). Fibers arising in the trigeminal motor nucleus emerge as a separate motor root and are then distributed peripherally with the mandibular division.

#### *Sensory nuclei*

Three sensory nuclei are associated with trigeminal afferents, and they form a long, almost continuous column of cells that extends from the rostral midbrain to the upper cervical spinal cord (see Figure 9-15). The *main* (or *principal*) *sensory nucleus* (Figure 9-12) forms an enlargement in this column in the midpons, slightly lateral to the trigeminal motor nucleus. The *spinal nucleus* extends cau-

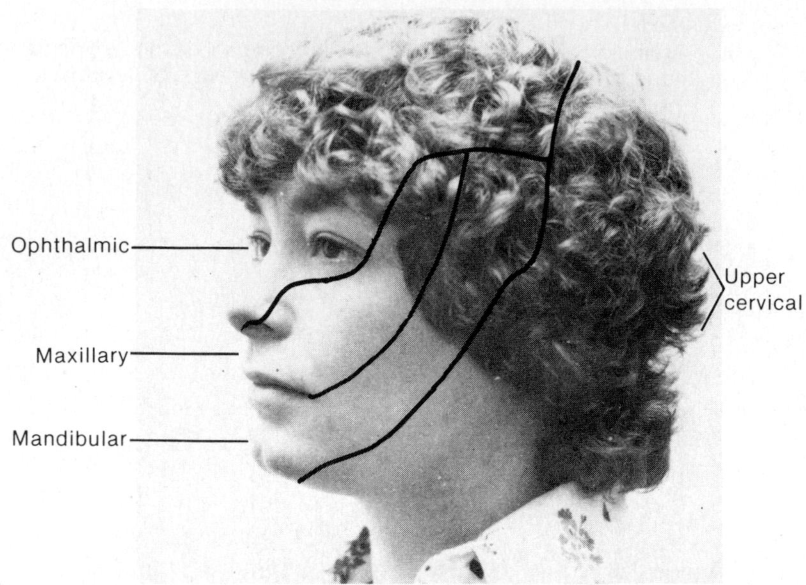


FIGURE 9-11
Peripheral distribution of the ophthalmic, maxillary, and mandibular branches of the trigeminal nerve.

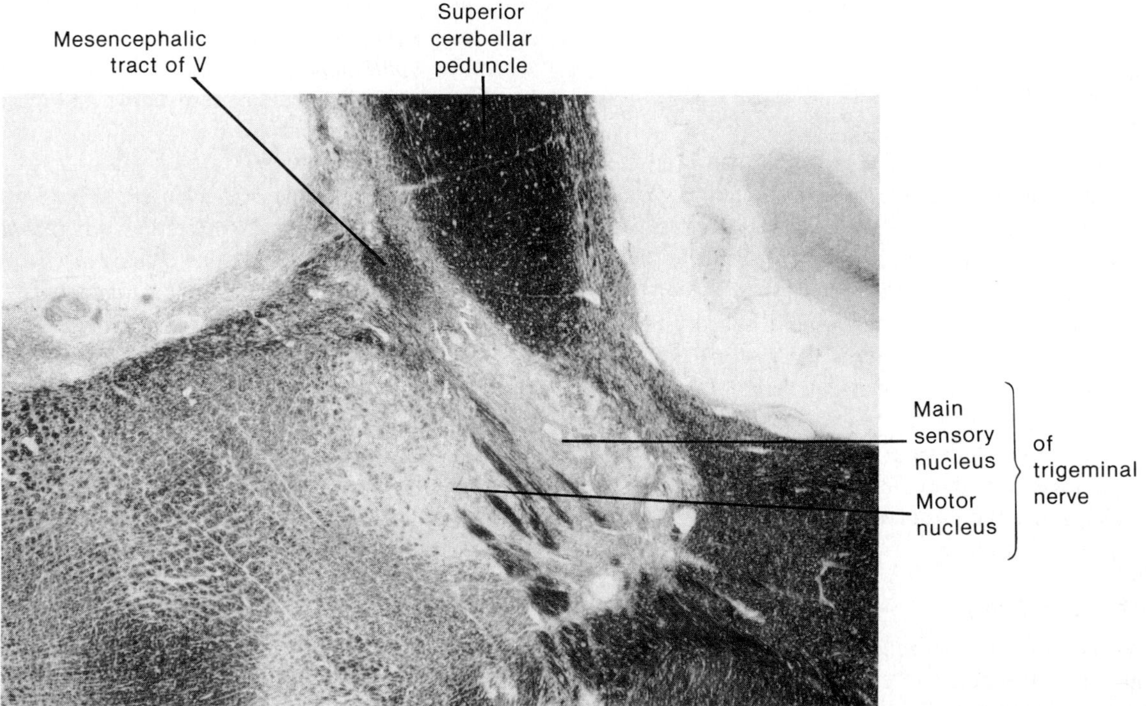


FIGURE 9-12
Section through the midpons showing the trigeminal motor and main sensory nuclei. This figure is an enlargement of part of a section similar to that shown in Figure 8-10.

dally from this level, and the very slender *mesencephalic nucleus* extends rostrally.

Entering trigeminal afferent (GSA) fibers, whose cell bodies are in the *trigeminal (gasserian* or *semilunar) ganglion,* do one of three things. (1) Most fibers bifurcate and send a very short ascending branch to the main sensory nucleus and a longer descending branch into the *spinal trigeminal tract,* which is just lateral to the spinal trigeminal nucleus. The remaining fibers do not bifurcate and either (2) terminate directly in the main sensory nucleus or (3) turn caudally and enter the spinal tract (see Figure 9-15).

*Spinal trigeminal nucleus.* The primary afferent collaterals of the spinal trigeminal tract are somatotopically arranged, with manidbular division fibers most dorsal, ophthalmic division fibers most ventral, and maxillary division fibers in between. They terminate in the medially adjacent spinal trigeminal nucleus. Both nucleus and tract extend caudally to about the third cervical segment of the spinal cord, the nucleus gradually blending with the posterior horn and the tract gradually blending with Lissauer's tract. This apparently peculiar arrangement allows for a smooth transition from spinal levels processing cutaneous information from the back of the head to brainstem levels processing similar cutaneous information from the face (see Figure 9-11).

The spinal trigeminal nucleus has been subdivided into three regions on the basis of its histology. The most caudal part, extending from the spinal cord to the obex, is the *caudal nucleus*. The most rostral part, extending from the main sensory nucleus to about the pontomedullary junction, is the *oral nucleus*. Between these two is the *interpolar nucleus* in the rostral medulla. Differences exist among these nuclei in terms of the types of afferents that terminate at each level and the types of secondary connections made from each level. The functional correlates of these differences are incompletely understood for the oral and interpolar nuclei, but the caudal nucleus is known to be particularly important for the processing of pain and temperature information from the head.* This fits nicely with its appearance (Figure 9-13): the caudal nucleus looks much like the posterior horn of the spinal cord, with a cap of cells resembling the substantia gelatinosa.

The caudal nucleus gives rise to a crossed ascending pain pathway analogous to the spinothalamic tract. It is called the *ventral trigeminal* (or *ventral trigeminothalamic) tract*. The exact position of this tract in the human brainstem is not known with certainty; it is often said to travel with the medial lemniscus, but clinical evidence suggests that it travels adjacent to the representation of cervical dermatomes in the spinothalamic tract (i.e., where it might be expected somatotopically). Fibers of the ventral trigeminal tract terminate in the *ventral posteromedial*

*The only exception is dental pain, which is also processed in the interpolar nucleus.

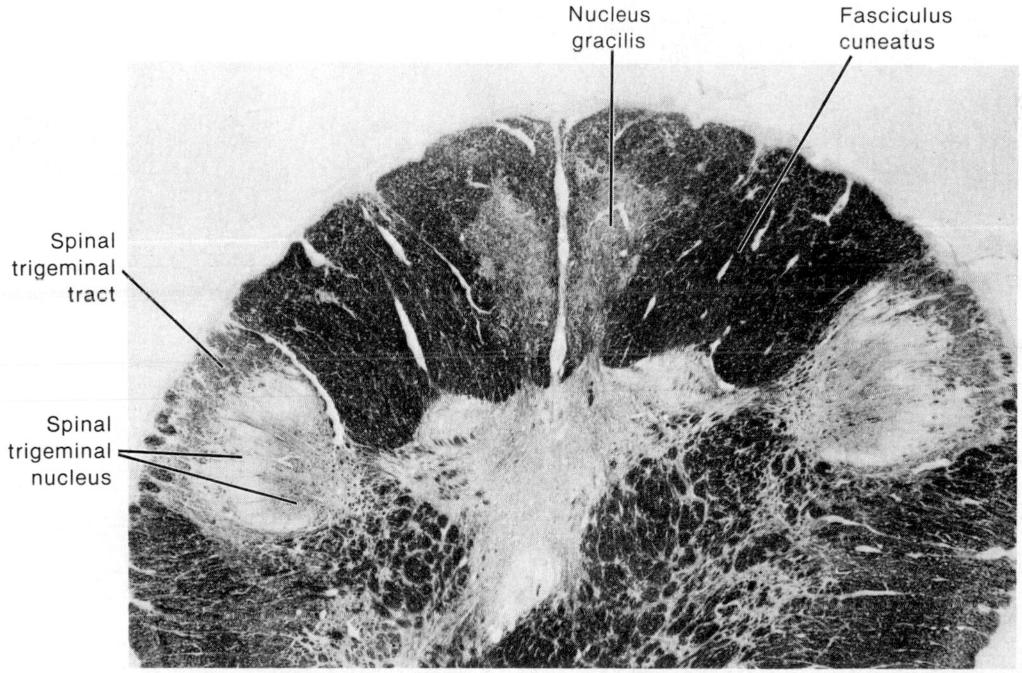


FIGURE 9-13
Section through the caudal medulla where the spinal trigeminal tract and nucleus have an appearance much like that of Lissauer's tract and the posterior horn in the spinal cord. At levels rostral to the obex (for example, Figure 9-10) the spinal trigeminal tract and nucleus do not have this appearance.

*(VPM) nucleus* of the thalamus, adjacent to the VPL (see Figure 9-16).* Trigeminal pain information also reaches the thalamus indirectly (via relays in the reticular formation) in a manner thought to be similar to spinoreticulothalamic projections. It is often assumed that this similarity holds in a functional sense as well (that is, that the ventral trigeminal tract is responsible for sharp, well-localized pain, whereas indirect trigeminal projections through the reticular formation are responsible for dull, aching pain). However, clinical evidence for such a functional similarity seems to be relatively scanty. Some pain fibers from all three divisions of the trigeminal nerve reach the upper cervical spinal cord, but most end at various levels in the causal medulla. There is a somatotopic arrangement in this rostral-caudal distribution of endings, so that in each trigeminal division pain fibers representing areas near the midline end near the obex, whereas fibers representing areas toward the back of the head end in the upper cervical cord (Figure 9-14). This makes sense, since the trigeminal fibers ending in the cervical cord are thereby overlapping spinal fibers that represent adjacent areas of skin (see Figure 9-11). This gives rise to a peculiar pattern of sensory loss, sometimes referred to clinically as an *onion-skin distribution,* when the spinal trigeminal tract is damaged; the farther caudally the lesion is located, the larger is the area surrounding the mouth that is spared from sensory loss.

The spinal trigeminal nucleus has other connections in addition to the direct and indirect pain pathways just described. Some fibers project to the cerebellum (through the inferior cerebellar peduncle), and some fibers carrying tac-

*VPL and VPM are sometimes referred to together as the *ventrobasal complex.*

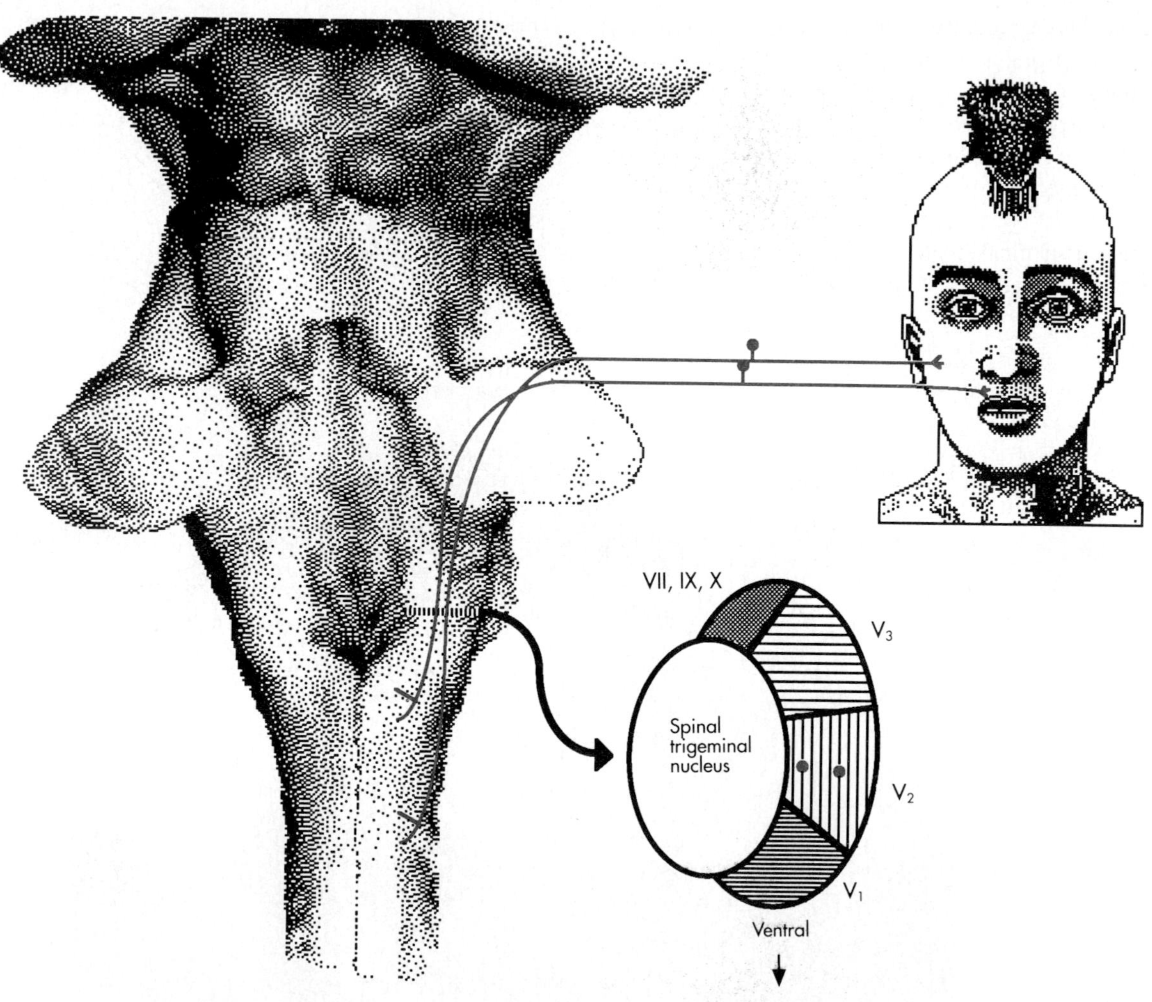


FIGURE 9-14
Somatotopic arrangement and termination pattern of trigeminal pain fibers. As shown in the schematic cross section from the indicated level, the face is represented upside-down in the spinal trigeminal tract and nucleus. Two fibers from the maxillary division are used for this example, but for each division, fibers carrying information from areas nearer the mouth end more rostrally.

tile information travel in the ventral trigeminal tract. These are presumably similar to spinocerebellar fibers and to the tactile component of the spinothalamic tract, respectively. There are also reflex connections within the brainstem involving the reticular formation and other cranial nerve nuclei. One of these, the *corneal reflex,* is of considerable clinical importance and is discussed in conjunction with the facial nerve. The relative contributions of the three portions of the spinal nucleus to these various functions are not completely understood.

*Main sensory nucleus.* The main sensory nucleus of the trigeminal nerve (Figure 9-12), located near the motor nucleus, is generally considered to be analogous to the posterior column nuclei. Thus it is primarily concerned with discriminative tactile and proprioceptive sensations. It receives large-diameter, heavily myelinated tactile afferents and gives rise to two ascending pathways. One is a collection of fibers that crosses the midline, joins the medial lemniscus adjacent to the representation of cervical dermatomes, and terminates in the VPM (Figure 9-15 and 9-16); these fibers are generally considered to be part of the ventral trigeminal tract (even though the pain fibers of the ventral trigeminal tract probably travel separately with the spinothalamic fibers). The other is a completely ipsilateral projection from the dorsomedial portion of the main sensory nucleus (an area that does not project through the ventral trigeminal tract). This is called the *dorsal trigeminal (dorsal trigeminothalamic) tract;* it travels through the dorsomedial part of the brainstem tegmentum and ends in its own separate portion of the VPM. The significance of this tract being uncrossed is unclear. However, it does end alongside the ascending taste pathway, which is also uncrossed; hence intraoral sensations from one side of the mouth are processed in adjacent areas of the thalamus.

Since tactile information from the head is processed in the main sensory nucleus as well as in the spinal trigeminal nucleus, lesions in the medulla affecting the spinal tract and nucleus leave the sense of touch relatively intact

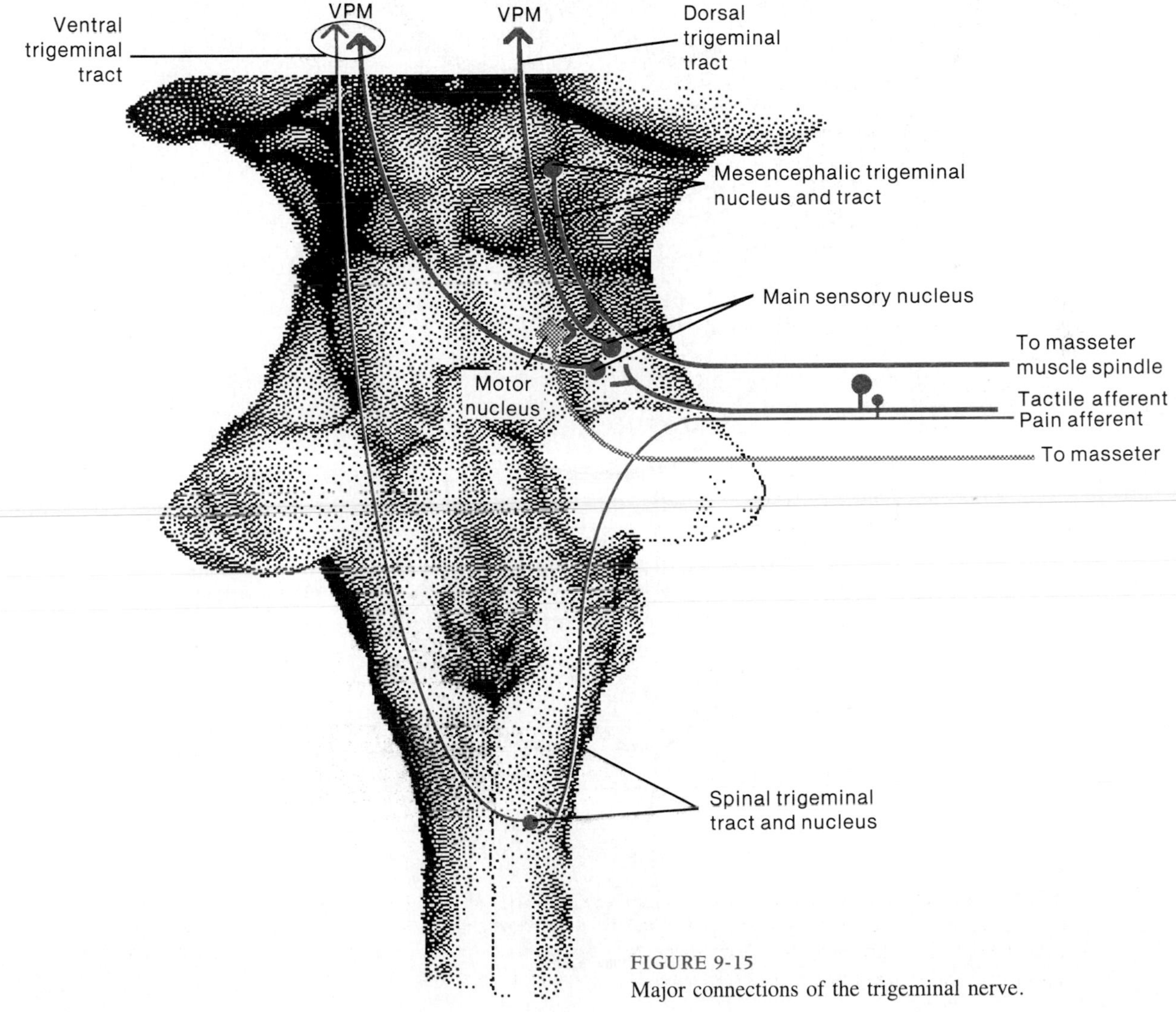


FIGURE 9-15
Major connections of the trigeminal nerve.

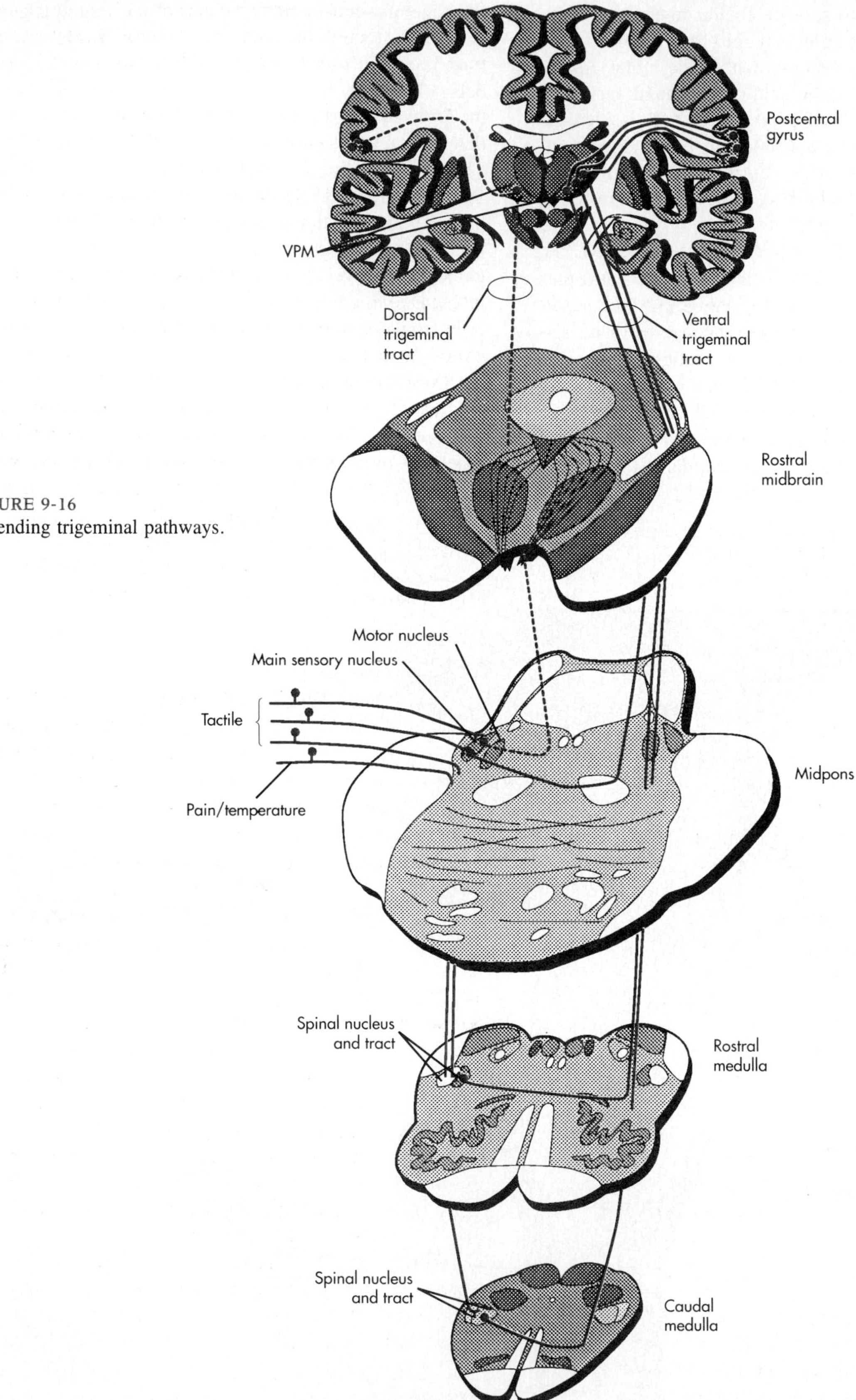


FIGURE 9-16
Ascending trigeminal pathways.

and cause a more or less selective impairment of pain sensation.

*Mesencephalic trigeminal nucleus.* Afferents from muscle spindles in the muscles of mastication and some from mechanoreceptors of the gums, teeth, and hard palate have their cell bodies not in the trigeminal ganglion but rather within the CNS. They are located in a slender column of cells called the *mesencephalic trigeminal nucleus* (Figure 9-15), which is quite unusual, since all other primary somatic sensory fibers have their cell bodies located in peripheral ganglia. The name of the nucleus refers to the fact that it extends rostrally all the way to the posterior commissure, although it is very small at midbrain levels. The cells of the mesencephalic nucleus are pseudounipolar (in every way analogous to dorsal root ganglion cells), and their myelinated processes collect in a bundle, called the *mesencephalic trigeminal tract* or *root,* adjacent to the nucleus (see Figure 8-12). The peripheral processes of these fibers are distributed through the trigeminal nerve to the structures mentioned previously. Central processes end in the motor and main sensory nuclei and a few other brainstem sites.

The function of the mesencephalic trigeminal nucleus is rather obscure. It is often assumed that it is important for the coordination of chewing movements, since its afferents carry relevant proprioceptive information. However, fairly discrete lesions of the mesencephalic nucleus in monkeys produce no gross abnormalities of chewing movements. Since this is a small but extended nucleus, it is unlikely to be selectively affected in disease processes, so no clinical observations on humans are available.

The one function definitely established for the mesencephalic trigeminal nucleus is its participation in the *jaw jerk reflex.* Stretching the masseter, typically by a downward tap on the chin, causes it to contract (bilaterally) in a reflex fashion. This is a monosynaptic reflex basically similar to the knee jerk reflex; the afferent limb is a mesencephalic trigeminal neuron whose peripheral process innervates a masseter muscle spindle and whose central process synapses on a trigeminal motor neuron; the efferent limb is the axon of the trigeminal motor neuron, which travels back to the masseter (Figure 9-15).

## Facial nerve (VII)

Cranial nerve VII, like IX and X, contains fibers belonging to several different functional components; certain aspects of all three nerves are described together in this section.

### *General afferents*

All three nerves contain general somatic afferent (GSA) fibers from the skin of the outer ear and its immediate vicinity. The exact distribution and the division of these fibers among the three nerves varies somewhat from one individual to another. These GSA fibers of nerves VII, IX, and X all enter the spinal trigeminal tract and thereafter behave exactly like trigeminal afferents. They are the most dorsomedial fibers in the spinal tract and occupy a position adjacent to those from the mandibular division of nerve V (see Figure 9-14).

Nerves VII, IX, and X also contain general visceral afferent (GVA) fibers. In the case of the facial nerve this is a small collection of afferents that innervate parts of the nasal cavity and soft palate; these fibers are seldom of clinical importance and are frequently omitted from accounts of the cranial nerves.

The GVA fibers from all three nerves enter a discrete bundle called the *solitary tract* (see Figures 9-10 and 9-18). This bundle received its name as a result of its unusual appearance, since it is a collection of afferents surrounded by the nucleus of termination of these afferents (the *solitary nucleus,* or the *nucleus of the solitary tract*) and looks isolated in cross sections. Both tract and nucleus extend through most of the medulla, dealing with facial afferents at rostral levels, vagal afferents at caudal levels, and glossopharyngeal afferents in between (although there is considerable overlap of these termination zones). The solitary nucleus in turn projects to the reticular formation, to brainstem visceral motor nuclei, and to the intermediolateral cell column of the spinal cord.

### *Taste*

This section deals with the *gustatory* sense, the sensations engendered by stimulated taste buds. We commonly assume that this is the same thing as the sense of taste, but taste is actually the result of the combination of three different kinds of input: direct chemical stimulation of taste buds, stimulation of olfactory receptors by vapors from food, and stimulation of chemical-sensitive free nerve endings of the trigeminal and other nerves in the mucous membranes of the oral cavity. The latter endings respond to qualities such as pungency and spiciness in food. We have difficulty appreciating the subtleties of food and wine using just our taste buds, and people with deficits in their sense of olfaction complain that things taste bland.

Taste buds are usually associated with the tongue, although they are also distributed widely over the palate and pharynx.* The pharyngeal and palatal taste buds may be more important for swallowing and for reflex responses to good or bad tastes than for conscious awareness of taste. Each taste bud is an ovoid collection of about 100 neuroepithelial taste receptor cells and supporting cells (Figure 9-17). At one end of the taste bud, the receptors send microvillar processes through a small opening, the *taste pore,* where they are exposed to chemical stimuli. At the deep end of the taste bud, the receptor cells make synapses on special visceral afferent (SVA) fibers from the facial,

*Fish even have taste buds on the external surface of their bodies, so they can "taste" the water through which they swim.

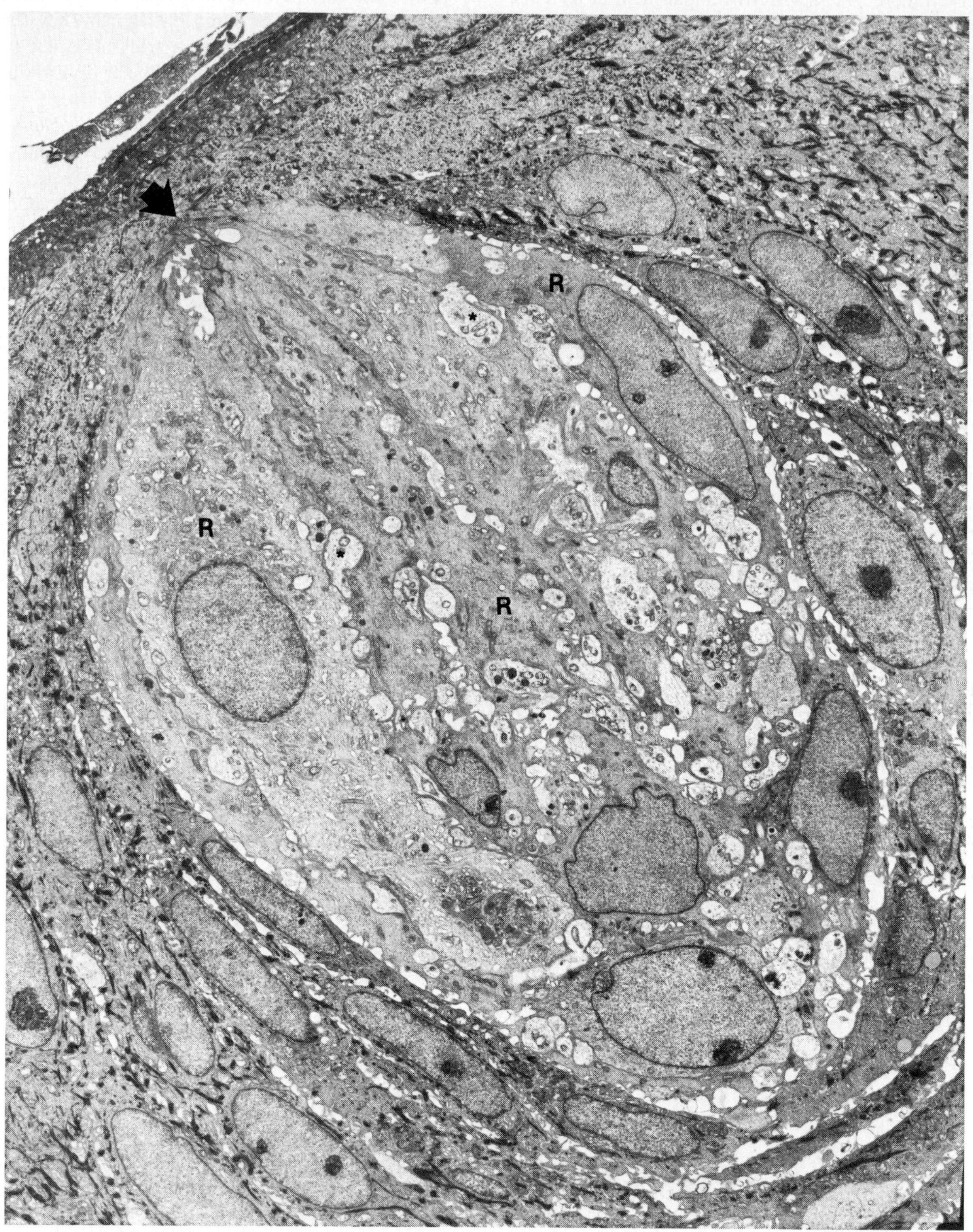


FIGURE 9-17
Electron micrograph of a taste bud from a human circumvallate papilla. The section is not quite through the middle of the taste bud, but the arrow indicates the apex where the taste pore would open in a nearby section. *R* indicates taste receptor cells. Discrete synapses of the receptor cells onto afferent fibers cannot be seen easily in this micrograph, but numerous glossopharyngeal nerve processes are apparent; two are indicated by asterisks.

Courtesy of Dr. David Moran and Pamela Eller, University of Colorado Health Sciences Center.

glossopharyngeal, and vagal nerves. Fibers from the facial nerve innervate taste buds in the palate and the anterior two thirds of the tongue; fibers from the glossopharyngeal nerve innervate those in the pharynx and posterior third of the tongue; and a few vagal fibers innervate those in the epiglottis.

The solitary nucleus is the principal visceral afferent nucleus of the brainstem and receives (via the solitary tract) gustatory afferents as well as the GVA fibers mentioned earlier. However, the SVA gustatory fibers, as well as the chemical-sensitive trigeminal fibers, end separately in lateral and rostral portions of the solitary nucleus (Figure 9-18).

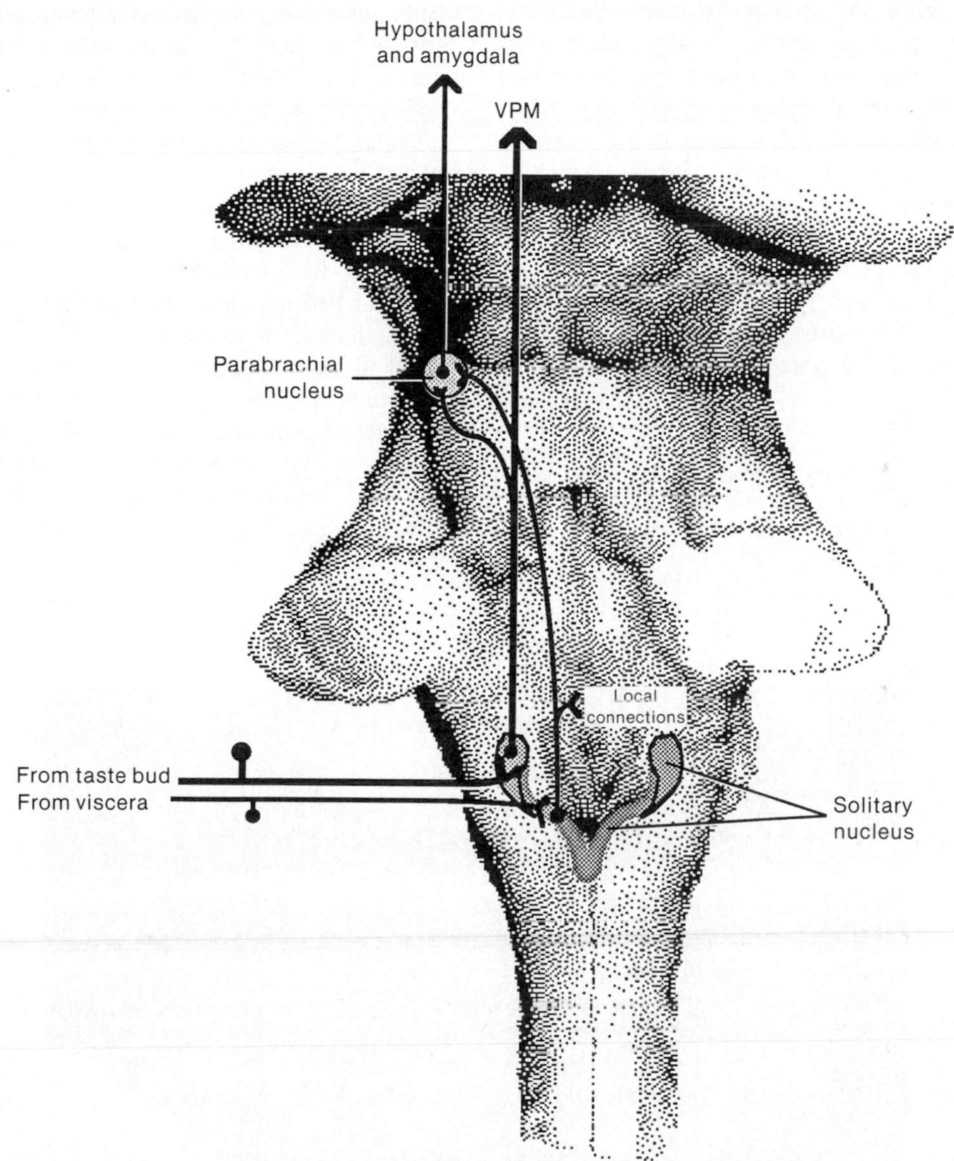


FIGURE 9-18
Brainstem connections of visceral afferents. All visceral afferents that enter the brainstem, whether from taste buds or from general viscera, end in the solitary nucleus. (They traverse the solitary tract, which runs down the middle of the nucleus, to reach their sites of termination; the tract was omitted from this diagram for the sake of simplicity.) Those from taste buds end preferentially in rostral and lateral parts of the nucleus. Some second-order fibers from the solitary nucleus, through local connections with the reticular formation and cranial nerve motor nuclei, participate in swallowing, chewing, and coughing. Others send information to the hypothalamus and amygdala, after a synapse in the parabrachial nucleus. Those carrying gustatory information that will reach consciousness end in the most medial part of the VPM.

Second-order taste fibers do three things (Figure 9-18). Some participate in reflex activities, such as swallowing or coughing, by way of motor nuclei of the branchiomeric nerves. Others, like sensory systems in general, project to the cerebral cortex by way of the thalamus. In this case, however, the projection is uncrossed. Fibers travel ipsilaterally through the central tegmental tract to the most medial part of the VPM (see Figure 10-9), where they end adjacent to the uncrossed fibers of the dorsal trigeminal tract (see Figures 9-15 and 9-16). This medial part of the VPM then projects to the gustatory cortex, which is adjacent to the somatosensory representation of the tongue and is located in the frontal-parietal operculum and the insula.* Finally, there is a hypothalamic-limbic projection of visceral and perhaps of gustatory information that presumably is involved in autonomic reflexes and in our subjective sense of the pleasantness (or unpleasantness) of things we ingest. This system, also uncrossed, includes a synapse in the *parabrachial nucleus* of the rostral pons, so named because it surrounds the superior cerebellar peduncle (brachium conjunctivum) as the peduncle joins the brainstem. The particular part of the parabrachial nucleus in which gustatory fibers end is sometimes referred to as the *pontine taste area,* although in primates the parabrachial nucleus deals primarily with general visceral information. The parabrachial nucleus then projects rostrally to the hypothalamus and amygdala.

### *Efferents*

A small collection of general visceral efferent (GVE) fibers, innervating the submandibular and sublingual salivary glands and the lacrimal gland, travel in the facial nerve. These fibers originate from a scattered group of cells called the *superior salivatory nucleus,* located in the reticular formation near the internal genu of the facial nerve.

Most of the fibers of the facial nerve are SVE fibers that innervate muscles derived from the second branchial arch. These are the muscles of facial expression and the stapedius, a small muscle in the middle ear. The large nucleus of origin of all these fibers, the *facial motor nucleus,* is located in the ventrolateral tegmentum of the caudal pons (Figure 9-19). The peculiar course of these fibers, through the internal genu of the facial nerve, was described earlier.

The facial motor nucleus is involved in a reflex of considerable clinical importance, the *corneal blink reflex.* If either cornea is touched by a foreign object (in testing sit-

*There are actually two separate cortical taste areas, one in the parietal operculum and a second in the frontal operculum and insula, extending onto the surface of the frontal lobe. The relative roles of these two areas in normal gustatory function are still being investigated.

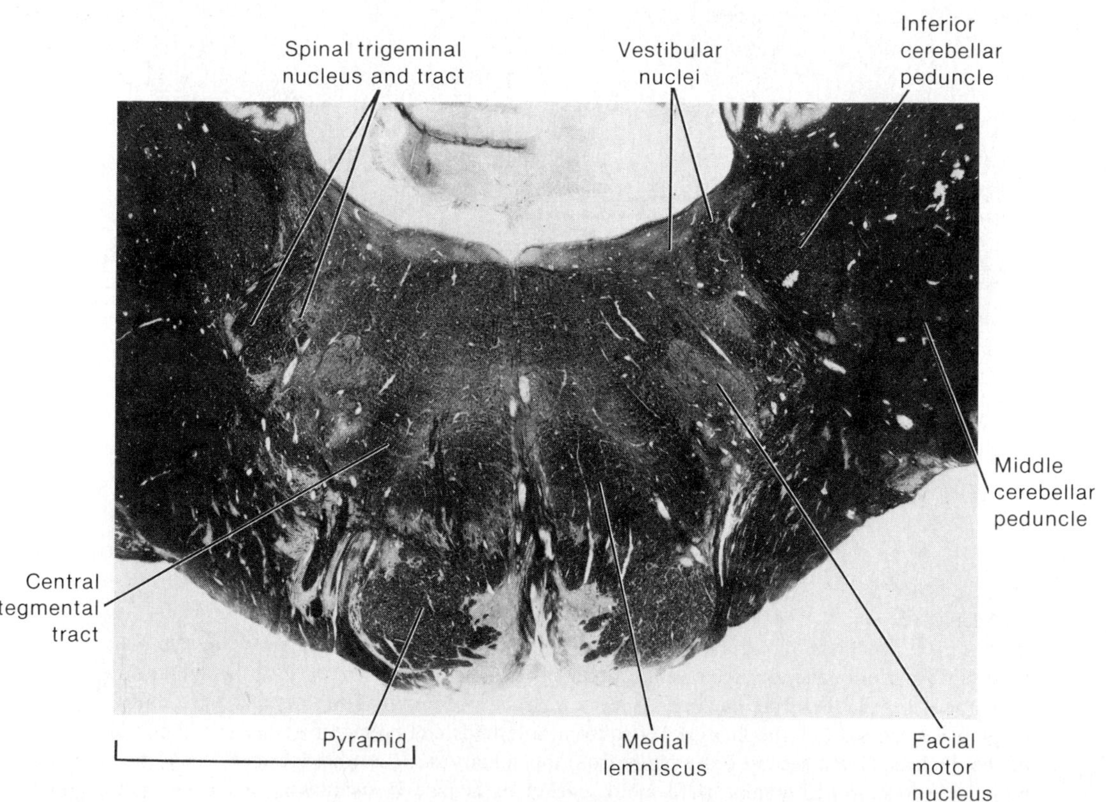


FIGURE 9-19
Section through the caudal pons showing the facial motor nucleus. Scale mark = 1 cm.

uations, typically a wisp of cotton), both eyes automatically blink. Sensory innervation of the cornea is by way of the ophthalmic division of the trigeminal nerve, so this is the afferent limb of the reflex. The afferents enter the spinal trigeminal tract and synapse on interneurons in the spinal trigeminal nucleus, mostly rostral to the obex, as well as on interneurons of the main sensory nucleus. These interneurons then project bilaterally to motor neurons of the facial motor nucleus, which form the efferent limb. Thus by touching each of an individual's corneas in turn and observing the resulting blinks, it is possible to test, in a crude fashion, the integrity of both trigeminal nerves, both facial nerves, and some of their central connections.

### Glossopharyngeal nerve (IX)

The glossopharyngeal nerve contains a number of general visceral afferent (GVA) fibers, among them afferents from the carotid body, carotid sinus, medial surface of the eardrum, posterior third of the tongue, and the walls of the pharynx. Most of these enter the solitary tract and synapse in the solitary nucleus. However, clinical evidence (described shortly) indicates that the fibers conveying information about pain from the pharynx and posterior part of the tongue (or at least collaterals of these fibers) enter the spinal trigeminal tract and terminate in the spinal nucleus. The same may be true of those fibers subserving tactile and temperature sensations; in addition, recent evidence indicates that glossopharyngeal afferents also reach the part of the main sensory nucleus concerned with intraoral sensation. This fits with common experience: even though the pharynx is technically a visceral structure, it "feels" like a somatic structure in the way in which we can localize and discriminate stimuli applied there. Thus it is not surprising that the afferents involved should enter the trigeminal system.

A small group of general visceral efferent (GVE) fibers supplying the parotid gland also travel with the glossopharyngeal nerve. These arise from scattered cells in the reticular formation of the rostral medulla, collectively called the *inferior salivatory nucleus*.

Finally, a number of special visceral efferent (SVE) fibers, partially responsible for the innervation of muscles of the pharynx, travel in cranial nerve IX. Specifically, they innervate the stylopharyngeus. Most or all of the remaining pharyngeal musculature is innervated by the vagus nerve. All these SVE fibers arise in the *nucleus ambiguus,* which is aptly named since it is embedded in the medullary reticular formation and is sufficiently noncompact that it is difficult to distinguish in myelin-stained sections. It is located in the ventrolateral medullary tegmentum just dorsal to and roughly coextensive with the inferior olivary nucleus (Figure 9-20).

The GSA (skin of outer ear) and SVA (taste buds) fibers of cranial nerve IX have connections similar to those of the facial nerve and were described in conjunction with that nerve.

### Vagus nerve (X)

Cranial nerve X has components and connections similar to and partially overlapping those of the glossopharyngeal nerve. GSA and SVA components were described in

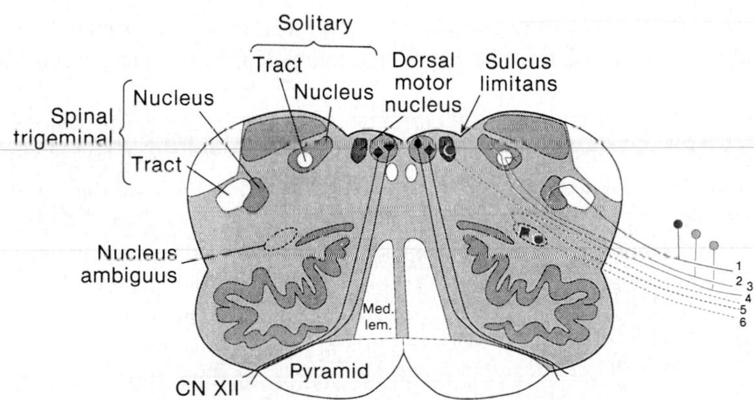


FIGURE 9-20
Contents of the vagus nerve as it leaves the brainstem. *1,* A few afferents from the skin of the outer ear (GSA) that travel through the most dorsomedial part of the spinal trigeminal tract and end in the spinal trigeminal nucleus. *2,* A few afferents from epiglottal taste buds (SVA) that travel through the solitary tract and end in lateral parts of the solitary nucleus. *3,* Afferents from thoracic and abdominal viscera (GVA) that travel through the solitary tract and end in caudal and medial parts of the solitary nucleus. *4* and *6,* Preganglionic parasympathetic efferents (GVE) to thoracic and abdominal viscera; most originate in the dorsal motor nucleus of the vagus, but some come from nucleus ambiguus. *5,* Efferents (SVE) to pharyngeal and laryngeal muscles.

the section on the facial nerve. The vagus also contains a large collection of GVA fibers innervating the thoracic and abdominal viscera, including pressure receptors and chemoreceptors of the aortic arch. Vagal GVA fibers innervating the larynx, esophagus, and lower pharynx, like similar fibers from the glossopharyngeal nerve, are thought to enter the spinal trigeminal tract and terminate in the spinal trigeminal nucleus. The remaining vagal GVA fibers enter the solitary tract and terminate in caudal portions of the solitary nucleus.

A major collection of GVE fibers travels in the vagus nerve to thoracic and abdominal viscera generally. Most of these arise in the *dorsal motor nucleus of the vagus,* which is the principal parasympathetic nucleus of the brain. It is located in the floor of the fourth ventricle just lateral to the hypoglossal nucleus (Figure 9-20), underlying the vagal trigone (see Figure 8-3). Other GVE fibers, particularly those to the heart, originate in the nucleus ambiguus.

Vagal SVE fibers arise in the nucleus ambiguus and innervate most of the striated muscles of the larynx and pharynx (which are of branchial arch origin). A clinically useful (though unpleasant for the patient) reflex is the *gag reflex.* Touching the wall of one side of the pharynx in a normal individual elicits the unpleasant bilateral response. The afferent limb is via the glossopharyngeal nerve, whereas the efferent limb is mainly via the vagus. The central connections are not entirely clear and may involve the spinal trigeminal tract and nucleus, the solitary tract and nucleus, or both, in addition to the nucleus ambiguus. Nevertheless, the gag reflex, like the blink reflex, can be used to test two cranial nerves (in this case IX and X) and some of their central connections.

### Accessory nerve (XI)

Cranial nerve XI consists of fibers that originate from the very caudal medulla and the anterior horn of the upper five cervical segments, exit just posterior to the dentate ligament, and innervate the sternocleidomastoid and part of the trapezius. These muscles are considered to be of branchial arch origin (although not all authors agree on this point), which would put accessory nerve fibers in the SVE category. In addition to these motor axons, the accessory nerve may include a few muscle afferent fibers.

## Some functional aspects of the branchiomeric nerves

### *Trigeminal neuralgia*

*Trigeminal neuralgia* (also called *tic douloureux*) is characterized by brief (usually less than a minute) attacks of excruciating pain in the distribution of one, or sometimes more than one, division of the trigeminal nerve. Between attacks, no significant sensory abnormalities can be found. There is frequently a "trigger zone" in the involved area, where tactile stimulation may precipitate an attack. The mechanism is unknown and could be peripheral (for example, in the trigeminal ganglion) or central (for example, in the spinal trigeminal nucleus). Most cases can be treated pharmacologically, but a number of surgical treatments are available if absolutely necessary. These include sectioning the involved nerve root and destroying or mechanically disturbing the trigeminal ganglion. The destructive procedures have a serious disadvantage in that the patient loses all tactile sensibility, in addition to pain, in the area. A more complex operation (but one that avoids this problem) is to section the trigeminal spinal tract slightly caudal to the obex. Tactile sensibility remains intact, and the corneal blink reflex is usually preserved. The fact that this operation abolishes pain sensations over one entire half of the face is a major piece of evidence that the caudal part of the spinal trigeminal nucleus deals with pain and that afferents from all three divisions of the trigeminal extend at least into the caudal medulla.

### *Glossopharyngeal neuralgia*

*Glossopharyngeal neuralgia* is rare but particularly distressing. The attacks of pain usually begin in the posterior tongue or walls of the pharynx and radiate to the vicinity of the ear. One reason this condition is so distressing is that the trigger zone is often on the tongue or pharyngeal wall, and attacks may be set off by simply swallowing or talking. Pharmacological relief is usually available, but if it is not, the dorsomedial portion of the spinal trigeminal tract may be sectioned in the caudal medulla. The fact that this surgical procedure is effective provides evidence that the involved pain fibers (technically GVA fibers) travel in the spinal trigeminal tract.

### *Facial paralysis*

Pyramidal system upper motor neurons originating in the cortex of the frontal lobe supply motor nuclei of the cranial nerves, much as corticospinal fibers supply alpha motor neurons of the spinal cord. These upper motor neurons are called *corticobulbar fibers (bulbar* is a loosely used term referring to just the medulla in some applications and to the medulla, pons, and midbrain in others).

There are a number of peculiarities about the organization of the corticobulbar fiber system that are discussed in some detail in Chapter 12; the pattern of innervation of the facial motor nucleus is a good example. Corticobulbar fibers from one frontal lobe contact three groups of facial motor neurons: those for both the ipsilateral and the contralateral upper face and those for the contralateral lower face (Figure 9-21). The consequence of this pattern is that a lesion of the corticobulbar fibers on one side produces weakness of only the lower facial muscles of the opposite side, since motor neurons to the upper face are bilaterally innervated. This can be useful in distinguishing facial weakness resulting from a supranuclear lesion from that resulting from a nuclear or root lesion, since the latter cause paralysis of the entire ipsilateral half of the face.

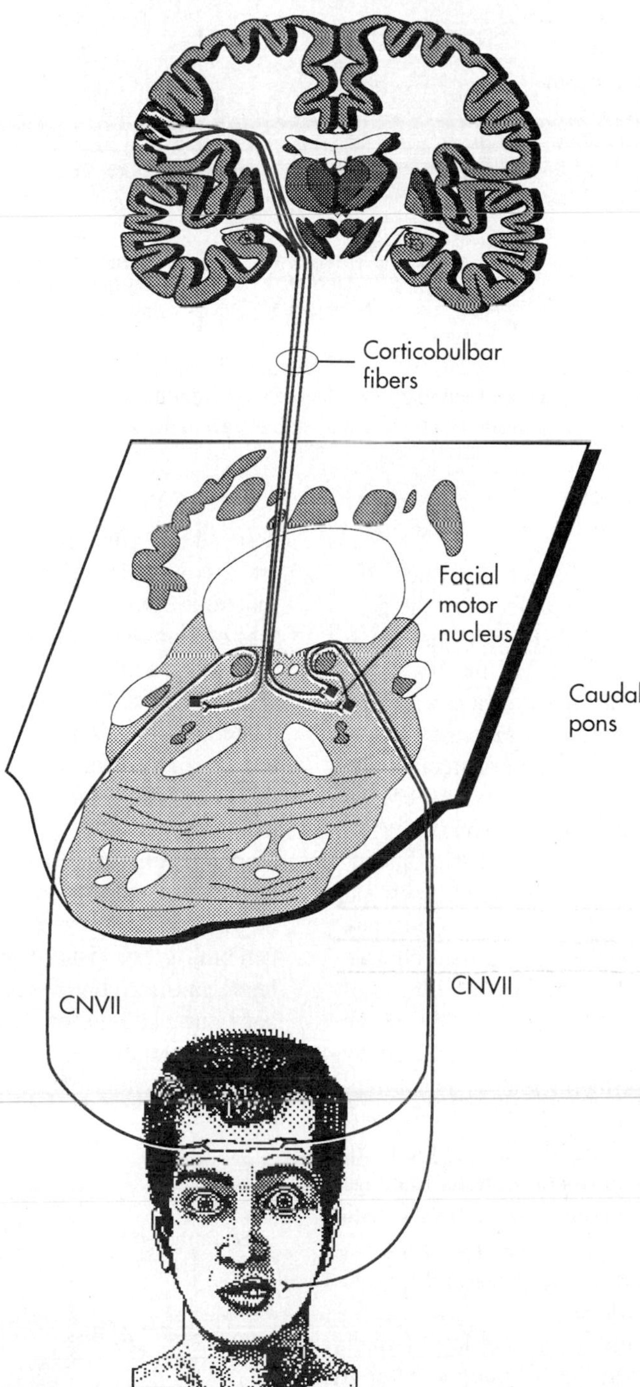


FIGURE 9-21
Corticobulbar fibers from one cerebral hemisphere to both facial motor nuclei can cause contraction of upper facial muscles bilaterally but of lower facial muscles only contralaterally.

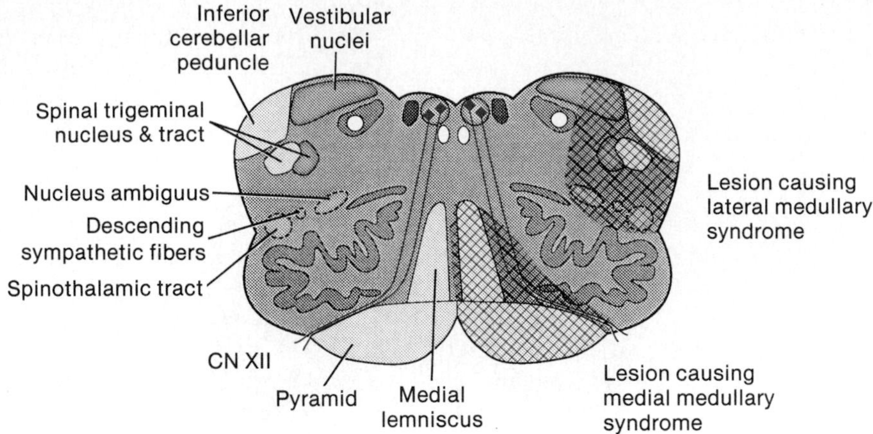


FIGURE 9-22
Lesions that would cause a lateral medullary (Wallenberg's) syndrome or a medial medullary syndrome. The structures whose damage leads to prominent symptoms are indicated on the left.

### *Other brainstem syndromes*

The Brown-Séquard syndrome (Chapter 7), which follows hemisection of the spinal cord, demonstrates the possibility of crossed or *alternating* syndromes, in which some symptoms are referred to one side of the body and others to the other side. In the brainstem, most descending pathways are contralateral to the side on which they terminate, and most ascending pathways are contralateral to the side on which they arise. However, all the exiting cranial nerves are *ipsilateral* to the side that they innervate;* in addition, most of the cranial nerve nuclei deal with ipsilateral structures. As a result, alternating syndromes, in which long tract symptoms are referred to one side and cranial nerve symptoms to the other side, are the hallmark of brainstem lesions. For example, consider the effects of a lesion involving the medial portion of one side of the rostral medulla (Figure 9-22), which could be caused by occlusion of a branch of one vertebral artery. The symptoms involved in the resulting *medial medullary syndrome* include contralateral spastic paralysis (damage to the pyramid), contralateral tactile and kinesthetic deficits (damage to the medial lemniscus), and ipsilateral paralysis with eventual atrophy of the tongue muscles (damage to the exiting hypoglossal nerve). This syndrome is also referred to as *alternating hypoglossal hemiplegia*.

More lateral damage at the same brainstem level (which can be caused by occlusion of branches of one vertebral or posterior inferior cerebellar artery) results in the *lateral medullary (*or *Wallenberg's) syndrome* (Figure 9-22). The damaged structures may include the spinothalamic tract, the spinal trigeminal tract, the nucleus ambiguus, and the descending sympathetic fibers. Symptoms of such damage are loss of pain and temperature sensations over the contralateral body (with relative sparing of tactile sensation), loss of pain and temperature sensations over the ipsilateral face, hoarseness and difficulty in swallowing (as a result of paralysis of the ipsilateral larynx and pharynx), and ipsilateral Horner's syndrome. If the inferior cerebellar peduncle and adjacent vestibular nuclei are included in the lesion, vertigo and ipsilateral cerebellar deficits such as ataxia may also result.

A final example involves a lesion of the cerebral peduncle on one side of the rostral midbrain (Figure 9-23) as might result from occlusion of branches of one posterior cerebral artery. This damages descending corticospinal fibers, causing contralateral spastic paralysis; it also damages one oculomotor nerve, causing ipsilateral ptosis, pupillary dilation, and lateral strabismus. This symptom complex is called *Weber's syndrome*.

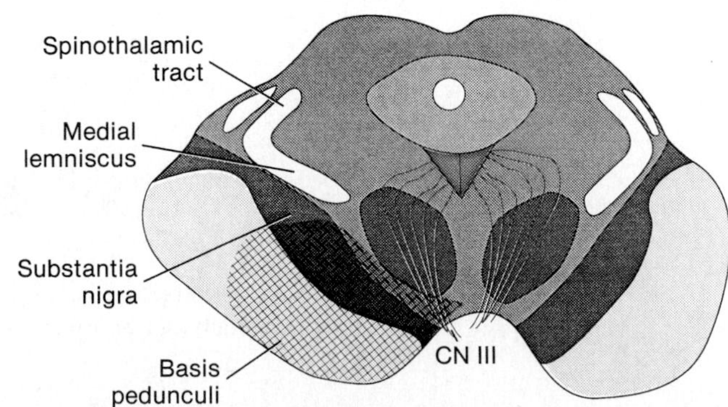


FIGURE 9-23
A lesion that would cause Weber's syndrome.

*Even in unusual cases like efferents to the superior rectus and superior oblique, the crossing occurs within the brainstem, near the cell bodies of origin.

## VESTIBULOCOCHLEAR NERVE (VIII)

The eighth cranial nerve carries two special somatic afferent (SSA) components, one in a *vestibular division* and one in a *cochlear division*. Both divisions innervate specialized sensory end organs containing ciliated mechanoreceptors (called *hair cells*), but the end organs are such that the two divisions carry different types of information. The vestibular division signals positions and movements of the head in space, whereas the cochlear division carries auditory information.

The structures innervated by the eighth nerve are embedded in the temporal bone (Figure 9-24), where the receptor cells form parts of the walls of a convoluted, membranous tube that is suspended within a bony tube (Figure 9-25). The walls of the bony tube are formed by a particularly dense portion of the temporal bone; since the tube consists of so many twists and turns, it is called the *bony labyrinth*. The membranous tube suspended within it, which follows most of its contours, is called the *membranous labyrinth*. The bony labyrinth is filled with *perilymph,* which is similar in composition to cerebrospinal fluid (and therefore to extracellular fluid generally; that is, low potassium concentration and high sodium concentration); the subarachnoid space around the brain is actually continuous with the perilymphatic space of the bony labyrinth through a tiny canal in the temporal bone. The membranous labyrinth, in contrast, is filled with *endolymph,* a peculiar fluid that is similar in ionic composition to intracellular fluids (that is, high potassium concentration and low sodium concentration). As might be expected from this different composition, the membranous labyrinth is a closed system and does not communicate with perilymphatic spaces. The resulting voltage and concentration gradients across the walls of the membranous labyrinth are important for the proper functioning of the receptors contained within these walls.

Fundamental aspects of the arrangement of receptor cells are the same in all parts of the labyrinth. The sensory

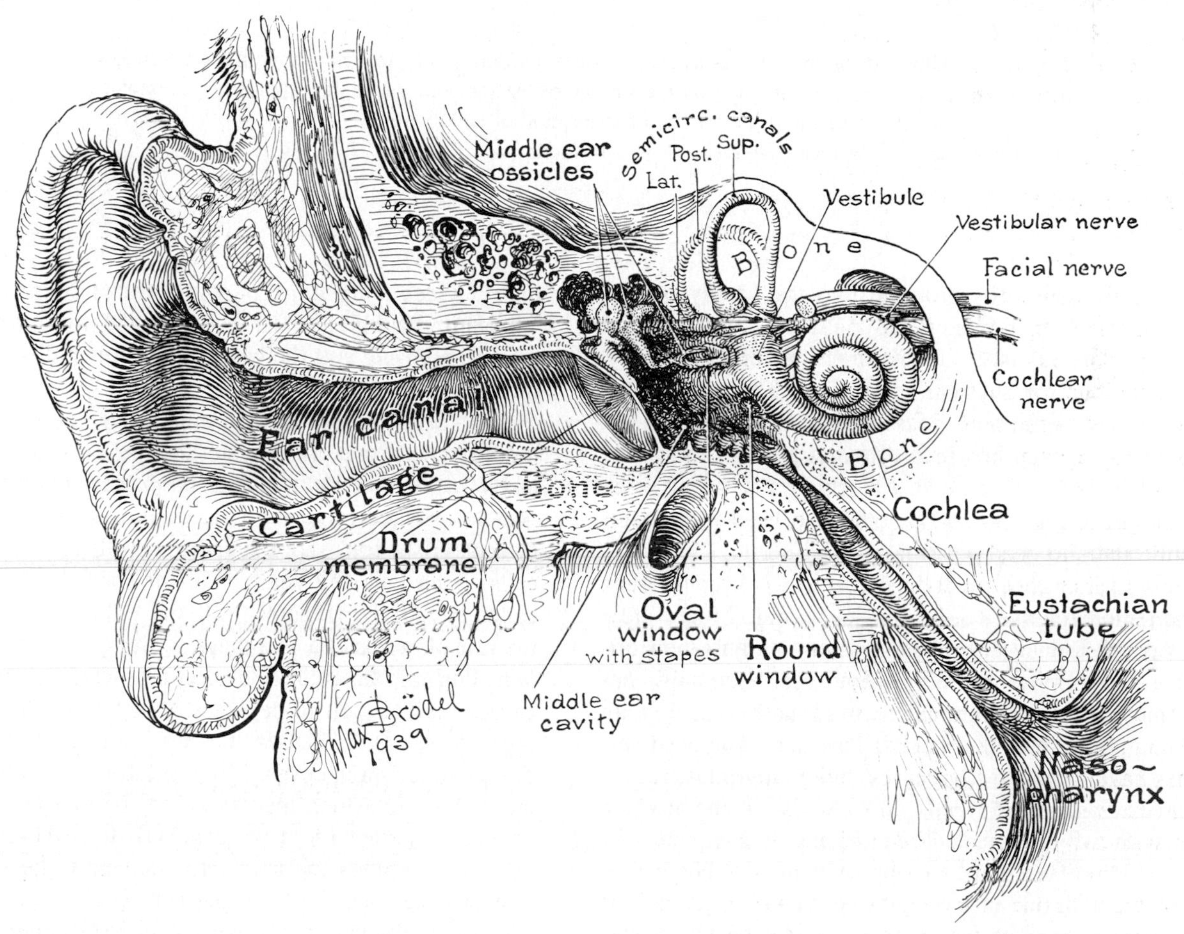


FIGURE 9-24
The outer, middle, and inner ears, showing the bony labyrinth embedded in the temporal bone. The lateral and superior semicircular canals in this drawing are called horizontal and anterior, respectively, in this chapter.
From Brödel M: Three unpublished drawings of the anatomy of the human ear, Philadelphia, 1946, WB Saunders Co.

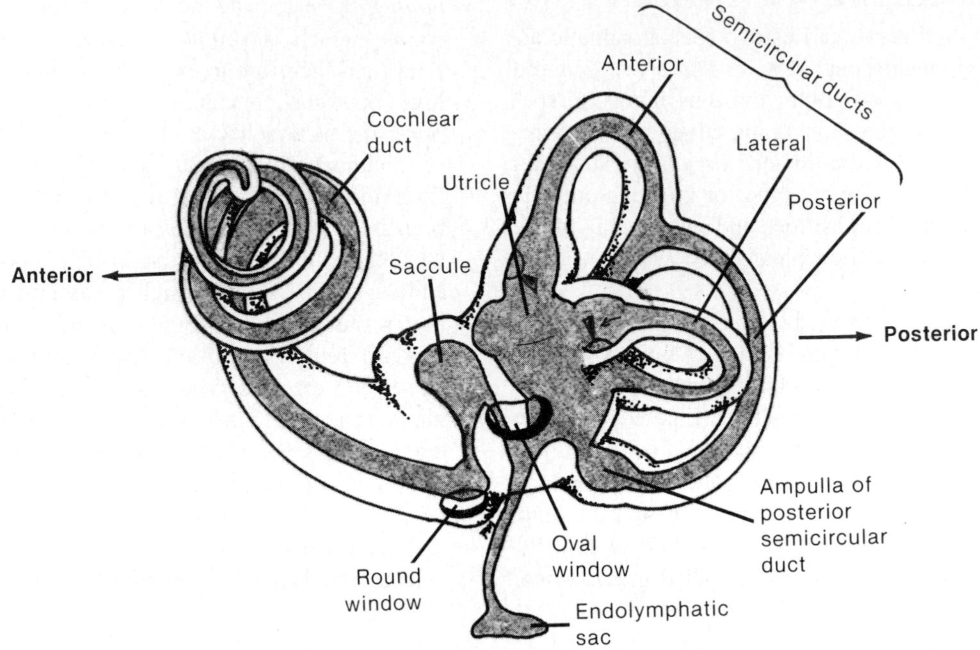


FIGURE 9-25

Membranous labyrinth of the left ear as seen through an outline of the bony labyrinth. The endolymphatic sac is located beneath the dura on the surface of the temporal bone. It contains no receptor cells but rather is thought to be the principal site of absorption of endolymph.

Modified from Warwick R, Williams PLW, editors: Gray's anatomy, Br. ed 35, Philadelphia, 1973, WB Saunders

"hairs" of the hair cells protrude into the endolymphatic space inside the membranous labyrinth and are associated with a specialized mass of gelatinous material; typically the association is a physical connection. The specifics of the way these gelatinous masses are made up and arranged, and the way in which different parts of the membranous labyrinth are suspended mechanically, allow some hair cells to respond to sound, others to head movement, and still others to head position.

One universal task for living creatures is keeping track of orientation relative to the outside world. Motile creatures have the added task of being able to adjust their orientation in response to self-generated or externally imposed movements. Vertebrates seem to have come up with an adaptation to meet these needs long ago. All jawed vertebrates have basically similar vestibular labyrinths, featuring three *semicircular canals* on each side of the head together with two or more *otolithic organs*. In every case the three semicircular canals are approximately orthogonal to each other, with one in a roughly horizontal plane and the other two in more or less vertical planes (Figure 9-26). The vestibular portion of the human bony labyrinth consists of a central area called the *vestibule* and three semicircular canals that are attached to the vestibule (Figure 9-27). Within each semicircular canal is a *semicircular duct**, which is the corresponding part of the membranous labyrinth. Within the vestibule are the two otolithic organs, the *utricle* and the *saccule*. Each is a dilation of the membranous labyrinth.

Each semicircular duct communicates at both ends with the utricle. At one end of each duct is a dilation called an *ampulla*. Each ampulla contains a *crista,* which is a transversely oriented ridge of tissue (Figure 9-28). The surface of each crista consists of supporting cells and sensory hair cells. Each hair cell bears a tuft of specialized microvilli called *stereocilia* (Figures 9-29 and 9-36). At one edge of the tuft of stereocilia is a single cilium called the *kinocilium*. Pushing the collection of cilia toward the kinocilium causes the hair cell to depolarize, whereas pushing in the opposite direction causes the hair cell to hyperpolarize. The entire crista is covered by a gelatinous partition called the *cupula,* in which the "hairs" of the hair cells are embedded. A deflection of the cupula distorts these hairs and excites or inhibits the hair cells, depending on the direction in which the hairs are pushed. The hair cells in turn synapse on the peripheral processes of vestibular afferents, and excitation or inhibition of the hair cells causes an in-

*The term semicircular canal is often used interchangeably to refer to either the bony semicircular canal or the membranous semicircular duct.

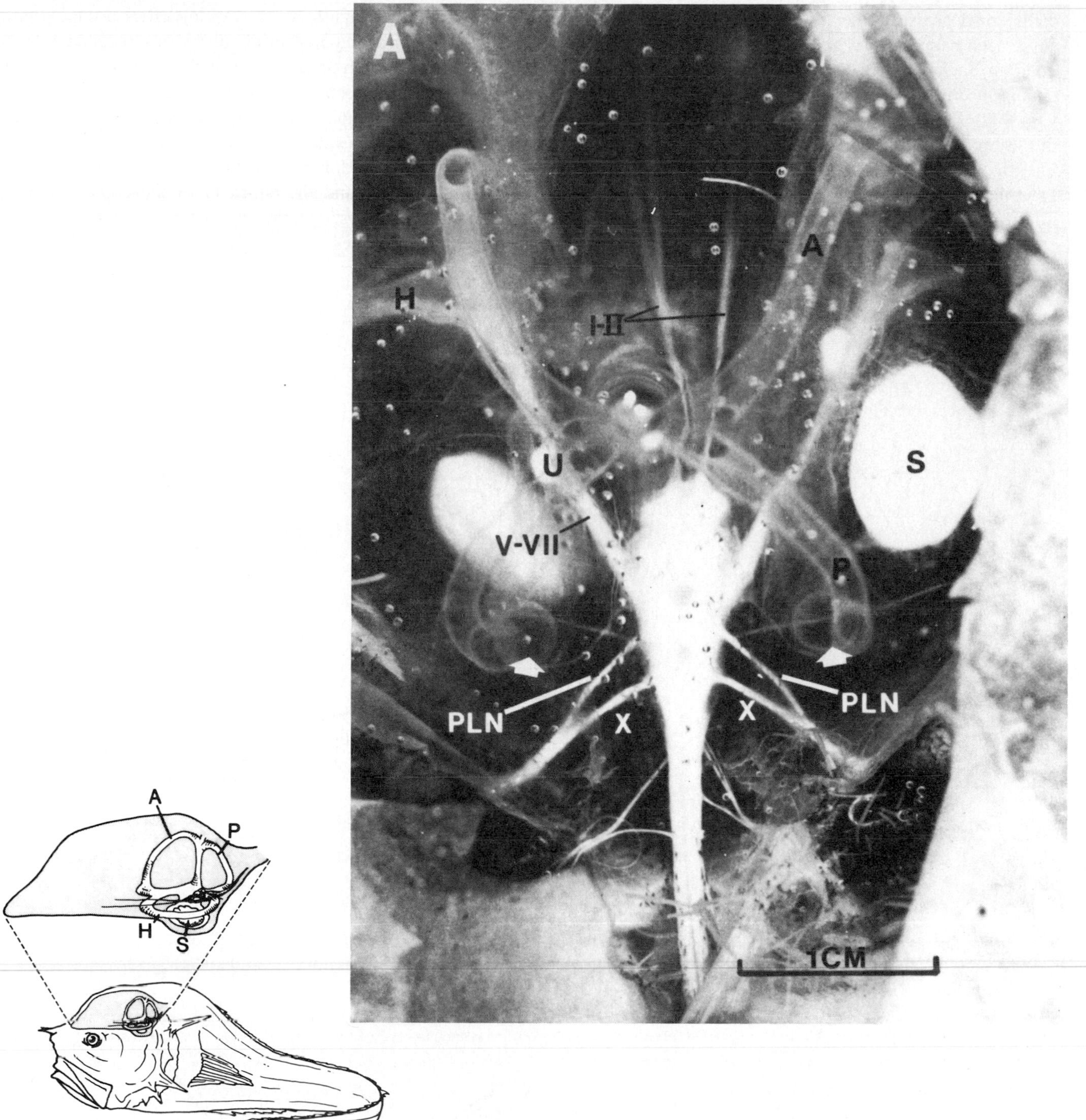


FIGURE 9-26
A striking illustration of the arrangement of vertebrate semicircular canals. *Acanthonus armatus* (drawn at the bottom left) is a species of small, deep-water fish that has particularly large semicircular canals and a particularly tiny brain. The photograph is a view into the cranial cavity from above; the orthogonally arranged anterior, posterior and horizontal semicircular canals (A, P and H) can be seen clearly. The large otoliths of the utricle (U) and especially the saccule (S) are also evident. Each saccular otolith weighed about four times as much as the fish's entire brain! Other abbreviations: I, II, V, VII and X are cranial nerves; PLN is the posterior lateral line nerve, which innervates sensory receptors along the fish's side.
From Fine ML et al., *Proc R Soc Lond* B230:257, 1987. Courtesy of Dr. M.L. Fine, Virginia Commonwealth University.

crease or decrease in the resting firing rate of these afferents. Each hair cell of a given crista is aligned with its kinocilium facing in the same direction, so deflection of the cupula in one direction causes all the afferents that innervate that crista to increase their firing rate, and deflection in the opposite direction causes them to decrease their firing rate. For example, the hair cells of the horizontal canal have their kinocilia facing the utricle, so deflecting the cupula of this canal toward the utricle causes an increased firing rate.

The most straightforward way to deflect a cupula is to rotate its semicircular duct about an axis perpendicular to it (like a wheel on an axle). As such a rotation begins, the endolymph lags behind because of inertia; this motion of duct and endolymph relative to one another deflects the cupula and stimulates the hair cells. However, as the rotation continues, the endolymph "catches up" because of factors such as friction and the elasticity of the cupula, and the stimulation ceases. At the end of the rotation, the endolymph continues to move for a short period of time

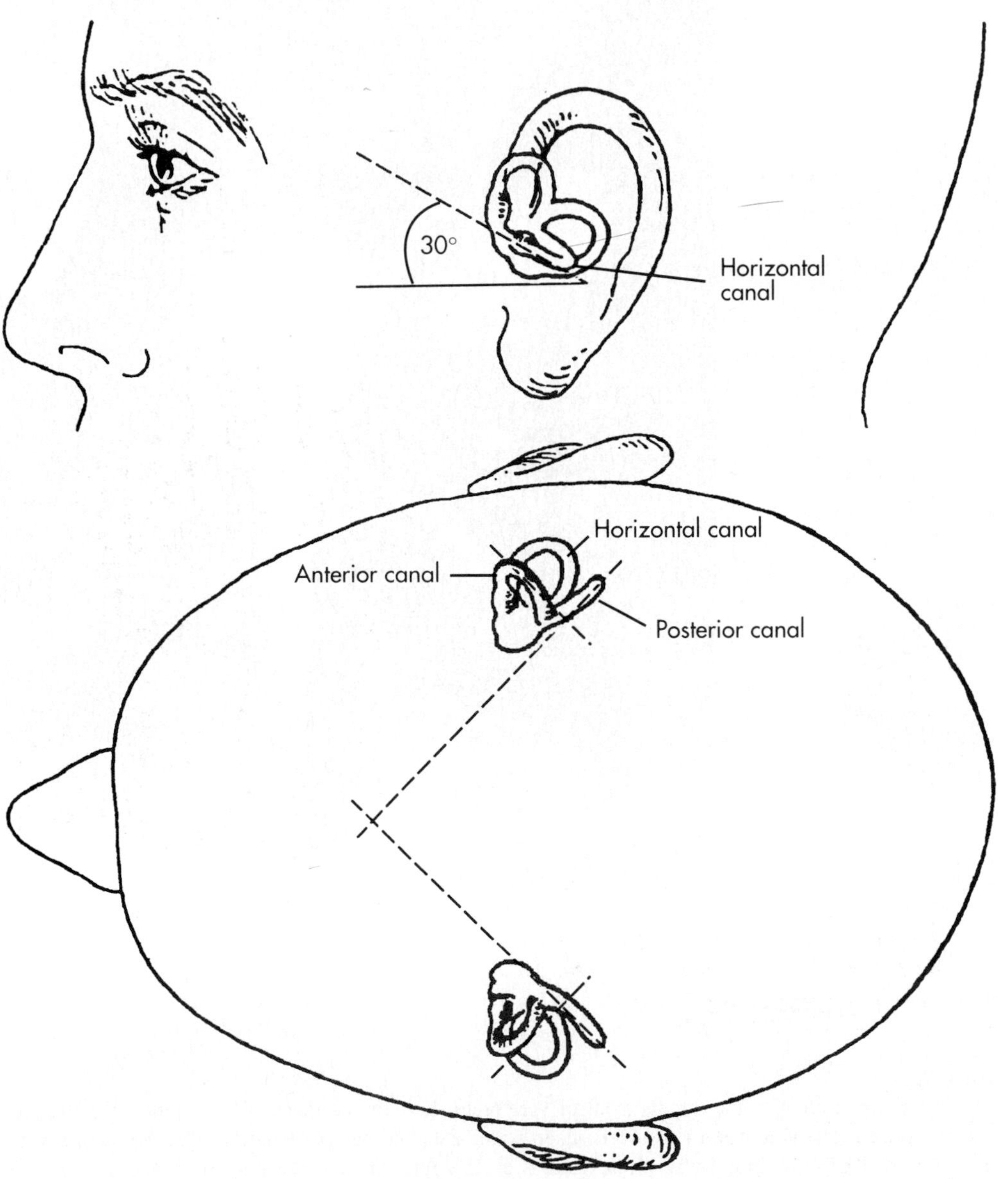


FIGURE 9-27
Orientation of the semicircular canals in the head. Note that the horizontal canals are actually tilted backward about 30°, and that the anterior canal of one side is in a plane parallel to the plane of the contralateral posterior canal.
Redrawn from Baloh RW, Honrubia V: *Clinical neurophysiology of the vestibular system,* ed 2, Philadelphia, 1990, F.A. Davis Company.

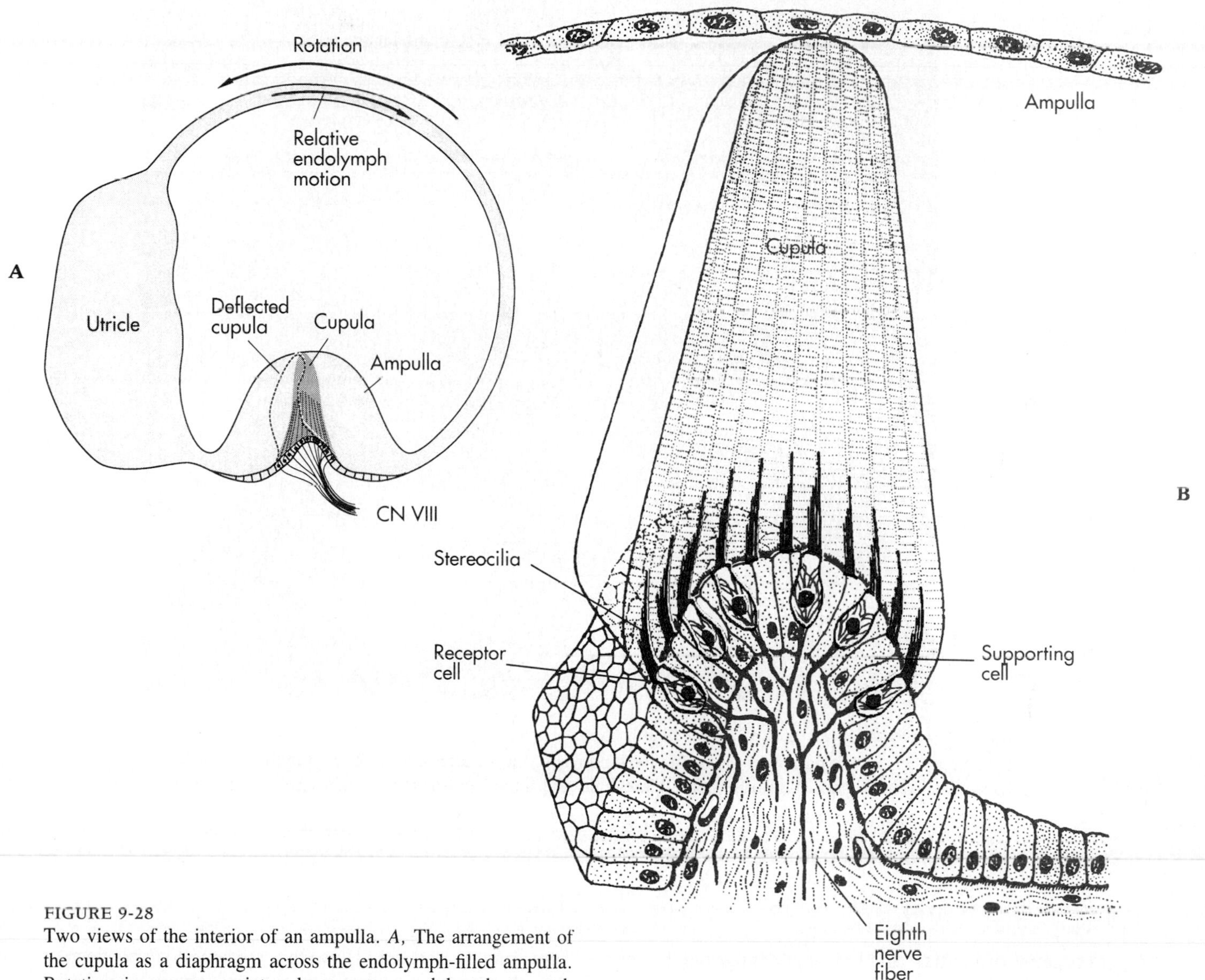


FIGURE 9-28

Two views of the interior of an ampulla. *A,* The arrangement of the cupula as a diaphragm across the endolymph-filled ampulla. Rotation in an appropriate plane causes endolymph to push against the cupula and deform it, which in turn causes deflection of hair cell stereocilia. *B,* An enlargement of a crista and cupula, showing the relationship of hair cells, their bundles of stereocilia, and the cupular diaphragm.

**A** Adapted from Bach-Y-Rita P et al.: *The control of eye movements,* New York, 1971, Academic Press. **B** Adapted from Berne RM, Levy MN: *Physiology,* ed 2, St. Louis, 1988, The C.V. Mosby Company.

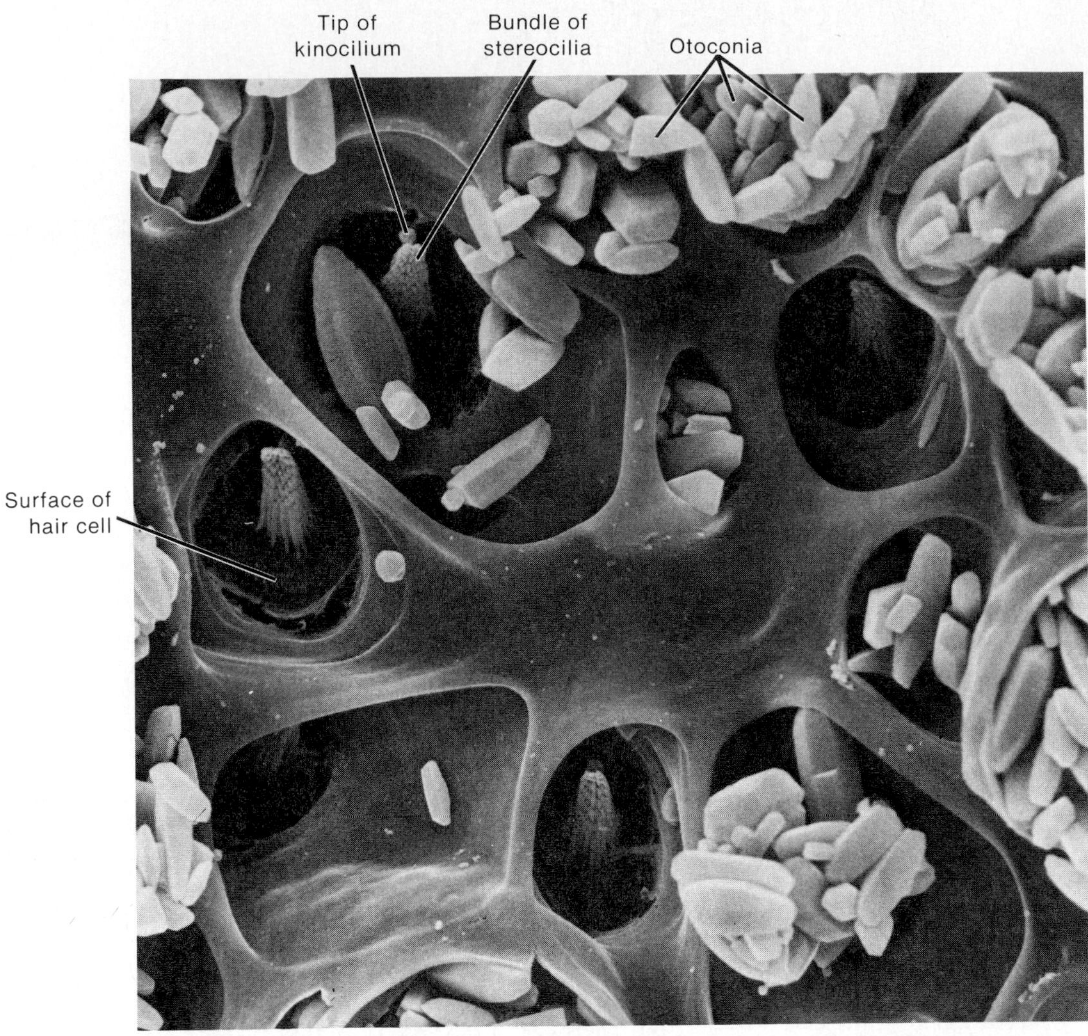


FIGURE 9-29
Scanning electron micrograph of the otolithic membrane of the saccule of a bullfrog. Bundles of sensory hairs, each bundle consisting of a single kinocilium and numerous stereocilia, can be seen projecting from individual hair cells into small holes in the otolithic membrane.

Courtesy of R Jacobs, DP Corey, AJ Hudspeth, California Institute of Technology. From Biophys J 26:499, 1979. Reproduced with the permission of Rockefeller University Press.

(again because of inertia), and the cupula bulges in the opposite direction. Thus each semicircular canal responds best to *changes* in the speed of rotation in a particular plane. Since the three semicircular canals are arranged in orthogonal planes, and since most head movements have a rotational component, movements in any direction can be detected. The fact that the semicircular canals cannot sense maintained rotation is not a great disadvantage, since (except at amusement parks) we usually do not experience maintained rotations.

The relative orientations of the three semicircular canals should be noted in Figure 9-27. One canal is roughly *horizontal* (actually, it is tilted backward about 30 degrees), whereas the other two (the *anterior* and *posterior* canals) are roughly vertical. However, the anterior and posterior canals are also arranged at an angle of about 45 degrees to the sagittal plane. The anterior canal of one side is therefore parallel to the posterior canal of the other side, so movements that stimulate one will stimulate the other. Thus the horizontal canals of the two sides form a functional pair, whereas the anterior canal of one side forms a functional pair with the posterior canal of the other side.

There are no cristae in the utricle and saccule, but each has in its wall a patch of supporting cells and hair cells called a *macula*. The utricular macula, lying at the bottom of the utricle, is roughly horizontal when one (or one's head) is in an upright posture. The saccular macula is on the medial wall of the saccule and is roughly vertical. The

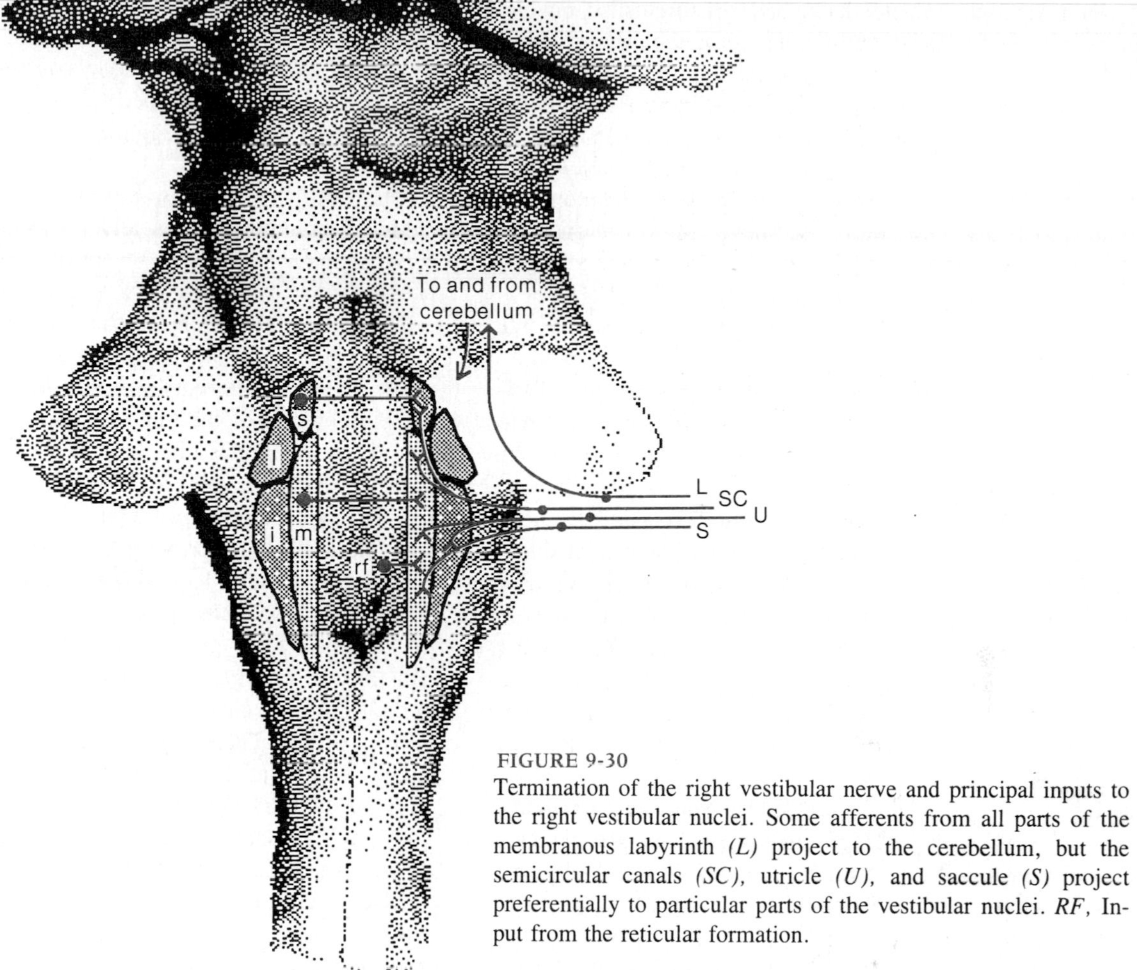


FIGURE 9-30
Termination of the right vestibular nerve and principal inputs to the right vestibular nuclei. Some afferents from all parts of the membranous labyrinth *(L)* project to the cerebellum, but the semicircular canals *(SC)*, utricle *(U)*, and saccule *(S)* project preferentially to particular parts of the vestibular nuclei. *RF*, Input from the reticular formation.

sensory hairs of the macular receptors are also embedded in a gelatinous membrane similar in composition to the cupula. However, in the case of the macula the gelatinous substance also contains minute crystals of calcium carbonate called *otoconia* or *otoliths** and so is called an *otolithic membrane* (Figure 9-29), from which the otolithic organs get their name. The otoconia make the otolithic membrane denser than the endolymph so the membrane flops around and stays flopped when the position of the head changes. This stimulates the hair cells, which then signal the new position of the head. In this case the macula is responding to the force of gravity, but it responds equally well to other accelerating forces, such as those experienced in elevators and automobiles.

As might be expected from the orientation of its macula, the utricle is most sensitive to tilts beginning from a head-upright position. The saccule, in contrast, is more sensitive to tilts beginning from a head-sideways position. The hair cells of a given macula are arranged with their kinocilia facing in several different directions, so any tilt stimulates some cells more than others. The result is that every different head position causes a unique pattern of activity in the branches of the eighth nerve that innervate the utricle and saccule.

### Central connections

Vestibular primary afferents have their cell bodies in the *vestibular* (or *Scarpa's)* ganglion in the internal auditory meatus. Their peripheral processes end about the hair cells just described. Their central processes enter the brainstem at the pontomedullary junction. Some proceed directly to the cerebellum, passing through the *juxtarestiform body,* which is located on the medial aspect of the inferior cerebellar peduncle. They end in the *flocculus, nodulus,* and nearby areas, as discussed in more detail in Chapter 14. Most primary vestibular afferents, however, end in the *vestibular nuclei* of the rostral medulla and caudal pons (Figure 9-30).

*Technically speaking, the very small crystals in the human otolithic membrane are otoconia (Greek for ear dust), whereas the somewhat larger concretions of some other vertebrates are otoliths (Greek for ear stones). However, the two terms are often used interchangeably.

Four vestibular nuclei have been distinguished on the basis of their histology and connections: the *inferior* (also called the *spinal* or *descending*), *medial*, *lateral* (or *Deiters'*), and *superior vestibular nuclei* (Figure 9-30). Each particular semicircular canal and otolithic organ has its own pattern of termination in the vestibular nuclei, and each vestibular nucleus has its own pattern of secondary connections. For the sake of simplicity, these patterns, for the most part, are ignored in this account and the vestibular nuclear complex treated as a uniform entity.

The connections of the vestibular nuclei are varied and widespread but not surprising in view of their function. We use the vestibular system principally to regulate posture and to coordinate eye and head movements; the anatomical substrates of these functions are connections with the spinal cord and with the motor nuclei of the extraocular muscles. The cerebellum is also involved in both these functions, and correspondingly there are substantial interconnections between it and the vestibular nuclei. We also have a conscious awareness of movement through space; there is a corresponding vestibular projection through the thalamus to cerebral cortex. Finally, there are connections between the vestibular nuclei and the reticular formation (including visceral centers of the reticular formation, as anyone who has been seasick can attest).

Inputs to the vestibular nuclei (in addition to primary vestibular afferents) include projections from the cerebellum (by way of the juxtarestiform body), the spinal cord, and the contralateral vestibular nuclei (Figure 9-30). The cerebellar projections arise directly from the flocculonodular lobe and indirectly from other cerebellar areas as well, as discussed further in Chapter 14. Input from the spinal cord makes reasonable sense, since it would be difficult to adjust posture properly in response to a movement or a tilt without knowledge of the current orientation of the body. A small amount of this information travels with the posterior spinocerebellar tract as direct spinovestibular fibers, but most of it reaches the vestibular nuclei indirectly via relays in the cerebellum or reticular formation. Finally, the left and right vestibular apparatus normally function together as a coordinated pair, and the vestibular nuclear complexes of the two sides are extensively interconnected.

Secondary fibers arising in the vestibular complex project to (1) the same cerebellar areas as do primary vestibular afferents (again, via the juxtarestiform body), (2) the spinal cord, in the lateral and medial vestibulospinal tracts, (3) the thalamus, (4) the motor nuclei of the extraocular muscles, and (5) the vestibular apparatus (Figure 9-31). (This is in addition to the previously mentioned projections to the reticular formation and the contralateral vestibular nuclei.)

The *lateral vestibulospinal tract* arises in the lateral vestibular nucleus and projects to all levels of the ipsilateral spinal cord, where it is located in the ventral part of the lateral funiculus. This is the principal route by which the vestibular system brings about postural changes to compensate for tilts and movements of the body. If as a child (or an adult) you ever spun yourself around until you felt dizzy and then proceeded to stagger, you have experienced the effects of exaggerated activity in your lateral vestibulospinal tract.

The *medial vestibulospinal tract* arises mainly in the medial vestibular nucleus and projects bilaterally to the cervical spinal cord. It is responsible for stabilizing head position as we do things like walk around.

Vestibular projections to the thalamus, and from there to the cerebral cortex, have been a matter of some controversy. The thalamic relay seems to be in a small nucleus in the inferior part of the thalamus near the VPL and VPM. Secondary vestibular fibers reach the thalamus bilaterally, some by traveling with the auditory fibers of the lateral lemniscus and others by traversing the reticular formation near the MLF. The primary vestibular cortical area is located in the parietal lobe at the junction between the intraparietal and postcentral sulci; this is adjacent to the portion of the postcentral gyrus where the head is represented. This makes sense, as the somatosensory cortex of the postcentral gyrus is concerned with conscious appreciation of body position. There may be an additional representation of the vestibular system in the superior temporal gyrus, near the auditory cortex.

Many secondary vestibular fibers project directly through the MLF to the motor neurons of the oculomotor, trochlear, and abducens nuclei. This forms much of the basis of the *vestibuloocular reflex,* by means of which a person's gaze can stay fixed on an object even though the head is moving or being moved. One might think that this is a form of visual tracking, but the reflex works even in the dark in normal individuals and works relatively poorly in individuals with bilateral vestibular damage (Figure 9-32); thus it seems clear that the vestibular division of cranial nerve VIII forms a major part of the afferent limb. Each semicircular canal has connections via the vestibular nuclei that are appropriate to cause eye deviation in its own plane. This is most easily understood in the case of the horizontal canal. Imagine rotating to the left about a vertical axis (Figure 9-40, *B*). This would cause the cupula of the left horizontal canal to bulge toward the utricle (Figure 9-27), hence depolarizing the hair cells of this canal and increasing the firing rate of the eighth nerve fibers that innervate them. Excitatory connections with the left vestibular nuclei and from there to the right abducens nucleus result in deviation of both eyes to the right (Figure 9-8), compensating for the rotation. Other combinations of semicircular canals and extraocular muscles are similarly straightforward, although more difficult to visualize. For example, rotating forward and to the right in the plane of the right anterior canal causes contraction of the right superior rectus and left inferior oblique, which in turn causes compensatory elevation and rotation of both eyes.

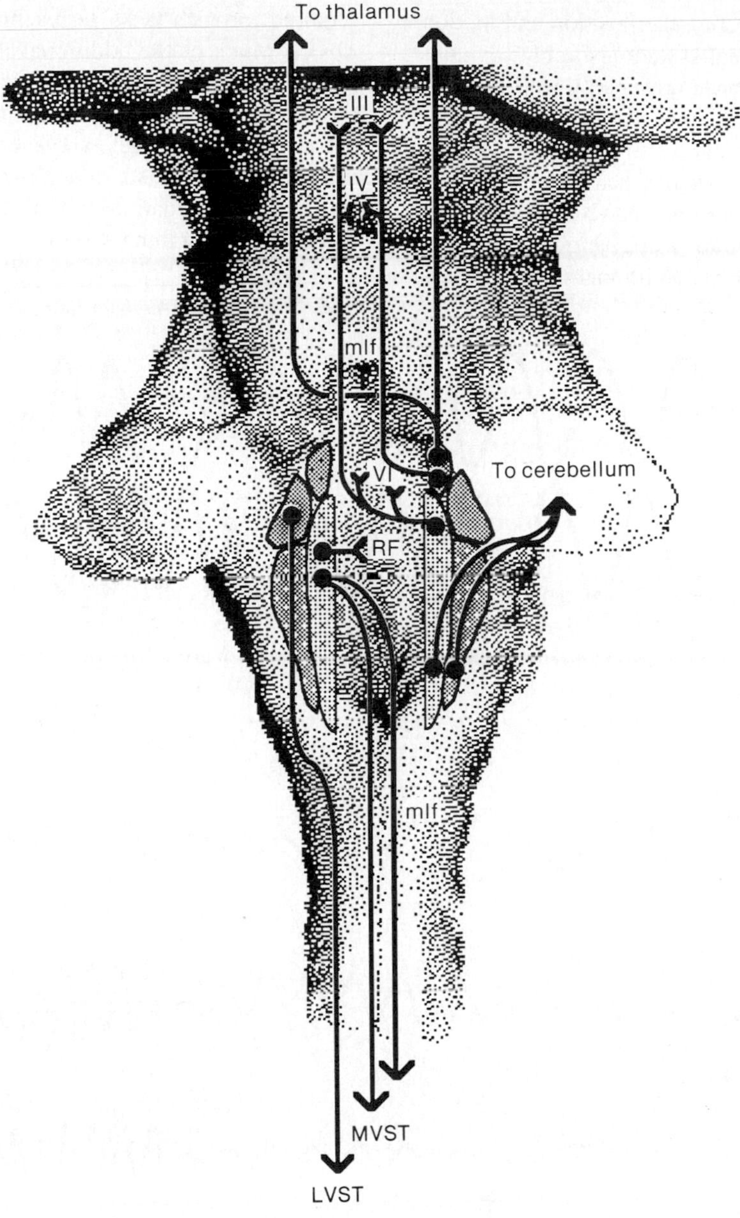


FIGURE 9-31
Some outputs from the vestibular nuclei. Projections to the contralateral vestibular nuclei are not shown but are extensive. *LVST,* Lateral vestibulospinal tract; *MVST,* medial vestibulospinal tract; *RF,* reticular formation.

Some fibers arising in or near the vestibular nuclei project back through the eighth nerve and end on the hair cells of the vestibular apparatus. These efferents are another example of the widespread phenomenon of feedback from a higher level to a lower level of a sensory system. The role of such efferents, in general, is poorly understood, and the vestibular system is no exception. One common suggestion is that the efferents could compensate for self-generated activity in the sensory system. For example, the horizontal semicircular canals receive the same stimulation if you rotate your head as they do if someone begins to rotate the chair in which you are sitting. However, the reflex postural adjustments to the two rotations are quite different. If the efferent system compensated for the hair cell response to self-generated rotation, the reflex postural adjustments would be eliminated. There is some experimental evidence that this may be the case, but there is also evidence that this is not the principal role of the efferents.

It should be noted that the vestibular system is not th

only means available for detecting the position and motion of the head in space. The visual system also plays a major role, and humans can compensate reasonably well for total loss of vestibular function, as long as visual cues are available. Most of us have experienced an illusion of movement when we were stationary and a nearby large object (such as a train on the next track) moved. It should also be noted that the vestibular apparatus can give no information about the position of the *body,* so additional information is required for such tasks as reaching with a hand for a seen object. Much of the additional information is provided by mechanoreceptors in the neck that detect the orientation of the head relative to the body. If the first three cervical dorsal roots of a monkey are anesthetized bilaterally, a remarkably severe disorientation results, involving not only eye-hand coordination but also such basic activities as walking and climbing.

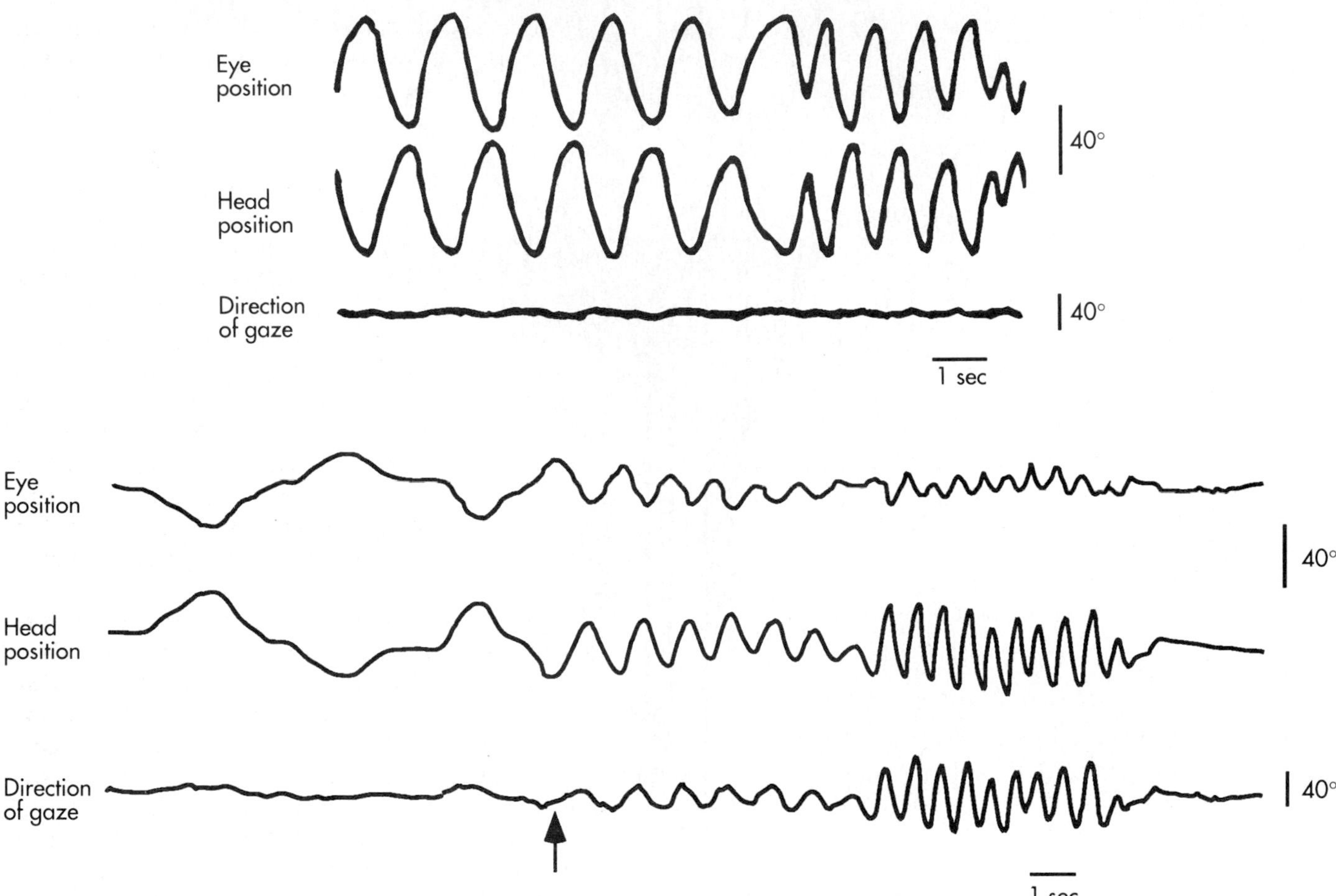


FIGURE 9-32
Normal and abnormal vestibuloocular reflexes. The surface of the cornea is electrically positive relative to the back of the eyeball, so deviation of an eye toward a nearby electrode will cause the electrode to become more positive relative to a distant electrode. This is used clinically to record eye movements. These traces show the position of the eyes in the horizontal plane, the position of the same individual's head, and (in color) the sum of these two positions, which corresponds to the net direction in which the individual is looking. *A,* A normal individual moved her head back and forth while trying to maintain her gaze fixed on a stationary target. Notice that as her head moves in one direction, her eyes move through an equal but opposite angle, so the direction of gaze does not change. This is the normal vestibuloocular reflex. *B,* A patient with bilateral loss of vestibular hair cells (caused by ototoxicity of the streptomycin used to treat her for pneumonia) attempts to do the same thing. At the slow head velocities at the beginning of the recording, she was able to use visual feedback to generate compensatory eye movements. However, once head velocity reached about 50°/sec (at the arrow), the lack of a vestibuloocular reflex made it impossible to generate large enough compensatory eye movements. As a result the direction of gaze began to oscillate in phase with head movement.
Redrawn from Atkin A, Bender MB, *Arch Neurol* 19:559, 1968.

## Cochlear division

### *Peripheral apparatus*

The auditory system faces a basic mechanical problem, since the sound vibrations that it must detect are propagated in air, whereas the auditory receptor cells (like other elements of the nervous system) live in a fluid-filled environment. Nearly all (99.9%) of the sound energy incident on an air-water interface is reflected, since water is harder to move than air. Therefore if the auditory receptor organ (the *organ of Corti*) and its fluid surroundings were mechanically coupled to the outside world by a simple membrane, it could utilize no more than 0.1% of the sound energy available to it. One major task of the air-filled *outer* and *middle ears* (Figure 9-24) therefore is to transfer sound as efficiently as possible to the fluid-filled *inner ear*.

The outer ear is basically a complicated funnel consisting of the *auricle* (or *pinna*) and the *external auditory meatus;* it conducts sound to the *tympanic membrane*. Sound-induced vibrations are transferred along a chain of three small bones or ossicles that traverse the middle ear cavity (a cavity in the temporal bone). The handle of the *malleus* is attached to the medial surface of the tympanic membrane, so movements of this membrane are transferred directly to the malleus. The malleus in turn is attached to the *incus,* which is attached to the *stapes*—so sound-induced vibrations eventually reach the oval-shaped footplate of the stapes. The footplate of the stapes occupies a hole in the temporal bone called the *oval window* (or *fenestra vestibuli*); on the other side of the oval window is the perilymph-filled vestibule of the bony labyrinth. The vestibule leads directly to the *cochlea,* which contains the organ of Corti. Thus vibration of the tympanic membrane ultimately results in vibration of the fluids of the inner ear.

The chain of middle ear ossicles acts as a lever system with a small mechanical advantage, so a given force at the tympanic membrane results in a slightly greater force at the footplate of the stapes. More important, the area of the tympanic membrane is about 15 times that of the footplate of the stapes. The net result of the mechanical advantage and the size difference is that stapedial vibrations have a much greater force *per unit area* of the footplate; this force is sufficient to move the perilymph, and more than 60% of the sound energy incident on the tympanic membrane is successfully transferred to the inner ear. The effectiveness of this system is quite extraordinary. At threshold at 3000 Hz (the frequency to which we are most sensitive) the tympanic membrane moves a distance somewhat less than the diameter of a single hydrogen atom. By the time such a threshold vibration of the tympanic membrane reaches the cochlear hair cells it deflects their stereocilia through an angle of only about 0.003°. Bending the Empire State Building through an angle of 0.003° would deflect its top by less than an inch!*

*An Americanization of an Eiffel Tower analogy presented by A.J. Hudspeth in *Nature* 341:397, 1989.

Two tiny muscles are attached to the middle ear bones. One, the *tensor tympani,* is attached to the handle of the malleus; when it contracts, it increases the tension on the tympanic membrane and decreases the transmission of vibrations through the ossicular chain. The other muscle, the *stapedius,* is attached to the neck of the stapes; it too decreases the transmission of vibrations when it contracts. The tensor tympani receives motor innervation from the trigeminal nerve and the stapedius from the facial nerve; both muscles are involved in certain auditory reflexes to be described shortly.

The auditory part of the inner ear, like the vestibular part, consists of a portion of the endolymph-filled membranous labyrinth suspended within a portion of the perilymph-filled bony labyrinth.

The bony part is the cochlea (Latin for snail), which coils through 2½ turns from its relatively broad base to its apex. The cochlea lies on its side in the temporal bone, with its base facing medially and posteriorly (Figures 9-24 and 9-25), but for the sake of simplicity it is usually discussed as though it sat upright on its base. The bony core of the cochlea is the *modiolus,* from which the *osseous spiral lamina* projects like the threads of a screw. A winding cavity within the modiolus houses the *spiral ganglion,* which contains the cell bodies of the primary auditory afferent fibers. The central processes of these cells collect at the base of the cochlea to form the cochlear division of the eighth nerve; the peripheral processes pass in bundles through a series of canals in the osseous spiral lamina to innervate the auditory receptors.

The *cochlear duct* (the auditory portion of the membranous labyrinth) is firmly anchored to the bony labyrinth in such a way that the duct is triangular in cross section (Figure 9-33). One corner of the triangle is attached to the edge of the osseous spiral lamina, and the other two corners are attached to the outer wall of the bony cochlea. The result is that the cochlear duct and osseous spiral lamina act as a partition separating two perilymphatic spaces from each other (except at the apex of the cochlea, where perilymph can pass from one space to the other through a small opening called the *helicotrema*). The perilymphatic space above the cochlear duct is called the *scala vestibuli* because it is directly continuous with the perilymph of the vestibule. The space below the cochlear duct is called the *scala tympani* because it ends blindly at the *secondary tympanic membrane* (or *round window membrane*). Vibrations reaching the stapedial footplate are transferred to the perilymph. Although perilymph is incompressible, the round window membrane is elastic, allowing these vibrations to enter the labyrinth. When the stapedial footplate moves inward, the round window membrane bulges out; when the footplate moves outward, the membrane is drawn inward. In the process, small quantities of perilymph oscillate within the cochlea. Most of this vibratory energy passes directly from the scala vestibuli to the scala tympani, deforming the cochlear duct. The cochlear duct

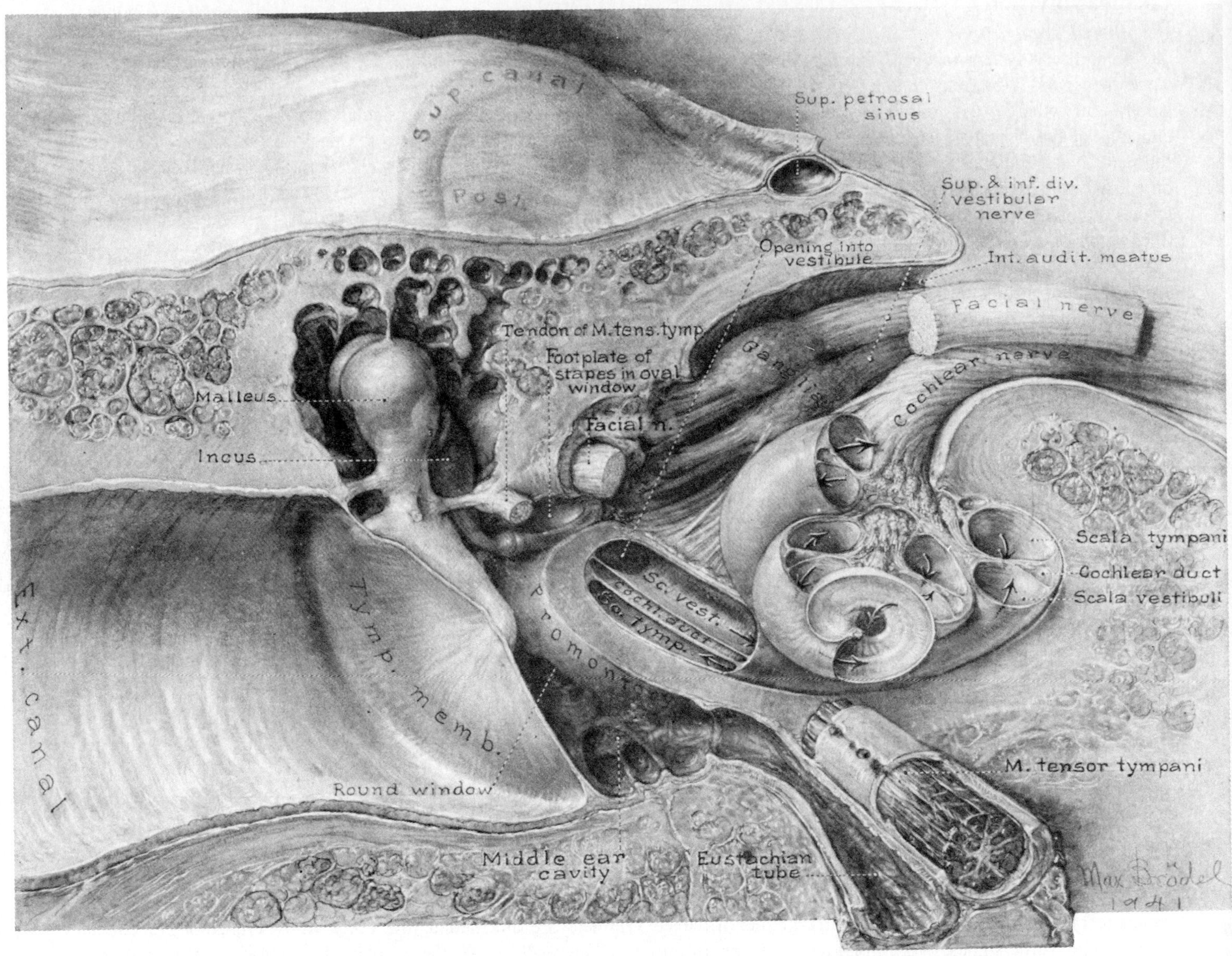


FIGURE 9-33
Drawing of a dissection of the right cochlea showing the continuous perilymphatic path from the vestibule into the scala vestibuli and from there into the scala tympani, finally ending at the round window membrane.
From Brödel M: Three unpublished drawings of the anatomy of the human ear, Philadelphia, 1946, WB Saunders.

contains the auditory receptors, and this deformation stimulates some of them.

The space enclosed by the cochlear duct is filled with endolymph and is called the *scala media*. As noted above, the scala media is triangular in cross section, and each of the three walls of the cochlear duct has a different structure. The thin *vestibular* (or *Reissner's*) *membrane* borders the scala vestibuli and probably serves mainly as a barrier between the endolymph and perilymph, playing no great role in the mechanical properties of the cochlea. The *stria vascularis* forms the second wall, adhering to the outer wall of the bony cochlea; it is a specialized area, rich in capillaries, that produces most of the endolymph in the membranous labyrinth. The *basilar membrane* completes the cochlear duct, separating the scala media from the scala tympani. Passing from the base to the apex of the cochlea, the osseous spiral lamina becomes narrower and the basilar membrane becomes broader. Because of this change in its width and progressive changes in its mechanical properties, the basilar membrane is vibrated most effi-

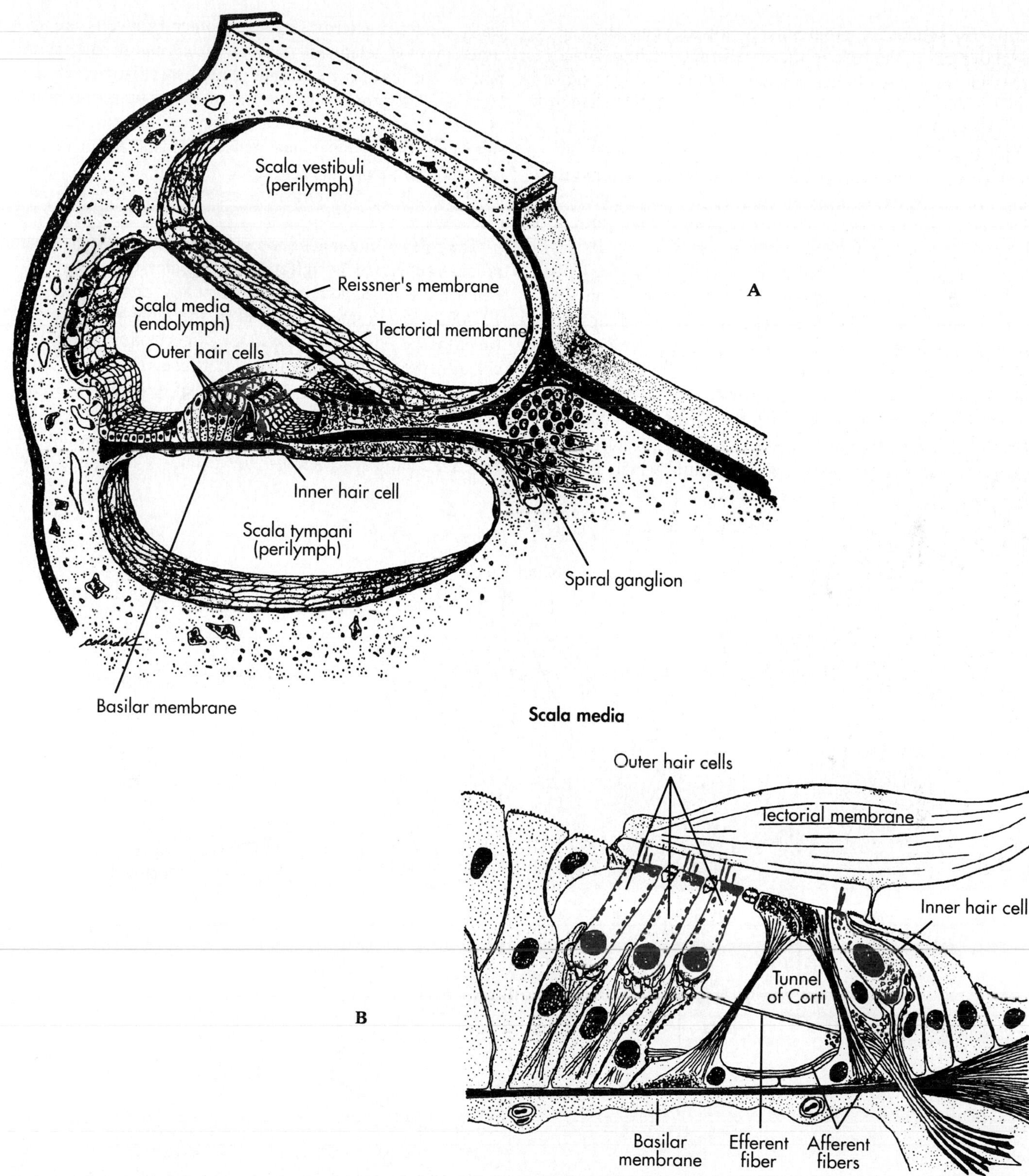


FIGURE 9-34
*A,* Cross section through one turn of the cochlea, showing the endolymphatic and perilymphatic spaces, as well as the organ of Corti and its inner and outer hair cells. *B,* Cross section through the organ of Corti.

**A** Redrawn from Fawcett DW: *A textbook of histology*, ed 11, Philadelphia, 1986, W.B. Saunders Company. **B** Redrawn from Northern JL: *Hearing disorders*, ed 2, Boston, 1984, Little, Brown & Co.

ciently by sounds of progressively lower frequencies as one moves from the base to the apex of the cochlea. Since the organ of Corti (which contains the auditory receptor cells) rests on the basilar membrane, different receptor cells respond best to sounds of different frequencies. This is the beginning of a *tonotopic organization* within the auditory system, quite analogous to the somatotopic organization of the somatosensory system; in this case particular frequencies are mapped in an orderly fashion onto particular areas of relay nuclei and auditory cortex.

The organ of Corti (Figures 9-34 and 9-35) is a long strip of hair cells and supporting cells that rests on the basilar membrane. The hair cells are arranged in two groups: a single row of *inner hair cells* near the osseous spiral lamina and a band of *outer hair cells* three to five cells wide. The two groups are separated by a space called the *tunnel of Corti,* through which the peripheral processes of auditory afferents must pass on their way to the outer hair cells. The sensory hairs (all stereocilia, which are actually modified microvilli) of the outer hair cells are inserted into the gelatinous *tectorial membrane* so that vibration of the basilar membrane causes oscillations of the hairs and therefore oscillation of the membrane potential of the hair cells. Anatomical evidence indicates that the stereocilia of the inner hair cells are not attached to the tectorial membrane and that these hair cells may be stimulated directly by movement of endolymph within the cochlear duct.

The roles of the inner and outer hair cells in the hearing process appear to be different. The outer hair cells outnumber the inner hair cells substantially; there are about 12,000 of the former and 3500 of the latter per cochlea. Nevertheless, most of the auditory information in the cochlear nerve is carried by fibers that innervate the less numerous inner hair cells. About 90% of all auditory afferents receive their entire input from single inner hair cells; one inner hair cell may make synapses on as many as 20 different auditory afferents. In contrast, the remaining

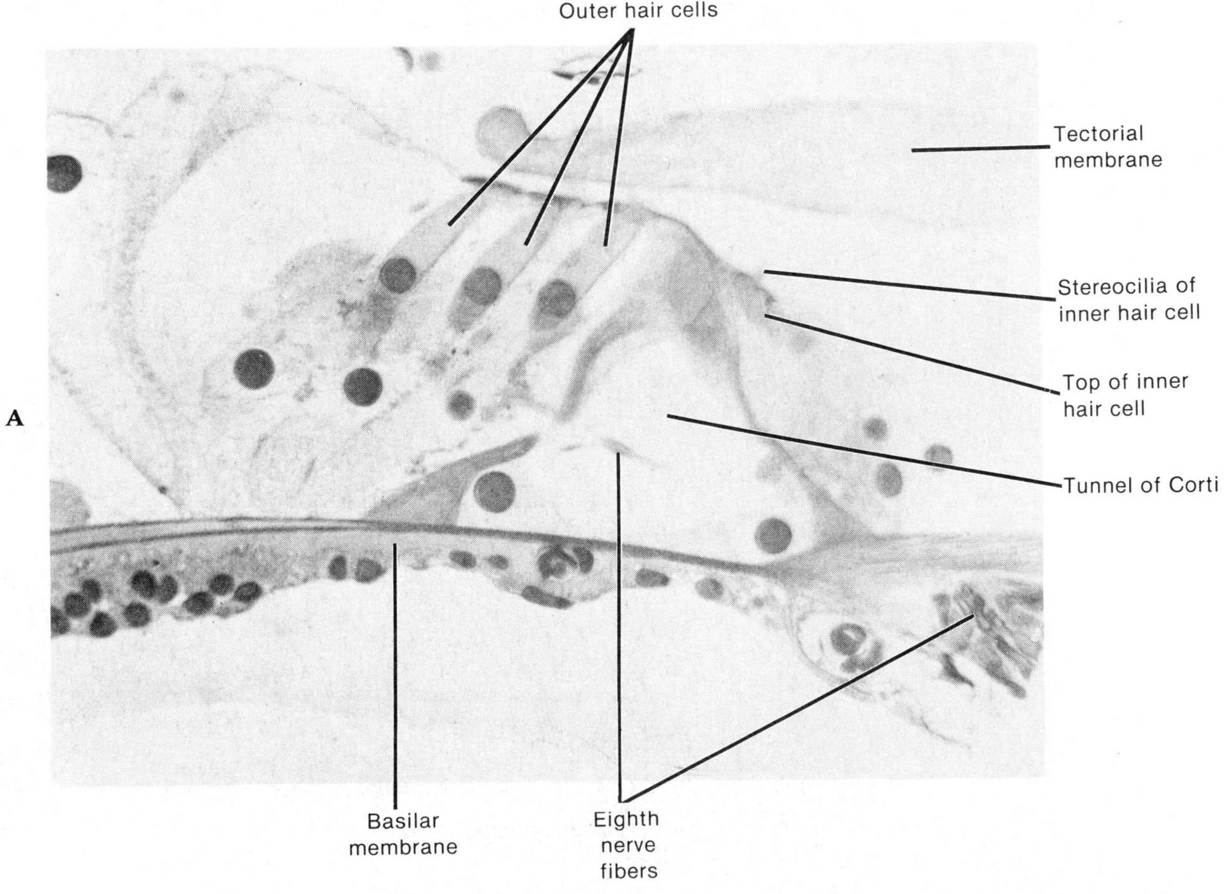


FIGURE 9-35
Micrographs of the organ of Corti. **A,** Light micrograph of the organ of Corti of a guinea pig; three outer hair cells can be seen, but only the top of an inner hair cell is present in this section.

**A** courtesy of Dr. David Asher; **B** with permission from Bredberg G. In Evans EF, Wilson JP, editors: Psychophysics and physiology of hearing, New York, 1977. Copyright by Academic Press, Inc. [London] Ltd.

10% of the auditory afferents branch repeatedly and innervate multiple outer hair cells. However, the outer hair cells seem to contribute substantially to the sensitivity of the inner hair cells; certain ototoxic drugs can be used to destroy the outer hair cells selectively, and this causes the auditory threshold to rise by a factor of $10^3$ to $10^4$. One possible mechanism is suggested by recent work indicating that the outer hair cells are contractile (Figure 9-36), so that oscillations of their membrane potential resulting from vibration of the basilar membrane cause the cells themselves to vibrate. This in turn could increase the vibratory stimulation of the inner hair cells, thus increasing their sensitivity.

In Figures 9-34, *B* and 9-35, *A,* it looks as though the organ of Corti is bathed in the endolymph of the scala media. However, it has long been reasoned that this is unlikely, since it would mean (among other things) that auditory afferents traversing the tunnel of Corti would be passing through endolymph. Endolymph has such a high potassium concentration that standard nerve fibers could not work in its presence. Recent evidence is consistent with this reasoning and indicates that the perilymphatic space of the scala tympani continues through the basilar membrane and into the organ of Corti. The real barrier between endolymph and perilymph is a series of tight junctions between hair cells and supporting cells at the surface of the organ of Corti so that only the stereocilia and upper surfaces of the hair cells are exposed to endolymph. Since perilymph is continuous with the cerebrospinal fluid of subarachnoid space, marker substances introduced into the cisterna magna infiltrate the organ of Corti and surround its hair cells, stopping only at the array of tight junctions (Figure 9-37).

### *Central connections*

Auditory primary afferents, whose cell bodies are located in the spiral ganglion of the modiolus, enter the brainstem at the pontomedullary junction. There each fiber bifurcates and sends one branch to the *dorsal cochlear nucleus* and one branch to the *ventral cochlear nucleus.* These cochlear nuclei form a continuous band of cells that covers the dorsal and lateral aspects of the inferior cerebellar peduncle.

Sensory systems characteristically analyze multiple aspects of a stimulus, such as the color and brightness of a visual stimulus or the shape and texture of a somatosensory stimulus. Similarly, the auditory system analyzes

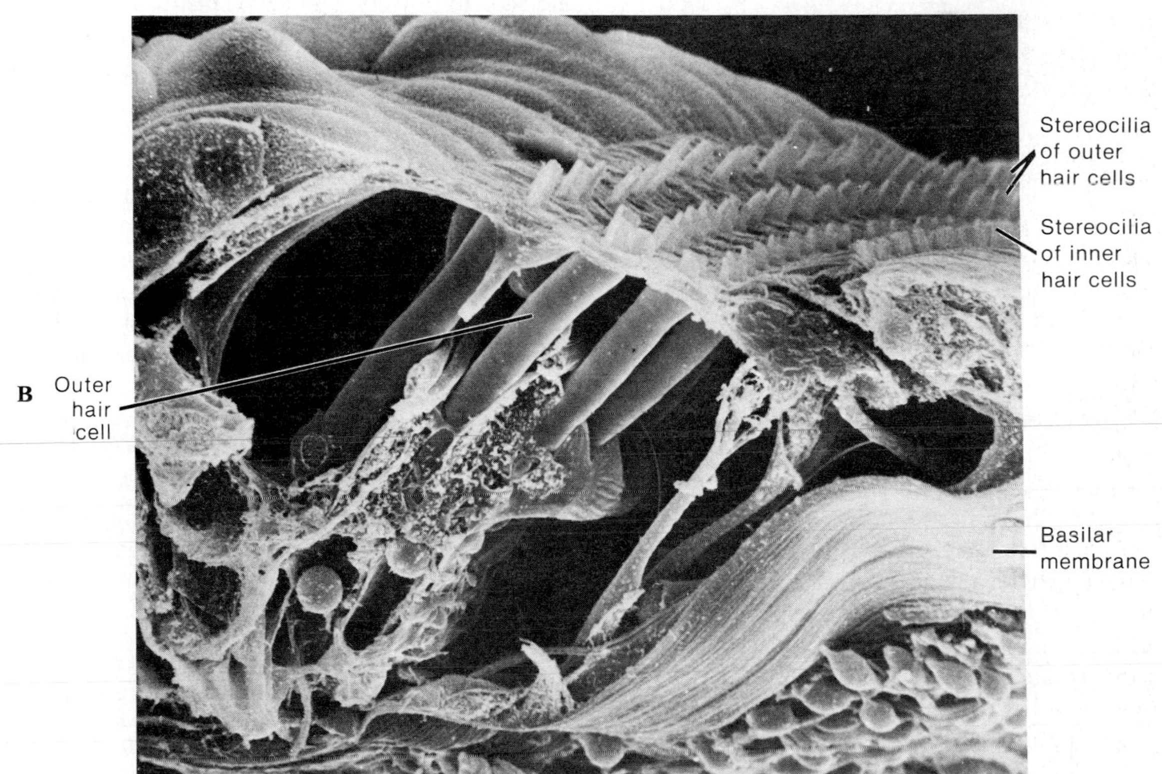


FIGURE 9-35, cont'd
**B,** Scanning electron micrograph of the organ of Corti of a guinea pig. The tectorial membrane has been removed, and the stereocilia of the three rows of outer hair cells can be seen protruding into the scala media; normally these stereocilia would be embedded in the tectorial membrane. No inner hair cells are present in this view, but their stereocilia can also be seen protruding into the scala media.

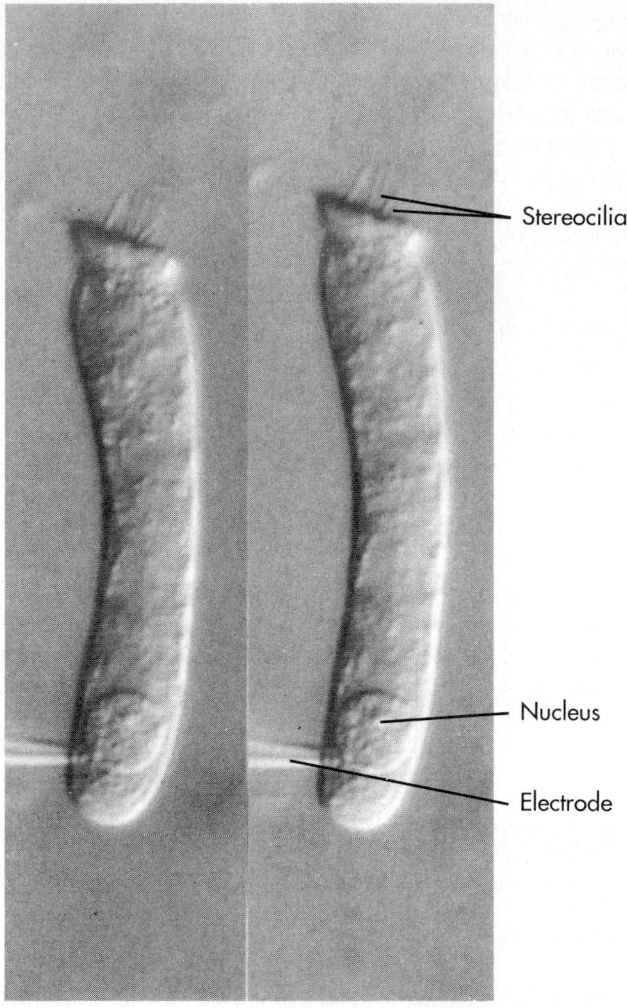


FIGURE 9-36
Electrically induced length changes in an isolated outer hair cell from a guinea pig. A microelectrode was used to depolarize (left) and hyperpolarize (right) the cell, causing it to shorten and lengthen. (Courtesy of Dr. M. Holley, University of Bristol.)

things like the frequency (pitch), loudness and location of a sound. Some aspects of this auditory analysis involve a fairly straightforward pathway (described shortly), but determining the location of a sound source involves some additional processing at the level of the brainstem.

Some fibers from the cochlear nuclei (mainly from the dorsal cochlear nucleus) loop over the top of the inferior cerebellar peduncle, cross the midline with a rostral inclination, and join the *lateral lemniscus,* the major ascending auditory pathway of the brainstem. The lateral lemniscus is somewhat diffuse as it forms in the caudal pons (Figure 9-38, *C*), but in the rostral pons it forms a flattened band (the Latin word *lemniscus* means ribbon) on the lateral surface of the tegmentum (see Figure 9-46). A smaller number of efferents from the cochlear nuclei do not cross the midline, but instead join the ipsilateral lateral lemniscus; hence each lateral lemniscus carries some information from both ears (Figure 9-38, *A*). Nearly all fibers of the lateral lemniscus terminate in the inferior colliculus. The inferior colliculus then gives rise to the *brachium* (Latin for arm) *of the inferior colliculus* (or *inferior brachium*), which assumes a superficial position and terminates in the *medial geniculate nucleus,* a portion of the thalamus that protrudes in a posterior direction, overlapping the midbrain. Fibers from the medial geniculate nucleus project to the primary auditory cortex, which is a portion of the superior temporal gyrus buried in the lateral sulcus (Figure 9-39). A few of these ascending auditory fibers, representing the contralateral ear, may forgo the stop in the inferior colliculus and proceed directly to the medial geniculate nucleus.

A much larger number of efferents from the cochlear nuclei, all from the ventral cochlear nucleus, pass beneath the inferior cerebellar peduncle. Some join the lateral lemniscus of each side and proceed to the inferior colliculus. Many, however, are involved in sound localization and end in the *superior olivary nucleus,* at the rostral end of the facial motor nucleus (Figure 9-38, *C*). There are two general strategies that can be used to localize sound, and the superior olivary complex contains a medial and a lateral subnucleus corresponding to these two strategies. A sound coming from the left reaches the left ear slightly before it reaches the right ear. In addition, because the head blocks some of the sound, it is a little bit louder in the left ear. Sound localization can therefore be accomplished by comparing the time of arrival and the intensity of a sound at the two ears.* The time-of-arrival comparison, which is begun in the medial superior olive, is more effective for terrestrial animals with relatively large heads (like us). We have a correspondingly large medial superior olive and small lateral superior olive. Fibers from the ventral cochlear nuclei of both sides converge on the medial superior olive of each side, providing the anatomical substrate for binaural comparison. Crossing from one cochlear nucleus to the contralateral superior olivary nucleus occurs in the *trapezoid body* (Figure 9-38, *A* and *C*), a large collection of second-order fibers that pass through and ventral to the medial lemnisci.† Each superior olivary nucleus then projects through the lateral lemniscus to the ipsilateral inferior colliculus.

*This method works well for determining the horizontal position of a sound, but is of little help in telling up from down or in front from behind. However, sounds coming from different directions in the sagittal plane are distorted in characteristic ways by the auricle. The CNS apparently compares what something sounds like to what it *ought* to sound like, and uses this comparison to help determine elevation.

†Historically, the term *trapezoid body* was used to refer to the trapezoid-shaped area of the brainstem containing both the medial lemnisci and the crossing auditory fibers. The term is now used in a functional sense, referring only to the crossing auditory fibers.

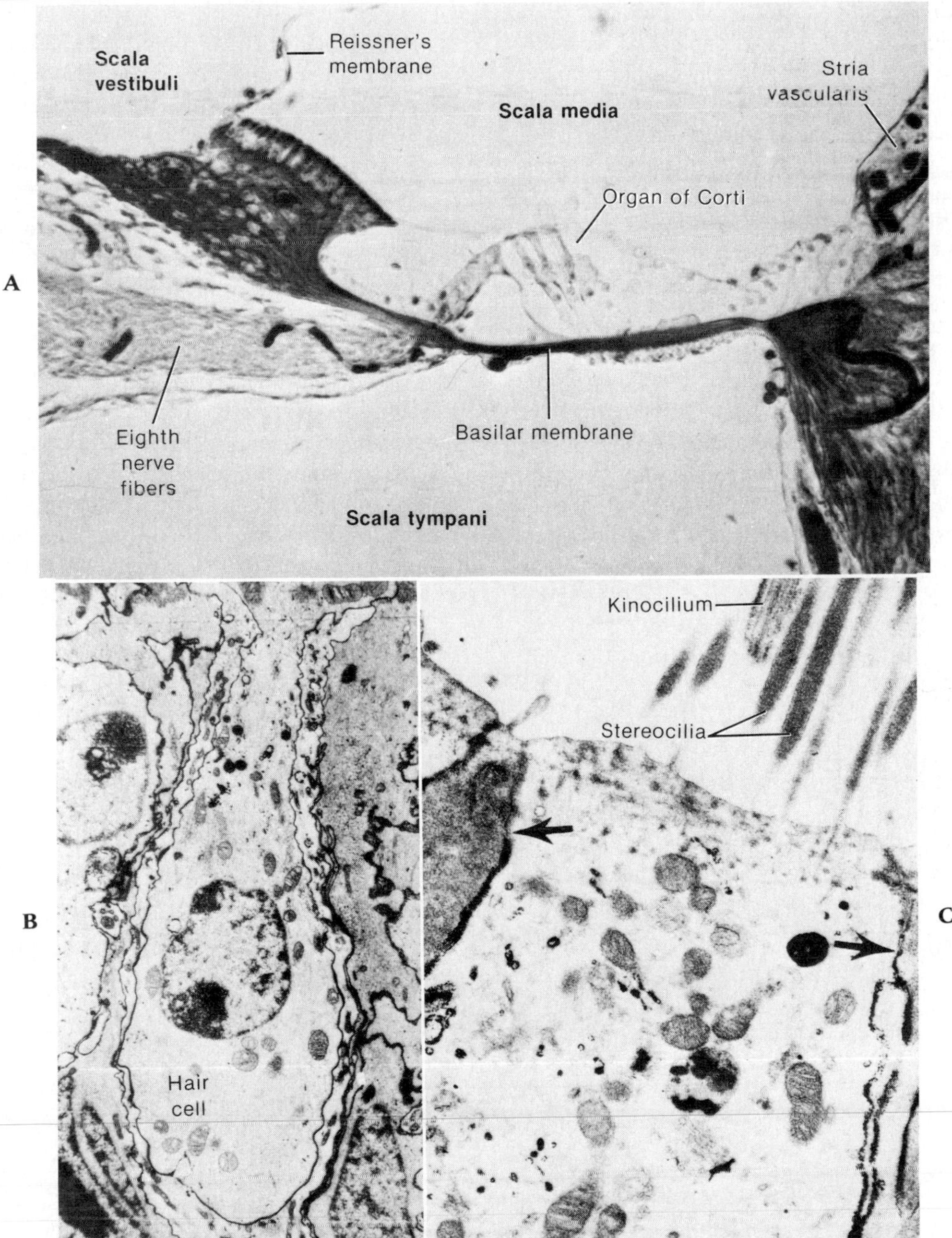


FIGURE 9-37
Portions of the membranous labyrinth of a guinea pig after a tracer substance (horseradish peroxidase) had been injected into the cisterna magna. **A,** Dark reaction product fills parts of the cochlea including, to some extent, the organ of Corti; the tectorial membrane cannot be seen because no tracer escaped from the organ of Corti into endolymphatic space. **B,** Electron micrograph of the saccular macula; dark reaction product outlines all the cellular elements of the macula. **C,** Higher magnification micrograph of the apical end of the hair cell shown in **B;** reaction product fills extracellular space up to, but not beyond, junctional complexes *(arrows)* that separate the perilymphatic from endolymphatic space.
Courtesy of Dr. David Asher.

Each lateral lemniscus conveys information from both ears, both because the cochlear nuclei project bilaterally and because the superior olive receives bilateral input (Figure 9-38, *A*). One consequence is that damage to the auditory pathway at any level rostral to the cochlear nuclei does not cause deafness in either ear. Rather, it causes problems with localizing sounds coming from the contralateral side and may cause some high-frequency hearing loss in the contralateral ear.

## Some functional aspects of the vestibulocochlear nerve

### *Nystagmus*

*Nystagmus* refers to involuntary rhythmic movements of one or both eyes; it can be of considerable diagnostic importance. The movements may be horizontal, vertical, or rotatory; they may have a faster component in one direction, or the movements in both directions may have the same speed. Nystagmus of certain types can be a normal physiological response to stimulation of the vestibular or visual system, but spontaneous or exaggerated nystagmus can be characteristic of some kinds of neuropathology. An example of normal physiological nystagmus is the horizontal nystagmus, with a fast component in one direction, induced by moving visual stimuli. In this case the nystagmus is named for the direction of rapid movement (that is, if the eyes move slowly to the left and then rapidly back to the right, it would be called *nystagmus to the right,* or *right-beating nystagmus*). Consider the reflex eye movements that occur when a person sits in a rapidly moving train, vaguely watching regularly spaced telephone poles fly by. The person's eyes tend to slowly follow a particular pole toward the rear of the train and then flick back toward the front of the train to find a new pole to fixate on. In the case of an individual seated on the right side of the train, this would constitute *nystagmus to the left* (Figure 9-40). Because it is induced by moving visual stimuli, it is called *optokinetic nystagmus (OKN)*. Fortunately it is not necessary to use trains and telephone poles to demonstrate optokinetic nystagmus clinically; a rotating striped drum or a moving piece of striped cloth usually suffices.

Nystagmus can also be induced by rotating a subject. It

*Text continued on p. 222.*

A

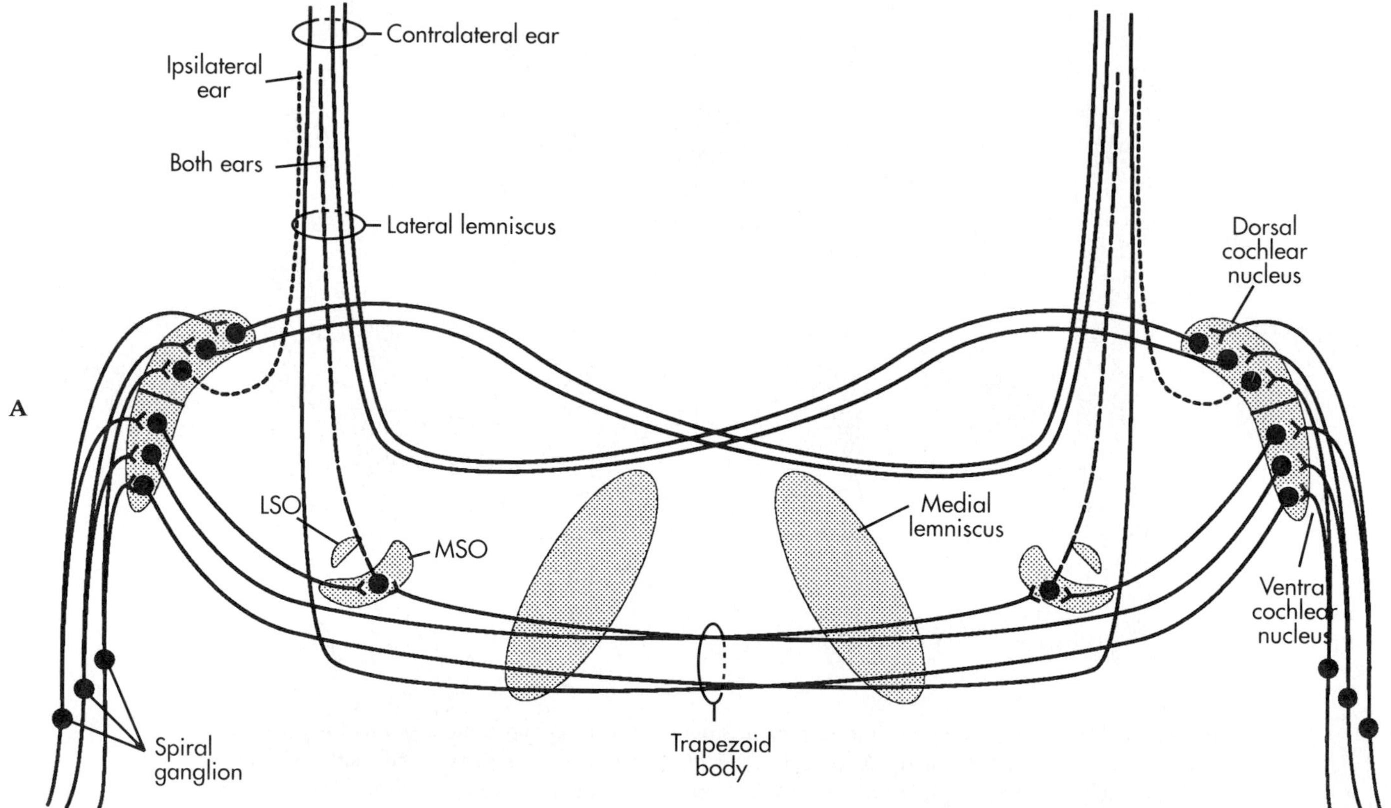


FIGURE 9-38
Formation of the lateral lemniscus, showing in a general sense how both ears become represented on each side of the brainstem. The cochlear nuclei project crossed and a few uncrossed fibers directly into the lateral lemniscus, so each lateral lemniscus contains a small representation of the ipsilateral ear. In addition, projections from the medial superior olivary nucleus (MSO) carry sound-localization information from both ears. Projections from the smaller lateral superior olivary nucleus (LSO) are not shown, but they also represent both ears. **A,** Initial synapses and some of the initial crossings of the midline by auditory fibers, showing how each ear becomes represented bilaterally at the level of the trapezoid body. This is a schematic diagram and is not strictly accurate anatomically, since the cochlear nuclei are located in a plane caudal to the trapezoid body.

B

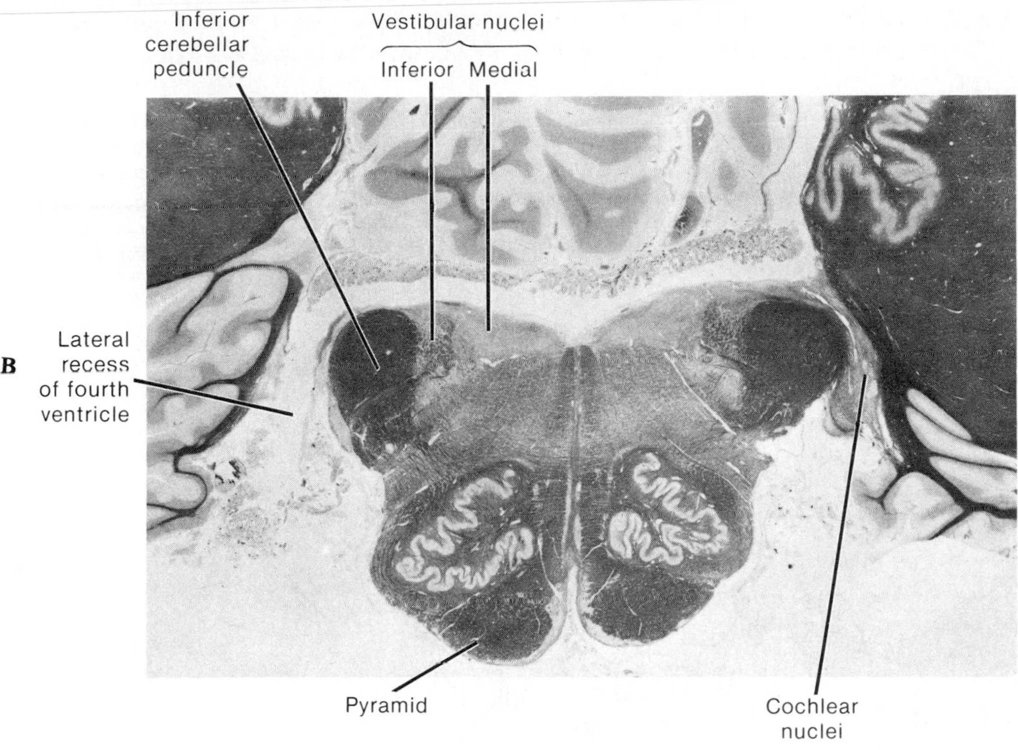


C

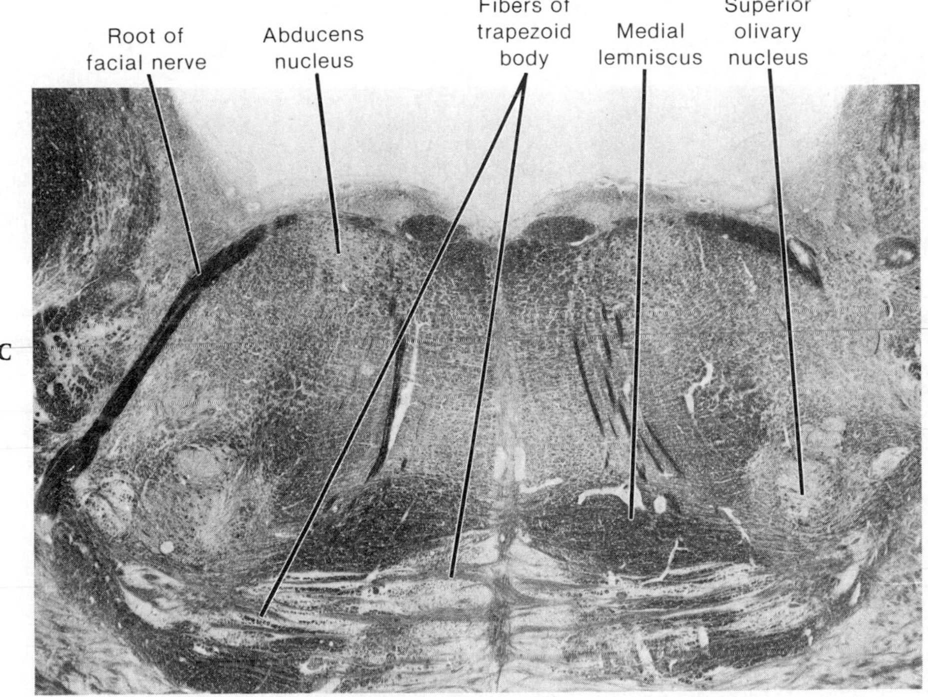


FIGURE 9-38, cont'd
**B,** Section through the pontomedullary junction showing the cochlear nuclei. **C,** Section through the caudal pons showing the superior olivary nuclei and the trapezoid body.

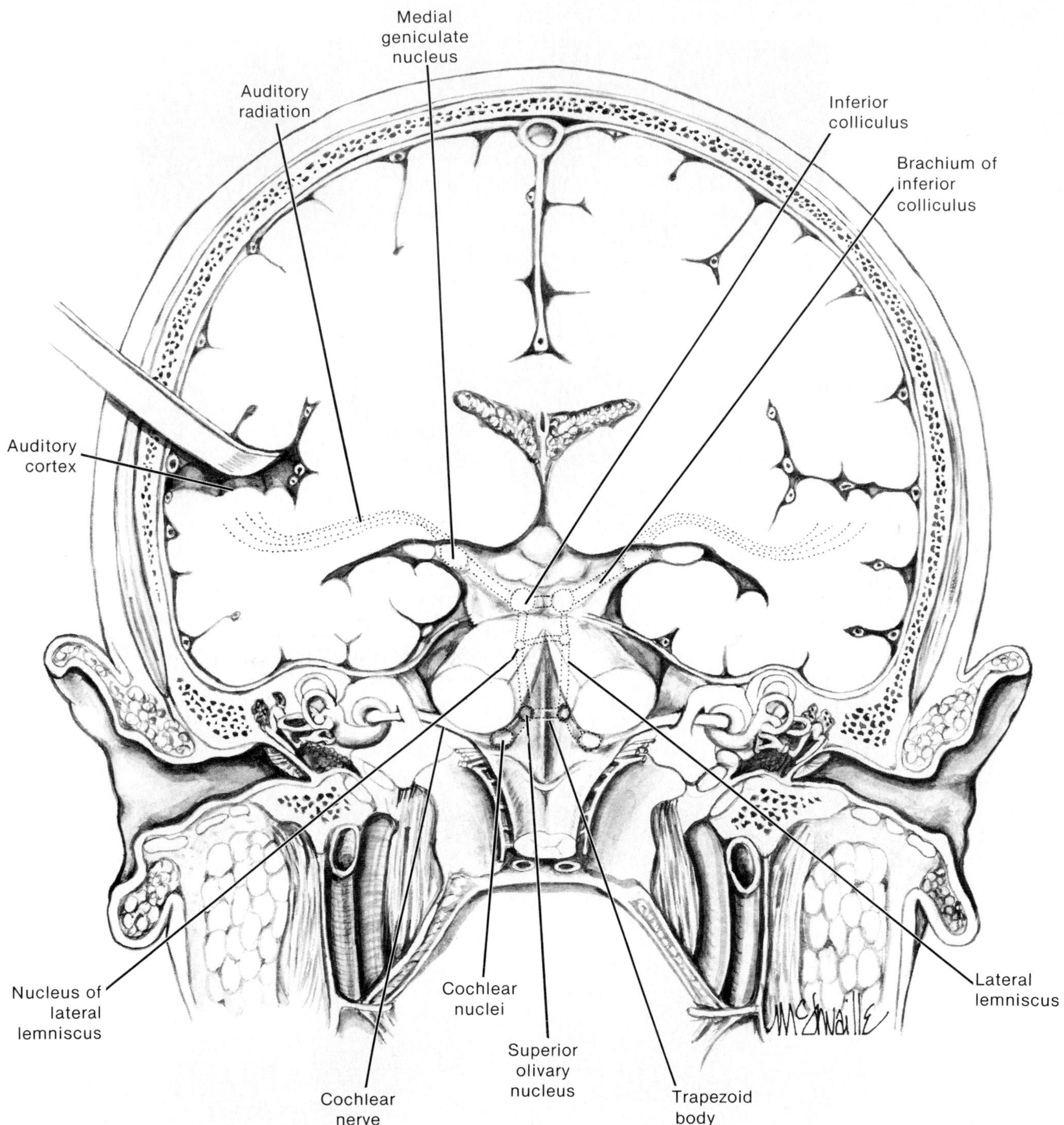


FIGURE 9-39
The ascending auditory pathway.

Modified from a drawing by Max Brödel. In Rothman L, Crowe SJ, editors: The 1940 year book of eye, ear, nose, and throat, Chicago, 1940, Year Book Medical Publishers, Inc.

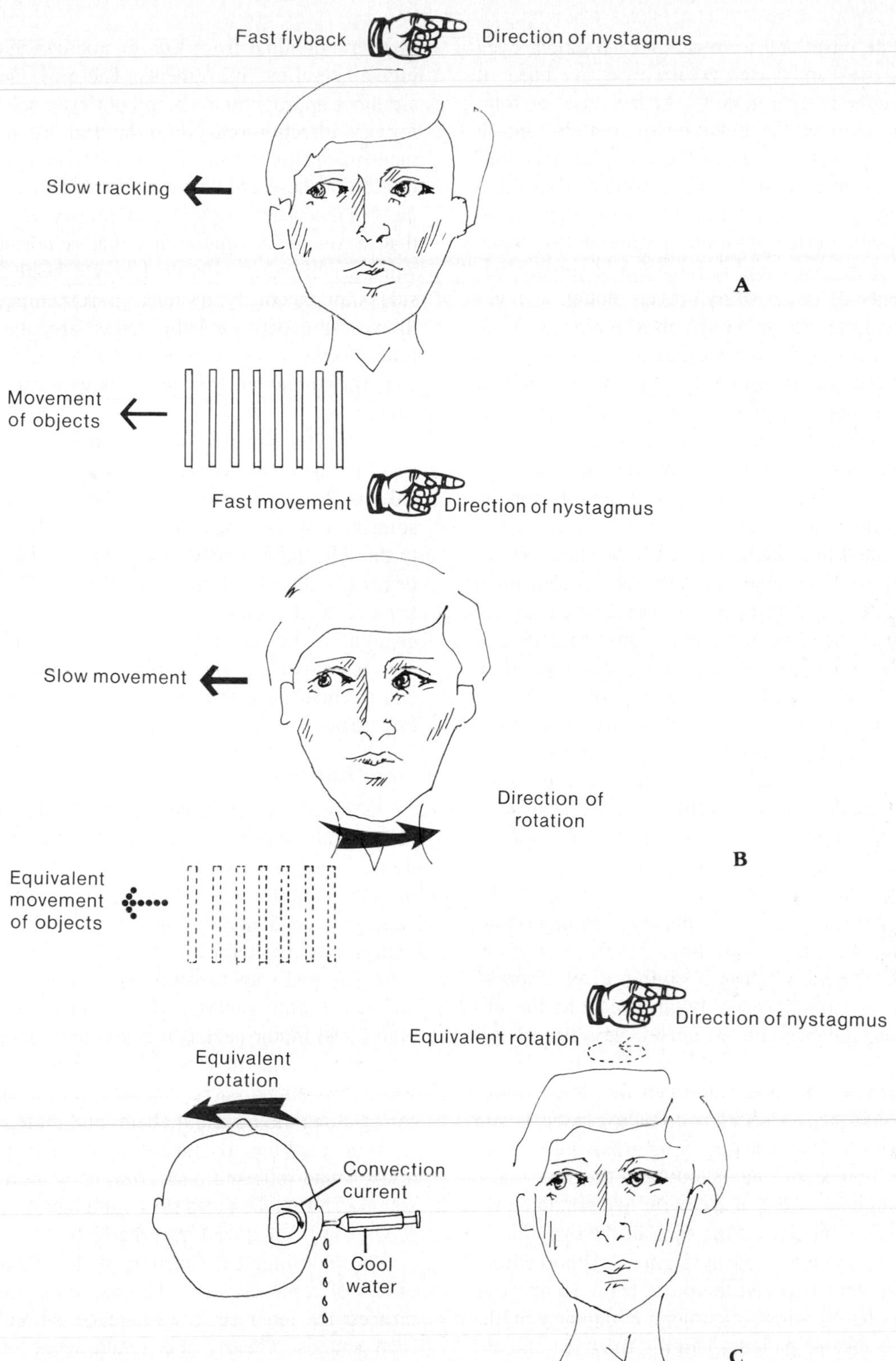


FIGURE 9-40
Three different ways to cause nystagmus with its fast phase to the left. **A,** Movement of a series of objects to an individual's right causes slow tracking eye movements to the right followed by rapid "reset" movements to the left. **B,** Rotation to the left is equivalent, as far as visual movement is concerned, to movement of objects around to the right. The result is nystagmus to the left, as in **A.** If the individual's eyes are open, visual movement continues throughout the rotation, and the nystagmus may persist. If the eyes are closed, the nystagmus is mediated by the vestibular system and is transient; its direction reverses at the end of rotation. **C,** Cool water instilled into the right ear causes the same movement of endolymph in the right horizontal semicircular duct as does the rotation in **B.** The result again is nystagmus to the left.

occurs at both the onset and termination of rotation, even if the subject's eyes are closed (if the eyes are open, it may occur throughout the rotation). At the onset of rotation the nystagmus is in the direction of rotation, and at the termination of rotation it is in the opposite direction. This makes reasonable sense if you consider what these movements correspond to in terms of reflex attempts to track visual stimuli during rotation (Figure 9-40). Since this nystagmus at the onset and termination of rotation occurs in the absence of visual stimuli (even though its function under normal conditions would be to maintain visual stability), it is called *vestibular nystagmus*. It corresponds to deflection of the cupula in one direction at the onset of rotation and in the opposite direction at the end of rotation.

The same movement of endolymph that underlies vestibular nystagmus can be produced by instilling cool or warm water into a subject's ear, causing endolymphatic convection currents that, in turn, induce nystagmus. Consider an individual whose head is tilted back about 60 degrees, bringing the horizontal semicircular canals into a vertical plane. Cool water instilled into the right ear causes the endolymph in the right horizontal canal to cool and sink, causing a convection current of endolymph in a clockwise direction (viewed from the top of the head). This movement of endolymph relative to the canal is the same movement that is produced at the onset of rotation of the individual to the left (Figure 9-40), and the response of this single semicircular canal is sufficient to cause nystagmus to the left. This is called *caloric nystagmus,* and its mechanism is the same as that of rotationally induced vestibular nystagmus.*

The pathway involved in vestibular nystagmus primarily involves the MLF for connections rostral to the abducens nucleus. The slow phase is simply a reflection of direct connections from the vestibular nuclei to the abducens, trochlear and oculomotor nuclei. The fast phase, like fast eye movements in general (see Chapter 12), requires timing signals that originate from the reticular formation. One consequence is that a comatose patient with depressed function of the reticular formation, but with an otherwise intact brainstem, may show only the slow phase of caloric nystagmus—that is, caloric stimulation produces only a tonic deviation of the eyes in the direction of the slow phase of the expected nystagmus. Abnormalities of this conjugate deviation can therefore be of some value in determining the location of structural damage in the brainstem of a comatose patient. Turning the head of a comatose individual from side to side can elicit similar conjugate lateral eye movements. The movements in this case are those appropriate to keep both eyes pointed in the same forward direction relative to the trunk (that is, head movement to the right causes contraversive eye movements to the left). These are called *doll's head eye movements* (or the *oculocephalic reflex*) and mostly represent no more than a vestibuloocular reflex that is normally suppressed when a conscious individual moves head and eyes to one side simultaneously to look at something. The afferent limb of the oculocephalic reflex probably also includes proprioceptors of the neck, since some reflex movement can still be elicited from patients with nonfunctional labyrinths.

At the termination of rotation to the left, nystagmus with its fast phase to the right is seen in a normal individual, as discussed above. In addition, trying to point at something with closed eyes results in deviation of the arm to the left; this is called *past pointing*. There is also a tendency to fall to the left when walking. The lateral vestibulospinal tract ordinarily is quite important in directing the changes in muscle tone that correspond to the postural changes involved in balance; postrotatory past pointing and a tendency to fall demonstrate exaggerated activity in this tract.

### *Stapedius reflex*

As noted earlier, contraction of the stapedius stiffens the ossicular chain and hampers the transmission of vibrations. When a loud sound enters one ear, both stapedius muscles contract in a reflex fashion; an individual with a damaged facial nerve may complain that sounds are too loud in the ipsilateral ear (a condition known as *hyperacusis*). The pathway involved is from one ventral cochlear nucleus to both superior olivary nuclei and from there to both facial motor nuclei. It is possible to test this reflex arc in a useful clinical procedure. When the stapedius contracts, less sound energy incident on the eardrum is transferred along the ossicular chain, and more is reflected back from the eardrum. By measuring changes in the amount of a test sound reflected back from one eardrum when a loud sound is introduced into the contralateral ear, the stapedius reflex can be analyzed quantitatively.

The physiological function of the stapedius reflex is a matter of some dispute. The most common view is that it protects the inner ear from damage caused by excessively loud sounds. Clearly this could work only for chronic noise, since a brief loud sound would be over before the stapedius could contract. A second view of the reflex is that it helps the inner ear extract meaningful sounds from noisy backgrounds. Stapedial contraction impedes the transmission of low frequencies more than high frequencies and so could selectively reduce the effects of low-frequency noise.

The function of the tensor tympani in auditory pro-

*This gravitational model seems so logical that it has been accepted without much question since caloric nystagmus was first described in 1908. However, the era of space flight has allowed demonstrations that caloric nystagmus can be elicited in orbiting astronauts, who are experiencing nearly zero gravity. However, its properties under these conditions are somewhat different from normal, and the current consensus is that caloric nystagmus is partly the result of convection currents and partly the result of a direct thermal effect of some sort.

cesses is also unclear. This muscle too is activated bilaterally in some individuals in response to a loud sound in one ear, but only if the sound is extremely loud. Thus for most individuals in most physiological situations, only the stapedius is active. The tensor tympani contracts bilaterally in response to startling stimuli whether they are auditory or not, but the function of this contraction as a part of the startle response is obscure.

### *Brainstem auditory evoked responses*

A brief sound causes a series of electrical waves, in the nanovolt range, that can be recorded from the surface of the head. The signals are so small that they are normally buried in the background electrical noise, but when the same brief stimulus is presented many times and the responses are averaged, the waves can be reproducibly measured. It is thought that the peaks of the waveform represent electrical activity at successive sites in the auditory pathway. Since this pathway extends from the pontomedullary junction to the temporal lobes, abnormalities in the *brainstem auditory evoked response* can be helpful in localizing lesions.

## ADDITIONAL READINGS


Baloh RW, Honrubia V: *Clinical neurophysiology of the vestibular system,* ed 2, Philadelphia, 1990, F. A. Davis Company.

Beckstead RM, Morse JR, Norgren R: The nucleus of the solitary tract in the monkey: projections to the thalamus and brain stem nuclei, *J Comp Neurol* 190:259, 1980.

Beckstead RM, Norgren R: An autoradiographic examination of the central distribution of the trigeminal, facial, glossopharyngeal and vagal nerves in the monkey, *J Comp Neurol* 184:455, 1979.

Bender MB, Feldman M: Visual illusions during head movement in lesions of the brain stem, *Arch Neurol* 17:354, 1967. *An interesting discussion of what happens if a patient's vestibular apparatus is damaged so that it is impossible to tell if movement of a visual image is caused by head movement or motion in the outside world.*

Bogousslavsky J, Meienberg O: Eye-movement disorders in brain-stem and cerebellar stroke, *Arch Neurol* 44:141, 1987. *A comprehensive, recent review.*

Borg E: On the neuronal organization of the acoustic middle ear reflex: a physiological and anatomical study, *Brain Res* 49:101, 1973.

Bracchi F et al: Multiday recordings from the primary neurons of the statoreceptors of the labyrinth of the bullfrog, *Acta Otolaryngol Suppl* 334, 1975. *Technically astonishing experiments in which continuous recordings were made from single utricular primary afferents of a bullfrog aboard a rocket that blasted off and put the frog in orbit for a few days.*

Brandt T, Daroff RB: The multisensory physiological and pathological vertigo syndromes, *Ann Neurol* 7:195, 1980. *Stimulation or dysfunction of the vestibular, visual, or somatosensory systems can cause illusions of movement.*

Bredberg G, Ades HW, Engström H: Scanning electron microscopy of the normal and pathologically altered organ of Corti, *Acta Otolaryngol Suppl* 301:3, 1972. *Pretty pictures from a variety of mammals.*

Brindley GS: How does an animal that is dropped in a nonupright posture know the angle through which it must turn in the air so that its feet point to the ground? *J Physiol* 180:20P, 1965. *Briefly, it remembers which way was up when you let go of it. The paper isn't much longer than its title.*

Brodal A: Central course of afferent fibers for pain in facial, glossopharyngeal and vagus nerves, *Arch Neurol Psychiatry* 57:292, 1947.

Brodal A: *Neurological anatomy in relation to clinical medicine,* ed 3, New York, 1981, Oxford University Press.

Büttner-Ennever JA et al: Vertical gaze paralysis and the rostral interstitial nucleus of the medial longitudinal fasciculus, *Brain* 105:125, 1982.

Carleton SC, Carpenter MB: Afferent and efferent connections of the medial, inferior and lateral vestibular nuclei in the cat and monkey, *Brain Res* 278:29, 1983.

Clark DL, Kreutzberg JR, Chee FKW: Vestibular stimulation influence on motor development in infants, *Science* 196:1228, 1977.

Cohen LA: Role of eye and neck proprioceptive mechanisms in body orientation and motor coordination, *J Neurophysiol* 24:1, 1961.

Dewson JH III: Efferent olivocochlear bundle: some relationships to stimulus discrimination in noise, *J Neurophysiol* 31:122, 1968.

Fernández C, Goldberg JM, Abend WK: Response to static tilts of peripheral neurons innervating otolith organs of the squirrel monkey, *J Neurophysiol* 35:978, 1972.

Fine ML, Horn MH, Cox B: *Acanthonus armatus,* a deep-sea teleost fish with a minute brain and large ears, *Proc R Soc Lond* B230:257, 1987. *"Acanthonus armatus, a deep-water benthopelagic fish, has, per unit body weight, the smallest brain and largest semicircular canals of any known teleost and possibly any vertebrate."*

Finger TE, Silver WL: *Neurobiology of taste and smell,* New York, 1987, John Wiley & Sons. *A modern, comprehensive review of the comparative anatomy and physiology of the chemical senses.*

Frederickson JM et al: Vestibular nerve projection to the cerebral cortex of the rhesus monkey, *Exp Brain Res* 2:318, 1966.

Fukushima T, Kerr FWL: Organization of trigeminothalamic tracts and other thalamic afferent systems of the brainstem in the rat: presence of gelatinous neurons with thalamic connections. *J Comp Neurol* 183:169, 1979.

Gauthier JM, Mommay D, Vercher JL: Ocular muscle proprioception and visual localization of targets in man, *Brain* 113:1857, 1990. *The use we make of information from the proprioceptors in extraocular muscles has long been a mystery; it isn't crucial for guiding eye movements. This paper presents one possibility.*

Goldberg JM, Fernández C: Efferent vestibular system in the squirrel monkey: anatomical location and influence on afferent activity, *J Neurophysiol* 43:986, 1980.

Goodwin GM, Luschei ES: Effects of destroying spindle afferents from jaw muscles on mastication in monkeys, *J Neurophysiol* 37:967, 1974.

Henkin RI, Christiansen RL: Taste localization on the tongue, palate and pharynx of normal man, *J Appl Physiol* 22:316, 1967.

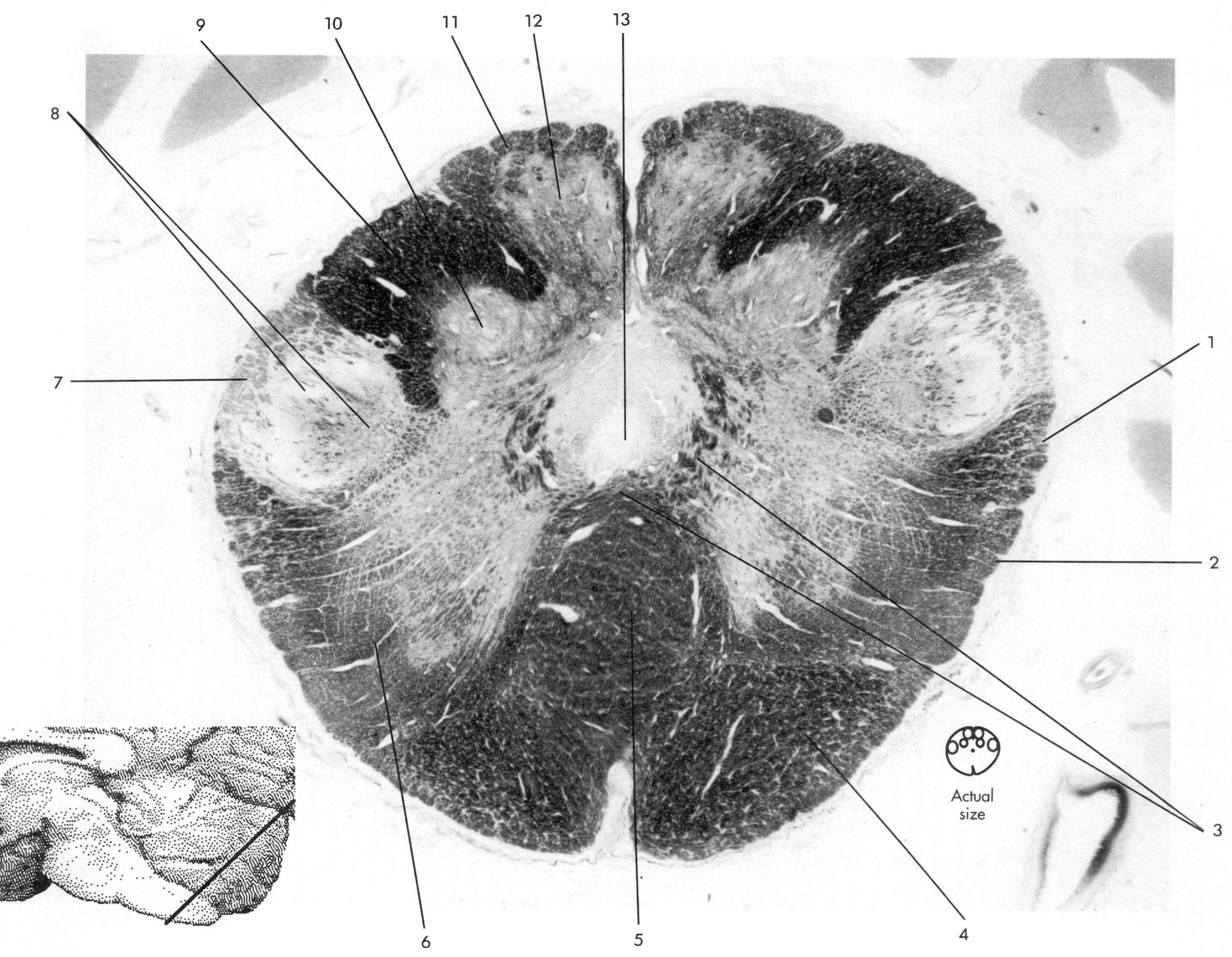
9
10
11
12
13
8
7
1
2
6
5
4
3
Actual size

## FIGURE 9-41 Claudal medulla

**1,** Posterior spinocerebellar tract. Uncrossed fibers from Clarke's nucleus, carrying proprioceptive information from the arm that will reach the ipsilateral half of the cerebellar vermis through the inferior cerebellar peduncle.

**2,** Anterior spinocerebellar tract. Crossed fibers from lumbosacral spinal gray matter, carrying proprioceptive and other information from the leg. This tract stays in approximately the same position until the rostral pons, where it moves over the surface of the superior cerebellar peduncle (Figures 9-45 and 9-46) and turns posteriorly into the cerebellum.

**3,** Crossing fibers from the gracile and cuneate nuclei forming the medial lemniscus, the principal ascending pathway for tactile and proprioceptive information.

**4,** Pyramid. Corticospinal fibers from the ipsilateral precentral gyrus and adjacent areas of cerebral cortex.

**5,** Pyramidal decussation. Fibers crossing from one pyramid into the opposite lateral corticospinal tract.

**6,** Location of the spinothalamic tract. Crossed fibers from the spinal posterior horns conveying pain and temperature information to the thalamus (ventral posterolateral [VPL] nucleus and other nuclei).

**7,** Spinal trigeminal tract. Primary afferents from the ipsilateral side of the face, at this level conveying information about pain and temperature.

**8,** Spinal trigeminal nucleus (caudal nucleus). Site of termination of part of the spinal trigeminal tract, and the origin of part of the ventral trigeminal tract. At this level, the nucleus has the appearance of the spinal posterior horn, has a component similar to the substantia gelatinosa, and processes pain and temperature information.

**9,** Fasciculus cuneatus. Uncrossed primary afferents, carrying tactile and proprioceptive information from the arm.

**10,** Nucleus cuneatus. Site of termination of fasciculus cuneatus and the origin of the arm portion of the medial lemniscus.

**11,** Fasciculus gracilis. Uncrossed primary afferents, carrying tactile and some proprioceptive information from the leg.

**12,** Nucleus gracilis. Site of termination of fasciculus gracilis and the origin of the leg portion of the medial lemniscus.

**13,** Central canal. Merges rostrally with the fourth ventricle and caudally with the central canal of the spinal cord.

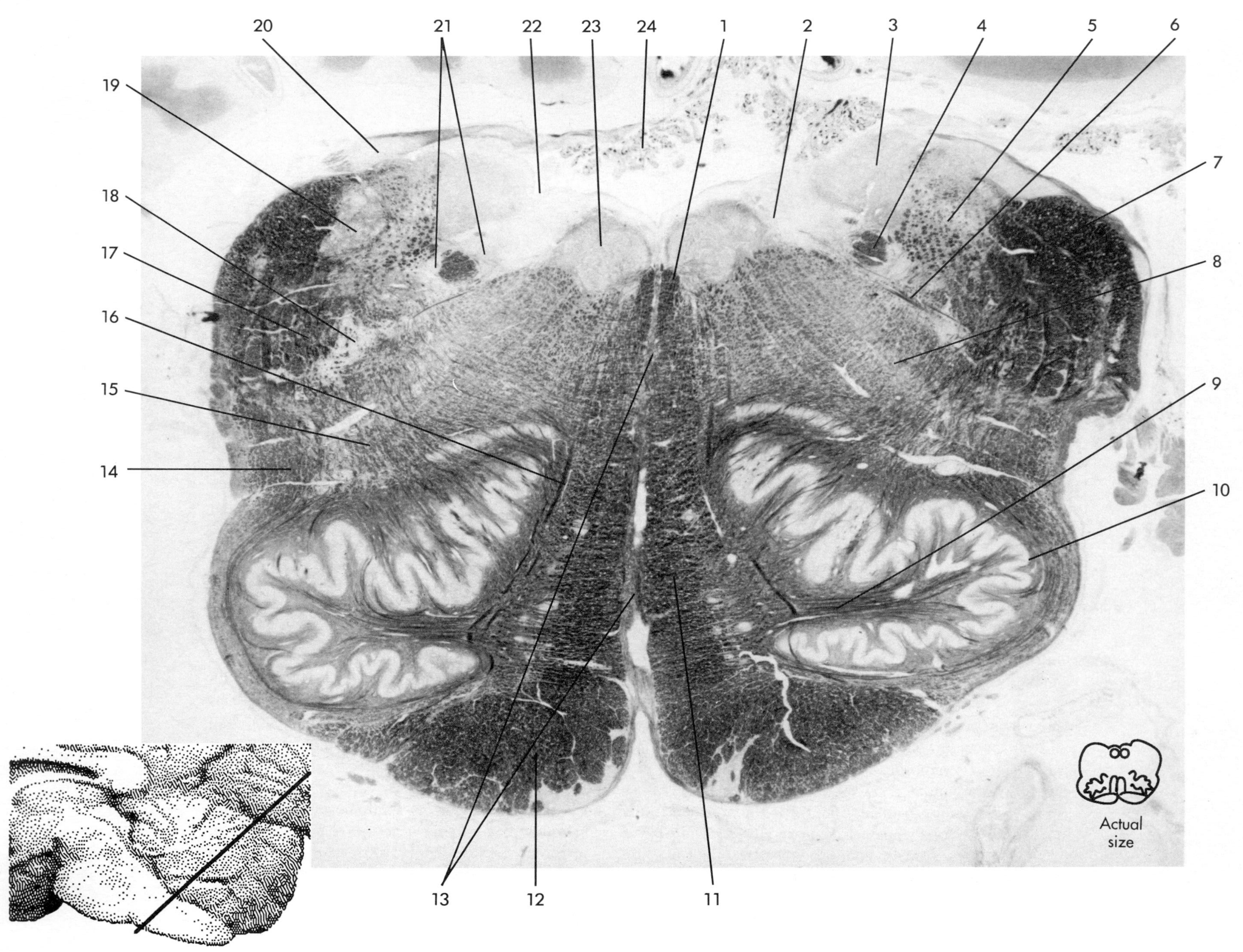

20
21
22
23
24
1
2
3
4
5
6
19
7
18
8
17
16
15
9
14
10
Actual size
13
12
11

**FIGURE 9-42 Rostral medulla.**

**1,** Medial longitudinal fasciculus (MLF). At this level, the fibers of the medial vestibulospinal tract.
**2,** Dorsal motor nucleus of the vagus. Most of the preganglionic parasympathetic neurons for thoracic and abdominal viscera.
**3,** Medial vestibular nucleus. Site of origin of the medial vestibulospinal tract (among other connections).
**4,** Solitary tract. Primary afferents conveying visceral information from cranial nerves VII, IX, and X (as well as some chemosensory information from the trigeminal nerve) to the surrounding nucleus of the solitary tract.
**5,** Inferior vestibular nucleus with bundles of vestibular primary afferents running through it.
**6,** Fibers of the vagus nerve (CN X).
**7,** Inferior cerebellar peduncle. Contains crossed olivocerebellar fibers, the uncrossed posterior spinocerebellar tract, vestibulocerebellar fibers, and other cerebellar afferents.
**8,** Location of nucleus ambiguus. Lower motor neurons for laryngeal and pharyngeal muscles and preganglionic parasympathetic neurons for the heart.
**9,** Olivocerebellar fibers. Cross the midline as internal arcuate fibers, join the inferior cerebellar peduncle, and end in the cerebellar cortex as climbing fibers.
**10,** Inferior olivary nucleus. Source of climbing fibers to contralateral cerebellar cortex.
**11,** Medial lemniscus, the principal ascending pathway for tactile and proprioceptive information. Originates in the contralateral posterior column nuclei and terminates in the thalamus (VPL).
**12,** Pyramid. Corticospinal fibers from the ipsilateral precentral gyrus and adjacent areas of cerebral cortex.
**13,** Raphe nuclei. Serotoninergic neurons that are one source of descending pain-control fibers to the spinal cord.
**14,** Location of the spinothalamic tract. Crossed fibers from the spinal posterior horns conveying pain and temperature information to the thalamus (VPL and others).
**15,** Location of some descending higher order sympathetic fibers from the hypothalamus to the intermediolateral cell column of the thoracic and lumbar spinal cord. Damage here causes ipsilateral Horner's syndrome.
**16,** Hypoglossal nerve fibers, on their way to the muscles of the ipsilateral half of the tongue.
**17,** Spinal trigeminal tract. Primary afferents from the ipsilateral side of the face, including those on their way to the caudal nucleus conveying information about pain and temperature.
**18,** Spinal trigeminal nucleus (interpolar nucleus). Some primary afferents of the spinal tigeminal tract, including those carrying information about dental pain, end here.
**19,** Lateral cuneate nucleus. Arm equivalent of Clarke's nucleus. Proprioceptive primary afferents travel through fasciculus cuneatus to reach the lateral cuneate nucleus, which then gives rise to uncrossed cuneocerebellar fibers that enter the cerebellum through the inferior cerebellar peduncle.
**20,** Dorsal cochlear nucleus. Site of termination of the cochlear nerve, and site of origin of some secondary auditory fibers that join the contralateral lateral lemniscus.
**21,** Nucleus of the solitary tract. Site of termination of the visceral primary afferents in the solitary tract.
**22,** Sulcus limitans. The groove separating motor nuclei (medial to it) and sensory nuclei (lateral to it).
**23,** Hypoglossal nucleus. Lower motor neurons for the ipsilateral half of the tongue.
**24,** Choroid plexus in the roof of the fourth ventricle.

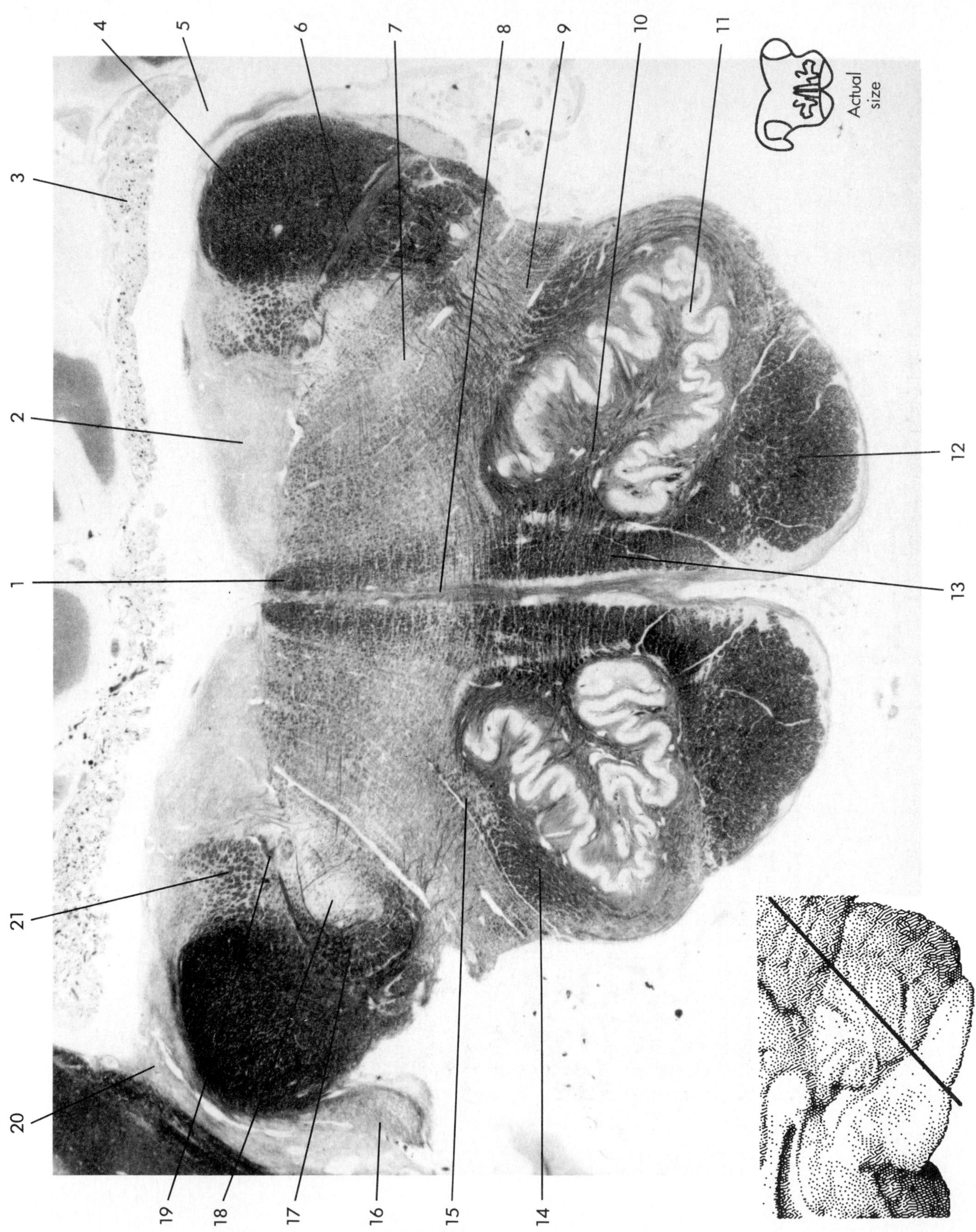
1
2
3
4
5
6
7
8
9
10
11
12
13
14
15
16
17
18
19
20
21
Actual size

## FIGURE 9-43 Pontomedullary junction.

**1,** Medial longitudinal fasciculus (MLF). Descending fibers of the medial vestibulospinal tract, ascending fibers for the vestibuloocular reflex.

**2,** Medial vestibular nucleus. Site of origin of the medial vestibulospinal tract (among other connections).

**3,** Choroid plexus in the roof of the fourth ventricle.

**4,** Inferior cerebellar peduncle. Contains crossed olivocerebellar fibers, the uncrossed posterior spinocerebellar tract, vestibulocerebellar fibers, and other cerebellar afferents.

**5,** Lateral recess of the fourth ventricle. Leads to the lateral aperture (foramen of Luschka), one of the three apertures through which cerebrospinal fluid passes from the ventricular system to subarachnoid space.

**6,** Fibers of the glossopharyngeal nerve (CN IX).

**7,** Location of nucleus ambiguus. Lower motor neurons for laryngeal and pharyngeal muscles, and preganglionic parasympathetic neurons for the heart.

**8,** Raphe nuclei. Serotoninergic neurons that are one source of descending pain-control fibers to the spinal cord.

**9,** Location of the spinothalamic tract. Crossed fibers from the spinal posterior horns conveying pain and temperature information to the thalamus (VPL and others).

**10,** Olivocerebellar fibers. Cross the midline as internal arcuate fibers, join the inferior cerebellar peduncle, and end in the cerebellar cortex as climbing fibers.

**11,** Inferior olivary nucleus. Source of climbing fibers to contralateral cerebellar cortex.

**12,** Pyramid. Corticospinal fibers from the ipsilateral precentral gyrus and adjacent areas of cerebral cortex.

**13,** Medial lemniscus. The principal ascending pathway for tactile and proprioceptive information. Originates in the contralateral posterior column nuclei and terminates in the thalamus (VPL).

**14,** Central tegmental tract ending in the inferior olivary nucleus. Most of these originate in the ipsilateral red nucleus.

**15,** Location of some descending higher order sympathetic fibers from the hypothalamus to the intermediolateral cell column of the thoracic and lumbar spinal cord. Damage here causes ipsilateral Horner's syndrome.

**16,** Ventral cochlear nucleus. Site of termination of cochlear nerve fibers and site of origin of some crossing fibers of the trapezoid body.

**17,** Spinal trigeminal tract. Primary afferents from the ipsilateral side of the face, including those on their way to the caudal nucleus conveying information about pain and temperature.

**18,** Spinal trigeminal nucleus (oral nucleus). Some primary afferents of the spinal trigeminal tract, particularly those carrying tactile information, end here.

**19,** Solitary tract. Primary afferents conveying visceral information from cranial nerves VII, IX, and X (as well as some chemosensory information from the trigeminal nerve) to the surrounding nucleus of the solitary tract.

**20,** Dorsal cochlear nucleus. Site of termination of the cochlear nerve and site of origin of some secondary auditory fibers that join the contralateral lateral lemniscus.

**21,** Inferior vestibular nucleus, with bundles of vestibular primary afferents running through it.

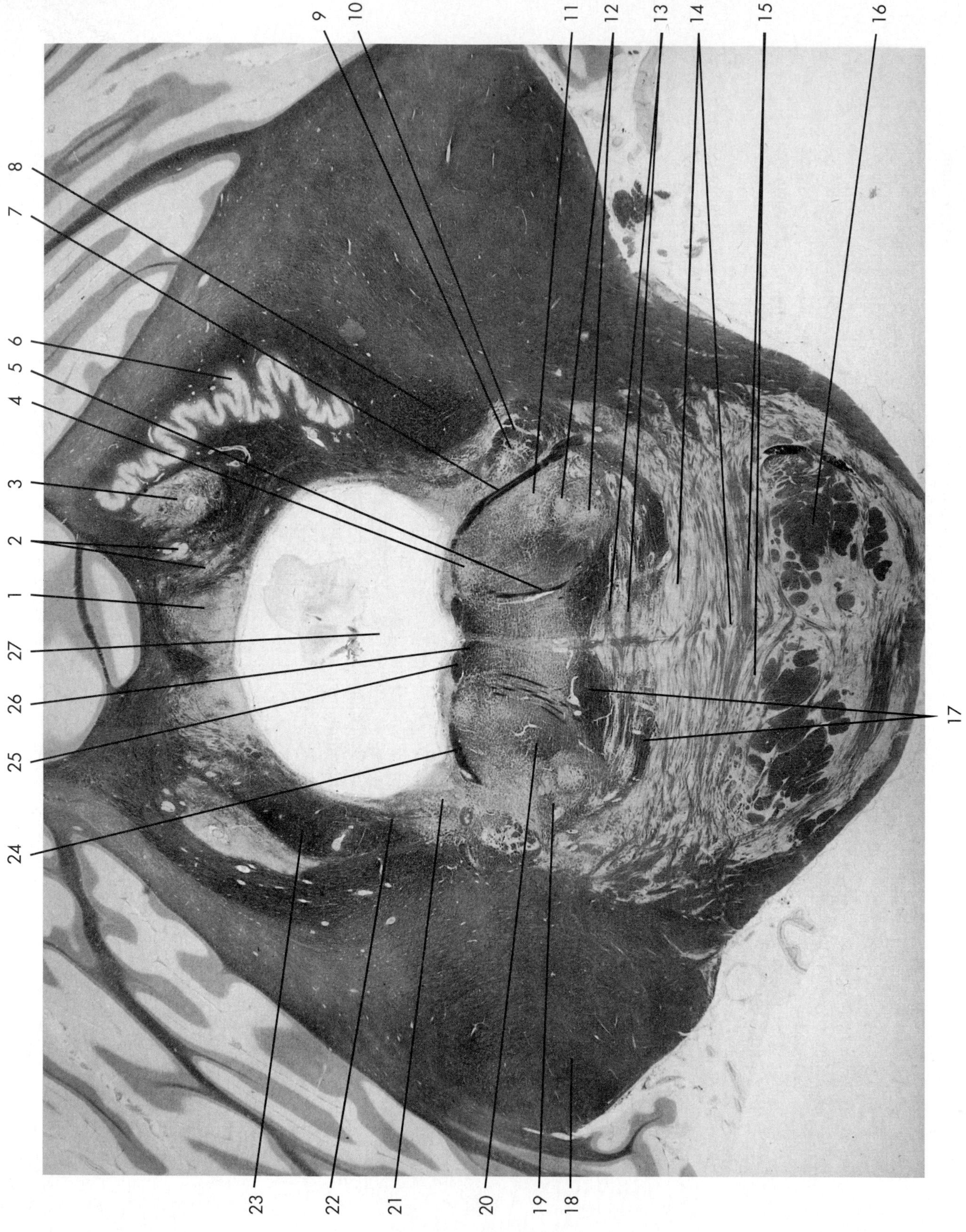

1
2
3
4
5
6
7
8
9
10
11
12
13
14
15
16
17
18
19
20
21
22
23
24
25
26
27

**FIGURE 9-44A Caudal pons.**

**1,** Fastigial nucleus. The deep cerebellar nucleus connected to the vermis.

**2,** Globose nucleus. Part of the interposed nucleus, which is the deep cerebellar nucleus connected to the paravermal or intermediate zone.

**3,** Emboliform nucleus. Part of the interposed nucleus, which is the deep cerebellar nucleus connected to the paravermal or intermediate zone.

**4,** Abducens nucleus. Contains the lower motor neurons for the ipsilateral lateral rectus, as well as the interneurons that project through the contralateral MLF to medial rectus motor neurons.

**5,** Abducens nerve fibers, on their way to the ipsilateral lateral rectus.

**6,** Dentate nucleus. The deep nucleus connected to the cerebellar hemisphere and the source of most of the fibers in the superior cerebellar peduncle.

**7,** Facial nerve fibers. Most of them are on their way to ipsilateral muscles of facial expression.

**8,** Inferior cerebellar peduncle. Contains crossed olivocerebellar fibers, the uncrossed posterior spinocerebellar tract, vestibulocerebellar fibers, and other cerebellar afferents.

**9,** Spinal trigeminal nucleus (oral nucleus). Some primary afferents of the spinal trigeminal tract, particularly those carrying tactile information, end here.

**10,** Spinal trigeminal tract. Primary afferents from the ipsilateral side of the face, including those on their way to the caudal nucleus conveying information about pain and temperature.

**11,** Facial motor nucleus. Lower motor neurons for ipsilateral muscles of facial expression.

**12,** Superior olivary nucleus. First site of convergence of fibers representing the two ears and the source of many of the fibers of the lateral lemniscus.

**13,** Trapezoid body. Crossing auditory fibers, primarily from the ventral cochlear nucleus.

**14,** Pontine nuclei. Source of pontocerebellar fibers that cross the midline and form the middle cerebellar peduncle.

**15,** Pontocerebellar fibers, from pontine nuclei of one side to the opposite middle cerebellar peduncle.

**16,** Corticospinal and corticopontine fibers, from ipsilateral cerebral cortex.

**17,** Medial lemniscus. The principal ascending pathway for tactile and proprioceptive information. Originates in the contralateral posterior column nuclei, terminates in the thalamus (VPL).

**18,** Middle cerebellar peduncle. Fibers from contralateral pontine nuclei that end as mossy fibers in all areas of cerebellar cortex.

**19,** Spinothalamic tract and lateral lemniscus. Crossed fibers from the spinal posterior horns conveying pain and temperature information to the thalamus (VPL and others), and ascending auditory fibers from the cochlear and superior olivary nuclei.

**20,** Central tegmental tract. Descending fibers from the red nucleus to the inferior olivary nucleus, together with fibers to and from the reticular formation.

**21,** Superior vestibular nucleus.

**22,** Juxtarestiform body. Fibers of the inferior cerebellar peduncle interconnecting the vestibular nuclei and cerebellum.

**23,** Superior cerebellar peduncle. Fibers from the deep cerebellar nuclei to the contralateral red nucleus and thalamus (ventral lateral nucleus [VL]).

**24,** Internal genu of the facial nerve. Facial nerve fibers, most of them on their way to ipsilateral muscles of facial expression.

**25,** Ascending root of the facial nerve. Facial nerve fibers just before they turn laterally in the internal genu.

**26,** Medial longitudinal fasciculus (MLF). At this level, the fibers are from vestibular nuclei and abducens interneurons, and are active in coordinating eye movements.

**27,** Fourth ventricle.

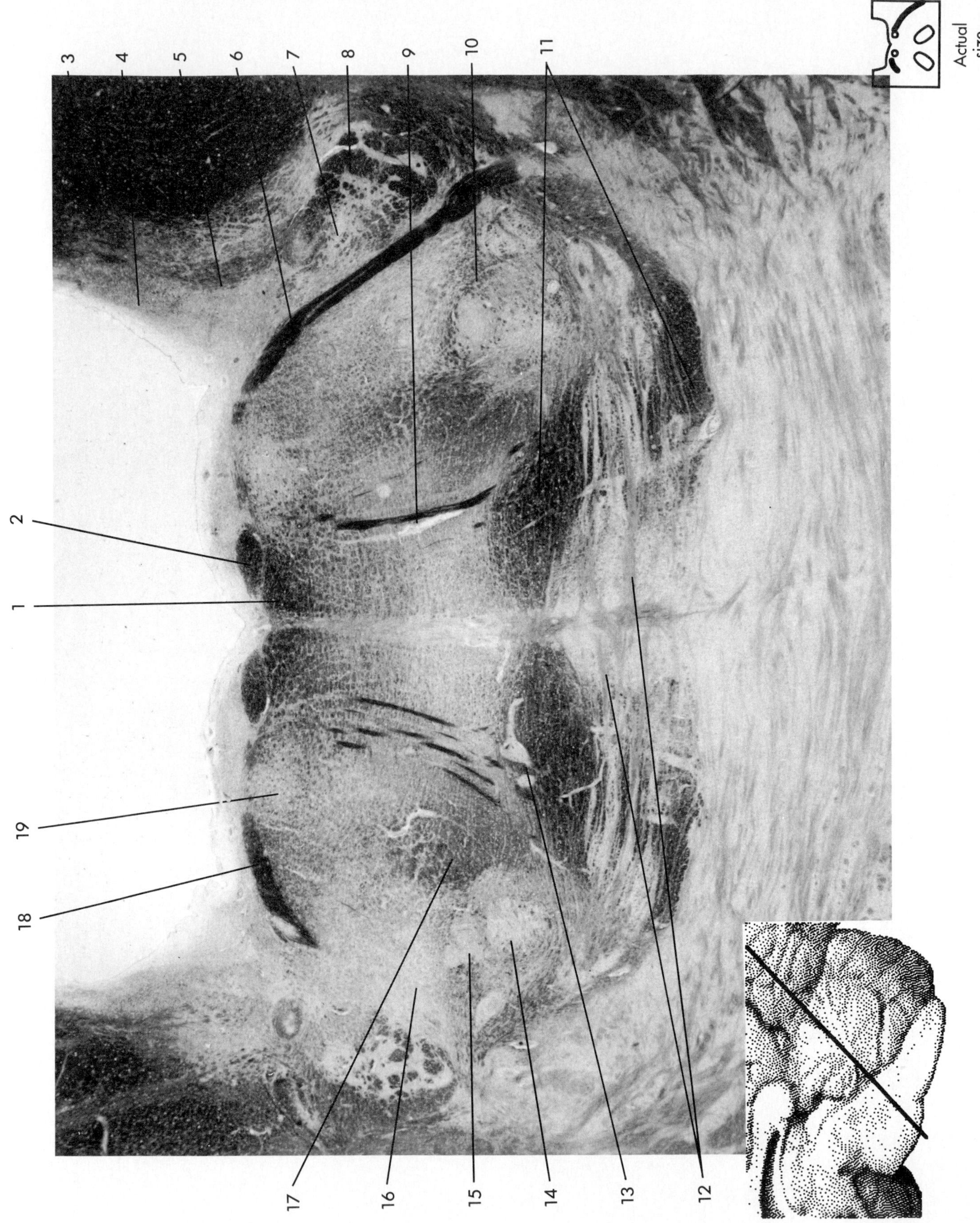
1
2
3
4
5
6
7
8
9
10
11
12
13
14
15
16
17
18
19
Actual size

## FIGURE 9-44B Caudal pons (enlarged)

**1,** Medial longitudinal fasciculus (MLF). At this level, fibers from vestibular nuclei and abducens interneurons, active in coordinating eye movements.

**2,** Ascending root of the facial nerve. Facial nerve fibers, just before they turn laterally in the internal genu.

**3,** The bulk of the inferior cerebellar peduncle. Contains crossed olivocerebellar fibers, the uncrossed posterior spinocerebellar tract, and other cerebellar afferents.

**4,** Superior vestibular nucleus.

**5,** Juxtarestiform body. Fibers of the inferior cerebellar peduncle interconnecting the vestibular nuclei and cerebellum.

**6,** Facial nerve fibers, most of them on their way to ipsilateral muscles of facial expression.

**7,** Spinal trigeminal nucleus (oral nucleus). Some primary afferents of the spinal trigeminal tract, particularly those carrying tactile information, end here.

**8,** Spinal trigeminal tract. Primary afferents from the ipsilateral side of the face, including those on their way to the caudal nucleus conveying information about pain and temperature.

**9,** Abducens nerve fibers, on their way to the ipsilateral lateral rectus.

**10,** Spinothalamic tract and lateral lemniscus. Crossed fibers from the spinal posterior horns conveying pain and temperature information to the thalamus (VPL), and ascending auditory fibers from the cochlear and superior olivary nuclei.

**11,** Medial lemniscus, the principal ascending pathway for tactile and proprioceptive information. Originates in the contralateral posterior column nuclei, terminates in the thalamus (VPL).

**12,** Trapezoid body. Crossing auditory fibers from the ventral cochlear nucleus and superior olivary nucleus.

**13,** Errant avian.

**14,** Medial superior olivary nucleus. Compares the relative times of arrival of sounds at the two ears and gives rise to many of the fibers of the ipsilateral lateral lemniscus.

**15,** Lateral superior olivary nucleus. Compares the relative intensities of sounds at the two ears and gives rise to some of the fibers of the ipsilateral lateral lemniscus.

**16,** Facial motor nucleus. Lower motor neurons for ipsilateral muscles of facial expression.

**17,** Central tegmental tract. Descending fibers from the red nucleus to the inferior olivary nucleus, together with fibers to and from the reticular formation.

**18,** Internal genu of the facial nerve. Facial nerve fibers, most of them on their way to ipsilateral muscles of facial expression.

**19,** Abducens nucleus. Contains the lower motor neurons for the ipsilateral lateral rectus, as well as the interneurons that project through the contralateral MLF to medial rectus motor neurons.

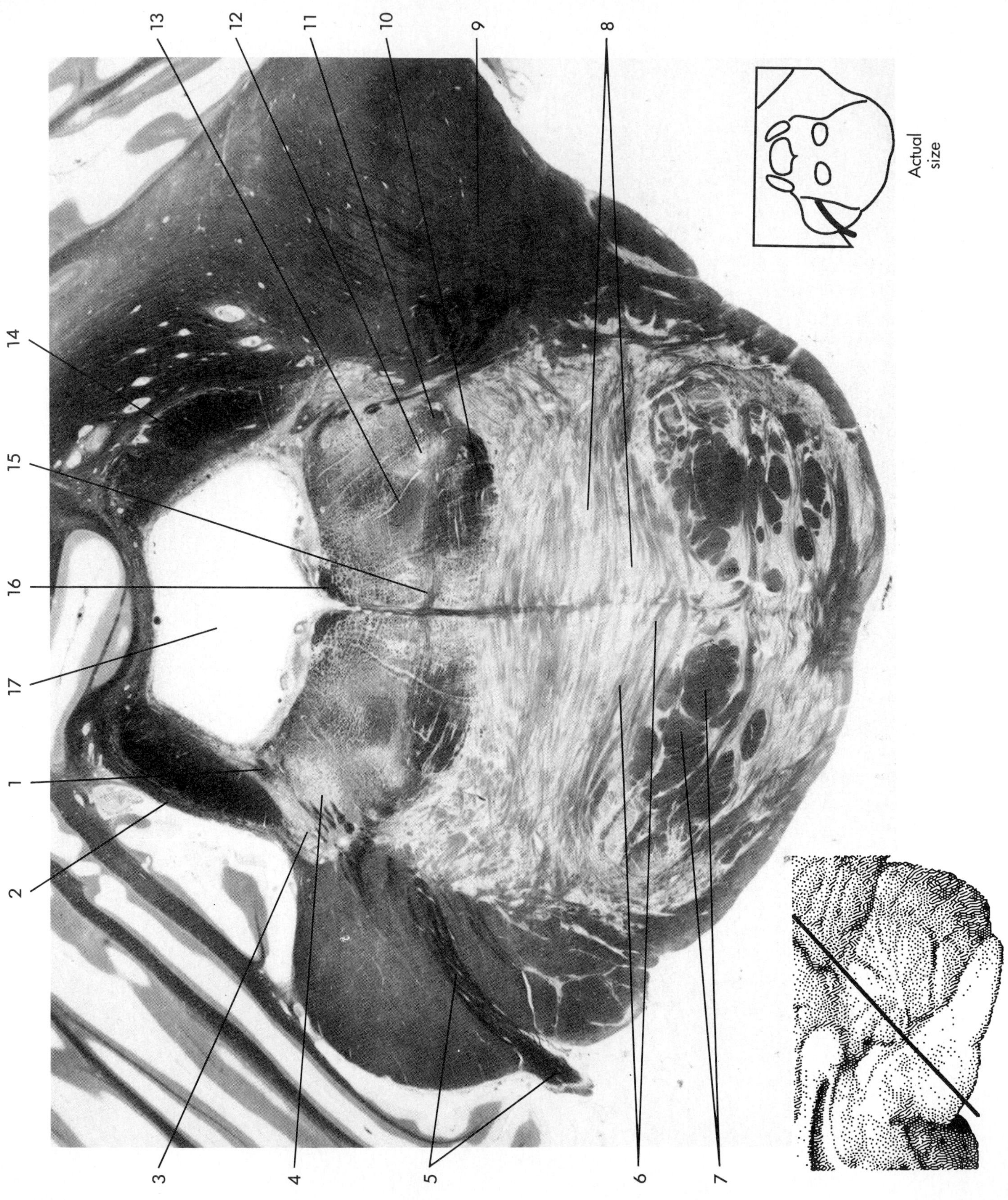

1
2
3
4
5
6
7
8
9
10
11
12
13
14
15
16
17
Actual size

**FIGURE 9-45 Midpons.**

**1,** Mesencephalic trigeminal tract. Processes of cell bodies in the adjacent mesencephalic trigeminal nucleus that innervate mechanoreceptors in and around the mouth.

**2,** Anterior spinocerebellar tract. Crossed fibers from lumbosacral spinal gray matter, carrying proprioceptive and other information from the leg.

**3,** Trigeminal main sensory nucleus. Site of termination of large diameter trigeminal afferents; site of origin of the uncrossed dorsal trigeminal tract and of part of the crossed ventral trigeminal tract.

**4,** Trigeminal motor nucleus. Lower motor neurons for ipsilateral muscles of mastication.

**5,** Trigeminal nerve. Somatosensory (and some chemosensory) fibers from the ipsilateral half of the head; efferents to ipsilateral muscles of mastication.

**6,** Pontocerebellar fibers, from pontine nuclei of one side to the opposite middle cerebellar peduncle.

**7,** Corticospinal and corticopontine fibers from ipsilateral cerebral cortex.

**8,** Pontine nuclei. Source of pontocerebellar fibers that cross the midline and form the middle cerebellar peduncle.

**9,** Middle cerebellar peduncle. Fibers from contralateral pontine nuclei that end as mossy fibers in all areas of cerebellar cortex.

**10,** Medial lemniscus. The principal ascending pathway for tactile and proprioceptive information. Originates in the contralateral posterior column nuclei and terminates in the thalamus (VPL).

**11,** Spinothalamic tract and lateral lemniscus. Crossed fibers from the spinal posterior horns, conveying pain and temperature information to the thalamus (VPL and others), and ascending auditory fibers from the cochlear and superior olivary nuclei.

**12,** Superior olivary nucleus. First site of convergence of fibers representing the two ears and the source of many of the fibers of the lateral lemniscus.

**13,** Central tegmental tract. Descending fibers from the red nucleus to the inferior olivary nucleus, together with fibers to and from the reticular formation.

**14,** Superior cerebellar peduncle. Fibers from the deep cerebellar nuclei to the contralateral red nucleus and thalamus (VL).

**15,** Trapezoid body. Crossing auditory fibers, primarily from the ventral cochlear nucleus.

**16,** Medial longitudinal fasciculus (MLF). At this level, the fibers are from vestibular nuclei and abducens interneurons and are active in coordinating eye movements.

**17,** Fourth ventricle.

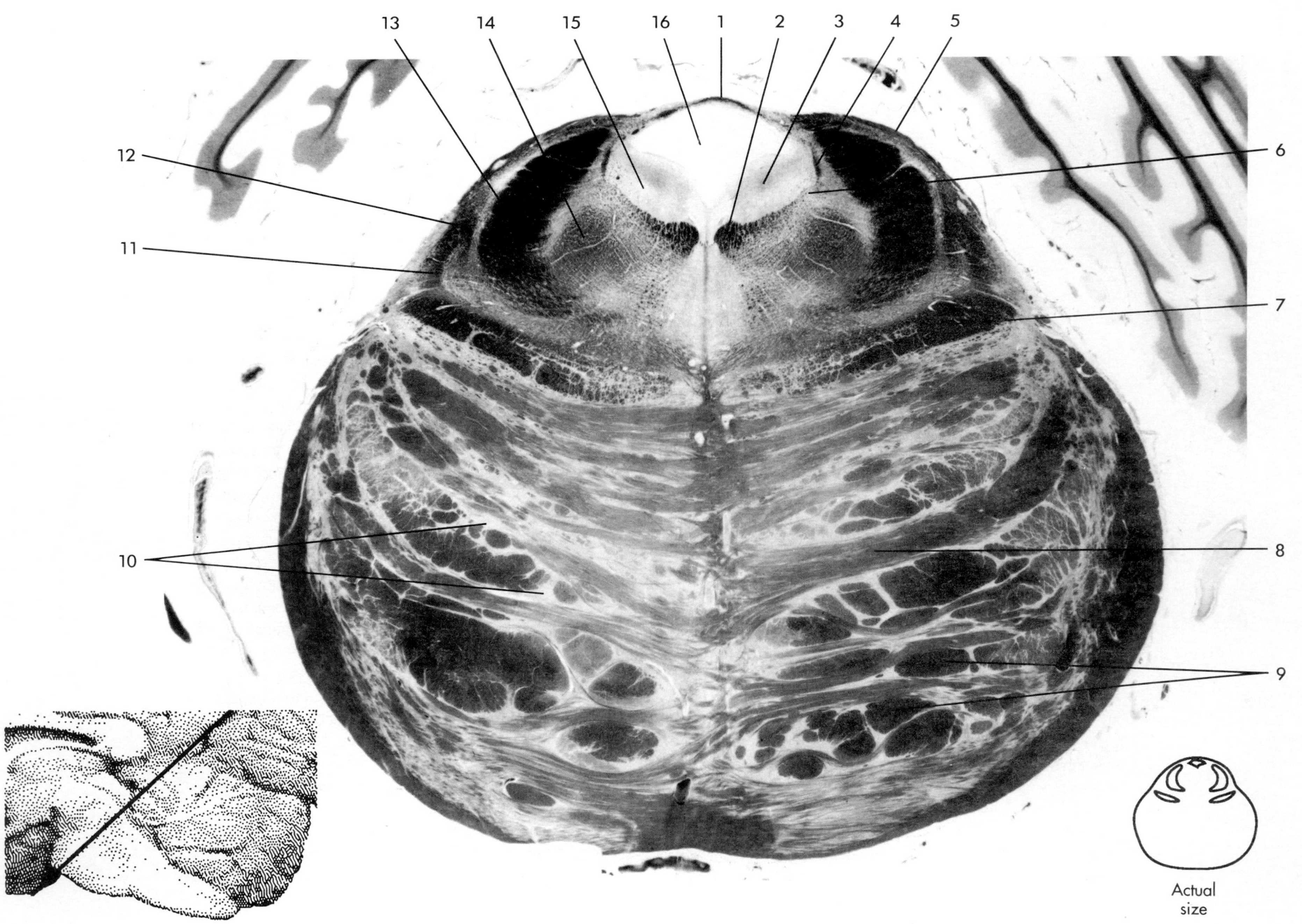
13
14
15
16
1
2
3
4
5
6
12
11
7
10
8
9
Actual size

## FIGURE 9-46 Pons-midbrain junction.

**1,** Decussation of the trochlear nerve. Fibers to the superior oblique muscles.

**2,** Medial longitudinal fasciculus (MLF). At this level, the fibers are from vestibular nuclei and abducens interneurons and are active in coordinating eye movements.

**3,** Dorsal longitudinal fasciculus. Descending hypothalamic fibers to the reticular formation and to preganglionic autonomic neurons.

**4,** Mesencephalic trigeminal tract. Processes of cell bodies in the adjacent mesencephalic trigeminal nucleus that innervate mechanoreceptors in and around the mouth.

**5,** Anterior spinocerebellar tract. Crossed fibers from lumbosacral spinal gray matter, carrying proprioceptive and other information from the leg.

**6,** Locus ceruleus. Noradrenergic neurons with widespread projections.

**7,** Medial lemniscus. The principal ascending pathway for tactile and proprioceptive information. Originates in the contralateral posterior column nuclei and terminates in the thalamus (VPL).

**8,** Pontocerebellar fibers from pontine nuclei on one side to the opposite middle cerebellar peduncle.

**9,** Corticospinal and corticopontine fibers, from ipsilateral cerebral cortex.

**10,** Pontine nuclei. Source of pontocerebellar fibers that cross the midline and form the middle cerebellar peduncle.

**11,** Spinothalamic tract. Crossed fibers from the spinal posterior horns conveying pain and temperature information to the thalamus (VPL and others).

**12,** Lateral lemniscus. Ascending auditory fibers from the cochlear and superior olivary nuclei, representing both ears.

**13,** Superior cerebellar peduncle. Fibers from the deep cerebellar nuclei to the contralateral red nucleus and thalamus (VL).

**14,** Central tegmental tract. Descending fibers from the red nucleus to the inferior olivary nucleus, together with fibers to and from the reticular formation.

**15,** Periventricular gray. Site of origin of the descending pain control pathway that relays in nucleus raphe magnus (among other connections).

**16,** Fourth ventricle.

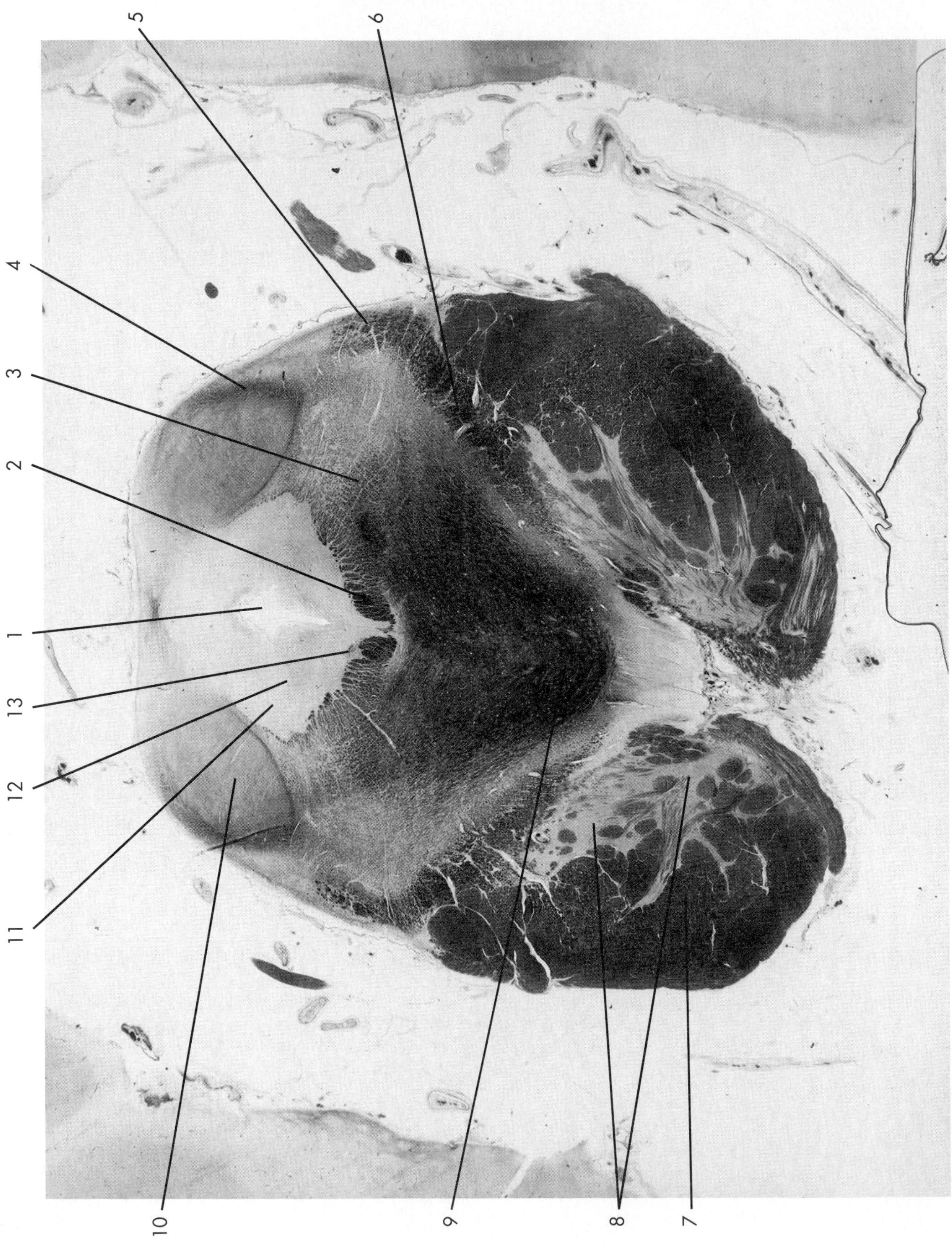
5
6
4
3
2
1
13
12
11
10
9
8
7

**FIGURE 9-47 Caudal midbrain.**

**1,** Cerebral aqueduct.

**2,** Medial longitudinal fasciculus (MLF). At this level, the fibers are from vestibular nuclei and abducens interneurons and are active in coordinating eye movements.

**3,** Central tegmental tract. Descending fibers from the red nucleus to the inferior olivary nucleus, together with fibers to and from the reticular formation.

**4,** Lateral lemniscus ending in the inferior colliculus, the next stop in the central auditory pathway.

**5,** Spinothalamic tract. Crossed fibers from the spinal posterior horns conveying pain and temperature information to the thalamus (VPL and others).

**6,** Medial lemniscus. The principal ascending pathway for tactile and proprioceptive information. Originates in the contralateral posterior column nuclei and terminates in the thalamus (VPL).

**7,** Basis pedunculi (of the cerebral peduncle). Descending corticospinal, corticobulbar, and corticopontine fibers from ipsilateral cerebral cortex.

**8,** Pontine nuclei. Source of pontocerebellar fibers that cross the midline and form the middle cerebellar peduncle.

**9,** Decussation of the superior cerebellar peduncles. Fibers from the deep cerebellar nuclei to the contralateral red nucleus and thalamus (VL).

**10,** Inferior colliculus. Site of termination of the lateral lemniscus and site of origin of the inferior brachium, which carries auditory information to the medial geniculate nucleus.

**11,** Periaqueductal gray. Site of origin of the descending pain control pathway that relays in nucleus raphe magnus (among other connections).

**12,** Dorsal longitudinal fasciculus. Descending hypothalamic fibers to the reticular formation and preganglionic autonomic neurons. These are thinly myelinated fibers that do not stand out from the gray matter through which they travel.

**13,** Trochlear nucleus. Lower motor neurons for the contralateral superior oblique muscle.

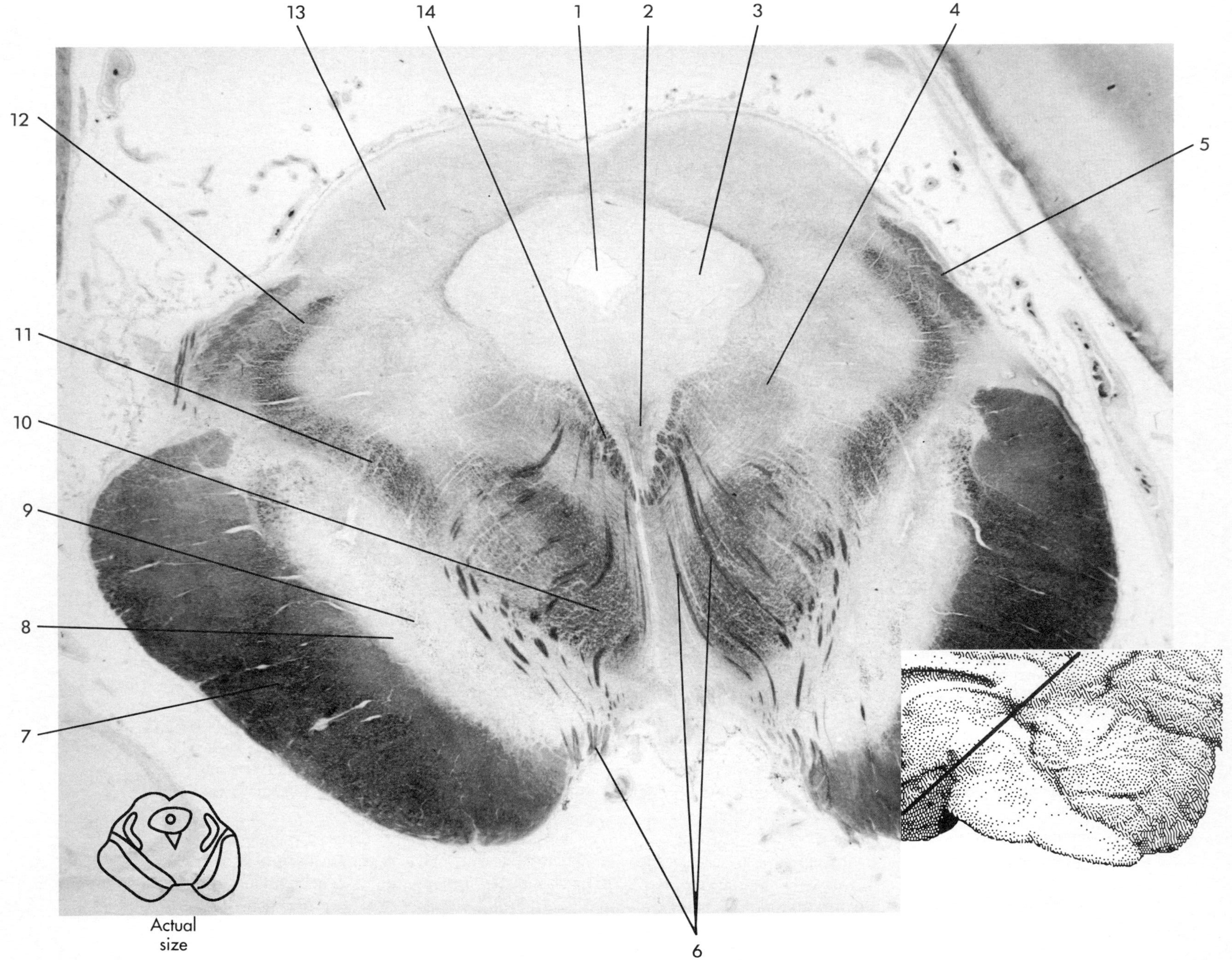
13
14
1
2
3
4
12
5
11
10
9
8
7
Actual size
6

**FIGURE 9-48 Rostral midbrain.**

**1,** Cerebral aqueduct.
**2,** Oculomotor nucleus. Lower motor neurons for the ipsilateral medial and inferior recti and inferior oblique muscles, the contralateral superior rectus muscle, and the levator palpebrae of both sides; preganglionic parasympathetic neurons for the pupillary sphincter and the ciliary muscle.
**3,** Periaqueductal gray. Site of origin of the descending pain control pathway that relays in nucleus raphe magnus (among other connections).
**4,** Central tegmental tract. Descending fibers from the red nucleus to the inferior olivary nucleus, together with fibers to and from the reticular formation.
**5,** Inferior brachium. Ascending auditory fibers on their way from the inferior colliculus to the medial geniculate nucleus.
**6,** Oculomotor nerve fibers. Axons of lower motor neurons and preganglionic parasympathetic neurons for the ipsilateral medial and inferior recti, inferior oblique, superior rectus, levator palpebrae, pupillary sphincter, and ciliary muscles.
**7,** Basis pedunculi (of cerebral peduncle). Descending corticospinal, corticobulbar, and corticopontine fibers from ipsilateral cerebral cortex.
**8,** Substantia nigra (reticular part). Site of termination of fibers from the caudate nucleus and putamen and site of origin of fibers to the thalamus, superior colliculus, and reticular formation.
**9,** Substantia nigra (compact part). Dopaminergic neurons whose axons terminate in the caudate nucleus and putamen.
**10,** Crossed superior cerebellar peduncle entering the red nucleus. Fibers from the deep cerebellar nuclei to the contralateral red nucleus and thalamus (VL).
**11,** Medial lemniscus. The principal ascending pathway for tactile and proprioceptive information. Originates in the contralateral posterior column nuclei and terminates in the thalamus (VPL).
**12,** Spinothalamic tract. Crossed fibers from the spinal posterior horns conveying pain and temperature information to the thalamus (VPL and others).
**13,** Superior colliculus. Involved in visual attention and eye movements and site of termination of most fibers of the superior brachium.
**14,** Medial longitudinal fasciculus (MLF). At this level, the fibers are from vestibular nuclei and abducens interneurons and are active in coordinating eye movements.

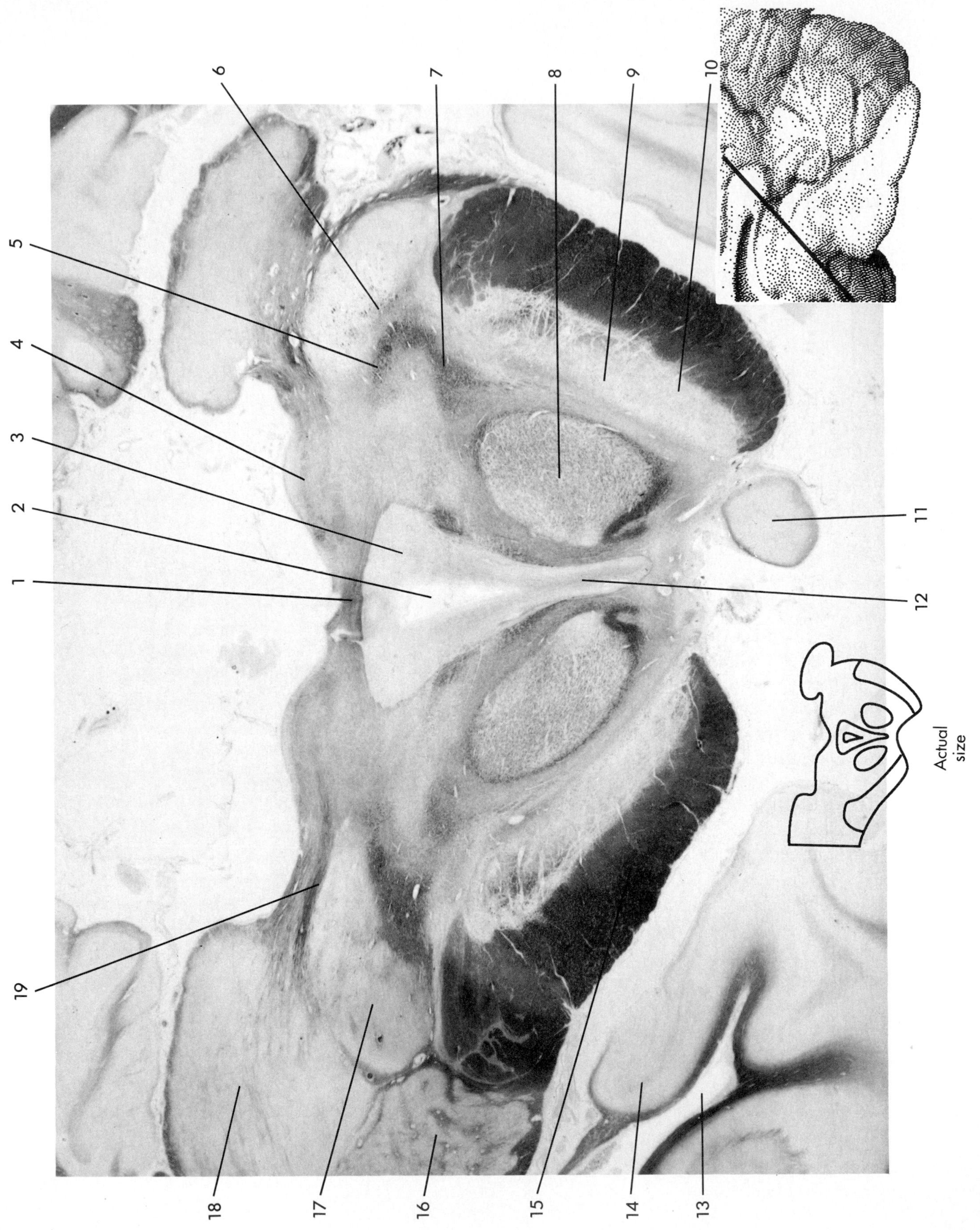
1
2
3
4
5
6
7
8
9
10
11
12
13
14
15
16
17
18
19
Actual size

**FIGURE 9-49 Midbrain-diencephalon junction.**

**1,** Posterior commissure. Crossing fibers involved in vertical eye movements and the pupillary light reflex.
**2,** Cerebral aqueduct, opening into the third ventricle.
**3,** Periaqueductal gray. Site of origin of the descending pain control pathway that relays in nucleus raphe magnus (among other connections).
**4,** Superior colliculus and pretectal area. Involved in visual attention, eye movements, and the pupillary light reflex and site of termination of superior brachium.
**5,** Spinothalamic tract. Crossed fibers from the spinal posterior horns conveying pain and temperature information to the thalamus (VPL and others).
**6,** Inferior brachium ending in the medial geniculate nucleus, the thalamic relay for hearing.
**7,** Medial lemniscus. The principal ascending pathway for tactile and proprioceptive information. Originates in the contralateral posterior column nuclei and terminates in the thalamus (VPL).
**8,** Red nucleus. Site of termination of part of the superior cerebellar peduncle and site of origin of uncrossed fibers to the inferior olivary nucleus and of the crossed rubrospinal tract.
**9,** Substantia nigra (compact part). Dopaminergic neurons whose axons terminate in the caudate nucleus and putamen.
**10,** Substantia nigra (reticular part). Site of termination of fibers from the caudate nucleus and putamen and site of origin of fibers to the thalamus, superior colliculus, and reticular formation.
**11,** Mammillary body. Part of the posterior hypothalamus; site of termination of much of the fornix and site of origin of the mammillothalamic tract.
**12,** Posterior hypothalamic nucleus, continuous with periaqueductal gray.
**13,** Inferior horn of the lateral ventricle.
**14,** Hippocampal formation.
**15,** Basis pedunculi (of the cerebral peduncle). Descending corticospinal, corticobulbar, and corticopontine fibers from ipsilateral cerebral cortex.
**16,** Lateral geniculate nucleus. The thalamic relay for vision and site of termination of most fibers of the optic tract.
**17,** Medial geniculate nucleus. The thalamic relay for hearing and site of termination of the inferior brachium.
**18,** Pulvinar. A large thalamic association nucleus connected with parietal, occipital, and temporal association cortex.
**19,** Superior brachium. Includes optic tract axons that bypass the lateral geniculate to reach the superior colliculus and pretectal area.

Hockman CH, Bieger D, Weerasuriva A: Supranuclear pathways of swallowing, *Prog Neurobiol* 12:15, 1979.

Hudspeth AJ: How the ear's works work, *Nature* 341:397, 1989. *A recent review of the biophysics of hair cells by one of the major investigators in this area.*

Jenkins WM, Masterton RB: Sound localization: effects of unilateral lesions in the central auditory system, *J Neurophysiol* 47:987, 1982.

Jones EG, Schwark HD, Callahan PA: Extent of the ipsilateral representation in the ventral posterior medial nucleus of the monkey thalamus, *Exp Brain Res* 63:310, 1986.

de Jong PTVM et al: Ataxia and nystagmus induced by injection of local anesthetics in the neck, *Ann Neurol* 1:240, 1977.

Kacher B et al: Electrokinetic shape changes of cochlear outer hair cells, *Nature* 322:365, 1986.

Kerr FWL: The divisional organization of afferent fibers of the trigeminal nerve, *Brain* 86:721, 1963.

Klinke R, Schmidt CL: Efferent influence on the vestigular organ during active movements of the body. *Pflügers Arch* 318:325, 1970. *Clever experiments giving a hint about a goldfish's use for the efferent fibers in its vestibular nerve.*

Korte GE: The brainstem projection of the vestibular nerve in the cat, *J Comp Neurol* 184:279, 1979.

Kunc Z: Treatment of essential neuralgia of the 9th nerve by selective tractotomy, *J Neurosurg* 23:494, 1965.

Lalonde ER, Eglitis JA: Number and distribution of taste buds on the epiglottis, pharynx, larynx, soft palate and uvula in a human newborn, *Anat Rec* 140:91, 1961.

Lang W, Büttner-Ennever JA, and Büttner U: Vestibular projections to the monkey thalamus: an autoradiographic study, *Brain Res* 177:3, 1979.

Lee D, Lishman R: Vision in movement and balance, *New Scientist* 65:59, 1975. *A popularized but fascinating account of how easy it is to confuse one's position sense by presenting conflicting visual and vestibular inputs.*

Lidén G, Peterson JL, Harford ER: Simultaneous recording of changes in relative impedance and air pressure during acoustic and non-acoustic elicitation of the middle-ear reflexes, *Acta Otolaryngol Suppl* 263:208, 1970.

Life without a balancing mechanism, *N Engl J Med* 246:458, 1962. *A first-hand account of the remarkable compensation we can achieve after bilateral damage to the vestibular apparatus.*

Lowe AA: The neural regulation of tongue movements, *Prog Neurobiol* 15:295, 1980.

Mahoney T, Vernon J, Meikle M: Function of the acoustic reflex in discrimination of intense speech, *Arch Otolaryngol* 105:119, 1979.

Martin MR, Mason CA: The seventh cranial nerve of the rat: visualization of efferent and afferent pathways by cobalt precipitation, *Brain Res* 121:21, 1977.

Matsumoto S, et al: A sensory level on the trunk in lower lateral brainstem lesions, *Neurol* 38:1515, 1988. *Clinical evidence about the relative locations of the spinothalamic and trigeminothalamic tracts in the brainstem.*

McCrea RA, Strassman A, Highstein SM: Morphology and physiology of abducens motoneurons and internuclear neurons intracellularly injected with horseradish peroxidase in alert squirrel monkeys, *J Comp Neurol* 243:291, 1986.

Mizuno N, Nomura S: Primary afferent fibers in the glossopharyngeal nerve terminate in the dorsal division of the principal sensory trigeminal nucleus, *Neurosci Lett* 66:338, 1986.

Moore JK: The human auditory brain stem: A comparative view, *Hearing Res* 29:1, 1987.

Moore JK: The human auditory brain stem as a generator of auditory evoked potentials, *Hearing Res* 29:33, 1987.

Norgren R: Gustatory system. In Paxinos G, editor: *The human nervous system,* San Diego, 1990, Academic Press.

Olszewski J: On the anatomical and functional organization of the spinal trigeminal nucleus, *J Comp Neurol* 92:401, 1950.

Ongerboer de Visser BW: Afferent limb of the human jaw reflex: electrophysiologic and anatomic study, *Neurology* 32:563, 1982.

Ongerboer de Visser BW, Kuypers HGJM: Late blink reflex changes in lateral medullary lesions, *Brain* 101:285, 1978.

Osterhammel P, Terkildsen K, Zilstorff K: Vestibular habituation in ballet dancers, *Adv Otorhinolaryngol* 17:158, 1970. *How do people who rotate for a living do it?*

Pickles JO: *An introduction to the physiology of hearing,* ed. 2 London, 1988, Academic Press.

Porter JD: Brainstem terminations of extraocular muscle primary afferent neurons in the monkey, *J Comp Neurol* 247:133, 1986.

Porter JD, Guthrie BL, Sparks DL: Innervation of monkey extraocular muscles: localization of sensory and motor neurons by retrograde transport of horseradish peroxidase, *J Comp Neurol* 218:208, 1983.

Raphan T, Cohen B: Brainstem mechanisms for rapid and slow eye movements, *Annu Rev Physiol* 40:527, 1978.

Rokx JTM, Jüch PJW, van Willigen JD: Arrangements and connections of mesencephalic trigeminal neurons in the rat, *Acta Anat* 127:7, 1986.

Rovit RJ, Murali R, Jannetta PJ, editors: *Trigeminal neuralgia,* Baltimore, 1990, Williams and Wilkins.

Rushton JG, Stevens JC, Miller RH: Glossopharyngeal (vagoglossopharyngeal) neuralgia: a study of 217 cases, *Arch Neurol* 38:201, 1981.

Ryan A, Dallos P: Effect of absence of cochlear outer hair cells on behavioral auditory threshold, *Nature* 253:44, 1975.

Scott TR et al: Gustatory responses in the nucleus tractus solitarius of the alert cynomolgus monkey, *J Neurophysiol* 55:182, 1986.

Shaw MD, Baker R: The locations of stapedius and tensor tympani motoneurons in the cat, *J Comp Neurol* 216:10, 1983.

Shigenaga Y et al: Oral and facial representation within the medullary and upper cervical dorsal horns in the cat, *J Comp Neurol* 243:388, 1986. *A detailed examination of the somatotopic arrangement of fibers and their terminations in the spinal trigeminal system.*

Simpson JI, Graf W: Eye-muscle geometry and compensatory eye movements in lateral-eyed and frontal-eyed animals, *Ann NY Acad Sci* 374:20, 1981. *Pitching to one side or the other requires vertical compensatory eye movements in rabbits but torsional eye movements in us, even though both species have semicircular canals arranged similarly. This fascinating paper provides an explanation.*

Smith RL: Axonal projections and connections of the principal sensory trigeminal nucleus in the monkey, *J Comp Neurol* 163:347, 1975.

Spoendlin H: The innervation of the organ of Corti, *J Laryngol Otol* 81:717, 1967.

Spoendlin H, Schrott A: Analysis of the human auditory nerve, *Hearing Res* 43:25, 1989.

Starr A, Schubert ED, Kitzes LM: *Binaural function.* In Asbury AK et al, editors: *Diseases of the nervous system,* Philadelphia, 1986, WB Saunders.

Steindler DA: Trigeminocerebellar, trigeminotectal and trigeminothalamic projections: a double retrograde axonal tracing study in the mouse, *J Comp Neurol* 237:155, 1985.

Stewart WA, King RB: Fiber projections from the nucleus caudalis of the spinal trigeminal nucleus, *J Comp Neurol* 121:271, 1963.

Stockard JJ, Stockard JE, Sharbrough FW: Detection and localization of occult lesions with brainstem auditory responses, *Mayo Clin Proc* 52:761, 1977.

Strominger NL, Nelson LR, Dougherty WJ: Second order auditory pathways in the chimpanzee, *J Comp Neurol* 172:349, 1977.

Tamai Y, Iwamoto M, Tsujimoto T: Pathway of the blink reflex in the brainstem of the cat: interneurons between the trigeminal nuclei and the facial nucleus, *Brain Res* 380:19, 1986.

Torvik A: The ascending fibers from the main trigeminal sensory nucleus, *Am J Anat* 100:1, 1957.

von Baumgarten R et al: Effects of rectilinear acceleration and optokinetic and caloric stimulations in space, *Science* 225:208, 1984.

Von Békésy G: *Experiments in hearing,* New York, 1960, McGraw-Hill. *A large collection of clever and skillful experiments by the grand master of auditory physiology.*

Wall M, Wray SH: The one-and-a-half syndrome—a unilateral disorder of the pontine tegmentum: A study of 20 cases and review of the literature, *Neurol* 33:971, 1983.

Warwick R: Representation of the extra-ocular muscles in the oculomotor nuclei of the monkey, *J Comp Neurol* 98:449, 1953.

Way JS: Evidence for the site of the superior salivatory nucleus in the guinea pig: a retrograde HRP study, *Anat Rec* 201:119, 1981.

Wilson VJ, Jones GM: *Mammalian vestibular physiology,* New York, 1979, Plenum Press.

Young RF: Effect of trigeminal tractotomy on dental sensation in humans, *J Neurosurg* 56:812, 1982. *Tractotomy near the obex causes facial analgesia but no change in dental pain.*

Young RF, Perryman KM: Neuronal responses in rostral trigeminal brain-stem nuclei of macaque monkeys after chronic trigeminal tractotomy, *J Neurosurg* 65:508, 1986. *Evidence that dental pain is processed rostral to the obex and facial pain caudal to the obex in the spinal trigeminal nucleus.*

Younge BR: Analysis of trochlear nerve palsies: diagnosis, etiology and treatment, *Mayo Clin Proc* 52:11, 1977.

Zee DS: The organization of the brainstem ocular motor subnuclei, *Ann Neurol* 4:384, 1978. *Speculation on why the motor axons to the superior oblique and superior rectus cross.*

# CHAPTER 10

# *Diencephalon*

The diencephalon, mostly hidden from view between the cerebral hemispheres, constitutes only about 2% of the central nervous system by weight. Nevertheless, it has extremely widespread and important connections, and the great majority of sensory, motor, and limbic pathways involve one or more relays in the diencephalon. Since most motor and limbic pathways also involve telencephalic structures that are discussed in later chapters, this chapter provides only a general overview of the connections of diencephalic nuclei. A more detailed consideration of these connections in terms of functional systems is provided in subsequent chapters. In addition, a series of sections demonstrating major structures of both the diencephalon and the telencephalon is provided as an appendix following Chapter 17.

The diencephalon is conventionally divided into four parts, each of which includes the term *thalamus* (from the Greek word meaning inner chamber) as part of its name. These parts are (1) the *epithalamus,* which includes the *pineal gland* and a few nearby neural structures; (2) the *dorsal thalamus,* which is usually referred to simply as the *thalamus;* (3) the *subthalamus;* and (4) the *hypothalamus.*

## EXTENT OF THE DIENCEPHALON

The only part of the diencephalon that can be seen on an intact brain is the inferior surface of the hypothalamus (see Figures 2-15 and 2-16), which includes the *mammillary bodies* and the *infundibular stalk.* However, the entire medial surface of the diencephalon, much of which forms each wall of the third ventricle, can be seen on a hemisected brain (Figure 10-1). Superiorly the diencephalon borders the subarachnoid space of the transverse cerebral fissure; inferiorly, as previously noted, it is also exposed to subarachnoid space. Laterally it is bounded by the internal capsule (see Figures 2-20 to 2-22). The caudal boundary of the diencephalon is a plane through the posterior commissure and the caudal edge of the mammillary bodies; the rostral boundary is a plane through the anterior commissure and the optic chiasm. These rostral and caudal boundaries are approximate and semiarbitrary and are used only for purposes of discussion. Functionally continuous neural tissue extends through both boundaries; in addition (as noted in earlier chapters), certain thalamic nuclei protrude through the posterior boundary to a position alongside the midbrain.

As a consequence of the cephalic flexure, the axis of the diencephalon is inclined about 100 degrees with respect to the axis of the brainstem (see Figure 2-1). This means that sections cut in a plane similar to that used in the last few chapters (that is, perpendicular to the axis of the brainstem) are at a peculiar angle to the diencephalon. Therefore in this and subsequent chapters, sections cut in horizontal and coronal planes are shown (Figure 10-2).*

## EPITHALAMUS

The epithalamus includes the *pineal gland* and the *habenular nuclei* and their connections.

### Pineal gland

The pineal gland is a midline, unpaired structure situated just rostral to the superior colliculi. It somewhat resembles a pine cone in shape—hence its name. Since each of us has only one pineal gland, which is located deep within the brain, it was thought for a time that this organ

*The horizontal sections are oriented with the anterior portion at the top of the picture, since this is the way CT and MRI scans are conventionally oriented. One result, which can sometimes cause confusion, is that anterior parts of the brainstem also are situated toward the top of the picture; this is upside down relative to the way the brainstem was pictured in Chapters 8 and 9.

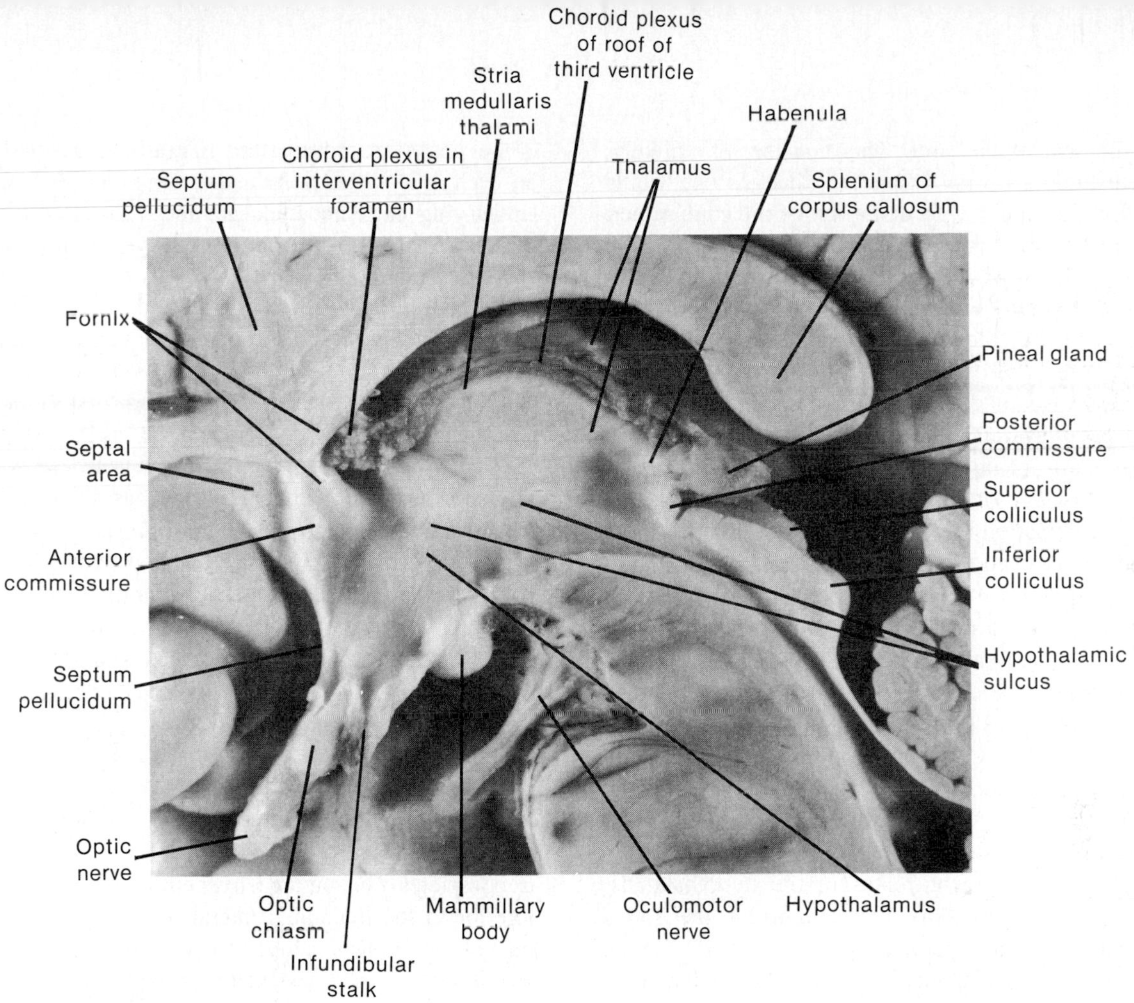

FIGURE 10-1
Close up photograph of the medial surface of the brain shown in Figures 2-14 and 10-2, illustrating parts of the diencephalon and some surrounding structures.

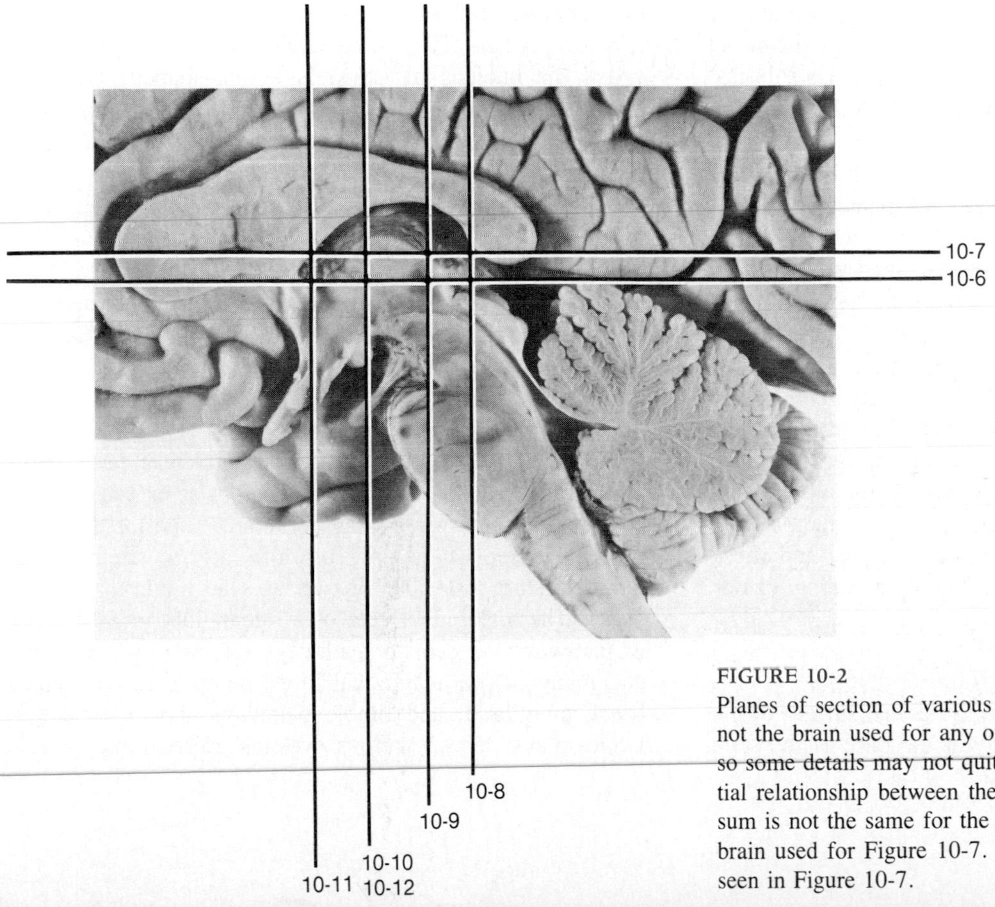

FIGURE 10-2
Planes of section of various photographs in this chapter. This is not the brain used for any of the sections shown in this chapter, so some details may not quite correspond. For example, the spatial relationship between the diencephalon and the corpus callosum is not the same for the brain shown in this figure as for the brain used for Figure 10-7. As a result, the splenium cannot be seen in Figure 10-7.

might be the seat of the soul. This now seems unlikely, since pineal tumors do not cause the changes one would expect to find associated with distortion of the soul; rather, these tumors compress the midbrain and cause the changes one would expect to find associated with distortion of this part of the brainstem. Early findings may include hydrocephalus (because of the squeezing shut of the aqueduct) and various defects of eye movements and pupillary reactions (because of damage to the oculomotor and trochlear nuclei and pathways ending in them). In addition, pineal tumors may cause changes in sexual development, giving a clue to at least one of its possible functions. The pineal arises as an evagination from the roof of the diencephalon; in fish, amphibians, and many reptiles, it contains photoreceptor cells similar to those of the eye. In these species it is suspected of monitoring day length and season and participating in the regulation of circadian and circannual rhythms (although there are probably other functions as well). The pineal gland of birds and mammals contains no photoreceptors and consists of a collection of secretory cells *(pinealocytes),* some glial cells, and a rich vascular network. Nevertheless, it still receives a light-regulated input by way of a circuitous pathway that begins in the retina and, after one or more relays in the hypothalamus, reaches the intermediolateral cell column of the spinal cord. Preganglionic sympathetic fibers from the spinal cord then synapse on postganglionic neurons of the superior cervical ganglion, which in turn send their axons to the pineal.

The mammalian pineal is an endocrine gland involved in reproductive cycles and has no known neural output. It secretes an antigonadotropic hormone called *melatonin* at relatively high rates during darkness. Light, by way of the neural pathway just described, causes a decrease in melatonin production. Thus increasing day lengths cause a decrease in melatonin production, which in turn causes an increase in gonadal function. This system is of considerable importance in mammals with prominent seasonal sexual cycles, but its effects in humans are not clear. It has been reported, however, that nonparenchymal pineal tumors, which presumably destroy pinealocytes, tend to be associated with precocious puberty, as though the production of some antigonadotropic substance had been halted. The converse has been reported as well—that parenchymal pineal tumors tend to be associated with hypogonadism. These tumors are quite rare, however, and the routine clinical importance of the pineal arises from the fact that after the age of 17 calcareous concretions accrue in it. This makes it opaque to x-rays and hence a useful radiological landmark, since it normally lies in the midline, and slight shifts in its position can be indicative of expanding masses of various types.

### Habenula

The pineal gland is attached to the dorsal surface of the diencephalon by a stalk. Caudally at the base of the stalk is the posterior commissure; rostrally is a small swelling on each side called a *habenula* (Figures 10-1 and 10-6). Underlying each habenula are the *habenular nuclei*. The two habenulae are interconnected by the small *habenular commissure*. Each habenula receives one major input bundle, the *stria medullaris thalami,* and gives rise to one major output bundle with the awesome name of *habenulointerpeduncular tract* (or *fasciculus retroflexus*). The stria medullaris thalami (Figures 10-1 and 10-9) underlies a horizontal ridge on the dorsomedial surface of the thalamus to which the roof of the third ventricle is attached. The habenulointerpeduncular tract, as its name implies, extends from the habenula to the *interpeduncular nucleus,* which is located between the cerebral peduncles in the reticular formation of the rostral midbrain. The fibers of the stria medullaris thalami originate in various limbic structures, so the pathway through the habenula is one route through which the limbic system can influence the brainstem reticular formation.

## SUBTHALAMUS

The midbrain tegmentum continues into the diencephalon as the *subthalamus,* or *subthalamic region*. This area is completely surrounded by neural tissue and is located inferior to the thalamus, lateral to the hypothalamus, and medial to the basis pedunculi and internal capsule (Figures 10-10 and 10-12). The subthalamus contains rostral portions of the red nucleus and substantia nigra and is traversed by somatosensory pathways on their way to the thalamus as well as by several pathways involving the cerebellum and basal ganglia (the latter pathways are discussed in Chapters 13 and 14). In addition, the subthalamus contains the *subthalamic nucleus* and *zona incerta* (Figure 10-12). The subthalamic nucleus (occasionally called the nucleus of Luys) is a lens-shaped, biconvex structure located just medial and superior to portions of the basis pedunculi and internal capsule. This nucleus is interconnected with the basal ganglia, as discussed in Chapter 13. The zona incerta is a small mass of gray matter intervening between the subthalamic nucleus and the thalamus. It appears to be a rostral continuation of the midbrain reticular formation and has rather widespread connections (including direct projections to the cerebral cortex). Its function is largely unknown.

## THALAMUS

The thalamus is a large egg-shaped nuclear mass, making up about 80% of the diencephalon. It extends anteriorly to the interventricular foramen, superiorly to the transverse cerebral fissure, and inferiorly to the hypothalamic sulcus; posteriorly it overlaps the midbrain (Figure 10-1). The thalamus is part of a remarkably large number of pathways; all sensory pathways relay in the thalamus, and many of the anatomical loops comprising cerebellar, basal ganglionic, and limbic pathways also involve thalamic relays. These various systems utilize more or less

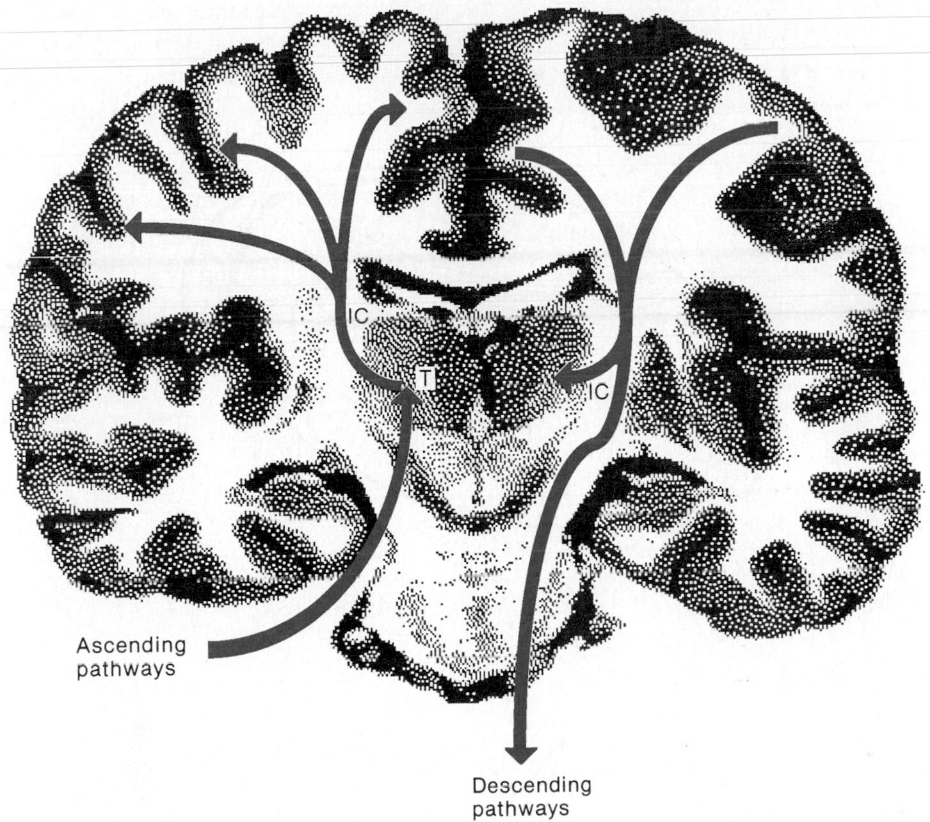


FIGURE 10-3
General arrangement of thalamic connections. Crossed fibers of ascending pathways end in the thalamus *(T),* which in turn projects through the internal capsule *(IC)* to areas of cerebral cortex. This example is a coronal section approximately at the level of the VPL and the postcentral gyrus, so the pathway illustrated might correspond to the medial lemniscus and the projection of the VPL to somatosensory cortex. Cortical areas project back to the thalamus, but this is not the origin of descending pathways such as the corticospinal tract. Rather, cortical areas project directly, through the internal capsule, to neural targets like the brainstem, spinal cord, and basal ganglia.

separate portions of the thalamus, which has therefore been subdivided into a series of nuclei. However, the overall pattern of thalamic connections is as indicated in Figure 10-3; each thalamic nucleus receives inputs from one or more subcortical sources, as well as feedback inputs from the cortical areas to which the nucleus projects. Although not much is known about the actual functional properties of the feedback pathways, these projections from the cortex to the thalamus appear to provide a means by which the cerebral cortex can control its own inputs.

Thalamic nuclei can be distinguished from each other both by their topographical locations within the thalamus and by the patterns of their connections with the cerebral cortex.

## Topographical subdivisions

The general organization of the thalamus is shown in Figures 10-4 and 10-5. A thin, curved sheet of myelinated fibers, the *internal medullary lamina,* divides most of the thalamus into medial and lateral groups of nuclei. Anteriorly the internal medullary lamina bifurcates and encloses the *anterior nucleus,* which borders on the interventricular foramen. The medial group similarly contains a single large nucleus, the *dorsomedial (DM) nucleus** (Figures 10-6, 10-7, 10-9, and 10-10).

The lateral group of nuclei composes the bulk of the thalamus and is further subdivided into a dorsal tier and a ventral tier. The dorsal tier consists of the large *pulvinar* (Figures 10-6, 10-7, and 10-8), the *lateral posterior (LP) nucleus* (Figure 10-9), and the *lateral dorsal (LD) nucleus* (Figure 10-9). The lateral posterior nucleus is continuous with the pulvinar; both nuclei have somewhat similar connections, so the two together are sometimes referred to as the pulvinar/LP complex. The ventral tier of the lateral nuclear group consists of three nuclei arranged along an anterior-posterior line: (1) the *ventral anterior (VA) nucleus*

*Also referred to by many authors as the *mediodorsal nucleus* (or *MD*).

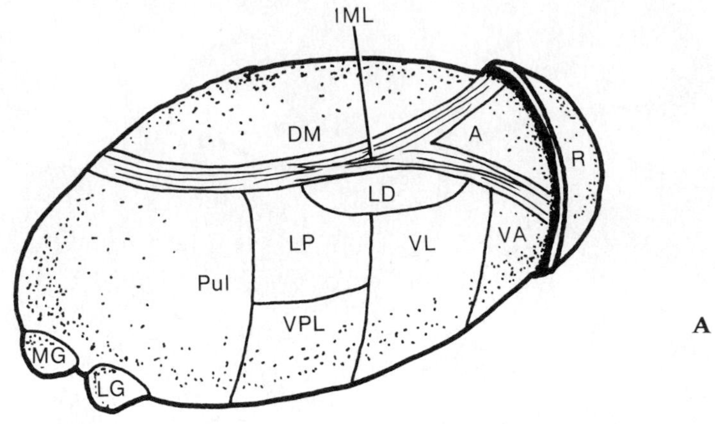


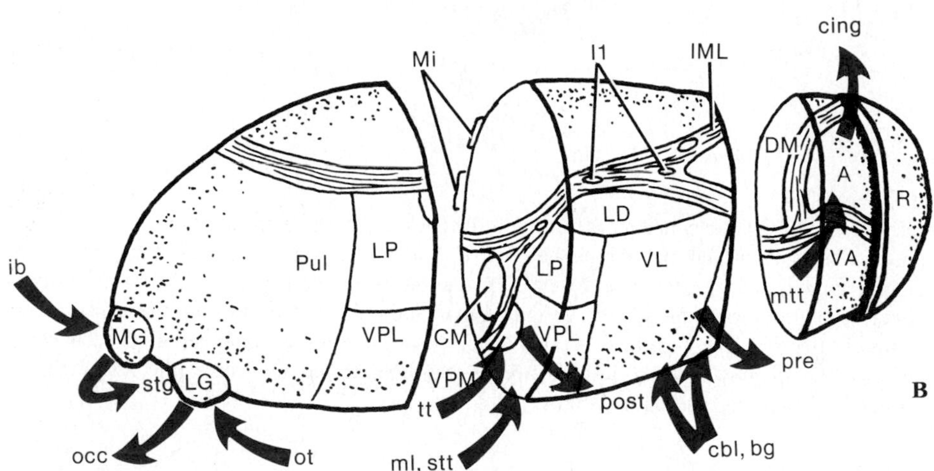


FIGURE 10-4
Diagrammatic illustration of the way in which the thalamus is subdivided. **A,** Lateral view of the right thalamus as seen from slightly above and behind. Most of the reticular nucleus has been removed; ordinarily it would cover the entire lateral surface. **B,** Same as **A** but exploded into three pieces to show certain aspects of the internal organization of the thalamus. Tracts ending in the specific relay nuclei are indicated, as are the destinations of the outputs from these nuclei. The more posterior sliced surface corresponds approximately to Figure 10-9; the more anterior sliced surface corresponds approximately to Figure 10-10. *A,* Anterior nucleus; *CM,* centromedian nucleus; *DM,* dorsomedial nucleus; *Il,* intralaminar nuclei; *IML,* internal medullary lamina; *LD,* lateral dorsal nucleus; *LG,* lateral geniculate nucleus; *LP,* lateral posterior nucleus; *MG,* medial geniculate nucleus; *Mi,* midline nuclei; *Pul,* pulvinar; *R,* reticular nucleus; *VA,* ventral anterior nucleus; *VL,* ventral lateral nucleus; *VPL,* ventral posterolateral nucleus; *VPM,* ventral posteromedial nucleus; *bg,* basal ganglia; *cbl,* cerebellum; *cing,* cingulate gyrus; *ib,* inferior brachium (brachium of the inferior colliculus); *ml,* medial lemniscus; *mtt,* mammillothalamic tract; *occ,* occipital lobe (visual cortex); *ot,* optic tract; *post,* postcentral gyrus (somatosensory cortex); *pre,* precentral gyrus and nearby cortex (motor, premotor, and supplementary motor cortex); *stg,* superior temporal gyrus (auditory cortex); *stt,* spinothalamic tract; *tt,* trigeminothalamic tracts.

Modified from Brodal A: Neurological anatomy in relation to clinical medicine, ed 3, New York, 1981, Oxford University Press.

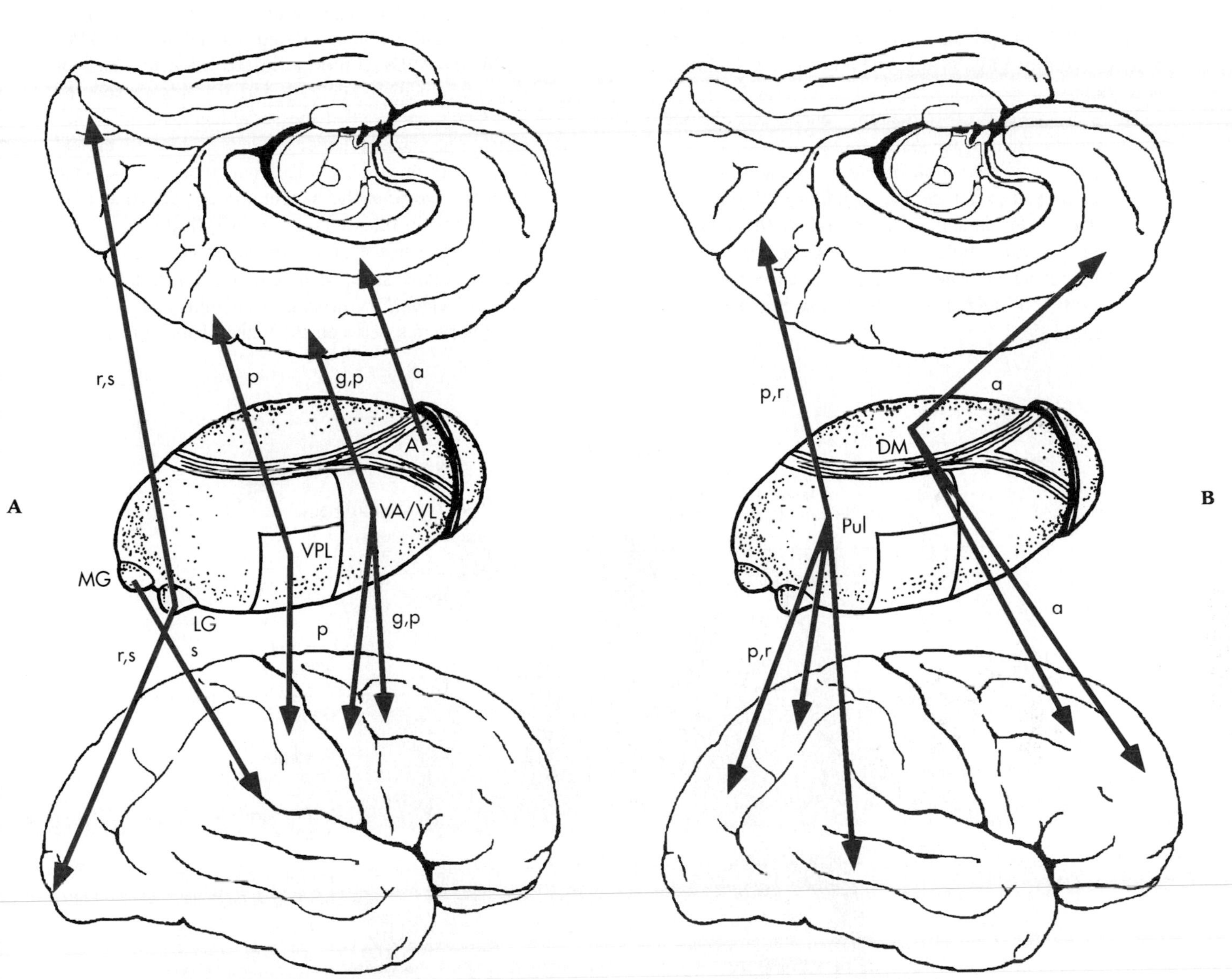


FIGURE 10-5
Major patterns of connections of thalamic nuclei. *A,* specific relay nuclei; *B,* association nuclei. The parts of the internal capsule utilized by each set of fibers are indicated: *a,* anterior limb; *g,* genu, *p,* posterior limb; *r,* retrolenticular part; *s,* sublenticular part. Other abbreviations: *A,* Anterior nucleus; *DM,* dorsomedial nucleus; *MG,* medial geniculate nucleus; *LG,* lateral geniculate nucleus; *Pul,* pulvinar; *VA/VL,* ventral anterior and ventral lateral nuclei; *VPL,* ventral posterolateral nucleus. (Portions adapted from Ono M et al: *Atlas of the cerebral sulci,* New York, 1990, Thieme Medical Publishers.)

(Figures 10-7 and 10-11), (2) the *ventral lateral (VL) nucleus* (Figure 10-10), and (3) the *ventral posterior (VP) nucleus* (Figure 10-9). The ventral posterior nucleus is customarily subdivided into the *ventral posterolateral (VPL) nucleus* and *ventral posteromedial (VPM) nucleus*. The VPL is the somatosensory relay nucleus for the body and the VPM for the head. The VA and VL are involved in motor control circuits that include the cerebellum and basal ganglia.

There are several other thalamic nuclei that do not fit neatly into the framework given above.

1. The *lateral geniculate nucleus* (visual system) and *medial geniculate nucleus* (auditory system) are located posterior and a bit ventral to the VPL/VPM and protrude posteriorly alongside the midbrain (Figure 10-8). These two nuclei are most conveniently considered as a posterior extension of the ventral tier.
2. At certain locations within the thalamus the internal medullary lamina splits and encloses groups of cells. These nuclei are collectively called the *intralaminar nuclei,* the two largest of which are the *centromedian (CM)* and *parafascicular (PF) nuclei* (Figures 10-6 and 10-9). The centromedian nucleus is a large, round nucleus located medial to the VPL/VPM; the VPM conforms to the rounded shape of the centromedian nucleus, and for this reason the VPM was once called the semilunar or arcuate nucleus. The parafascicular nucleus is located medial to the centromedian nucleus and received its name from the fact that the habenulointerpeduncular tract (fasciculus retroflexus) passes through it.
3. The lateral surface of the thalamus is covered by a second curved sheet of myelinated fibers called the *external medullary lamina.* The thin shell of cells that intervenes between the external medullary lam-

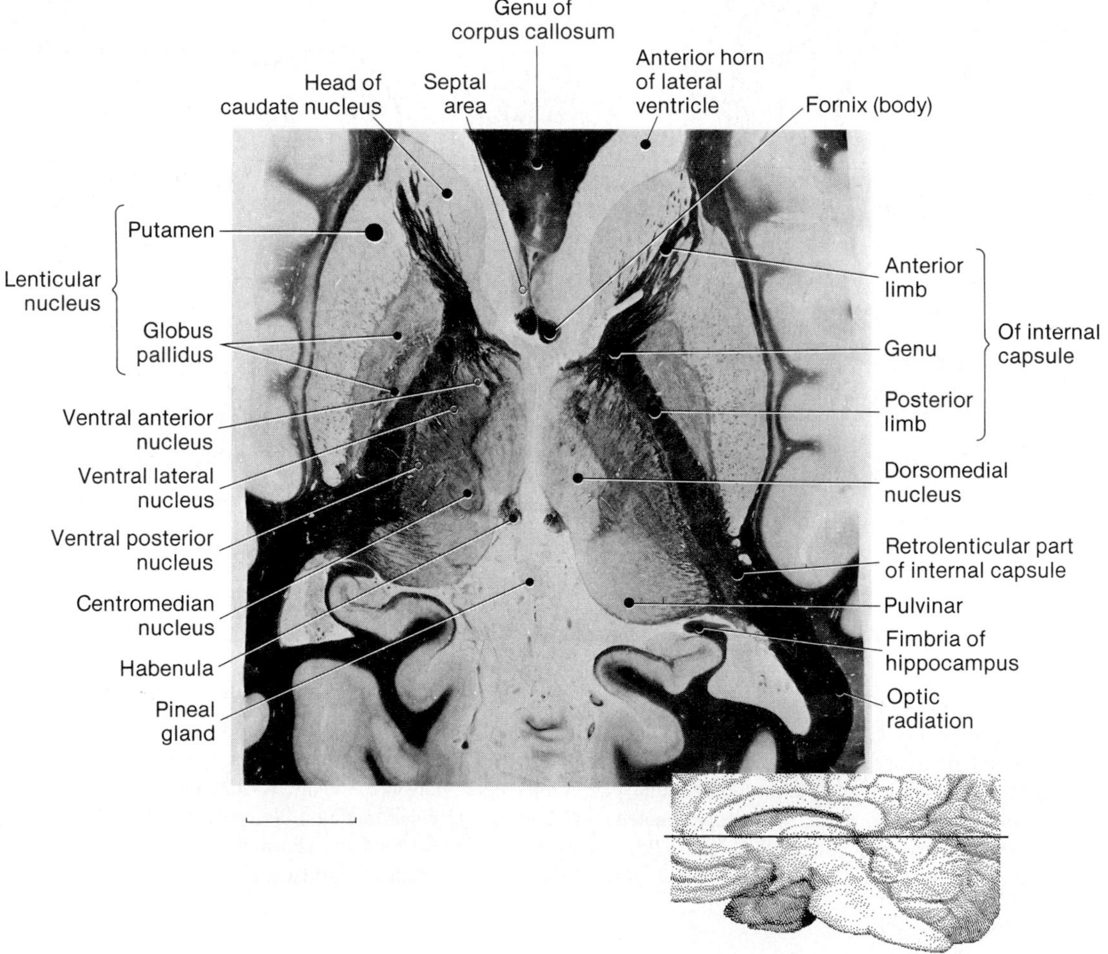


FIGURE 10-6
Horizontal section through the thalamus at the level of the centromedian nucleus. Scale mark = 1 cm. At this magnification and with this staining technique, the VPL/VPM, VL, and VA can be distinguished from one another only by location and not by appearance.

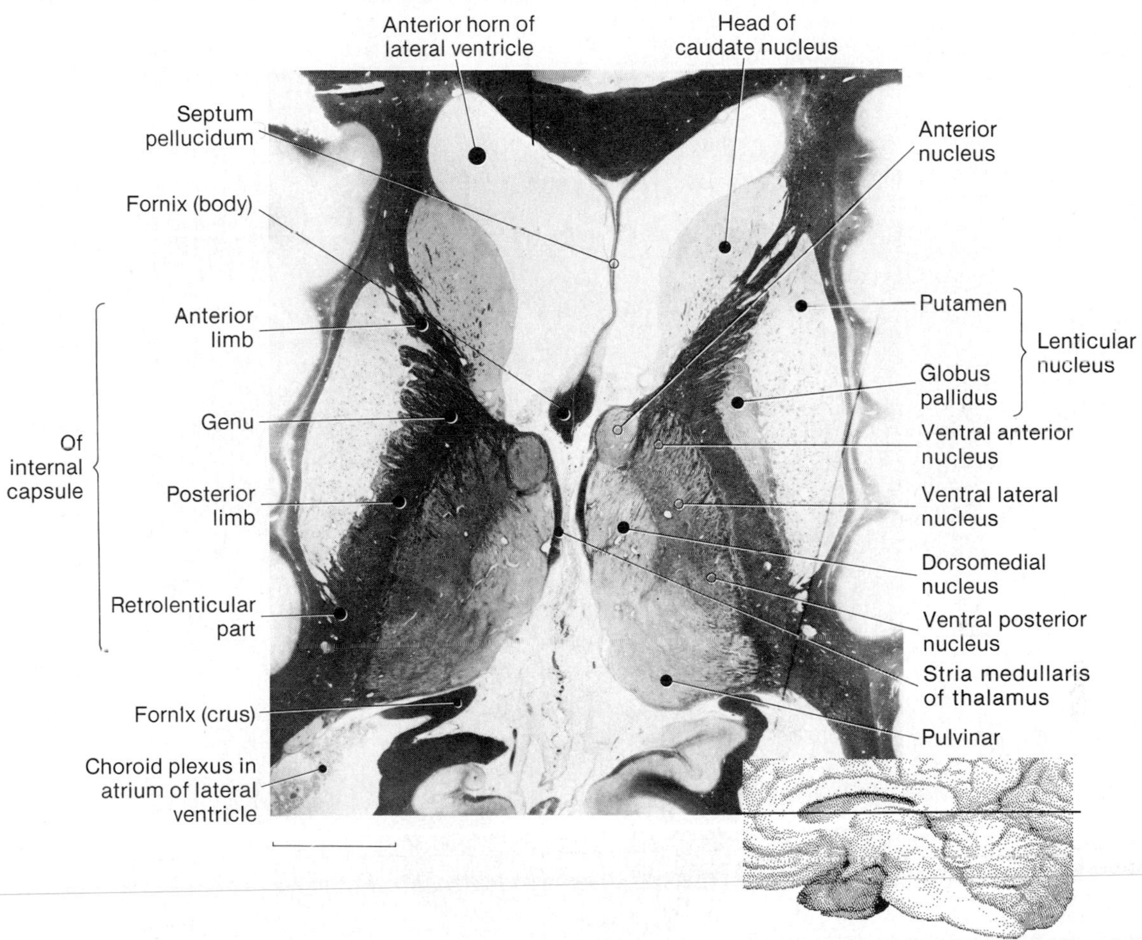


FIGURE 10-7
Horizontal section through the thalamus at a level slightly superior to that of Figure 10-6. Scale mark = 1 cm.

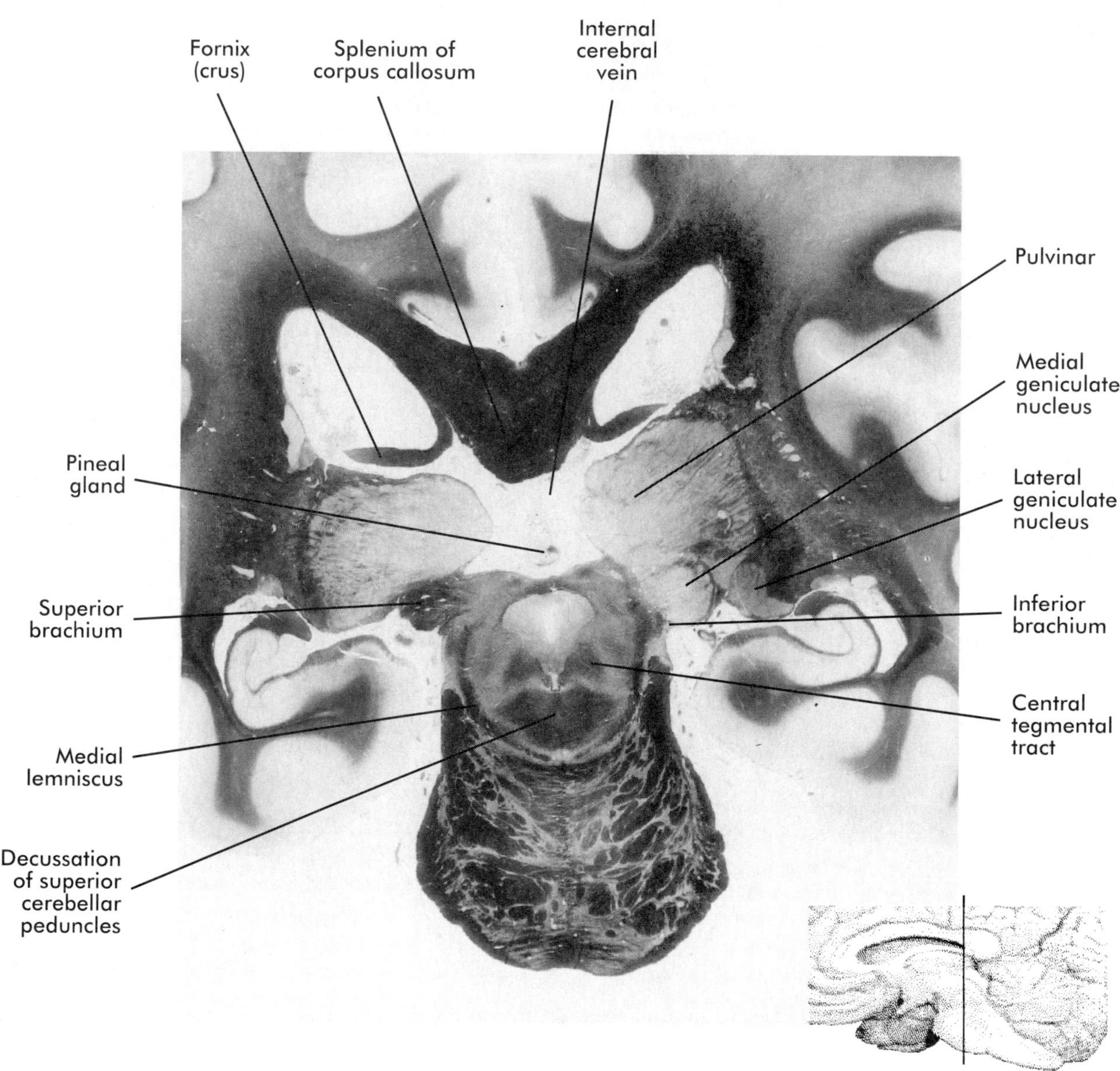


FIGURE 10-8
Coronal section through the posterior thalamus. Scale mark = 1 cm.

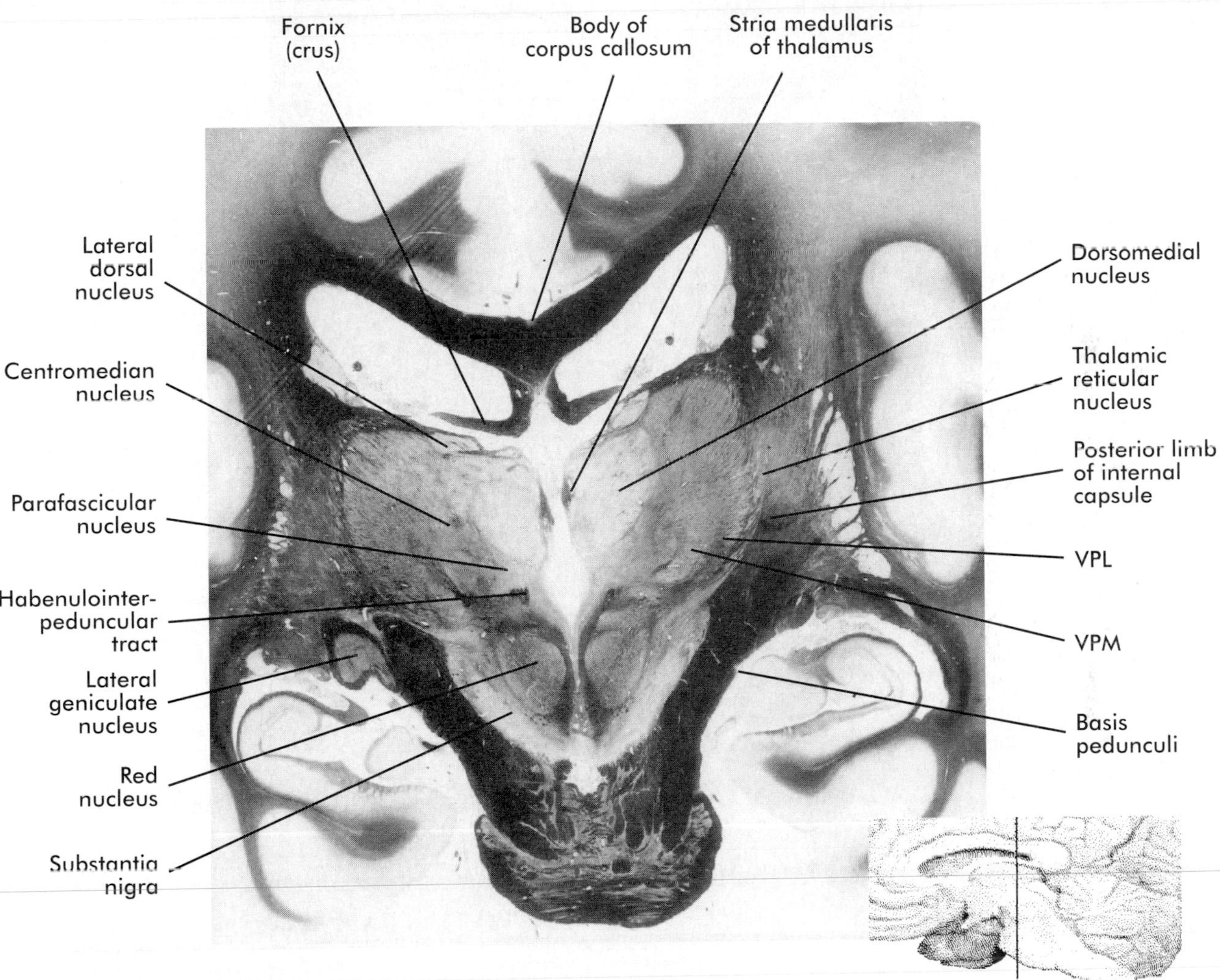


FIGURE 10-9
Coronal section through posterior thalamus. Scale mark = 1 cm.

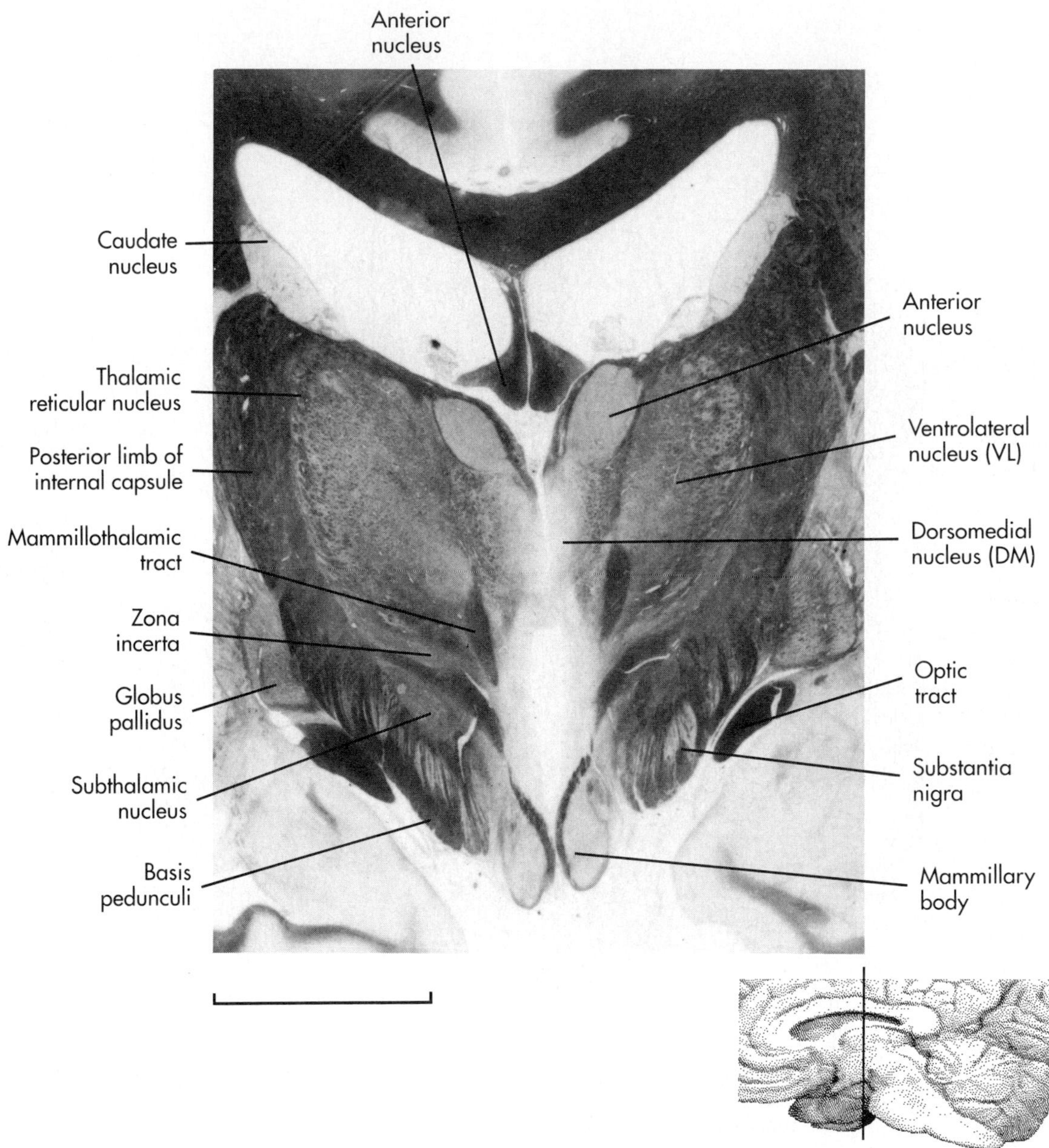


FIGURE 10-10
Coronal section through anterior thalamus. Scale mark = 1 cm.

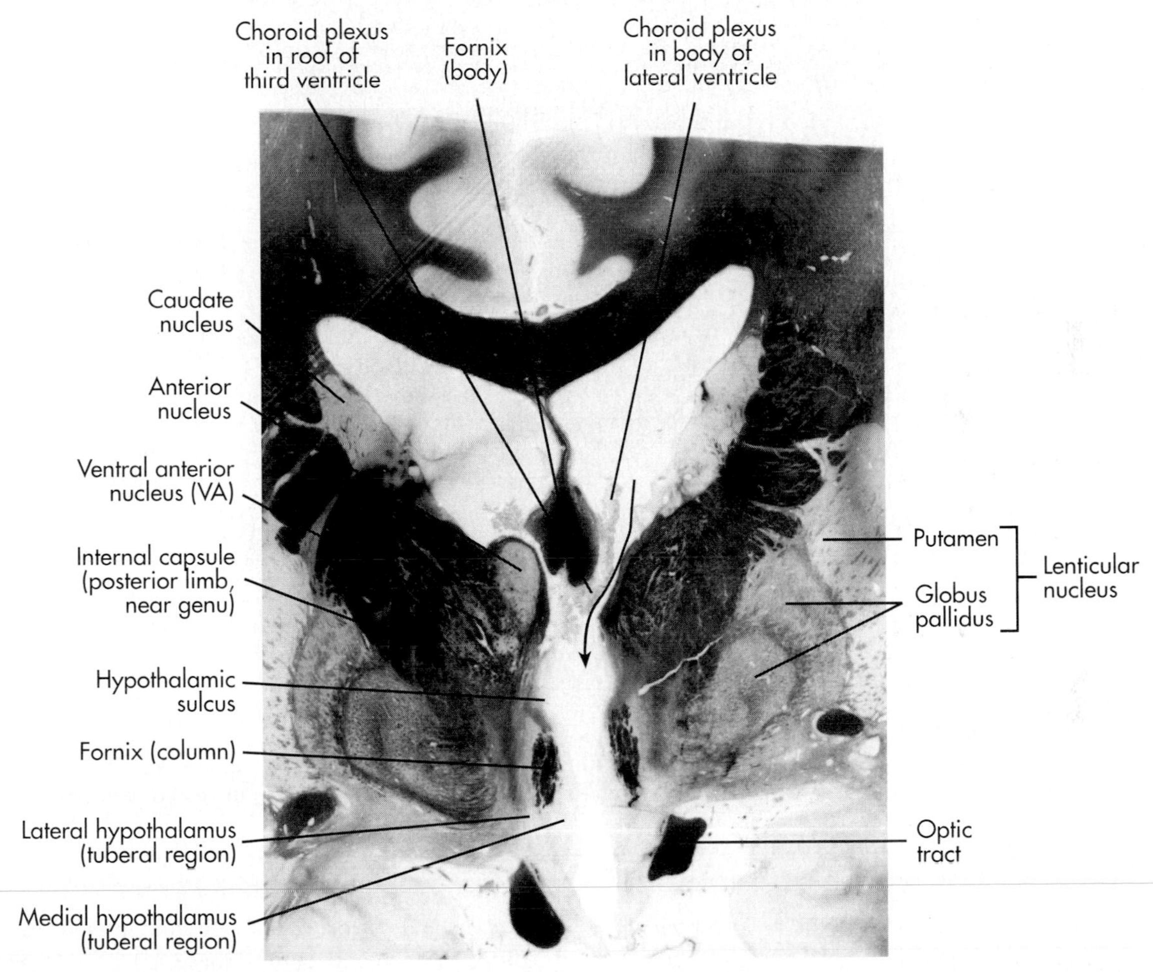


FIGURE 10-11
Coronal section through anterior thalamus at the interventricular foramen. An arrow passes through this foramen on the right. Scale mark = 1 cm.

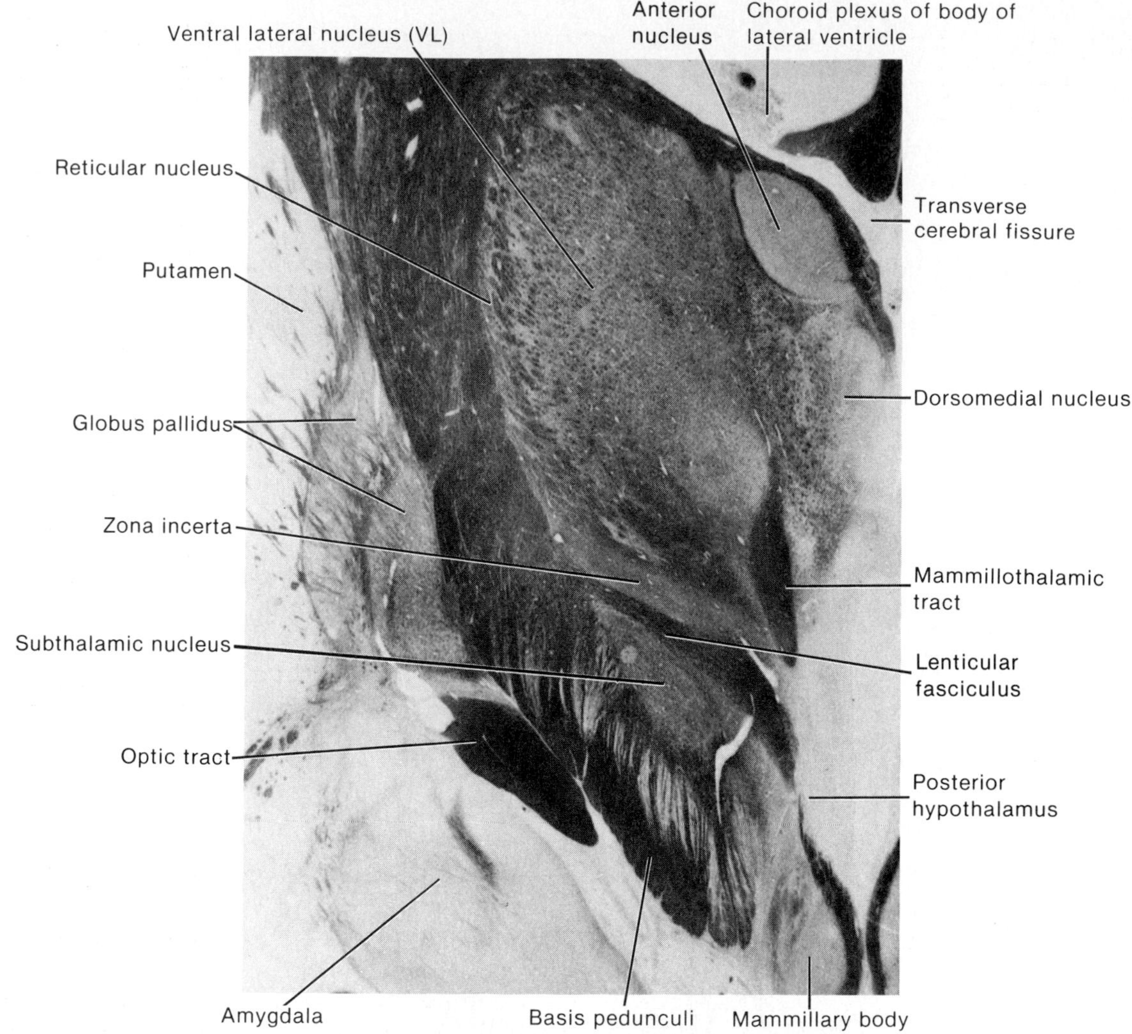


FIGURE 10-12
Enlargement of the section shown in Figure 10-10 to demonstrate the subthalamic region more clearly. The lenticular fasciculus is an output bundle from the basal ganglia on its way from the globus pallidus to the VL and VA.

ina and the internal capsule is the *reticular nucleus* of the thalamus (Figures 10-6, 10-7, 10-9, and 10-12). The reticular nucleus looks continuous inferiorly with the zona incerta (Figure 10-12), but this continuity is of no apparent functional significance.

4. A thin layer of cells, essentially a rostral continuation of parts of the periaqueductal gray, covers portions of the medial surface of the thalamus. These cells constitute the *midline nuclei* of the thalamus (not to be confused with the dorsomedial nucleus). The midline nuclei of the two sides fuse in the interthalamic adhesion, when it is present.

### Functional subdivisions

Thalamic nuclei are interconnected with the cerebral cortex in various ways. Some receive well-defined bundles of fibers and project specifically to particular functional areas of the cerebral cortex; these are called *specific relay nuclei*. A good example of a specific relay nucleus is the medial geniculate nucleus, which receives the inferior brachium and projects to auditory cortex in the temporal lobe. Other nuclei receive their inputs from a variety of places and project to fairly broad areas of association cortex (explained in Chapter 15); these are appropriately called *association nuclei*. Still other nuclei, called *nonspecific nuclei,* project to extremely widespread areas of the cortex, frequently via fibers that are collaterals of fibers on their way to someplace else. Finally, one nucleus has no projections to the cerebral cortex at all; it is naturally called a *subcortical nucleus*.

The cortical connections of thalamic nuclei are often described as though they were one-way affairs (for exam-

**TABLE 7** *Thalamic nuclei*

| *Type* | *Name of nucleus* | *Major subcortical input* | *Major output* |
|---|---|---|---|
| Specific relay | Lateral geniculate | Optic tract | Visual cortex |
| | Medial geniculate | Inferior brachium | Auditory cortex |
| | Ventral posterolateral (VPL) | Medial lemniscus, spinothalamic tract | Somatosensory cortex |
| | Ventral posteromedial (VPM) | Trigeminothalamic tracts | Somatosensory cortex |
| | Ventral lateral, ventral anterior (VL/VA*) | Cerebellum, basal ganglia | Motor/premotor cortex |
| | Anterior | Mammillothalamic tract | Cingulate gyrus |
| Association | Pulvinar | Retina, superior colliculus | Parietal-occipital-temporal association cortex |
| | Lateral posterior (LP) | Superior colliculus | Parietal association cortex |
| | Lateral dorsal (LD) | Few | Cingulate gyrus |
| | Dorsomedial (DM)† | Amygdala, septal area, olfactory cortex | Prefrontal cortex |
| Nonspecific | Part of VA | Other thalamic nuclei? | Prefrontal cortex |
| | Intralaminar | Reticular formation, basal ganglia, cerebellum, somatosensory pathways | Collaterals to widespread cortical areas |
| Subcortical | Reticular | Thalamus | Thalamus |

*The part of the ventral anterior nucleus in which motor fibers end is included as part of the ventral lateral nucleus by some authors. However, as the terms are used in this account, cerebellar efferents end primarily in the VL and pallidal efferents primarily in part of the VA.
†Referred to by many authors as the mediodorsal nucleus (MD).

ple, inferior brachium → medial geniculate nucleus → auditory cortex). However, as a general rule these connections are reciprocal (see Figure 10-3). In addition, thalamic nuclei may receive inputs from cortical areas to which they do not project.

### *Specific relay nuclei*

The specific relay nuclei and their connections are indicated in Figures 10-4 and 10-5 and Table 7. They include the sensory relay nuclei (the VPL/VPM and the geniculate nuclei) and several others as well, since parts of the motor and limbic systems also have thalamic relays. The VL and VA are the motor relay nuclei, receiving the superior cerebellar peduncle and various outputs from the basal ganglia and projecting to motor and premotor cortex. The anterior nucleus is the principal relay nucleus for the limbic system, receiving the *mammillothalamic tract* and projecting to the cingulate gyrus. The mammillothalamic tract, as its name implies, arises in the mammillary body (Figure 10-10). The cingulate gyrus is a prominent component of the limbic lobe (see Figure 2-8). The way in which this pathway fits into the limbic system as a whole is detailed in Chapter 16. It was thought for a time that the lateral dorsal (LD) nucleus was an association nucleus connected to association cortex in the parietal lobe. However, more recent evidence indicates that, in projecting to the cingulate gyrus, it closely resembles the anterior nucleus. Therefore, in spite of the fact that a discrete input tract does not end in it, some authors have begun to refer to the LD as a relay nucleus. As might be expected from the uncertainty surrounding its connections, the function of this nucleus is unknown.

One should not get the impression from the preceding description or from Table 7 that a thalamic relay nucleus does no more than pass along to the cortex an unaltered copy of its input. The lateral geniculate nucleus provides a well-studied example showing that this is not the case. Fewer than 25% of the synapses on the thalamocortical neurons of the lateral geniculate actually come from optic tract axons. The rest come from places like visual cortex, the reticular formation, and geniculate interneurons. The reticular inputs are able to cause substantial changes in the response properties of geniculate neurons, and the cortical inputs are probably critical for focusing visual attention.

### *Association nuclei*

There are two great areas of association cortex in the human brain (see Figure 15-13). One is the prefrontal cortex, anterior to the motor areas of the frontal lobe. The second is the parietal-occipital-temporal association cortex occupying the area surrounded by the primary somatosensory, visual, and auditory cortices. Corresponding to these two areas are two large association nuclei or nuclear complexes (Figure 10-5). The dorsomedial nucleus is reciprocally interconnected with the prefrontal cortex and is involved in prefrontal functions such as affect and foresight, as described further in Chapters 15 and 16. Bilateral damage to the dorsomedial nucleus or to its connections with the frontal lobe has effects similar in some ways to those of prefrontal lobectomy. Major inputs to the dorsomedial nucleus, in addition to those from prefrontal cortex, come from various elements of the limbic system, such as the amygdala.

The pulvinar/LP complex is reciprocally interconnected with the parietal-occipital-temporal association cortex. The major inputs to this complex, aside from those arising in association cortex, come from parts of the visual system. The pulvinar is the largest nucleus in the human thalamus and is better developed in humans than in any other mammal. One would expect that a nucleus this large and this highly developed in humans would have an important, well-defined function. Unfortunately, the role of the pulvinar (and of the LP) is almost entirely unknown at this time. There are hints that it may be involved in some aspects of visual perception, and there are occasional reports of language deficits following damage to it, but in general no particular syndrome and no obvious sensory deficits follow damage to the pulvinar/LP complex.

### *Nonspecific nuclei*

The midline and intralaminar nuclei and a portion of the VA form a nonspecific system that projects to widespread areas of the cerebral cortex. The precise connections of individual nuclei vary, but with the exception of the centromedian nucleus, they are treated as a group in the following account. Inputs to these nuclei are from diverse sources, including the basal ganglia, cerebellum, brainstem reticular formation, and spinothalamic and spinoreticulothalamic fibers carrying information about dull, aching pain. The efferent projections have long been a matter of controversy. For a time they were regarded as having projections to other thalamic nuclei and to the basal ganglia but none to the cerebral cortex, since retrograde degeneration was not seen in them following removal of large areas of cortex. This finding was at odds with physiological studies showing that stimulation of the nonspecific nuclei causes changes in the electrical activity of broad cortical areas. Anatomical studies using newer tracing techniques have resolved the problem. The major output projections of the nonspecific nuclei are to noncortical targets such as the basal ganglia, but these efferents also send collaterals to the cerebral cortex. The damage caused by destruction of these collaterals during cortical removal in the older anatomical experiments was presumably insufficient to cause retrograde degeneration.

The broad extent of the cortical connections of the nonspecific nuclei makes them suitable for general roles such as regulating the level of cortical excitability; they are considered to be one route through which the ascending reticular activating system affects the cortex.

Although the centromedian nucleus is one of the intralaminar nuclei, it has a special relationship with the basal ganglia and probably has a role different from that of other nonspecific nuclei. The centromedian nucleus, like the pulvinar, is disproportionately large in primates, and its growth parallels the increase in size of the caudate nucleus and putamen. As discussed further in Chapter 13, its major connections are with the basal ganglia and motor areas of the cortex.

### *Subcortical nuclei*

With the cortical projections of the nonspecific nuclei confirmed, the reticular nucleus became the principal representative of the subcortical thalamic nuclei. Inspection of Figures 10-6 and 10-7 reveals that most of the fibers reciprocally connecting the thalamus and cortex must traverse the reticular nucleus. As they do so, these fibers give off collaterals to the reticular nucleus. Thus, for example, the portion of the reticular nucleus adjacent to the VPL/VPM receives convergent inputs from somatosensory fibers on their way to the postcentral gyrus, and from descending fibers on their way from the postcentral gyrus to the VPL/VPM. The output of each portion of the reticular nucleus goes to that thalamic nucleus from which it receives its input. This puts the reticular nucleus in an anatomical position suitable for controlling thalamic output, and there are some indications that it may have a major role in modulating transmission from thalamus to cortex during different phases of the sleep-wake cycle.

## Blood supply

Inspection of a hemisected brain (see Figure 5-6) reveals that the anterior and middle cerebral arteries and their branches near the circle of Willis are anterior to most of the thalamus. The blood supply of the thalamus is therefore mostly from branches of the posterior cerebral artery. Specifically branches of the posterior choroidal artery supply some dorsomedial regions, and most of the rest of the thalamus is supplied by small ganglionic or perforating arteries arising from the posterior cerebral and posterior communicating arteries. These ganglionic arteries are sometimes divided into two groups: a *posteromedial* group arising within the circle of Willis and a *posterolateral* group arising distal to the circle. The posteromedial group tends to supply medial and anterior portions of the thalamus as well as the subthalamus. The posterolateral group (sometimes also called *thalamogeniculate arteries*) supplies most of the posterior and lateral thalamus. Finally, the anterior choroidal artery often sends a few small branches to the subthalamus and to ventral regions of the thalamus, particularly the lateral geniculate nucleus.

## Some functional aspects of the thalamus

As a general rule, the cerebral cortex is more important for the proper functioning of sensory systems in humans than it is in other mammals. For example, cats deprived of somatosensory cortex or visual cortex retain a significant portion of their previous somatosensory or visual capabilities, and rats treated similarly retain even more. Nevertheless, it is sometimes claimed that sensory stimuli, particularly somatosensory stimuli, "enter consciousness" in humans at the level of the thalamus. When the somatosensory cortex in humans is destroyed, the remaining awareness of stimuli is very crude, consisting mainly of an ability by the individual to recognize the fact of being touched or receiving a painful stimulus. The individual's ability to localize the stimulus or to discriminate its intensity is severely impaired. These conclusions are based mainly on studies of humans who have sustained damage to one parietal lobe, but it seems doubtful that the remaining sensory capabilities are in fact a result of consciousness at the level of the thalamus ipsilateral to the lesion. In most cases it appears that the remaining capabilities could be a result of slight bilaterality in the function of the contralateral thalamus and parietal lobe.

Damage to the thalamus most often occurs as a result of vascular accidents, particularly involving the thalamogeniculate arteries. Occasionally tumors may encroach on the thalamus. The damage almost always involves other structures in addition to the thalamus (for example, the adjacent internal capsule), and a large collection of deficits with far-reaching consequences may result from relatively small lesions in this area. Characteristically a type of dysesthesia results from damage more or less restricted to the posterior thalamus. The condition is somewhat similar to trigeminal neuralgia in that paroxysms of intense pain may be triggered by somatosensory stimuli. This pain may spread to involve one entire half of the body. It is usually resistant to pain-killing drugs and is called *thalamic pain*. In addition, those stimuli that do not cause a pain attack may be perceived abnormally; their intensity (and even their modality) may be distorted, and they may seem unusually uncomfortable or pleasant. As mentioned previously, some pain syndromes following damage to more caudal levels of the nervous system are thought to result from an imbalance between the activities of the fast-pain and slow-pain systems. A similar mechanism may be involved in thalamic pain, since the fast-pain spinothalamic fibers end in the VPL/VPM, whereas many of the slow-pain spinothalamic and spinoreticulothalamic fibers end in the intralaminar and other nuclei (excluding the centromedian nucleus). Thus it would be possible for a posterior thalamic lesion to preferentially damage the fast-pain system, just as mesencephalic tractotomy does (see Chapter 8).

Extensive damage to the posterior thalamus also causes total (or nearly total) loss of somatic sensation in the contralateral head and body. After a period of time, some appreciation of painful, thermal, and gross tactile stimuli usually returns. Functions customarily associated with the medial lemniscus tend to be more severely and permanently impaired. Discriminative tactile sensibility may be abolished, position sense may be greatly impaired, and a sensory type of ataxia (resulting from the loss of proprioception) may persist. The combination of thalamic pain, hemianesthesia, and sensory ataxia, all contralateral to a posterior thalamic lesion, is called the *thalamic syndrome*. It is often accompanied by mild and transient paralysis (a result of damage to corticospinal fibers in the adjacent internal capsule) and by various types of residual involuntary movements (a result of damage to nearby basal ganglia).

## INTERNAL CAPSULE

The large collection of thalamocortical and corticothalamic fibers just described need a route by which to travel from their origins to their destinations. This route is provided by the *internal capsule,* a compact bundle of fibers through which almost all the neural traffic to and from the cerebral cortex passes. As Figures 10-6 and 10-7 indicate, the internal capsule is in a convenient location for fibers entering or leaving the thalamus. In addition to these, other fibers descend from the cortex through the internal capsule and then through the cerebral peduncle to reach pontine nuclei *(corticopontine fibers),* motor nuclei of cranial nerves *(corticobulbar fibers),* and spinal cord motor neurons and interneurons *(corticospinal fibers)*. Still other fibers project from the cerebral cortex through the internal capsule to additional subcortical targets, such as various nuclei of the extrapyramidal system (for example, the putamen and the caudate nucleus).

The three-dimensional shape of the internal capsule is a bit difficult to visualize, but the beautiful dissections shown in Figures 10-13 and 10-14 should help. The internal capsule is a continuous sheet of fibers that forms the medial boundary of the lenticular nucleus (Figure 10-13) and then continues around posteriorly and inferiorly to partially envelop this nucleus (Figure 10-14). Inferiorly many of the fibers in the internal capsule funnel down into the cerebral peduncle. Superiorly they all fan out into the *corona radiata* (Figures 10-13 and 10-14), in which they travel through the cerebral white matter to reach their cortical origins or destinations. Thus the entire fiber system is shaped like a trumpet with a large notch cut out of its bell (Figure 10-14); the flared-out bell corresponds to the region where the fibers of the internal capsule spread out to form the corona radiata, and the notch corresponds to the location where this continuous sheet of fibers is interrupted in an intact brain by the lateral sulcus. The narrowest part of the trumpet corresponds to the cerebral peduncle, and in an intact brain the lenticular nucleus sits where a mute would sit in a trumpet.

The internal capsule is divided into five regions on the basis of the relationship of each part to the lenticular nucleus (Figures 10-6 and 10-7). The *anterior limb* is the portion between the lenticular nucleus and the head of the caudate nucleus. The *posterior limb* is the portion between the lenticular nucleus and the thalamus. The *genu* is the

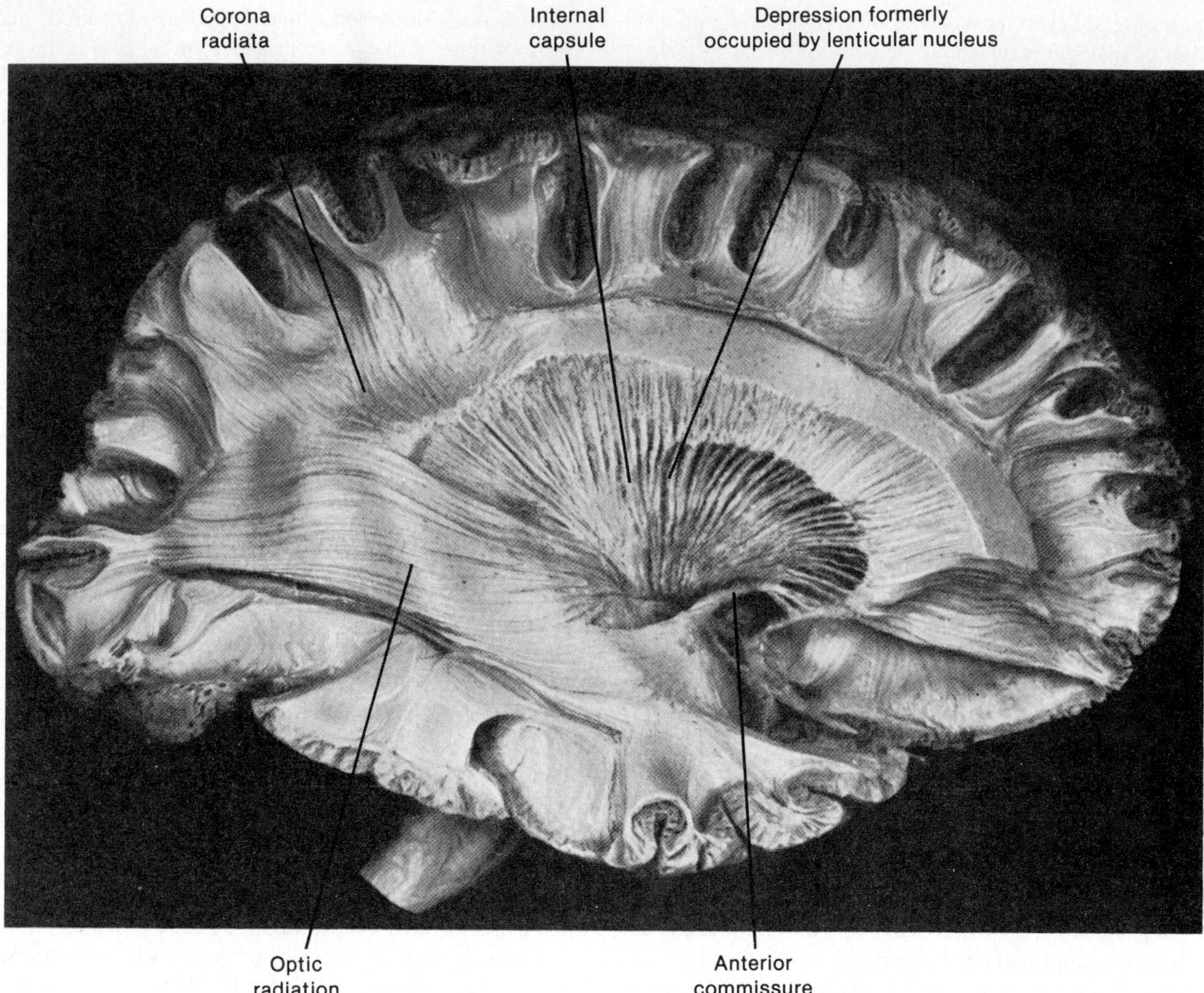


FIGURE 10-13
Dissection of the right cerebral hemisphere from its lateral aspect. Most of the cerebral cortex, including that of the insula, was removed. The lenticular nucleus (putamen and globus pallidus) was then removed, revealing the internal capsule. The internal capsule outlines the former location of the lenticular nucleus, and its fibers then continue into the corona radiata. The fibers of the anterior commissure can also be seen collecting from the temporal lobe and projecting toward the midline.
From Ludwig E, Klingler J: Atlas cerebri humani, Boston, 1956, Little Brown & Co.

portion at the junction of the anterior and posterior limbs; since this junction occurs at the anterior end of the thalamus, the genu is adjacent to the interventricular foramen (Figures 10-6 and 10-11) and to the venous angle (see Figure 5-21). The *retrolenticular part* is the portion posterior to the lenticular nucleus. The *sublenticular part* is the portion inferior to the lenticular nucleus. The demarcation of the anterior and posterior limbs is distinct at the genu, but the transition from the posterior limb to the retrolenticular part to the sublenticular part is gradual, and dividing lines between these portions are somewhat arbitrary. Since the internal capsule is a continuous, curved sheet of fibers, it is not possible to see all of its parts in any one section, no matter what the plane of the section is. It is possible to see the first four parts mentioned above in a single horizontal section (Figures 10-6 and 10-7), but to get a clear idea of the sublenticular part, it is usually necessary to use coronal sections.

By and large, the contents of each portion of the internal capsule can be inferred from its anatomical location. Major components are as follows:

1. The anterior limb contains the fibers interconnecting

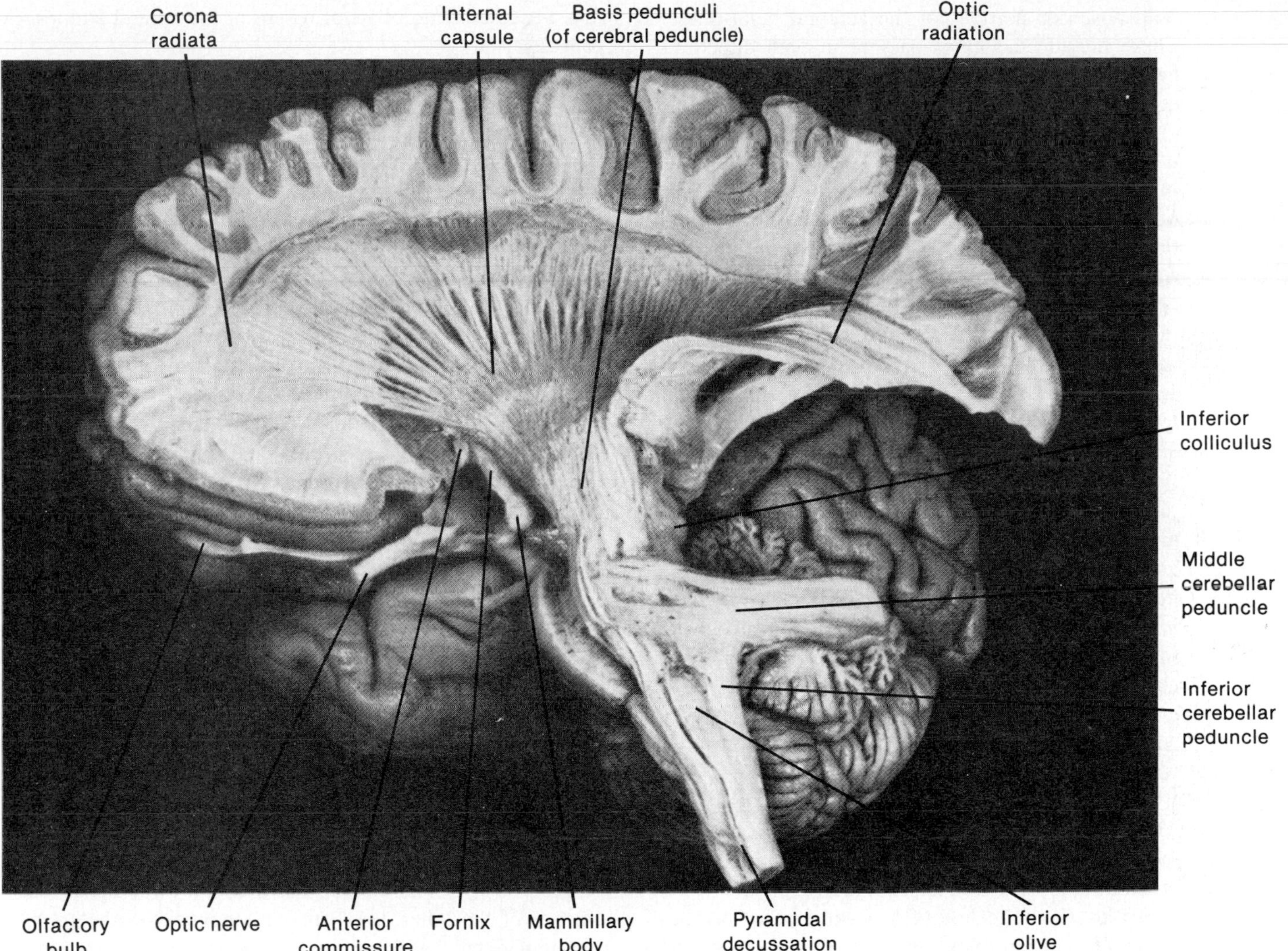


FIGURE 10-14
Dissection of the left cerebral hemisphere from its lateral aspect. This dissection is similar to that of Figure 10-13 except that the temporal lobe has also been removed so that the continuity of the internal capsule and the cerebral peduncle can be seen. The flared-out, trumpet-shaped progression from the cerebral peduncle, through the internal capsule, and into the corona radiata is shown here about as well as it can be. The entire course of the pyramidal tract from the corona radiata through the medullary pyramid can also be seen, as can the origin of the middle cerebellar peduncle in the basal part of the pons.
From Ludwig E, Klingler J: Atlas cerebri humani, Boston, 1956, Little, Brown & Co.

the anterior nucleus and the cingulate gyrus and those interconnecting the dorsomedial nucleus and prefrontal cortex. Also included are some of the fibers projecting from the frontal lobe to the ipsilateral pontine nuclei *(frontopontine fibers)*.

2. The posterior limb contains fibers interconnecting the VA and VL with the motor and premotor cortex. It also contains the corticospinal and corticobulbar fibers and the somatosensory fibers projecting from the VPL/VPM to the postcentral gyrus. It was thought for many years that the corticospinal and corticobulbar fibers were located in the anterior portion of the posterior limb near the genu. For most of their course, however, these fibers are actually located in the posterior third of the posterior limb adjacent to the somatosensory projections.
3. The genu is a transition zone between the anterior and posterior limbs and contains some frontopontine fibers as well as many of the fibers interconnecting the VA and VL with the motor and premotor cortex.
4. The retrolenticular part of the internal capsule contains most of the fibers interconnecting the thalamus

with posterior portions of the cerebral hemisphere. These include the fibers passing in both directions between the parietal-occipital-temporal association cortex and the pulvinar/LP complex. They also include part of the *optic radiation*. The optic radiation is the large collection of visual system fibers projecting from the lateral geniculate nucleus to the banks of the calcarine sulcus. The portion in the retrolenticular part of the internal capsule ends in the superior bank of the calcarine sulcus. As explained in the next chapter, these are the fibers conveying information from inferior portions of the visual fields. Finally, the retrolenticular part also contains additional corticopontine fibers, principally from the parietal lobe.

5. The sublenticular part of the internal capsule is continuous with the retrolenticular part and contains the remainder of the optic radiation (that is, those fibers ending in the inferior bank of the calcarine sulcus and carrying information about superior visual fields). The sublenticular part also contains the *auditory radiation,* whose fibers pass laterally from the medial geniculate nucleus under the lenticular nucleus and lateral sulcus and then turn superiorly to end in the superior temporal gyrus (see Figures 9-39 and 10-9).

### Blood supply

The blood supply of the internal capsule is from two principal sources, the *lateral striate arteries* and the *anterior choroidal artery*. The lateral striate (or *lenticulostriate*) arteries are the collection of fine ganglionic branches of the proximal portion of the middle cerebral artery and supply most of the anterior limb, genu, and posterior limb. The anterior limb and genu also receive part of their supply from ganglionic branches of the anterior cerebral and anterior communicating arteries, particularly from a relatively large one called the *recurrent artery (of Heubner),* or *medial striate artery*. The anterior choroidal artery supplies inferior and posterior regions of the internal capsule. It overlaps the lateral striate arteries in supplying the posterior limb and provides most of the supply of the retrolenticular and sublenticular parts. Ganglionic branches of the posterior cerebral artery also help supply the retrolenticular and sublenticular parts.

Small strokes in the internal capsule could obviously have major consequences. Hemorrhage of a lateral striate artery in the vicinity of the posterior limb can result in contralateral spastic paralysis and hemianesthesia. If the retrolenticular and sublenticular parts are also involved, visual deficits would be added to the symptoms (and would indicate that the damage was almost certainly in the internal capsule). The auditory radiations would be damaged as well, but this would produce relatively minor deficits because of the bilateral nature of the central auditory pathways.

## HYPOTHALAMUS

The hypothalamus is a small portion of the diencephalon (weighing only about 4 g) but is important as a nodal point in pathways concerned with autonomic, endocrine, emotional, and somatic functions. For example, stimulation of appropriate hypothalamic areas in experimental animals can cause vasodilation, rage, feeding behavior, or alterations of pituitary function. Accordingly the connections of the hypothalamus are widespread and complex, but they fall into three principal categories: (1) interconnections with various components of the limbic system, (2) outputs that influence the pituitary gland, and (3) interconnections with various visceral and somatic nuclei, both motor and sensory, of the brainstem and spinal cord. The hypothalamus is divided into a number of nuclei and areas, as described shortly. Each of these different nuclei and areas has more or less distinctive connections, but for the sake of simplicity these connections are discussed here as though the hypothalamus were by and large a uniform structure.

### Extent and subdivisions of the hypothalamus

The inferior surface of the hypothalamus (see Figures 2-15 and 2-16), exposed directly to subarachnoid space, is bounded by the optic chiasm, the optic tracts, and the posterior edge of the mammillary bodies. This area, exclusive of the mammillary bodies, is called the *tuber cinereum* (Figure 10-15). The *median eminence,* a swelling on the surface of the tuber cinereum, is continuous with the infundibular stalk, which in turn is continuous with the posterior lobe of the pituitary. The median eminence, infundibular stalk, and posterior lobe together constitute the *neurohypophysis*.

The medial surface of the hypothalamus (Figure 10-1) extends anteriorly to the lamina terminalis, superiorly to the hypothalamic sulcus, and posteriorly to the caudal edge of the diencephalon. As mentioned previously, the longitudinal boundaries are semiarbitrary. For example, the anterior border of the hypothalamus technically is the plane through the anterior edge of the optic chiasm and the posterior edge of the anterior commissure. However, the neural tissue immediately in front of this formal boundary is structurally and functionally continuous with the hypothalamus. Therefore this region (the *preoptic area*), traditionally considered to be part of the telencephalon, is usually treated instead as part of the anterior hypothalamus.

The hypothalamus can be subdivided longitudinally into *anterior, tuberal,* and *posterior* regions. The anterior region is the part above the optic chiasm, the tuberal region is the part above and including the tuber cinereum, and the posterior region is the part above and including the mam-

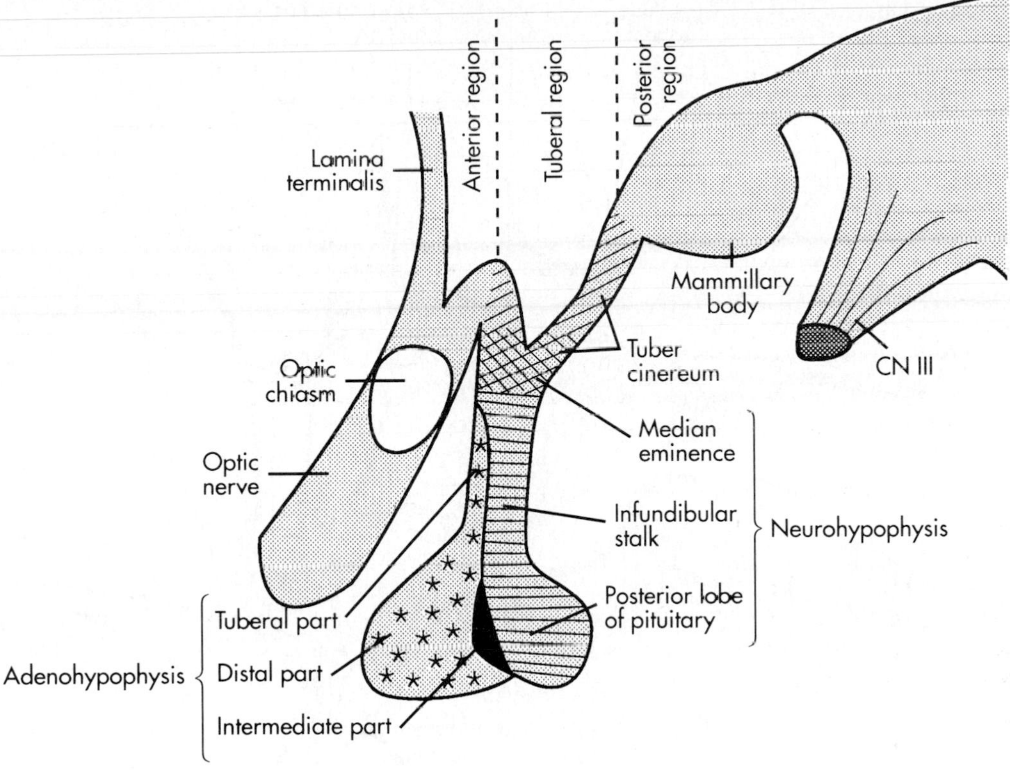


FIGURE 10-15
Regions of the hypothalamus and pituitary in midsagittal view. The entire area filled with diagonal lines is the tuber cinereum. The crosshatched portion of the tuber cinereum is the median eminence.

millary bodies. In addition, the entire hypothalamus of each side is divided into *medial* and *lateral* zones* by a parasagittal plane through the fornix as this fiber bundle traverses the hypothalamus (Figures 10-11 and 10-16). Thus the hypothalamus consists of six parts on each side: the medial and lateral zones of the anterior, tuberal, and posterior regions. The principal nuclei of these areas are indicated in Table 8 and Figure 10-16.

The lateral zone consists mainly of scattered cells interspersed among the longitudinally running fibers of the *medial forebrain bundle*. Anteriorly it is continuous with the lateral preoptic nucleus, and caudally it is continuous with the midbrain tegmentum. Part of the supraoptic nucleus intrudes into it, as do clumps of cells called *lateral tuberal nuclei,* but otherwise it is undivided.

The medial zone, on the other hand, contains a number

*The part of the medial hypothalamus immediately adjacent to the wall of the third ventricle is often considered separately as a *periventricular* zone.

**TABLE 8** *Hypothalamic nuclei*

| *Region* | *Medial area* | *Lateral area* |
|---|---|---|
| Anterior | Medial preoptic nucleus | Lateral preoptic nucleus |
| | Supraoptic nucleus | Lateral nucleus |
| | Paraventricular nucleus | Part of supraoptic nucleus |
| | Anterior nucleus | |
| | Suprachiasmatic nucleus | |
| Tuberal | Dorsomedial nucleus | Lateral nucleus |
| | Ventromedial nucleus | Lateral tuberal nuclei |
| | Arcuate (infundibular) nucleus | |
| Posterior | Mammillary body | Lateral nucleus |
| | Posterior nucleus | |

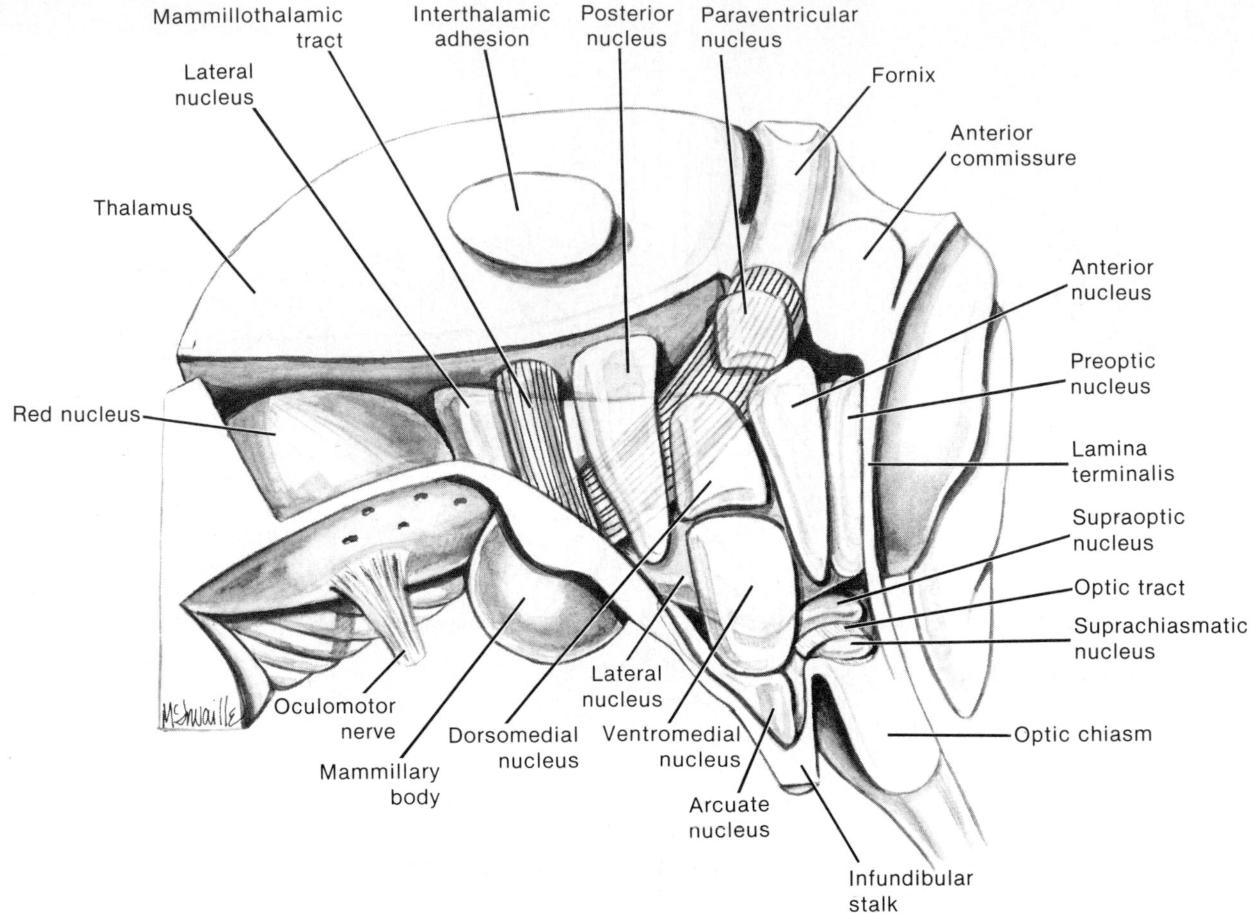


FIGURE 10-16
Principal nuclei of the hypothalamus.
Modified from Nauta WJH, Haymaker W: The hypothalamus, 1969. Courtesy of Charles C Thomas, Publisher, Springfield, Illinois.

of nuclei. The supraoptic region contains two distinctive nuclei containing large neurosecretory cells, the *supraoptic* and *paraventricular nuclei*. The supraoptic nucleus sits astride the optic tract, extending into the lateral hypothalamic zone; the paraventricular nucleus is higher up in the wall of the third ventricle, adjacent to the anterior commissure. Most cells of the supraoptic nucleus and many cells of the paraventricular nucleus secrete hormones that travel down the axons of these cells and are released in the neurohypophysis. The hormones involved and the pathway traversed by them are discussed later in this chapter (see Figure 10-19). The supraoptic region also contains a small *suprachiasmatic nucleus* and a larger *anterior nucleus*. The suprachiasmatic nucleus, as described in the next chapter, receives direct projections from the retina and is important in the regulation of diurnal rhythms. The anterior nucleus is continuous anteriorly with the medial preoptic nucleus.

The medial tuberal region is subdivided into dorsal and ventral portions called the *dorsomedial* and *ventromedial nuclei*, respectively. In addition, cells in the floor of the infundibular recess of the third ventricle constitute the *arcuate* (or *infundibular*) *nucleus*.

The medial mammillary region contains the mammillary body (actually a complex of several nuclei) and the *posterior hypothalamic nucleus,* which is continuous with the periaqueductal gray matter of the midbrain.

## Afferents to the hypothalamus

Hypothalamic inputs arise in two general areas (Figure 10-17); (1) various parts of the forebrain, particularly components of the limbic system, and (2) the brainstem and spinal cord. Afferents from the brainstem and spinal cord convey visceral and somatic sensory information, whereas those from limbic structures convey information relevant to the role of the hypothalamus in mediating many of the autonomic and somatic aspects of affective states. The connections of limbic components with each other and with the hypothalamus are discussed in Chapter 16 and are only mentioned briefly here.

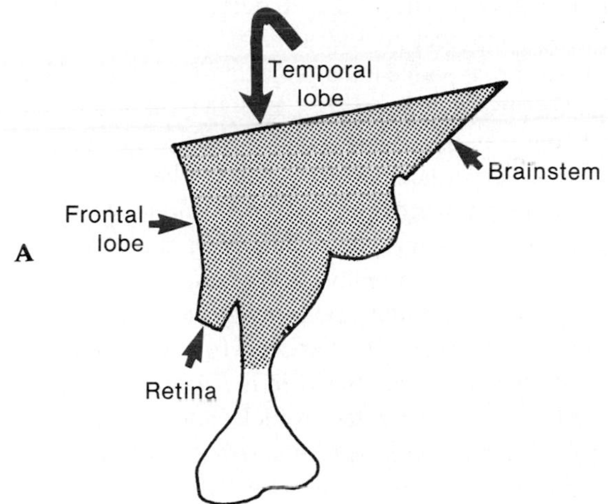


FIGURE 10-17
Major inputs to the hypothalamus. **A,** Schematic indication of the directions from which these inputs come. Those labeled "frontal lobe" arise in the orbital cortex of the frontal lobe and also from limbic structures near the hypothalamus such as the septal area. Inputs from the temporal lobe arise in the hippocampal formation and amygdala. **B,** More detailed depiction of hypothalamic afferents. The medial forebrain bundle includes afferents arising in both the septal area and the brainstem. Some inputs from the amygdala travel through the stria terminalis, which follows a path parallel to the lateral ventricle; others take a more direct route (indicated but unlabeled in this figure) under the lenticular nucleus, referred to as the *ventral amygdalofugal pathway*. *AM,* Amygdala; *DLF,* dorsal longitudinal fasciculus; *F,* fornix; *H,* hippocampus; *MFB,* medial forebrain bundle; *MP,* mammillary peduncle; *O,* orbital cortex of frontal lobe; *OT,* optic tract; *S,* septal area; *ST,* stria terminalis.

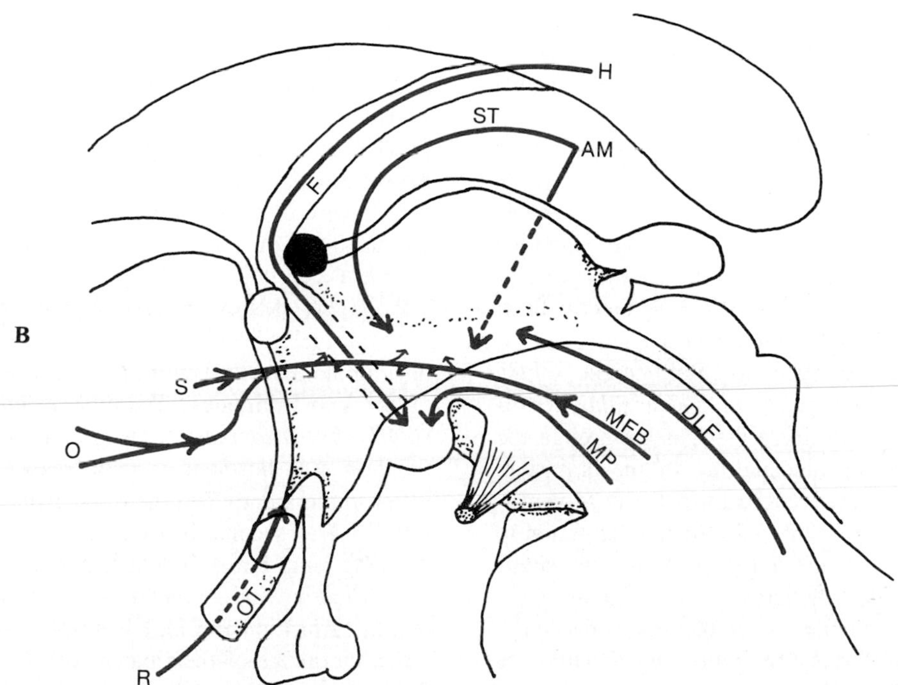

### *Afferents from the forebrain*

Major forebrain afferents to the hypothalamus arise in (1) the septal area and nearby parts of the basal forebrain, (2) the hippocampal formation, (3) the amygdala, (4) the orbital cortex of the frontal lobe, and (5) the retina. The *septal area,* a prominent component of the limbic system located adjacent to the septum pellucidum, projects fibers to the hypothalamus through the *medial forebrain bundle.* The medial forebrain bundle is built like a frayed rope, with fibers entering and leaving it at many levels as it traverses the lateral hypothalamic zone and extends into the brainstem tegmentum. This is a bidirectional bundle, containing afferents from the brainstem to the hypothalamus as well as hypothalamic efferents passing both rostrally and caudally and fibers interconnecting different hypothalamic levels.

The major output from the hippocampal formation is contained in the fornix. This fiber bundle arches around under the corpus callosum and through the hypothalamus, where most of its fibers reach the mammillary body (see Figure 16-10).

The amygdala projects fibers to the hypothalamus by two different routes. Some travel through the *stria terminalis,* a long, curved fiber bundle that accompanies the caudate nucleus. Others take a shorter course and pass under the lenticular nucleus directly to the hypothalamus.

Finally, there are direct projections from the cerebral cortex to the hypothalamus. These arise mainly in the orbital cortex of the frontal lobe and in the insula and join the medial forebrain bundle.

### *Afferents from the brainstem and spinal cord*

An assortment of sensory inputs reaches the hypothalamus by routes that are incompletely understood. Some involve synapses in various portions of the reticular formation and periaqueductal gray; others arrive directly from sites such as the solitary and parabrachial nuclei. Some of these afferents travel in the medial forebrain bundle, others are contained in the *dorsal longitudinal fasciculus,* a collection of thinly myelinated fibers that passes through the periventricular and periaqueductal gray of the brainstem and then fans in the hypothalamic wall of the third ventricle. Others travel from the midbrain reticular formation to the mammillary body and other parts of the hypothalamus by way of the *mammillary peduncle;* many of these fibers join the medial forebrain bundle once they reach the hypothalamus. Still other afferents enter the hypothalamus as collaterals of fibers in other pathways such as the spinothalamic tract.

### *Physical inputs*

In addition to receiving various types of visceral and somatic information through the brainstem pathways just mentioned, the hypothalamus contains cells that are directly responsive to physical stimuli. Some of these cells are sensitive to the temperature of the hypothalamus itself, whereas the activity of others is sensitive to such things as the concentration of glucose or certain hormones in the hypothalamus.

## Efferents from the hypothalamus

Efferent pathways from the hypothalamus are, to a great extent, reciprocal to the afferent pathways (Figure 10-18). Thus the hypothalamus projects to the septal area, the hippocampus, the amygdala, and the brainstem and spinal cord by way of the same fiber bundles that carry afferents to the hypothalamus (the mammillary peduncle, however, is thought to contain no hypothalamic efferents). In addition, a few pathways are totally or predominantly efferent in nature. The prominent *mammillothalamic tract* passes from the mammillary body to the anterior nucleus of the thalamus (Figures 10-10 and 16-14). Some fibers in the mammillothalamic tract travel in the opposite direction as well (that is, from the anterior nucleus to the mammillary body). The *mammillotegmental tract* branches from the mammillothalamic tract near the latter's origin and projects to the midbrain reticular formation.

### *Outputs to the pituitary gland*

The final efferent pathways from the hypothalamus are of great functional importance because they control the *pituitary gland* (or *hypophysis*). This control is accomplished by two means: a neural projection to the neurohypophysis and a vascular link with the adenohypophysis.

The supraoptic and paraventricular nuclei, as mentioned previously, contain large neurosecretory cells. (The paraventricular nucleus also contains numerous smaller cells, many of which project as hypothalamic efferents to the dorsal motor nucleus of the vagus nerve, the intermediolateral cell column of the spinal cord, and other sites.) The larger, neurosecretory cells of the supraoptic and paraventricular nuclei produce two peptide hormones, each nine amino acids in length; a given cell produces only one of the two hormones. The first is *antidiuretic hormone* (*ADH,* or *vasopressin*), whose principal physiological function as a hormone is to increase the reabsorption of water in the kidney and thereby decrease the production of urine.* The second is *oxytocin* (from the Greek words meaning rapid birth), a similar peptide that causes contraction of uterine and mammary smooth muscle and is important in parturition and milk ejection. Both hormones travel down the axons of their parent cell bodies by axoplasmic flow, bound to a carrier protein *(neurophysin).* These neurosecretory cells are electrically excitable, and the passage of action potentials down their axons causes release of their hormones from bulbous endings adjacent to capillar-

*Both vasopressin and oxytocin, like the hypothalamic releasing factors, are also thought to serve as neurotransmitters or neuromodulators, so their total physiological roles extend beyond their functions as hormones.

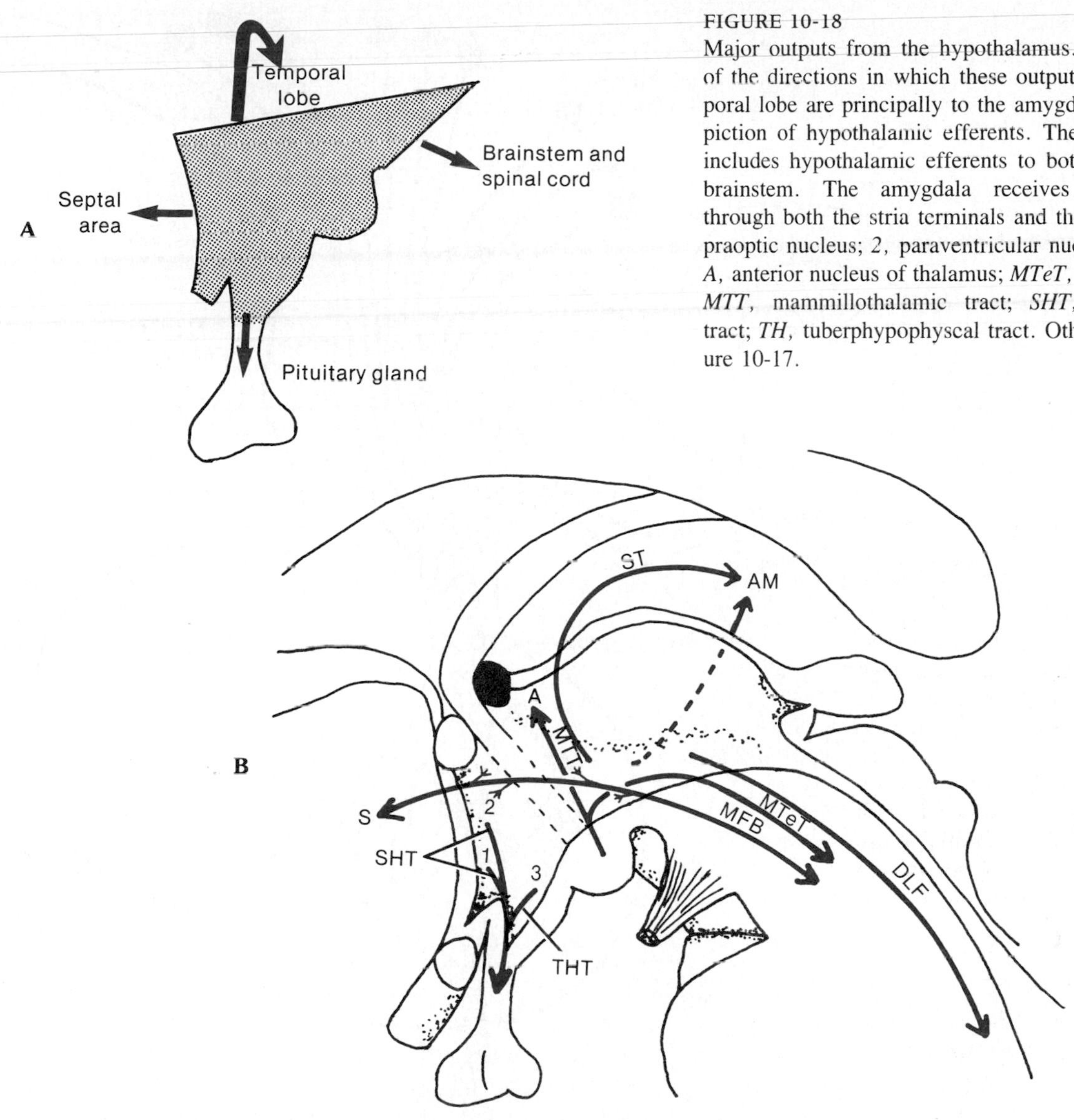


FIGURE 10-18
Major outputs from the hypothalamus. **A,** Schematic indication of the directions in which these outputs go. Outputs to the temporal lobe are principally to the amygdala. **B,** More detailed depiction of hypothalamic efferents. The medial forebrain bundle includes hypothalamic efferents to both the septal area and the brainstem. The amygdala receives hypothalamic efferents through both the stria terminals and the ventral pathway. *1,* Supraoptic nucleus; *2,* paraventricular nucleus; *3,* arcutate nucleus; *A,* anterior nucleus of thalamus; *MTeT,* mammillotegmental tract; *MTT,* mammillothalamic tract; *SHT,* supraopticohypophyseal tract; *TH,* tuberphypophyseal tract. Other abbreviations: see Figure 10-17.

ies in the median eminence, infundibular stalk, and posterior lobe of the pituitary (Figure 10-19). Most of the axons arise in the supraoptic nucleus, so this pathway is called the *supraopticohypophyseal tract*.

The adenohypophysis secretes a multitude of hormones whose discussion is beyond the scope of this book. It has been known for some time that electrical stimulation of certain areas of the hypothalamus can modulate the rates of secretion of these hormones, but no neural connections are known that could explain this modulation. This drew attention to the *hypophyseal portal system* as a vascular connection between the hypothalamus and the adenohypophysis (Figure 10-19). The *superior hypophyseal artery,* a branch of the internal carotid, breaks up into a capillary bed in the median eminence and proximal part of the infundibular stalk. Blood in these capillaries then re-collects into *hypophyseal portal vessels,* which travel down the infundibular stalk and break up into a second capillary bed in the adenohypophysis. Abundant evidence has now shown that small peptides, called *hypothalamic releasing factors* and *inhibiting factors,* are secreted by cells of the arcuate nucleus and nearby sites in the wall of the third ventricle,* travel down the axons of these cells, and are released into the bloodstream in the first capillary bed (recall that the median eminence is one of the circumventricular organs [Figure 5-14] and its capillaries are fenestrated [Figure 5-15]). From there the releasing and inhibiting fac-

*Some of these are located in the paraventricular nucleus, which therefore contains three distinct cell types—large neurons that secrete oxytocin or vasopressin, smaller neurons that secrete releasing or inhibiting factors, and neurons that project to the brainstem and spinal cord.

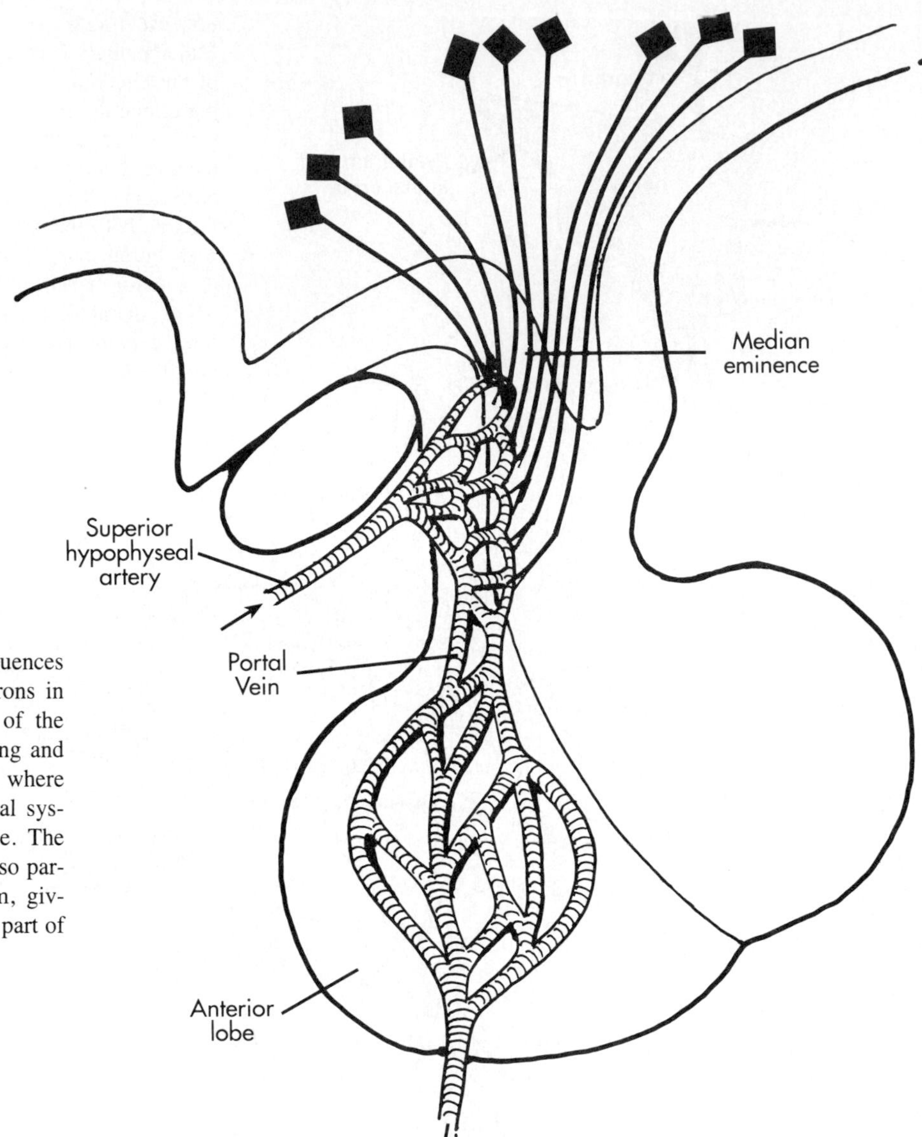


FIGURE 10-19
Routes by which the hypothalamus influences the pituitary gland. *A,* Parvocellular neurons in the arcuate nucleus and nearby regions of the walls of the third ventricle secrete releasing and inhibiting factors in the median eminence, where they gain access to the hypophyseal portal system and through it reach the anterior lobe. The inferior hypophyseal artery (not shown) also participates in the hypophyseal portal system, giving rise to capillary sinusoids in the lower part of the infundibulum.

tors travel down the hypophyseal portal vessels to the adenohypophysis, where they act. As their names imply, releasing factors promote the release of particular hormones, whereas inhibiting factors prevent this release. The entire collection of axons carrying these releasing and inhibiting factors is called the *tuberoinfundibular* or *tuberohypophyseal tract.*

The relatively small cells that secrete releasing and inhibiting factors are commonly referred to as the *parvocellular neurosecretory system,* as distinguished from the *magnocellular neurosecretory system* of larger neurons in the supraoptic and paraventricular nuclei that secrete oxytocin and vasopressin.

A great deal of interest has been generated by the recent discovery that these small hypothalamic peptides are also found in other neurons in widespread areas of the CNS and in other cells of the body as well. This is reminiscent of the situation with enkephalins and endorphins, briefly discussed in Chapter 8. A slowly emerging picture is that in some respects the brain is a much more "distributed" organ than it is normally considered to be—that is, it may use the same chemical both as a neurotransmitter acting locally on a postsynaptic neuron and as a hormone acting at a distance, both actions working toward the same physiological goal.

### Blood supply

Inspection of Figure 5-2 reveals that the infundibular stalk is located just about in the middle of the circle of Willis, and the inferior surface of the entire hypothalamus is more or less surrounded by the circle. The arterial supply of the hypothalamus is derived from a series of small

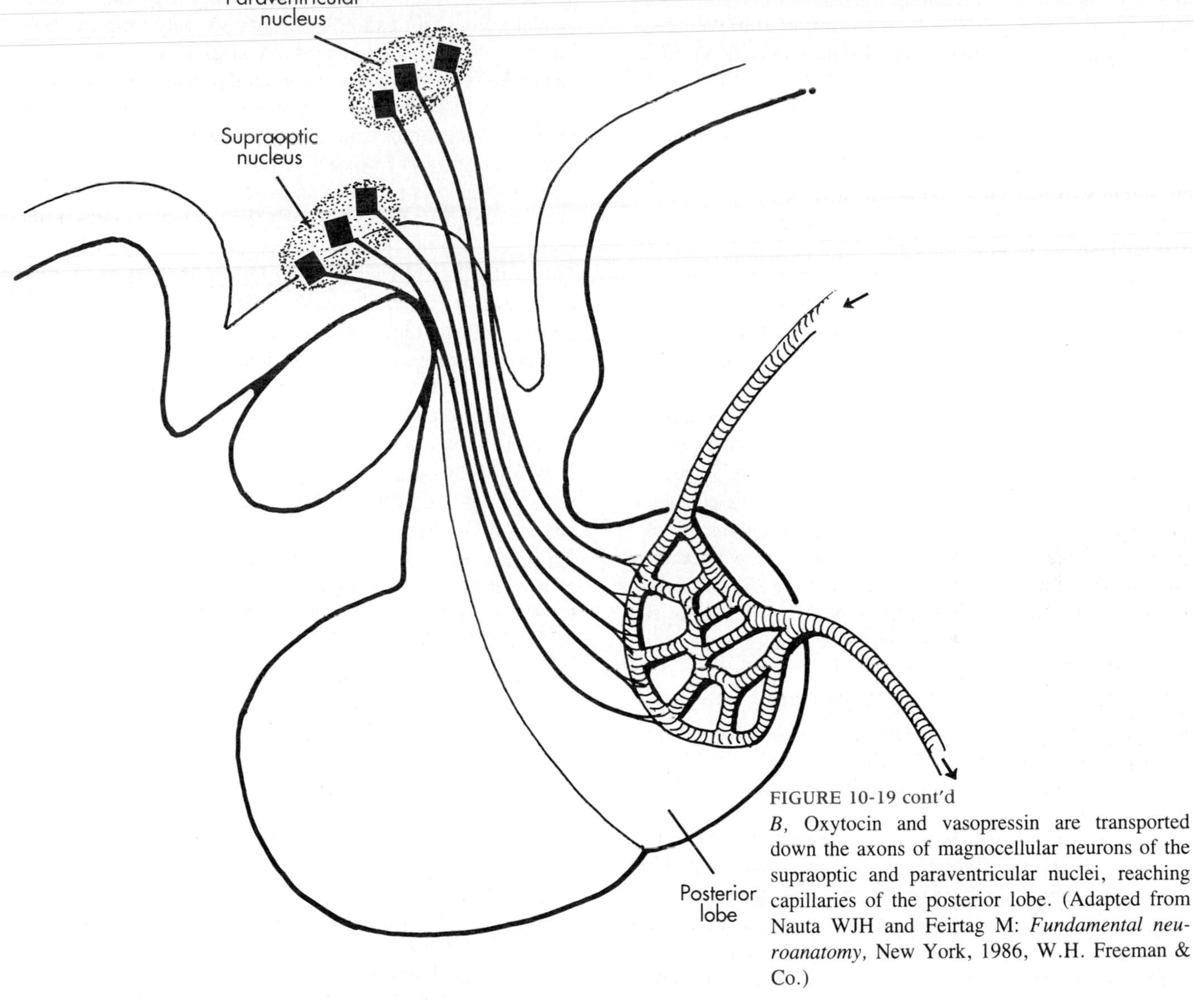


FIGURE 10-19 cont'd
*B,* Oxytocin and vasopressin are transported down the axons of magnocellular neurons of the supraoptic and paraventricular nuclei, reaching capillaries of the posterior lobe. (Adapted from Nauta WJH and Feirtag M: *Fundamental neuroanatomy,* New York, 1986, W.H. Freeman & Co.)

ganglionic or perforating arteries arising from arteries in and adjacent to the circle of Willis. Specifically the *anteromedial* group of ganglionic arteries, arising from the anterior cerebral and anterior communicating arteries, supplies the preoptic and supraoptic regions; the *posteromedial* group, arising from the posterior communicating arteries and the proximal portions of the posterior cerebral arteries, supplies the tuberal and mammillary regions; the *anterolateral* group (or lateral striate arteries), arising from proximal portions of the middle cerebral arteries, helps supply the lateral hypothalamus.

## Some functional aspects of the hypothalamus

The connections of the hypothalamus with the limbic system, pituitary, and brainstem make it eminently suitable for controlling various visceral functions and activities involved in drives and emotional states. Consistent with this, many hypothalamic "centers" have been described that are concerned with feeding and drinking behavior, temperature regulation, gut motility, sexual activity, and numerous other functions. In most cases, however, fragments of a behavior pattern elicited by stimulating a hypothalamic location can be elicited by stimulating appropriate sites in the brainstem. Thus many of the hypothalamic sites associated with particular behaviors may really be trigger points that, when stimulated, initiate neural activity in other parts of the CNS, which in turn causes the behavior pattern. Furthermore, many parts of the hypothalamus are organized loosely enough that electrical stimulation of only a certain part of a certain nucleus is impossible. For example, the medial forebrain bundle runs through the lateral hypothalamus, so if a particular behavior were elicited by stimulating a particular site in the lateral hypothalamus, it could be the result of stimulating either a portion of the lateral hypothalamic nucleus or some fibers of the medial forebrain bundle.

Given these caveats, it has nevertheless been found that certain types of changes consistently follow stimulation of or damage to particular hypothalamic areas in experimental animals. Since the hypothalamus is so small, discrete lesions affecting individual functional areas of the human hypothalamus are quite rare; in addition, lesions must be bilateral to disrupt most hypothalamic functions. However, the clinical findings in humans with hypothalamic damage are generally consistent with what would be expected from work on experimental animals. Only a few examples are cited here.

The hypothalamus is in overall control of the autonomic nervous system in the sense that practically any type of autonomic response can be elicited by stimulating some hypothalamic site. Although the sites overlap to a considerable degree, those associated with parasympathetic responses tend to be located anteriorly, and those associated with sympathetic responses tend to be located posteriorly. Appropriate somatic motor activity accompanies these autonomic responses, as the example of hypothalamic control of temperature regulation demonstrates. Stimulation of the anterior hypothalamus and preoptic area induces panting (or sweating in humans) and cutaneous vasodilatation, which in turn causes body temperature to fall. In contrast, stimulation of the posterior hypothalamus causes cutaneous vasoconstriction and shivering, which in turn causes an increase in body temperature. The hypothalamus thus acts as a thermostat, monitoring the temperature of blood passing through it and activating heat-dissipation or heat-production mechanisms as necessary to maintain the desired value. Bilateral lesions of the anterior hypothalamus make an animal unable to dissipate heat in a warm environment. (Such lesions may also cause diabetes insipidus, in which large amounts of dilute urine are produced as a result of destruction of the supraoptic nuclei.) Bilateral lesions of the posterior hypothalamus may make an animal unable to regulate its body temperature in either a warm or a cold environment, since the destruction involves not only the area concerned with the production and conservation of heat but also the fibers descending from the more anterior heat-dissipation areas.

The role of the hypothalamus in more complex activities is demonstrated by its involvement in feeding behavior. Here again, two areas with opposing influences have been found. Bilateral destruction of the ventromedial nucleus ("satiety center") produces animals that overeat and get fat, whereas destruction of the lateral hypothalamus in the tuberal region ("feeding center") produces animals that do not eat and may actually starve to death unless force-fed during the postoperative weeks. The complete mechanism of these effects is not known, but they are probably not as simple as they sound. The obesity following ventromedial lesions, for example, results not only from overeating but also from decreased physical activity and from metabolic changes favoring the accumulation of fat.

One should not get the impression that discrete lesions in the hypothalamus cause single changes such as hypothermia or obesity. The case of bilateral lesions of the ventromedial nucleus provides an instructive example not only of multiple effects from discrete lesions but also of the involvement of the hypothalamus in emotional behavior. Cats with bilateral ventromedial lesions overeat and get fat and are also extremely nasty.* They respond with full-blown, hissing rages to the most innocuous of stimuli. Similar rage responses can be elicited by stimulation of the lateral hypothalamus adjacent to the ventromedial nucleus of an intact cat. The attacks are coordinated and well directed but cease the moment the stimulus does. The ways in which such emotional responses are related, under normal circumstances, to activity in the limbic system are discussed in Chapter 16.

*"One of my own most striking memories is of huge, fat, and extremely hostile cats with ventromedial hypothalamic lesions. When they observed laboratory visitors through the bars, thankfully strong bars, of their cages, they appeared to have a singular interest in attack. They gave every sign of dedication to the goal of destroying the visitor. Their great size made the threat something not to be taken lightly." (From Isaacson RL: The limbic system, New York, 1974, Plenum Press, p. 85)

## ADDITIONAL READINGS


Adams JH, Daniel PM, Prichard MML: Observations on the portal circulation of the pituitary gland. *Neuroendocrinology* 1:193, 1965/66.

Albe-Fessard D et al: Diencephalic mechanisms of pain sensation, *Brain Res Rev* 9:217, 1985.

Allen LS et al: Two sexually dimorphic cell groups in the human brain, *J Neurosci* 9:497, 1989. *Both are contained in the preoptic/anterior hypothalamus, a region known to be involved in the production of gonadotropin-releasing factor.*

Bergland RM, Page RB: Pituitary-brain vascular relations: a new paradigm, *Science* 204:18, 1979. *Results that indicate that the pituitary portal system may not be so straightforward; for example, it may at times function in reverse, transporting adenohypophyseal hormones to the brain.*

Braak H, Braak E: The hypothalamus of the human adult: chiasmatic region, *Anat Embryol* 175:315, 1987.

Dierickx K: Immunocytochemical localization of the vertebrate cyclic nonapeptide neurohypophyseal hormones and neurophysins, *Int Rev Cytol* 62:120, 1980.

Dietrichs E, Haines DE: Interconnections between hypothalamus and cerebellum, *Anat Embryol* 179:207, 1989.

Duggan JP, Booth DA: Obesity, overeating, and rapid gastric emptying in rats with ventromedial hypothalamic lesions, *Science* 231:609, 1986. *A satisfyingly simple partial explanation for why rats with ventromedial hypothalamic lesions eat too much. These authors propose that autonomic regulation of stomach emptying is disturbed, that the stomach empties too quickly, and that the rat doesn't feel full for long. Consequently it eats again sooner than a normal rat.*

Eisenman JE, Masland WS: *The hypothalamus.* In Goldensohn ES, Appel SH, editors: *Scientific approaches to clinical neurology,* Philadelphia, 1977, Lea & Febiger. *A good, concise review of hypothalamic anatomy and physiology.*

Erlich SS, Apuzzo MLJ: The pineal gland: anatomy, physiology and clinical significance, *J Neurosurg* 63:321, 1985.

Flynn FG, Cummings JL, Tomiyasu U: Altered behavior associated with damage to the ventromedial hypothalamus: a distinctive syndrome, *Behav Neurol* 1:49, 1988.

Giguere M, Goldman-Rakic PS: Mediodorsal nucleus: areal, laminar, and tangential distribution of afferents and efferents in the frontal lobe of rhesus monkeys, *J Comp Neurol* 277:195, 1988.

Gillilan LA: The arterial and venous blood supplies to the forebrain (including the internal capsule) of primates, *Neurol* 18:653, 1968.

Groothius DR, Duncan GW, Fisher CM: The human thalamocortical sensory path in the internal capsule: evidence from a small capsular hemorrhage causing a pure sensory stroke, *Ann Neurol* 2:328, 1977.

Guillemin R: Peptides in the brain: the new endocrinology of the neuron, *Science* 202:390, 1978.

Hardy JD, Hellon RF, Sutherland K: Temperature-sensitive neurones in the dog's hypothalamus, *J Physiol* 175:242, 1964.

Haymaker WE, Anderson E, and Nauta WJH, editors: *The hypothalamus,* Springfield, Ill., 1969, Charles C Thomas.

Hayward JN: Functional and morphological aspects of hypothalamic neurons, *Physiol Rev* 57:574, 1977.

Heller HC, Crawshaw LI, Hammel HT: The thermostat of vertebrate animals, *Sci Am* 239(2):102, 1978.

Ilinsky IA, Kultas-Ilinsky K: Sagittal cytoarchitectonic maps of the *Macaca mulatta* thalamus with a revised nomenclature of the motor-related nuclei validated by observations on their connectivity, *J Comp Neurol* 262:331, 1987.

Jones EG: Some aspects of the organization of the thalamic reticular complex, *J Comp Neurol* 162:285, 1975.

Jones EG: *The thalamus,* New York, 1985, Plenum Press. *A recent, well-written, profusely illustrated review of the comparative anatomy and physiology of the thalamus.*

Jones EG, Leavitt RY: Retrograde axonal transport and the demonstration of non-specific projections to the cerebral cortex and striatum from thalamic intralaminar nuclei in the rat, cat, and monkey, *J Comp Neurol* 154:349, 1974.

Katter JT, Burstein R, Giesler GJ, Jr: The cells of origin of the spinohypothalamic tract in cats, *J Comp Neurol* 303:101, 1991.

Kievit J, Kuypers HGJM: Organization of the thalamocortical connections to frontal lobe in the rhesus monkey, *Exp Brain Res* 29:299, 1977. *An indication, based on experiments using newer anatomical tracing techniques, that thalamocortical projections are highly ordered topographically but not necessarily in the traditionally accepted pattern: strips of cortex receive inputs from thalamic slabs that sometimes run right through conventional nuclear boundaries.*

Krieger DT, Brownstein MJ, Martin JB: *Brain peptides,* New York, 1983, John Wiley & Sons.

Krieger DT, Liotta AS: Pituitary hormones in brain: where, how, and why? *Science* 205:366, 1979.

Langworthy OR, Fox HM: Thalamic syndrome. Syndrome of the posterior cerebral artery: a review, *Arch Intern Med* 60:203, 1937.

Lin C-S et al: A major direct GABAergic pathway from zona incerta to neocortex, *Sci* 248:1553, 1990.

Loewy AD, Spyer KM: *Central regulation of autonomic function,* New York, 1990, Oxford University Press.

Ludwig E, Klingler J: *Atlas cerebri humani,* Boston, 1956, Little, Brown & Co., Inc. *A collection of remarkable dissections of human brains. Formalin-fixed brains were frozen and thawed once or twice, which for some reason makes dissection much easier. (This accounts for the spongy appearance of the cortex in Figures 10-13 and 10-14.) The actual dissections were done with jeweler's forceps and wooden probes.*

Martin JB, Barchas JD: Neuropeptides in neurologic and psychiatric disease, *Res Publ Assoc Res Nerv Ment Dis,* vol 64, New York, 1986, Raven Press.

Mikol J et al: Connections of laterodorsal nucleus of the thalamus. II. Experimental study in *Papio papio, Brain Res* 138:1, 1977.

Morgane PJ, Panksepp J: *Handbook of the hypothalamus.* Vol. 1. *Anatomy of the hypothalamus,* New York, 1979, Marcel Dekker.

Mosko SS, Moore RY: Neonatal suprachiasmatic nucleus lesions: effects on the development of circadian rhythms in the rat, *Brain Res* 164:17, 1979.

Mountcastle VB, Henneman E: The representation of tactile sensibility in the thalamus of the monkey, *J Comp Neurol* 97:409, 1952. *An early physiological demonstration of the mapping of the body surface onto the VPL/VPM.*

Nathan PW, Smith MC: The location of descending fibres to sympathetic neurons supplying the eye and sudomotor neurons supplying the head and neck, *J Neurol Neurosurg Psychiatry* 49:187, 1986.

Plets C et al: The vascularization of the human thalamus, *Acta Neurol Belg* 70:687, 1970. *Long and detailed.*

Price JL, Slotnick BM: Dual olfactory representation in the rat thalamus: an anatomical and electrophysiological study, *J Comp Neurol* 215:63, 1983.

Pritchard TC et al: Projections of thalamic gustatory and lingual areas in the monkey, *Macaca fascicularis, J Comp Neurol* 244:213, 1986.

Raisman G, Brown-Grant K: The "suprachiasmatic syndrome": endocrine and behavioural abnormalities following lesions of the suprachiasmatic nucleus in the female rat, *Proc R Soc Lond* B198:297, 1977.

Reichlin S, Baldessarini RJ, Martin JB: The hypothalamus, *Res Publ Assoc Res Nerv Ment Dis,* vol 56, New York, 1978, Raven Press. *A volume principally about hypothalamic involvement in neuroendocrine function but including an interesting chapter by Fred Plum on human hypothalamic disorders.*

Reiter RJ, editor: *The pineal and reproduction: progress in reproductive biology,* vol 4, Basel, 1978, S. Karger.

Rinvik E: The corticothalamic projection from the pericruciate and coronal gyri in the cat: an experimental study with silver-impregnation methods, *Brain Res* 10:79, 1968.

Robertson RT, Thompson SM, Kaitz SS: Projections from the pretectal complex to the thalamic lateral dorsal nucleus of the cat, Exp *Brain Res* 51:157, 1983.

Ross ED: Localization of the pyramidal tract in the internal capsule by whole brain dissection, *Neurology* 30:59, 1980.

Russchen FT, Amaral DG, Price JL: The afferent input to the magnocellular division of the mediodorsal thalamic nucleus in the monkey, *Macaca fascicularis, J Comp Neurol* 256:175, 1987.

Sandson TA et al: Frontal lobe dysfunction following infarction of the left-sided medial thalamus, *Arch Neurol* 48:1300, 1991.

Schally AV, Kastin AJ, Arimura A: Hypothalamic hormones: the link between brain and body, *Am Sci* 65:712, 1977.

Sherman SM, Koch C: The control of retinogeniculate transmission in the mammalian lateral geniculate nucleus, *Exp Brain Res* 63:1, 1986. *A large majority of the synapses in the lateral geniculate nucleus come from places other than the retina. This paper presents some ideas about what they might be doing.*

Singer W: Control of thalamic transmission by corticofugal and ascending reticular pathways in the visual system, *Physiol Rev* 57:386, 1977.

Sugitani M: Electrophysiological and sensory properties of the thalamic reticular neurones related to somatic sensation in rats, *J Physiol* 290:79, 1979.

Swanson LW, Sawchenko PE: Hypothalamic integration: organization of the paraventricular and supraoptic nuclei, *Annu Rev Neurosci* 6:269, 1983.

Ulrich DJ, Tamamaki N, Sherman SM: Brainstem control of response modes in neurons of the cat's lateral geniculate nucleus, *Proc Nat Acad Sci* 87:2560, 1990.

Walker AE: *The primate thalamus,* 1938, University of Chicago Press. *An early (and historically important) exposition of the thalamic terminology commonly used today.*

Wasman M, Flynn JP: Directed attack elicited from hypothalamus, *Arch Neurol* 6:220, 1962.

Whitsel BL et al: Thalamic projections to S-I in macaque monkey, *J Comp Neurol* 178:385, 1978. *The microarchitecture of the projection from the VPL/VPM to the cortex, giving some idea of how remarkably detailed this projection is.*

Wilkins RH, Brody IA: The thalamic syndrome, *Arch Neurol* 20:560, 1969. *A brief introduction to (and excerpted translation of) the original work (Dejerine J, Roussy G: Le syndrome thalamique, Rev Neurol* 14:*521, 1906).*

# CHAPTER 11

# Visual System

It is clear from everyday experience that we are a visually oriented species. While it is arguable which of our senses is the most important, loss of the visual sense is certainly a greater handicap for humans than loss of, for example, the olfactory or gustatory sense. Partly because of its importance (and partly for anatomical and technical reasons to be discussed later), a great deal of research has been done on the visual system. At the present time we probably know more about the visual system than about any other sensory system, and there is considerable promise that with further study we will be able to understand in some detail how this portion of the central nervous system actually works.

Some lizards, fish, and amphibians have a photosensitive pineal organ that constantly stares up at the sky as a sort of "third eye." In mammals, however, all photic information originates in the *rods* and *cones* of the retina and then is conveyed to the brain by way of the axons of the output cells (called *ganglion cells*) of the retina. These axons, together with the axons of higher order cells on which they synapse, form a visual pathway that begins in the eyes anteriorly and ends in the occipital lobes posteriorly. Throughout this course a precise *retinotopic* arrangement of fibers is maintained so that particular small regions of the retina are represented in particular small regions of more central parts of the pathway. Damage at many different locations within this system can result in visual deficits, and a knowledge of the anatomy involved makes it possible to understand these deficits. Conversely, the same knowledge is frequently helpful in deducing the site of a lesion.

## RETINAL HISTOLOGY

The retina is a two-part structure, reflecting its origin from the two layers of infolded optic cup (Figure 11-1). The outer portion, adjacent to the choroid, is the *retinal pigment epithelium,* whereas the inner portion, adjacent to the vitreous, is the *neural retina*. Under normal conditions no space exists between the pigment epithelium and the neural retina in the adult. However, the mechanical connections between the two are not very strong, and under certain circumstances this potential space opens, constituting *retinal detachment*. Retinal receptors are metabolically dependent on pigment epithelial cells, so detached areas stop working.

### Cell types

One reason so much research has been done on the visual system is the overall anatomical simplicity of the neural retina relative to other parts of the nervous system. Although it contains hundreds of millions of cells, there are only five basic types involved in the processing of visual information, and their patterns of interconnections are fundamentally the same throughout the retina.

The five cell types have their somata neatly arranged in three layers and make most of their synapses in two additional layers. In each synaptic zone, one cell type brings visual information in, another type carries information out, and a third type serves as a laterally interconnecting element.

A simplified, schematic illustration of these basic connection patterns is shown in Figure 11-2, *B*. Starting peripherally, the photoreceptor cells, stimulated by light, project to the first layer of synapses where they terminate on the aptly named *bipolar* and *horizontal cells*. The bipolar cells then project to the next layer of synapses, while the horizontal cells spread laterally and interconnect receptors, bipolar cells, and other horizontal cells. In the second layer of synapses, bipolar cells terminate on ganglion cells and *amacrine cells*. Axons of the ganglion cells leave the

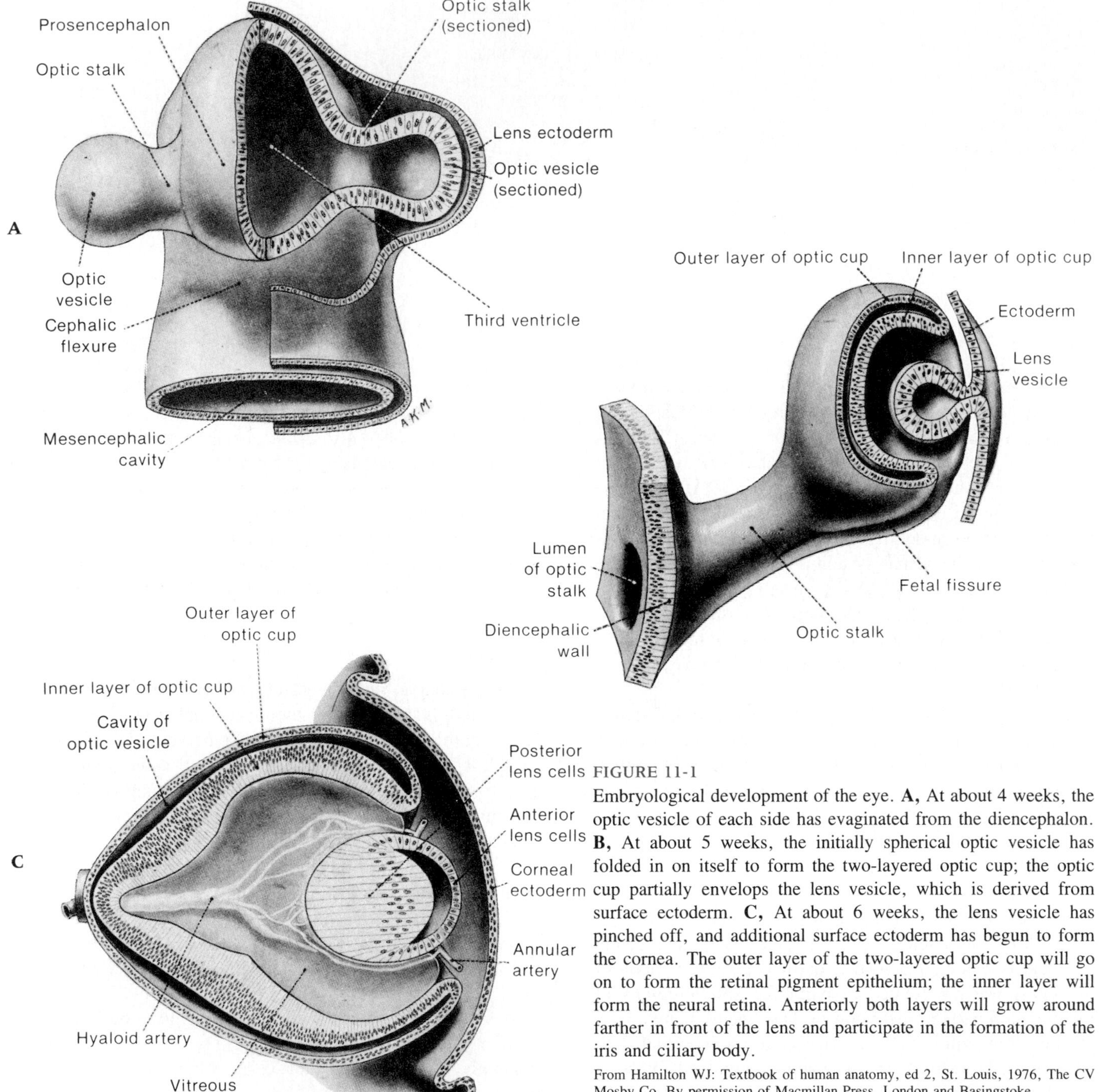


FIGURE 11-1

Embryological development of the eye. **A,** At about 4 weeks, the optic vesicle of each side has evaginated from the diencephalon. **B,** At about 5 weeks, the initially spherical optic vesicle has folded in on itself to form the two-layered optic cup; the optic cup partially envelops the lens vesicle, which is derived from surface ectoderm. **C,** At about 6 weeks, the lens vesicle has pinched off, and additional surface ectoderm has begun to form the cornea. The outer layer of the two-layered optic cup will go on to form the retinal pigment epithelium; the inner layer will form the neural retina. Anteriorly both layers will grow around farther in front of the lens and participate in the formation of the iris and ciliary body.

From Hamilton WJ: Textbook of human anatomy, ed 2, St. Louis, 1976, The CV Mosby Co. By permission of Macmillan Press, London and Basingstoke.

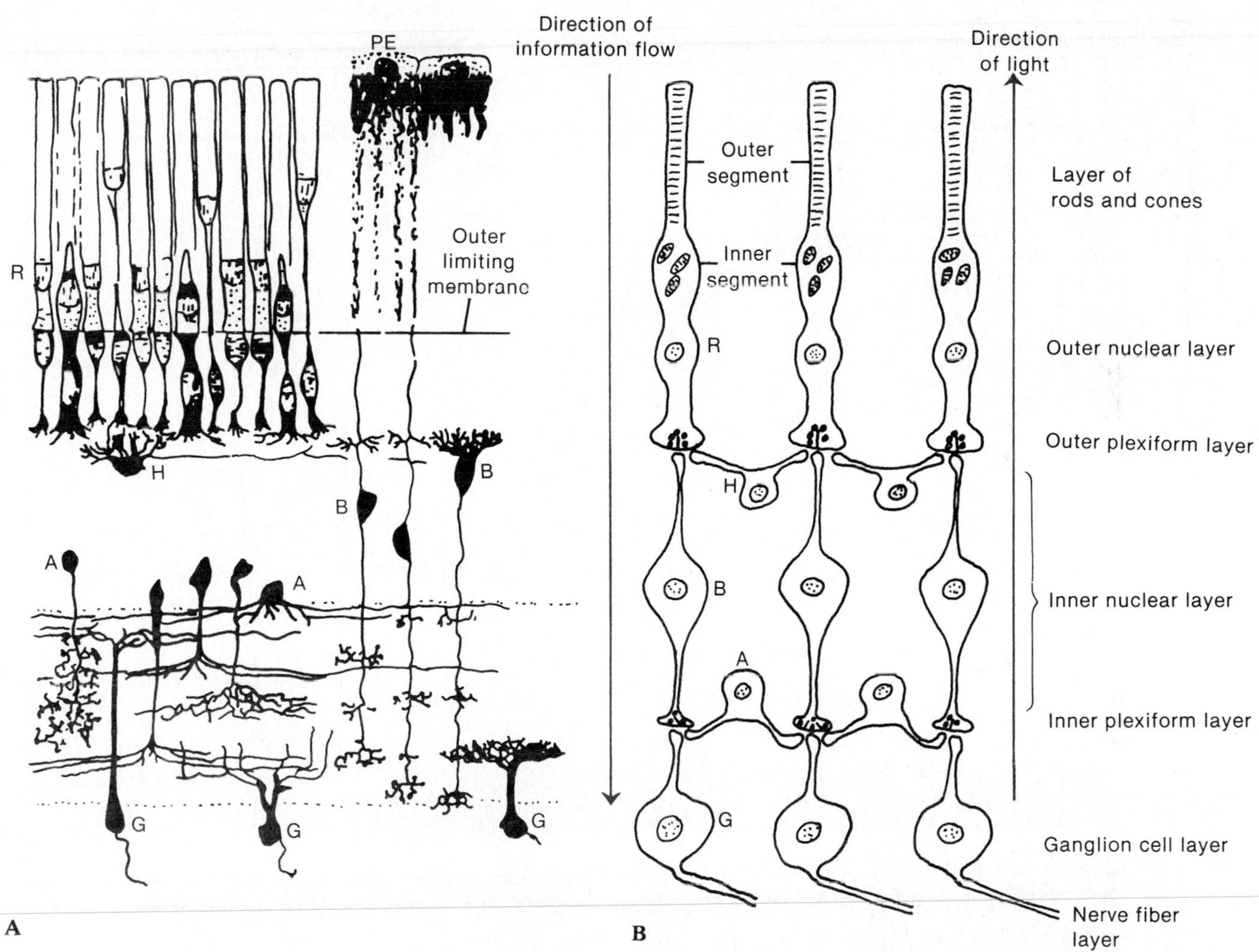


FIGURE 11-2

Cell types and their arrangement in the retina. **A,** Drawing of Golgi-stained cells of the frog retina. (Modified from Ramón y Cajal, S.: Histologie due système nerveux, vol. 2, Paris, 1911, Libraire Maloine.) **B,** Schematic illustration of a generalized vertebrate retina showing retinal layers. *A,* Amacrine cell; *B,* bipolar cell; *G,* ganglion cell; *H,* horizontal cell; *PE,* pigment epithelium; *R,* receptor cell (rod or cone).

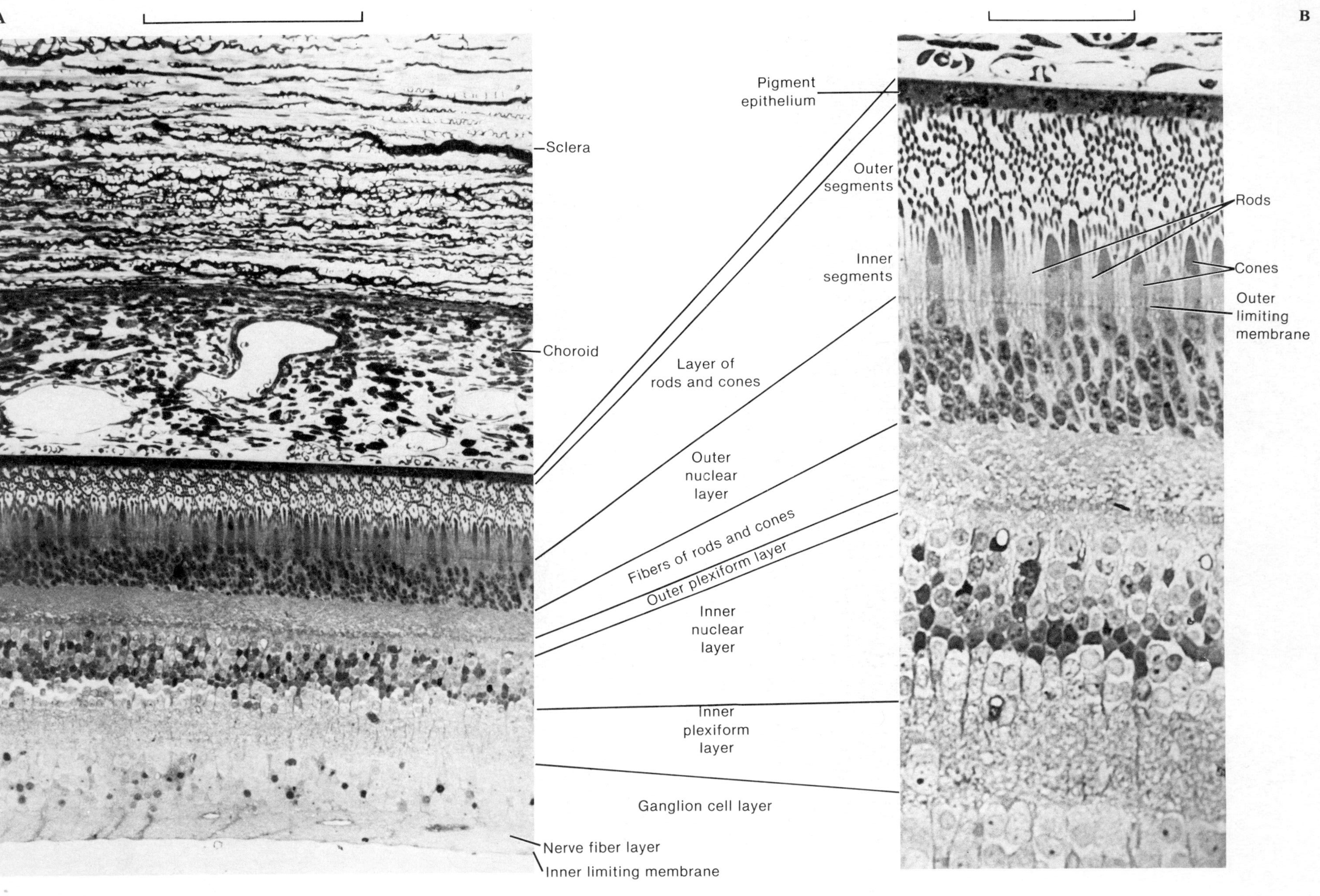


FIGURE 11-3
**A,** Section through the entire wall of an eye of a rhesus monkey near the fovea, showing the sclera, choroid, and retina; scale mark = 200 μm. **B,** Enlarged view of part of **A,** showing the retina; the plane of section is not quite parallel to the outer segments of the rods and cones, so they are cut transversely and appear as dots. Scale mark = 50 μm.

Courtesy of Fay Eldred and Virginia Miller, University of Colorado Health Sciences Center.

eye as the *optic nerve,* while processes of the amacrine cells spread laterally and interconnect bipolar cells, ganglion cells, and other amacrine cells.

### Retinal layers

The entire retina is conventionally described as a 10-layered structure, beginning with the pigment epithelium (Figure 11-3); five of these layers are the layers of cell bodies and synapses mentioned above. In naming these layers, the term *nuclear* refers to cell bodies and the term *plexiform* to synaptic zones. *Inner* and *outer* refer to the number of synapses by which a structure is separated from the brain, so that, for example, receptors are "outer" with respect to bipolar cells. The 10 layers of the retina are as follows.

1. The *pigment epithelium* is a single layer of polygonal, pigmented cells. One side of each cell adjoins the choroid, whose capillaries supply the avascular first two layers of the retina. The other side of each cell forms numerous fine processes that partially surround the outer portions of the receptor cells and obliterate the space that existed embryonically within the wall of the optic cup. Pigment epithelial cells are intimately involved metabolically with the receptors. They also play a role in absorbing light that has passed through the retina.

2. *Rods* and *cones* are the two different types of vertebrate photoreceptor. Each consists of several regions (Figures 11-4 — 11-6): an *outer segment,* an *inner segment,* a cell body, and a synaptic terminal. Strictly speaking, "rod" or "cone" refers to only the outer segment plus the inner segment of a photoreceptor cell, but in common usage these terms are often used to refer to entire receptors.

The outer segment of a rod is relatively long and cylindrical, whereas that of a cone is shorter and tapered (Figures 11-4 and 11-5). Each type of outer segment is filled with flattened membranous sacs, or *disks.* In cones, the interior of many of these disks is continuous with extracellular space, but in rods, almost all of the disks have pinched off from the external membrane and are wholly intracellular. The major protein constituent of the outer segment membranes of both rods and cones is the visual pigment, which is called *rhodopsin* in rods. (There is no universally accepted name for the visual pigments of cones, and they are often called rhodopsins as well, or simply *cone pigments*). Hence photons traversing the outer segment of a rod or cone must pass through hundreds or thousands of

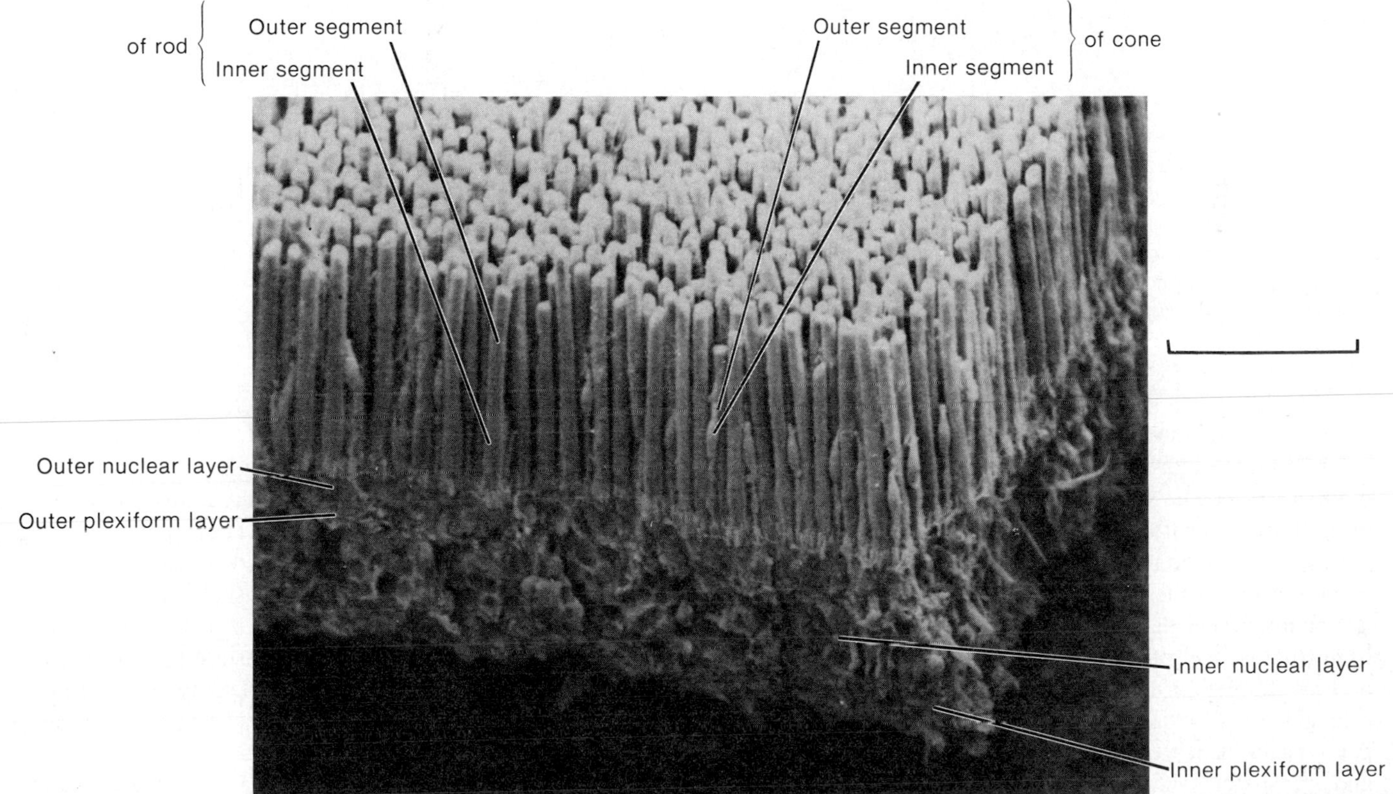


FIGURE 11-4
Scanning electron micrograph of the retina of a bullfrog. Scale mark = 50 μm.

Courtesy of Dr. Roy H. Steinberg, University of California at San Francisco. From Steinberg RH: Scanning electron microscopy of the bullfrog's retina and pigment epithelium, *Z Zellforsch* 143:451, 1973.

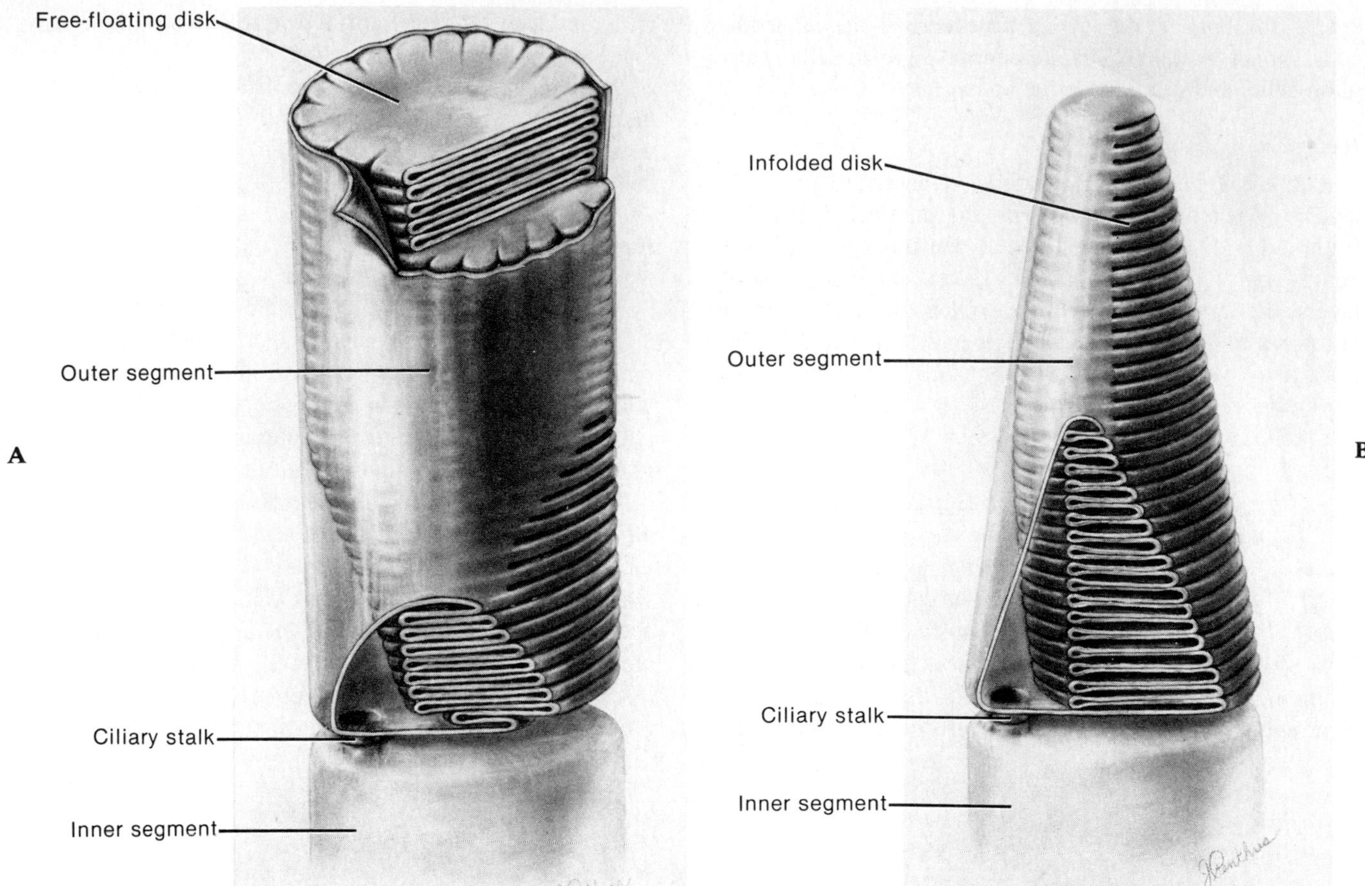


FIGURE 11-5
Ultrastructural differences between the outer segment of rods and cones. **A,** Rod outer segment (cut off toward the top to be the same length as the cone outer segment in **B**); note that some disks toward the base of the outer segment are open to the outside world but that most disks are pinched off and completely surrounded by cytoplasm. **B,** Cone outer segment; note that this outer segment tapers toward its apex (hence its name) and that all of its disks are infoldings of the plasma membrane with their interiors still continuous with extracellular space.
Courtesy of Dr. Richard W. Young, University of California at Los Angeles.

sheets of membrane, each full of visual pigment molecules. As one might expect from this localization of visual pigment, the outer segment is the site of visual transduction; photons absorbed here cause a receptor potential that then spreads to the rest of the cell. Note that the photosensitive portion of the receptor cells is located in the part of the neural retina that is farthest removed from incoming light (that is, the retina is inverted with respect to the path of light through it). This curious situation is universally true among vertebrates. However, this does not detract from visual sensitivity or acuity, since the retina is thin and transparent and since other anatomical modifications (discussed shortly) are found in the retinal area of greatest acuity.

Each outer segment is connected to its inner segment by a narrow ciliary stalk. The inner segments contain, among other organelles, a very prominent collection of mitochondria. These mitochondria are thought to supply the energy necessary for processes associated with transduction and for the synthesis of visual pigments. These pigments are continually renewed, being synthesized in the inner segment, transported through the ciliary stalk, and incorporated into disk membranes. "Old" disks at the apical ends of the outer segments of rods and cones are then phagocytosed by the pigment epithelium. (Certain types of retinal degeneration are probably caused by a defect in this renewal-phagocytosis process.)

Rods are considerably more sensitive than cones and are the receptors used in dim light. However, there is a great deal of convergence in rod pathways, so the spatial acuity mediated by them is relatively poor. In addition, there is only one type of rod in the human retina, so color

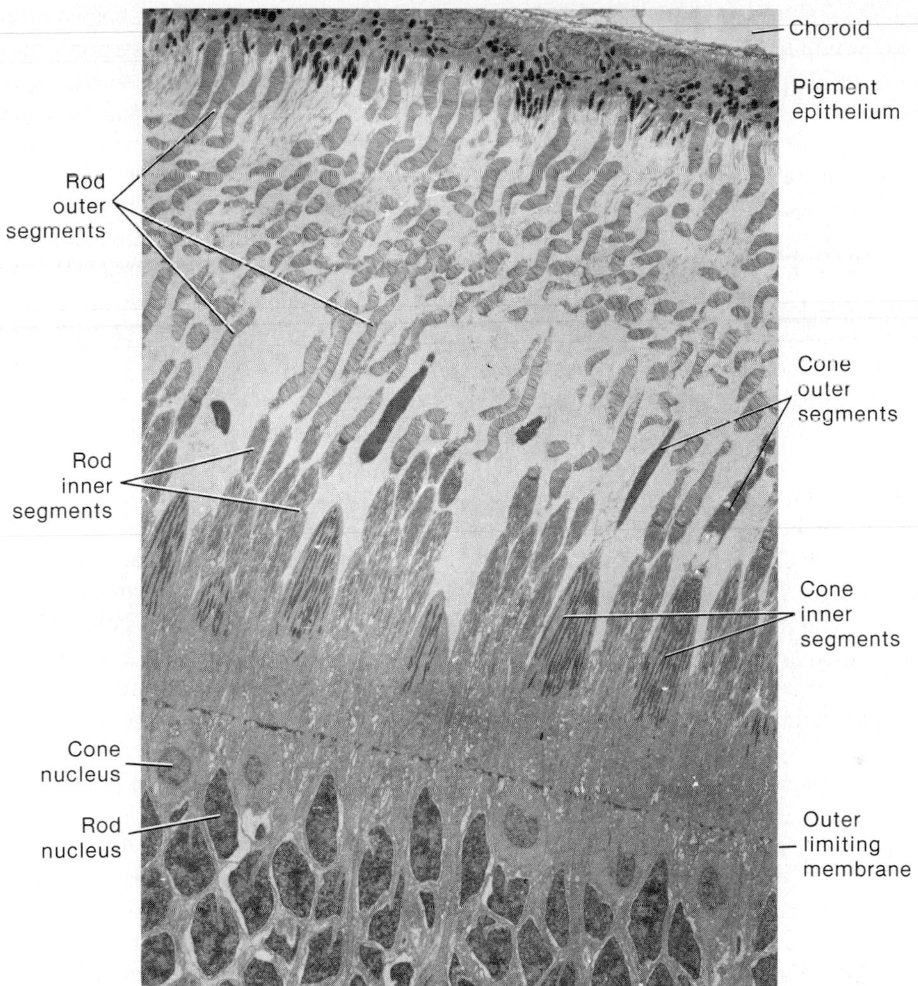


FIGURE 11-6
Electron micrograph of the photoreceptor layer of a rhesus monkey's retina. This section was taken from a region near the fovea but not in it, so both rods and cones are plentiful. The outer limiting membrane is actually a row of intercellular junctions. The insertion of the tips of rod outer segments into the pigment epithelial layer is apparent.
Courtesy of Dr. David Moran and Pamela Eller, University of Colorado Health Sciences Center.

vision is not possible when only rods are active. On the other hand, we have three types of cones (red- yellow-, and blue-sensitive), so information about the colors of objects can be extracted by the cone system if the illumination is bright enough. There is also relatively little convergence in the cone pathway, so spatial acuity is good.

3. The *outer limiting membrane* was so named because it has the appearance of a distinct line when viewed with a light microscope. However, electron microscopy has revealed it to be a row of intercellular junctions (Figure 11-6). Elongated specialized glial cells called *Müller cells* span almost the entire retina, ending distally at the bases of the inner segments of the rods and cones. Here adjacent Müller processes and inner segments are joined by junctional complexes, which collectively form the outer limiting membrane.

4. The *outer nuclear layer* consists of the cell bodies of the rods and cones.

5. The *outer plexiform layer* is the relatively thin synaptic zone in which receptors terminate on horizontal and bipolar cells and in which processes of horizontal cells spread laterally. The actual pattern of interconnections is somewhat more complex than that shown in Figure 11-2, *B*. For example, there are differences between the synaptic complexes of rods and cones, and there are several subpopulations of bipolar cells. Other types of junctions are either known or inferred. For example, there are receptor-receptor connections and feedback synapses of horizontal cells onto receptors.

6. The *inner nuclear layer* contains the cell bodies of all the retinal interneurons as well as those of the Müller cells. The nuclei of horizontal cells are found near its dis-

tal edge, those of bipolar cells in the middle, and those of amacrine cells near its proximal edge. Bipolar cells conduct visual information through this layer, projecting to the second synaptic zone.

7. The *inner plexiform layer* is the relatively thick synaptic zone in which bipolar cells terminate on amacrine and ganglion cells, and processes of amacrine cells spread laterally. Here again, the actual pattern of interconnections is somewhat more complex than that shown in Figure 11-2, *B*. The amacrine cells provide one example of this added complexity: based on neurochemical and anatomical characteristics, more than 30 different types, each presumed to have a somewhat distinctive function, have been described.

8. The *ganglion cell layer* contains the cell bodies of the ganglion cells, whose dendrites ramify in the inner plexiform layer and whose axons leave the eye as the optic nerve. This cell layer is considerably thinner than either the outer or the inner nuclear layer in most retinal locations, reflecting the fact that there are about 5 million cones and about 100 million rods in a human retina but only about 1 million ganglion cells. Clearly a good deal of convergence is involved in retinal processing, but the convergence is not uniform across the retina. As discussed shortly, some regions are specialized for high acuity and have little convergence, whereas other regions are specialized for high sensitivity and have a great deal of convergence.

It has now become apparent that visual information travels in several parallel streams, just as somatosensory information travels rostrally through the spinal cord and brainstem in multiple parallel pathways. In the case of the visual system, the axons of several anatomically and functionally distinct classes of ganglion cells share the same optic nerve in their course toward the brain. In the primate visual system, approximately 80% of all ganglion cells form a single class of small cells that are particularly responsive to the colors of visual objects and to details of their shapes. Some general aspects of the distinctive connections of this and other ganglion cell classes are mentioned later in this chapter.

9. The *nerve fiber layer* is the collection of axons of ganglion cells, which converge like spokes toward the *optic disk* or *optic papilla* (located posteriorly and slightly medial to the midline of the eye) where they form the optic nerve.

10. The *inner limiting membrane* is a thin basal lamina that intervenes between the vitreous and the proximal ends of the Müller cells.

## RETINAL TOPOGRAPHY

Cross sections through the retina do not have the same appearance at all locations. For example, no photoreceptors, interneurons, or ganglion cells are present at the optic disk, where the axons of ganglion cells leave the eye to form the optic nerve. These axons originate near the vitreous, so they must turn posteriorly and traverse the retina before passing through the sclera. Since there are no photoreceptors at the optic disk, we are blind to any object whose image falls on this part of the retina. Although the *blind spot* can easily be demonstrated (Figure 11-7), we have no awareness as we walk around of a blank spot in visual space. One might think this is because the left eye can see the part of the visual field that falls on the right eye's blind spot, and vice versa. This cannot be the explanation, though, since we are unaware of the blind spot even with one eye closed. The real reason is that our nervous system simply "fills it in." We are actually quite skillful at this, and patients with damage to their visual systems can become blind in surprisingly large areas of their visual fields without being aware of it.

Beginning near the lateral edge of the optic disk is a circular portion of the retina, about 1 cm in diameter, in which many of the cells contain a yellow pigment. This gives the area a yellowish color when examined with appropriate illumination and has led to its being called the *macula lutea* (Latin for yellow spot), often shortened to *macula*. In the center of the macula is a depression about 1.5 mm in diameter, called the *fovea*, which is particularly rich in cones. In the central part of the fovea is a pit, only about 350 μm across, which contains only elongated cones (no rods) and is directly in line with the visual axis (Figure 11-8). The central fovea is specialized for vision of the highest acuity; all the neurons and capillaries that are present elsewhere (and that light would otherwise traverse before reaching the receptors) are collected around the edges of the fovea. Specialized interneurons called *midget bipolar cells* receive their inputs from individual foveal cones. These bipolars in turn contact individual *midget ganglion cells*, so that an anatomical basis for highly detailed foveal vision is maintained.*

The fovea is one extreme in a changing rod/cone distribution across the retina (Figure 11-9). The packing density of cones decreases sharply outside the fovea, whereas that of the rods increases, reaching a maximum just outside the macula. From here to the edge of the retina, the cone density remains at a low level, and the rod density slowly declines as well (Figure 11-10). Given the known properties of rods and cones, it follows from these distributions that the fovea is used for high-acuity color vision in reasonably

*One might think it advantageous to continue the anatomical specializations of the fovea, such as small, tightly packed photoreceptors and no convergence, throughout the retina; this would give us highly detailed vision over our entire field of view. However, as Wässle and Boycott point out (*Physiol Rev* 71:447, 1991), foveal vision requires so much cerebral cortex (e.g., Figures 11-15 and 11-16) that using foveal specializations throughout the retina would necessitate 100 times as much cerebral cortex as we presently have available in our entire cerebrum! Hence, we use a very small fovea, together with precisely controlled eye movements that allow us to aim it at objects of interest (see Chapter 12).

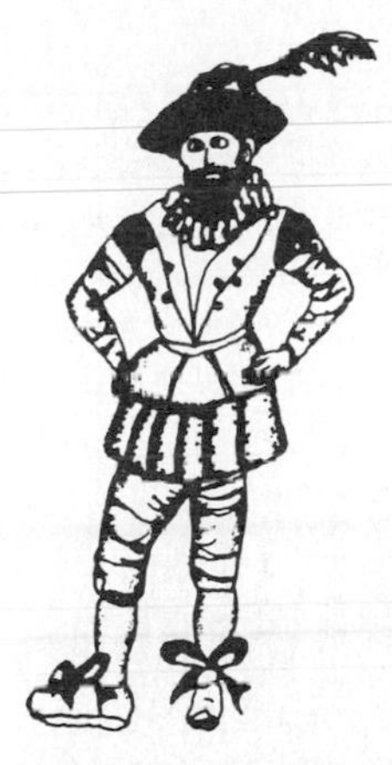


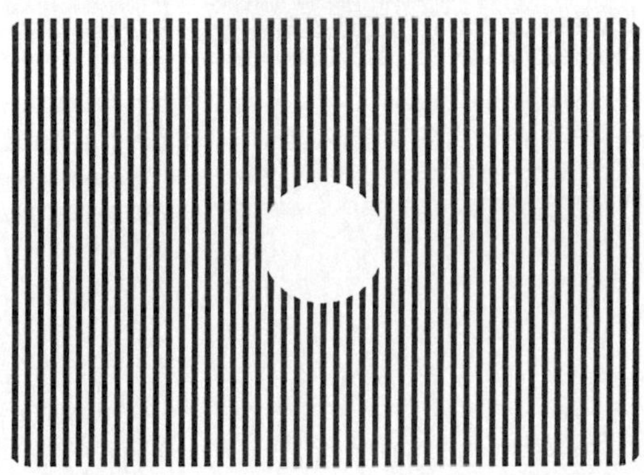


FIGURE 11-7
How to demonstrate your right eye's blind spot to yourself. **A,** Close your left eye, hold the book at arm's length, stare fixedly at the spot on the left side of the figure, and slowly move the book toward you. At some point about a foot from your face, the bearded gentleman will lose his head. **B,** Demonstration of how the central nervous system "fills in" the blind spot. As in part **A** above, close your left eye, stare at the black spot with your right eye, and move the book slowly toward you. When the image of the hole in the striped pattern falls on your blind spot, your brain will try to convince you that there are stripes where none exist.

**A** based on a technique of King Charles II, as recounted by Rushton WAH: *Vision Res* 19:255, 1979.

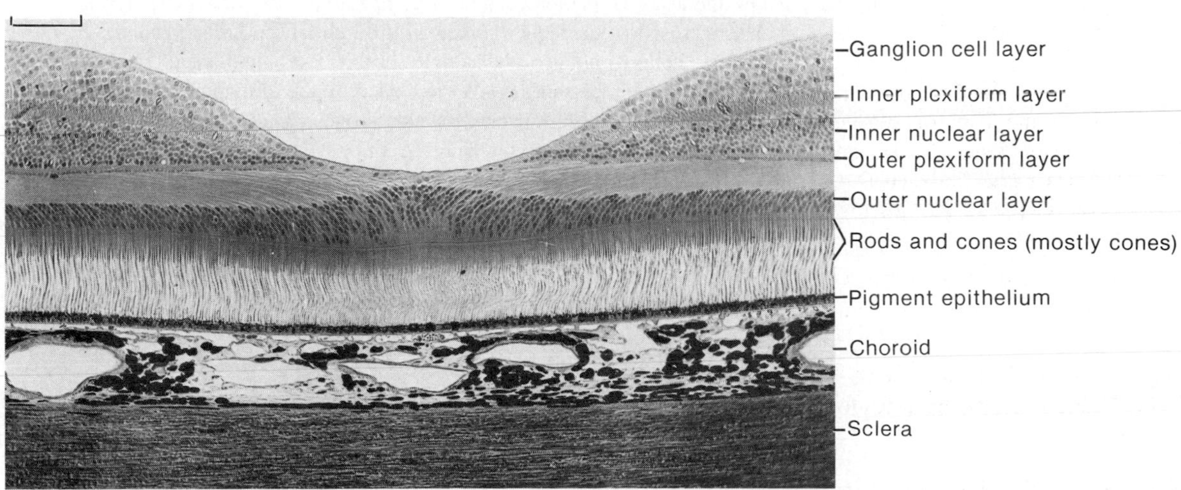


FIGURE 11-8
Fovea of a rhesus monkey. Note that all retinal elements (except the photoreceptors, which are all cones in the center of the fovea) are displaced to either side so that light only needs to pass through the outer nuclear layer before reaching the cones. The nerve fiber layer is scanty in this region because the axons of more laterally placed ganglion cells arc around the fovea on their way to the optic disk. Scale mark = 100 μm.

From Fine BS, Yanoff M: Ocular histology, ed 2, New York, 1979, Harper & Row, Publishers.

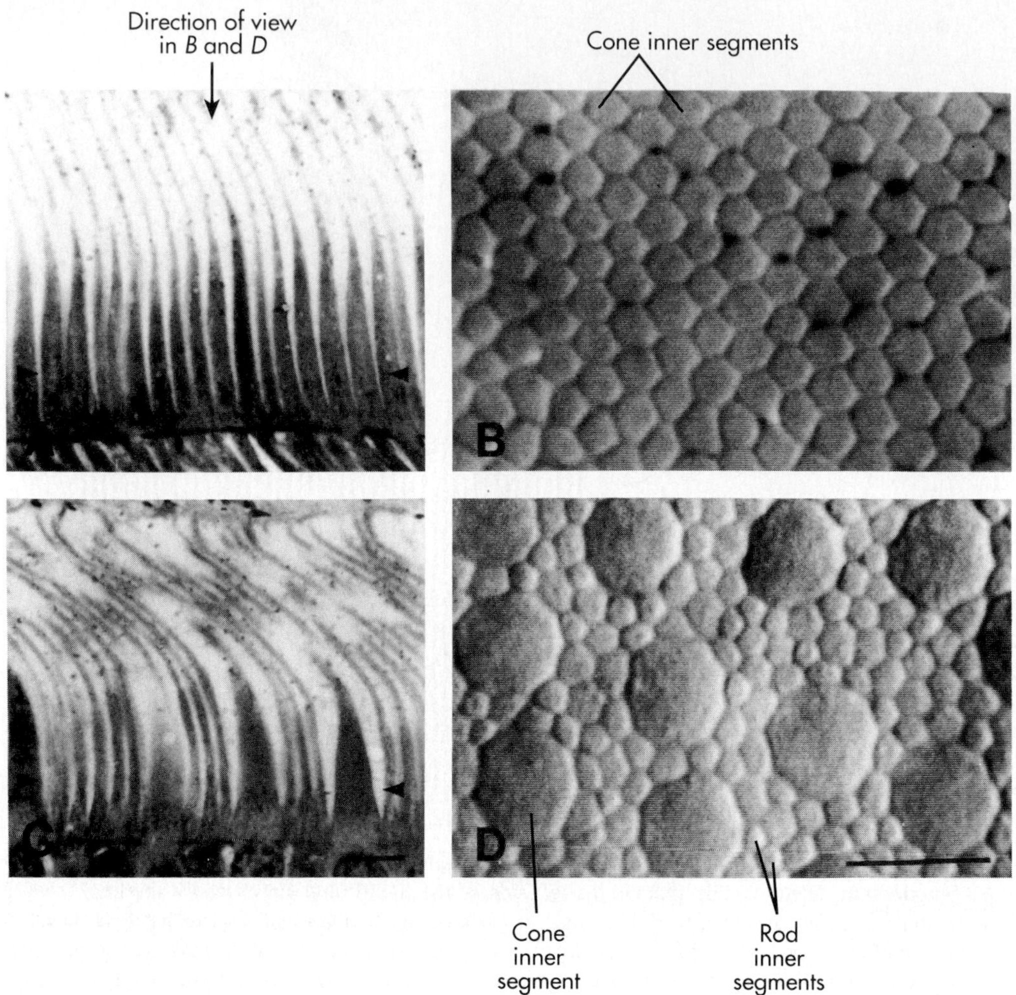


FIGURE 11-9
Differential distribution of rods and cones in the human retina. *A* and *C* show standard histological sections parallel to the long axes of photoreceptor inner and outer segments in the fovea (A) and the midperipheral retina (C). *B* and *D* show the array of photoreceptors in comparable areas of another retina viewed end-on, using a special video microscopy technique (Nomarski differential interference contrast) that allows focusing on a particular cross-sectional plane of the sample. In this case, the plane of focus is one that cuts through the photoreceptor inner segments at the level indicated by the arrowheads in A and C. In the fovea *(B)* all the inner segments are of closely packed, slender cones, whereas in the midperipheral retina *(D)* the inner segments of fatter cones are interspersed among the rod inner segments. Scale marks in C and D = 10μm. From Curcio CA et al, *J Comp Neurol* 292:497, 1990. Courtesy of Dr. Christine A. Curcio, Departments of Biological Structure and of Ophthalmology, University of Washington.

bright light, whereas extrafoveal regions function at lower light levels.

## CENTRAL VISUAL PATHWAYS

Ganglion cell axons travel in the optic nerve to the *optic chiasm,* where they undergo a partial decussation and enter one or the other *optic tract*. Most of the fibers in each optic tract then terminate in the *lateral geniculate nucleus,* which is the thalamic relay nucleus for vision. Geniculate fibers travel through the internal capsule and corona radiata to the primary visual cortex in the banks of the calcarine sulcus. In addition, a considerable number of optic tract fibers project to the midbrain and a few to the hypothalamus. Throughout this pathway, the numbers of fibers and areas of representation for the macula are disproportionately large for the macula's actual size. This reflects

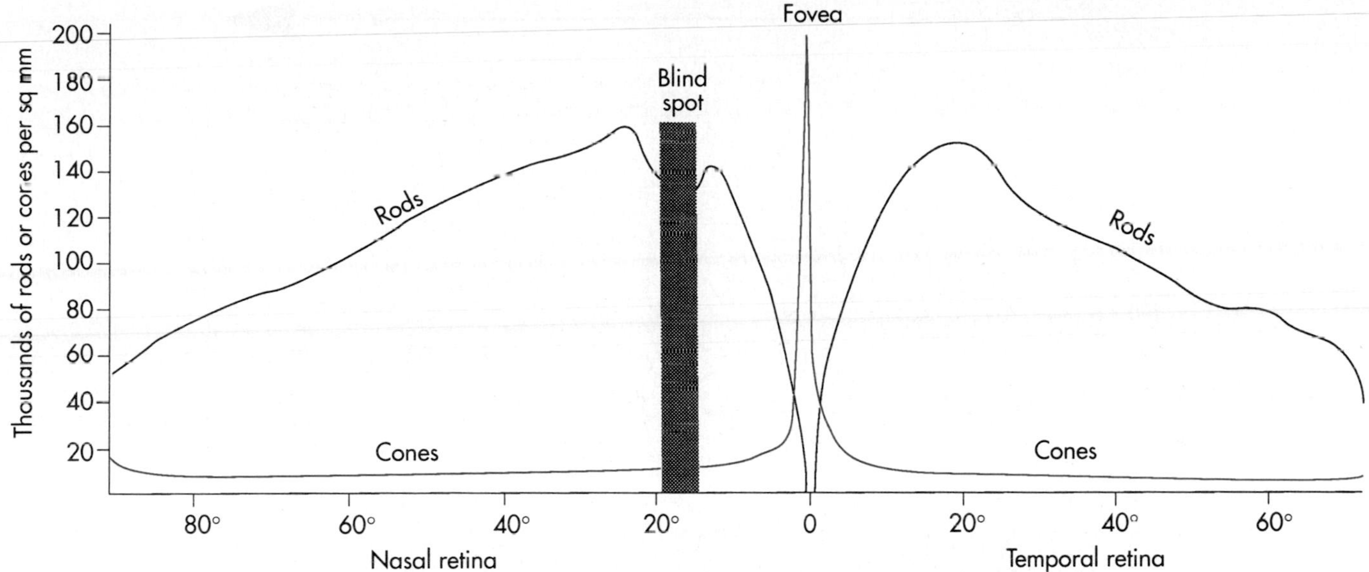


FIGURE 11-10
Packing densities of rods and cones in the human retina along a horizontal band passing through the fovea.
Modified from Østerberg GA: *Acta Ophthalmol Suppl* 6, 1935 and Curcio CF et al.: *J Comp Neurol*. 292:497, 1990.

the relatively small amount of convergence in the macula, which in turn reflects its specialization for high acuity.

## Optic nerve, chiasm, and tract

The unmyelinated axons of ganglion cells collect at the optic disk, pierce the sclera in a region called the *lamina cribrosa,* and acquire myelin sheaths, forming the optic nerve. The optic nerve is, by embryology and adult anatomy, actually a tract of the CNS and as such has meningeal coverings much like other areas. The sclera continues as its dural sheath, lined in turn by arachnoid and pia. The subarachnoid space around the optic nerve communicates with subarachnoid space generally; increases in intracranial pressure are transmitted to the optic nerve. Such an increase in pressure can cause detectable swelling of the optic disk. This swelling, called *papilledema,* can be a valuable diagnostic sign.

Just anterior to the infundibular stalk, the two optic nerves partially decussate in the optic chiasm. All fibers from the nasal half of each retina cross to the contralateral optic tract; all fibers from the temporal half of each retina pass through the lateral portions of the chiasm without crossing and enter the ipsilateral optic tract. The result is that each optic tract contains the fibers arising in the temporal retina of the ipsilateral eye and the nasal retina of the contralateral eye. As indicated in Figure 11-11, this apparently curious partial decussation is exactly appropriate for delivering all the information from the contralateral visual field to each optic tract. Also since much of the basis for depth perception involves a comparison of the slightly different views seen by our two eyes, it is necessary to bring together information from comparable areas of the two retinas, which the optic chiasm accomplishes.

In the optic tract, fibers arising in corresponding areas of the two retinas (that is, fibers carrying information about the same area in the visual field) are located near each other.* This relationship continues throughout the remainder of the visual pathway so that damage to the optic tract or more central parts of the pathway tends to cause comparable visual deficits in both eyes.

## Lateral geniculate nucleus

The optic tract curves posteriorly around the cerebral peduncle, and most of its fibers terminate in the lateral geniculate nucleus (Figure 11-12). This is a six-layered, dome-shaped nucleus in which the optic fibers terminate in a precise retinotopic pattern. The pattern is about the same in each layer so that a given point in the visual field is represented in a column of cells extending through all six layers. However, each layer receives input from only one eye: layers 1 (most inferior), 4, and 6 (most superior) from the contralateral eye and layers 2, 3, and 5 from the ipsi-

*The retinotopic arrangement in the optic nerve and tract is only approximate, because fibers sort themselves not only by retinal origin but also by functional type. This may be the basis of occasional clinical reports of deficits involving only some aspects of visual function, such as color vision, following optic tract lesions.

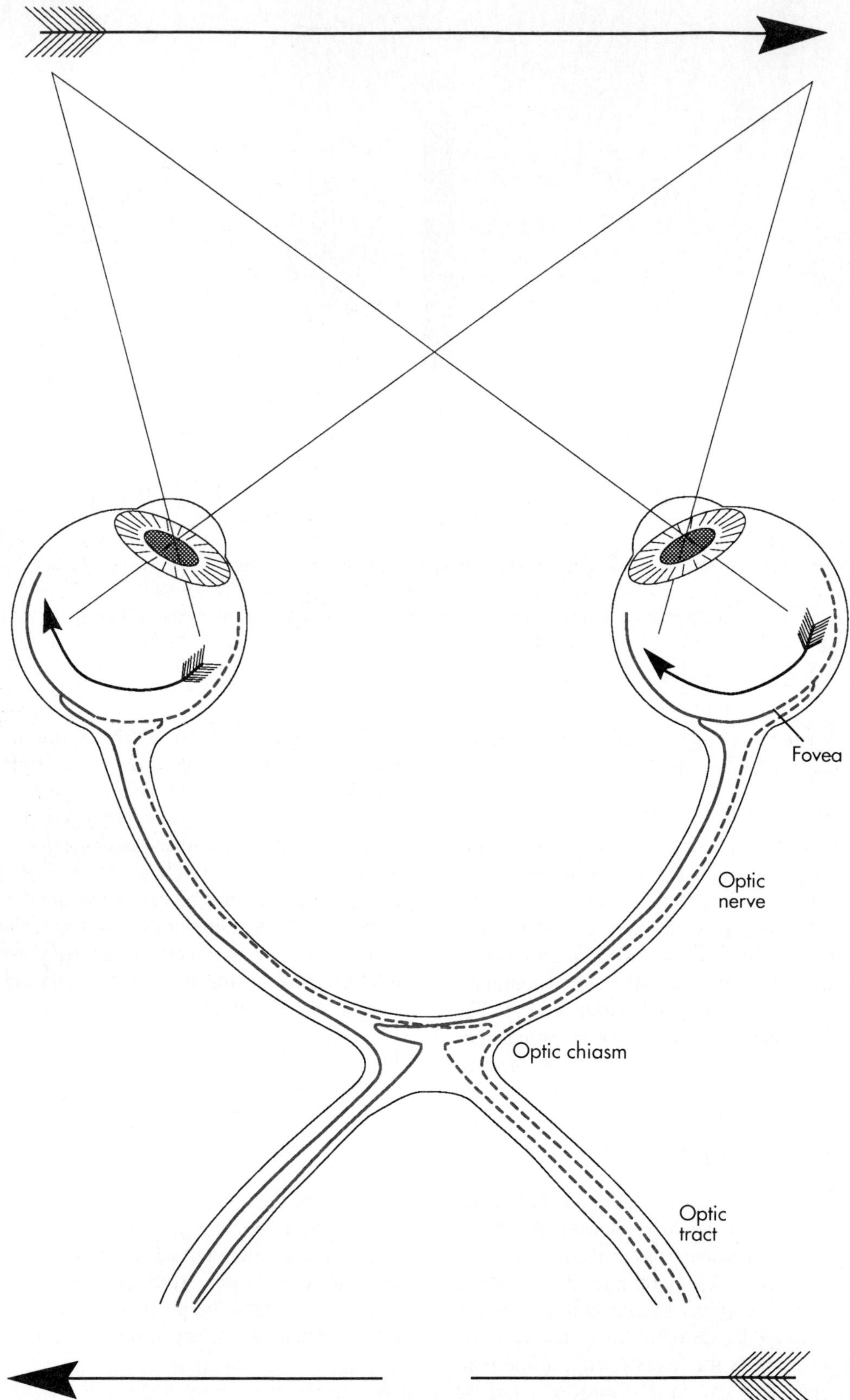


FIGURE 11-11
Schematic diagram illustrating the formation of the optic chiasm and tracts. All information from the temporal side of a vertical line passing through a given fovea enters the ipsilateral optic tract; all information from the nasal side crosses in the chiasm and enters the contralateral optic tract. The result, as indicated, is that each optic tract "looks" at the contralateral visual field.

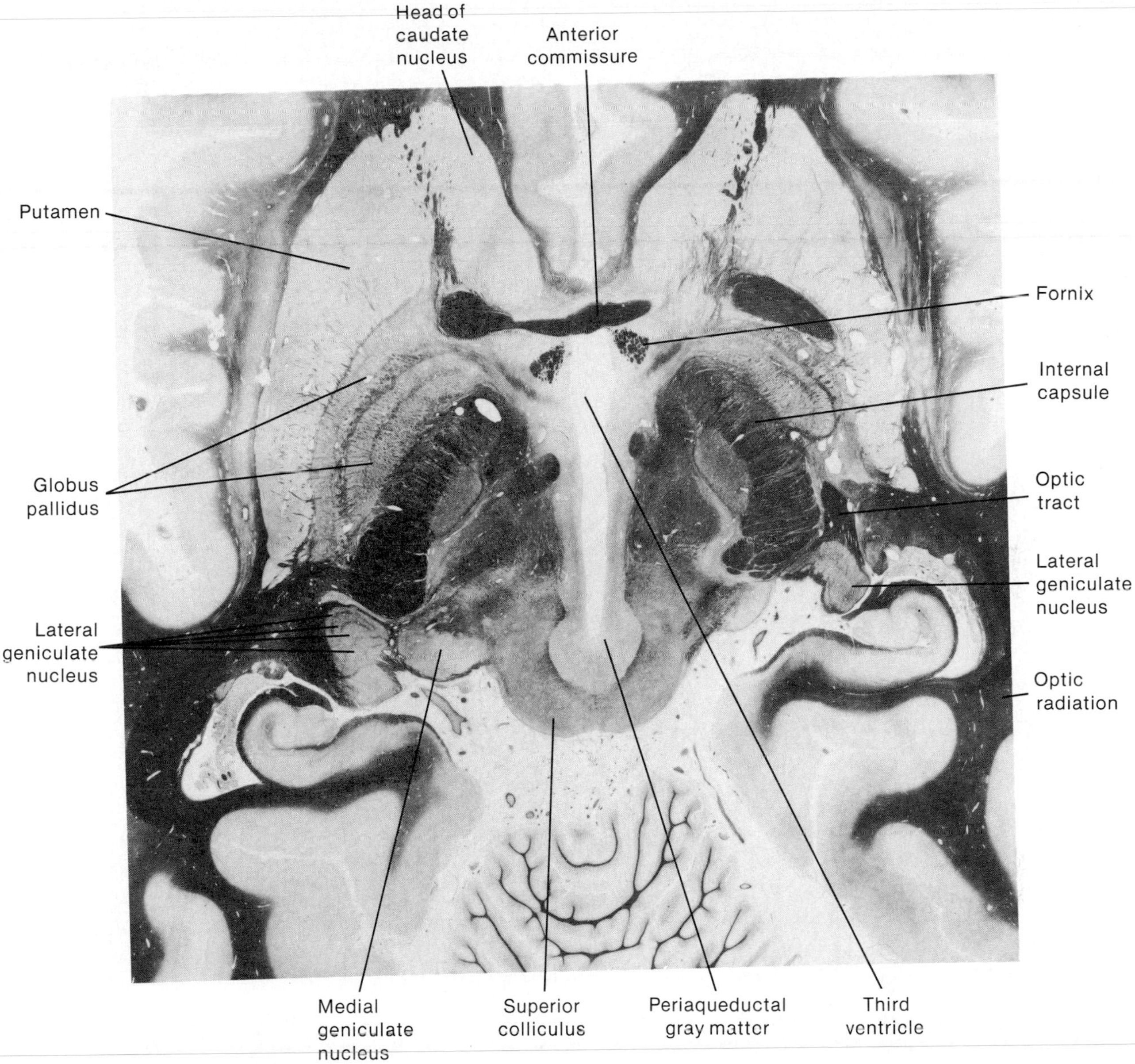

Head of caudate nucleus
Anterior commissure
Putamen
Fornix
Internal capsule
Globus pallidus
Optic tract
Lateral geniculate nucleus
Lateral geniculate nucleus
Optic radiation
Medial geniculate nucleus
Superior colliculus
Periaqueductal gray matter
Third ventricle

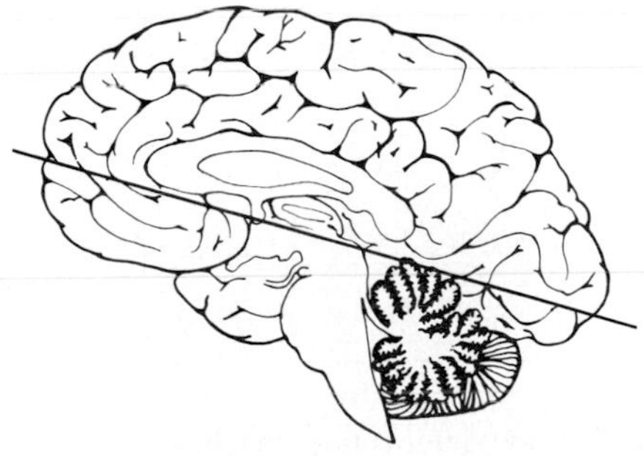

FIGURE 11-12
Horizontal section showing the optic tract entering the lateral geniculate nucleus on one side. The continuity of the cerebral aqueduct (surrounded by periaqueductal gray) and the third ventricle is shown nicely in this section. Notice the layering of the lateral geniculate nucleus (seen clearly on the left).

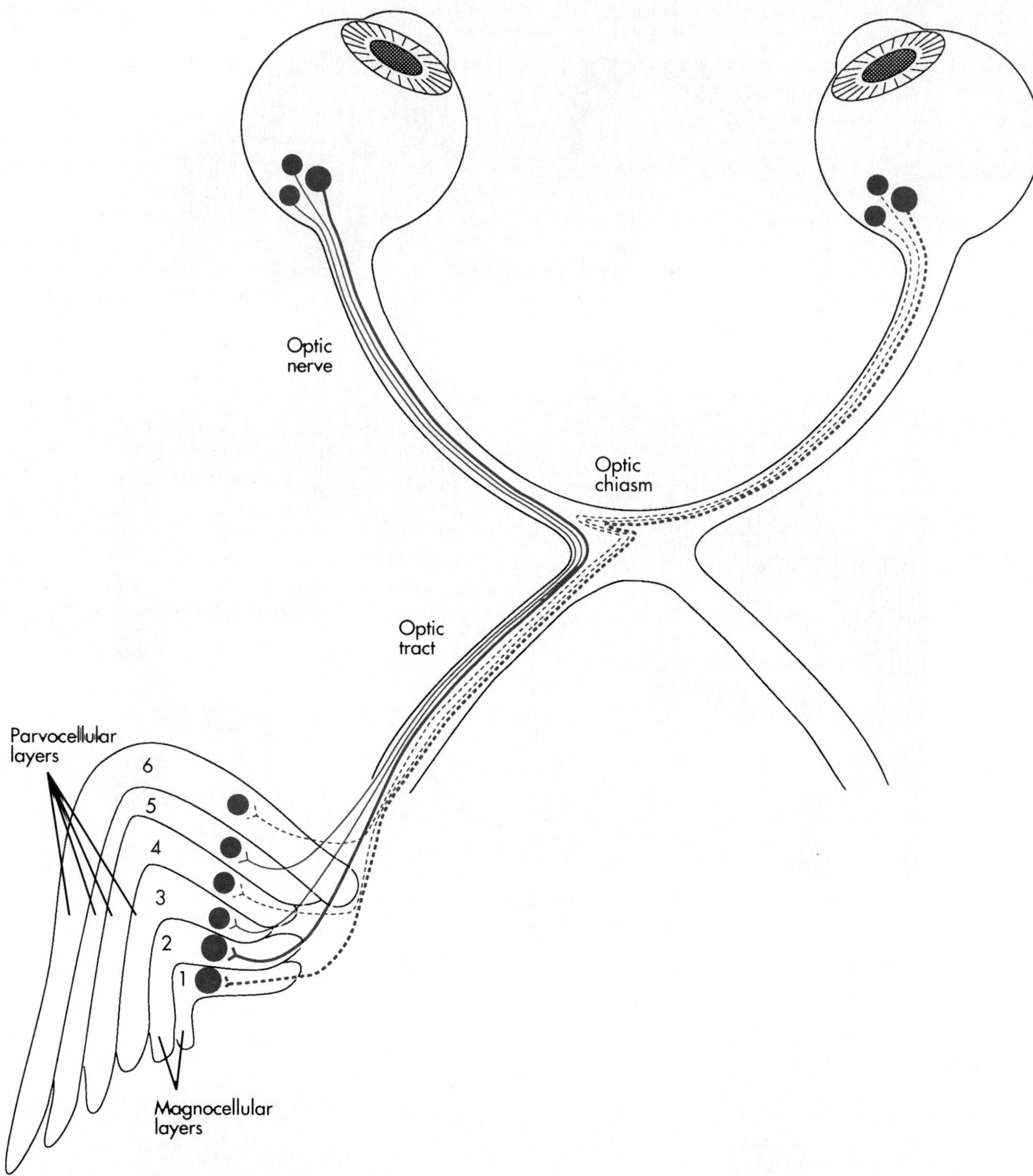


FIGURE 11-13
The projection from the retina to the lateral geniculate nucleus, indicating how information traveling in the magnocellular and parvocellular pathways, as well as information from the two eyes, remains segregated at the level of the lateral geniculate. Notice, however, that all information from a given point in the visual field ends up in a column that extends through all six geniculate layers.

lateral eye (Figure 11-13). Consistent with this anatomical arrangement, electrical recordings from the lateral geniculate nucleus reveal few cells that can be activated by both eyes.

Layers 3-6 contain small neurons that receive their inputs from the numerically dominant class of small ganglion cells sensitive to color and form. In view of its small neurons these layers are referred to as the *parvocellular layers* and this entire subdivision of the visual system as the *parvocellular system*. Layers 1 and 2 contain larger neurons that receive their inputs from a separate class of larger ganglion cells that are more sensitive to movement and contrast. This subdivision, including the *magnocellular layers* (1 and 2) of the lateral geniculate nucleus, is referred to as the *magnocellular system*.

## Optic radiation

Fibers arising in the lateral geniculate nucleus project through the retrolenticular and sublenticular parts of the internal capsule, curve around the lateral wall of the lateral ventricle (Figure 11-12 and 11-14), and terminate in the cortex adjacent to the calcarine sulcus. The optic radiation is often called the *geniculocalcarine tract,* reflecting its origin and termination. Not all of these fibers pass directly backward to the occipital lobe. Rather, they form a broad sheet covering much of the posterior and inferior horns of the ventricle. Fibers representing superior visual quadrants (that is, those representing inferior *retinal* quadrants) loop out into the temporal lobe *(Meyer's loop)* before turning posteriorly (Figure 11-14, *A*). As a result, temporal lobe damage can somewhat surprisingly produce a visual deficit.

A retinotopic organization is maintained in the optic radiation. Fibers representing inferior visual fields are most superior, whereas those representing superior visual fields loop farthest out into the temporal lobe. Macular fibers occupy a broad middle area. The visual pathway is more dispersed in the optic radiation than elsewhere, and individual fibers still carry information from only one eye, so damage here sometimes results in deficits that are slightly different for the two eyes.

The visual pathway ends retinotopically in the cortex above and below the calcarine sulcus (*area 17;* this numerical nomenclature, with which the cerebral cortex is divided into a series of areas called *Brodmann's areas,* is discussed in Chapter 15). Inferior visual fields project to the cortex above the calcarine sulcus and superior fields to the cortex below the sulcus. The macula is represented more posteriorly and peripheral fields more anteriorly (Figures 11-15 and 11-16). Numerous myelinated fibers ramify within this cortex in a discrete layer that can be seen as a thin white stripe (the *line of Gennari*) with the naked eye.

*Text continued on p. 296.*

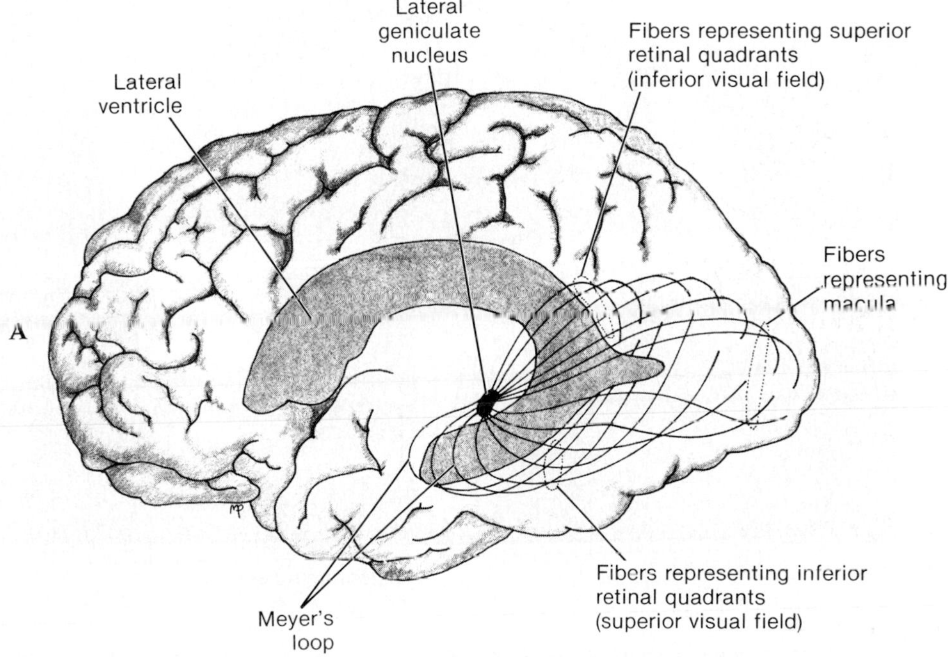


FIGURE 11-14

Three different views of the optic radiation. **A,** Schematic illustration of the course of geniculocalcarine fibers as they loop over the lateral aspect of the lateral ventricle and then turn posteriorly to end in the banks of the calcarine fissure on the medial surface of the hemisphere; note that the fibers representing inferior visual fields end in the upper bank, fibers representing superior visual fields end in the lower bank, and fibers representing the macula end most posteriorly.

*continued.*

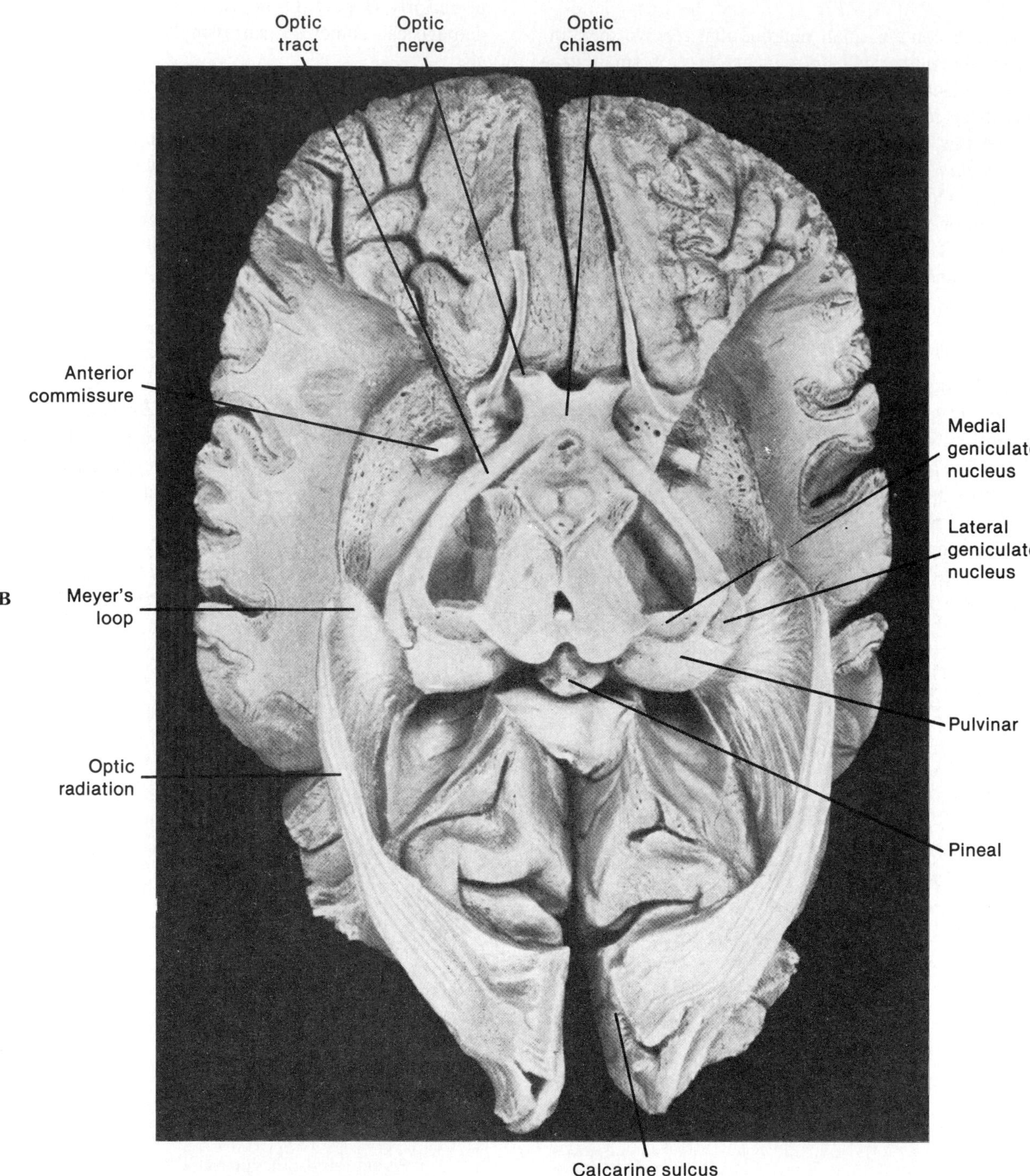


FIGURE 11-14, cont'd.
**B,** Inferior aspect of a brain dissected to show the entire visual pathway from optic nerve to striate cortex.

**B** from Ludwig E, Klingler J: Atlas cerebri humani, Boston, 1956, Little, Brown & Co.

C

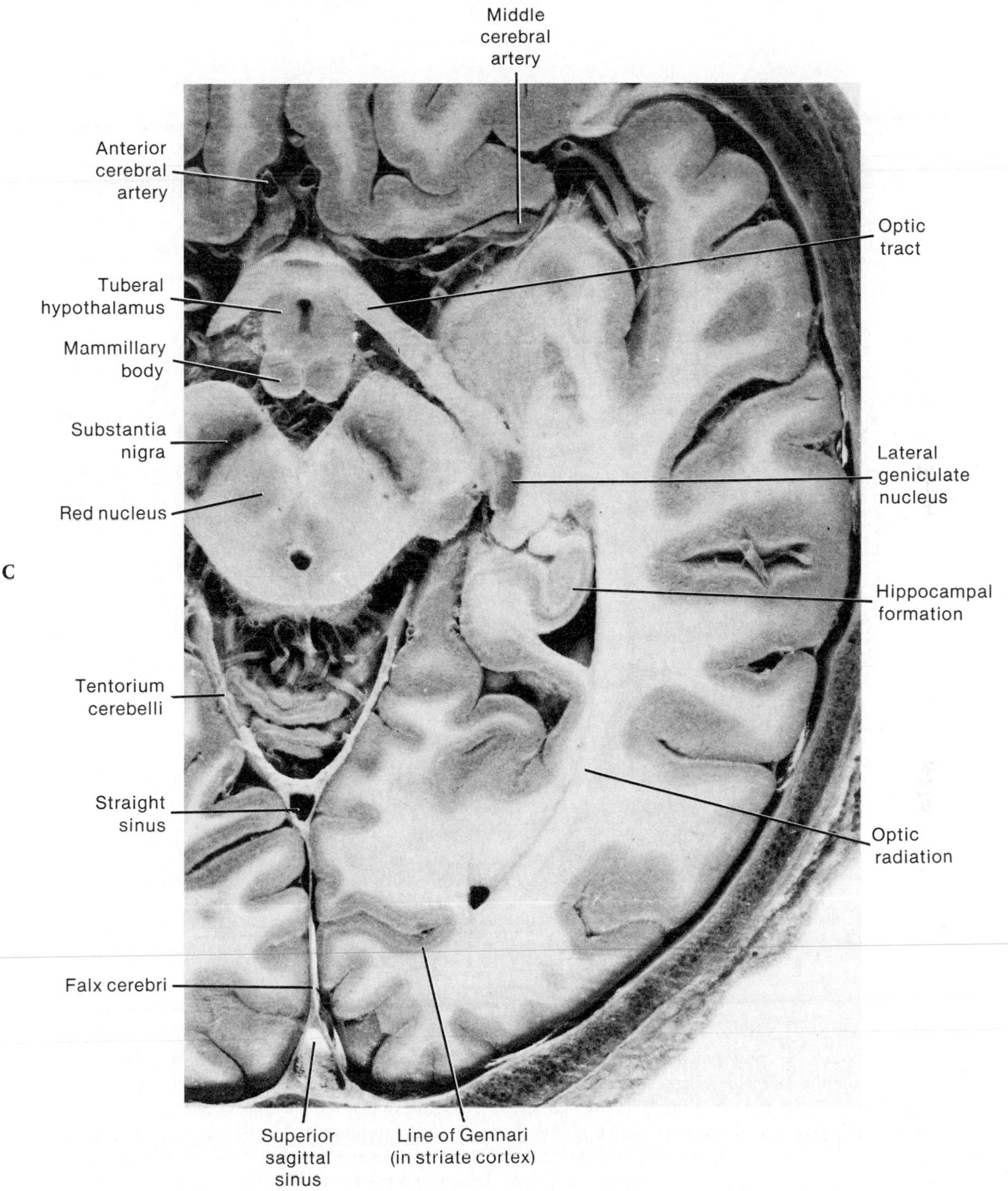


FIGURE 11-14, cont'd.

**C,** Enlargement of a portion of Figure 3-4 to show the visual pathway in a section approximately perpendicular to the long axis of the brainstem.

C courtesy of Dr. John T. Willson, University of Colorado Health Sciences Center.

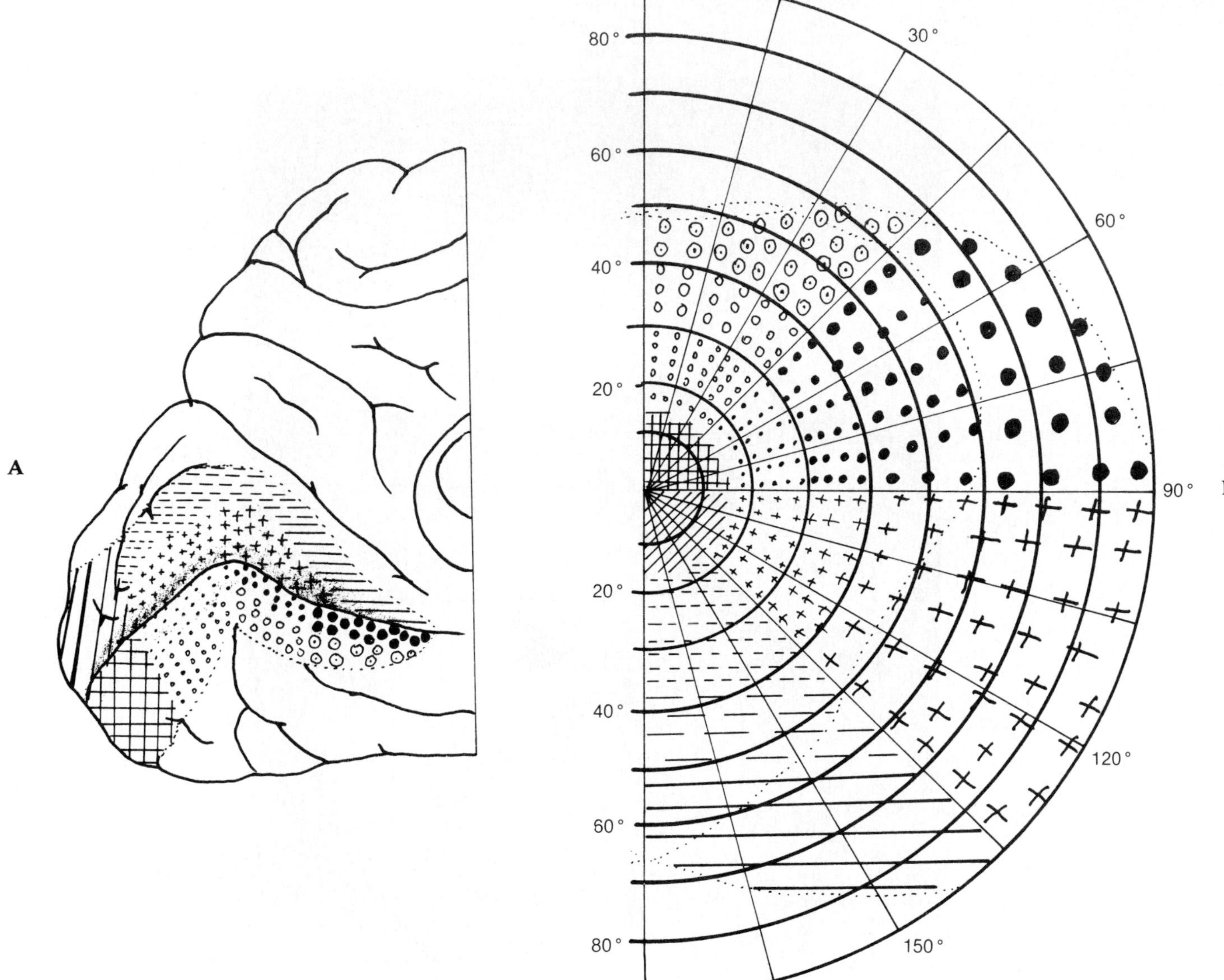


FIGURE 11-15

Mapping from the right visual field (**B, D**) to the striate cortex of the left hemisphere (**A, C**). In **A**, imagine that the calcarine sulcus has been pried open so that the map extends into its depths. In **B**, the inner dotted line outlines the area seen by both eyes; the right eye can see the edge of the area outlined by the outer dotted line (compare Figure 11-21). Note the disproportionately large area of striate cortex devoted to the representation of the macula (hatched and cross-hatched regions). More recent work (**C** and **D**), based on comparisons between visual field deficits and the extent of infarcts seen in magnetic resonance images, suggest that the representation of the macula is even larger than that depicted in the "classic" map shown in **A**. **C** and **D** also show clearly how the map of the visual field becomes distorted in the transition from retina to visual cortex, so that the vertical meridians end up in a roughly horizontal orientation. (**A** and **B** from Holmes G, *Proc R Soc Lond* B132:348, 1945. **C** and **D** adapted from Horton JC, Hoyt WF, *Arch Ophthalmol* 109:816, 1991.

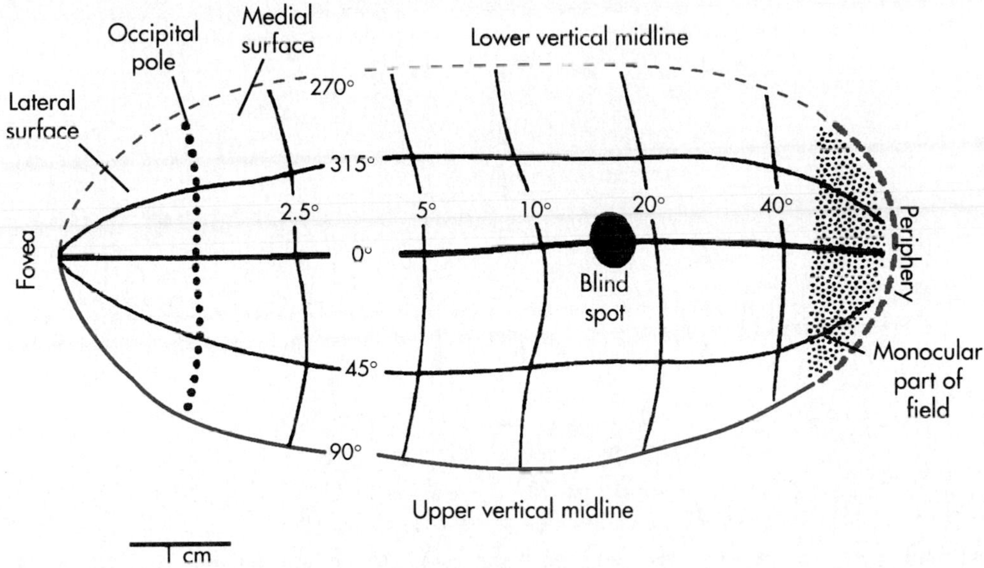


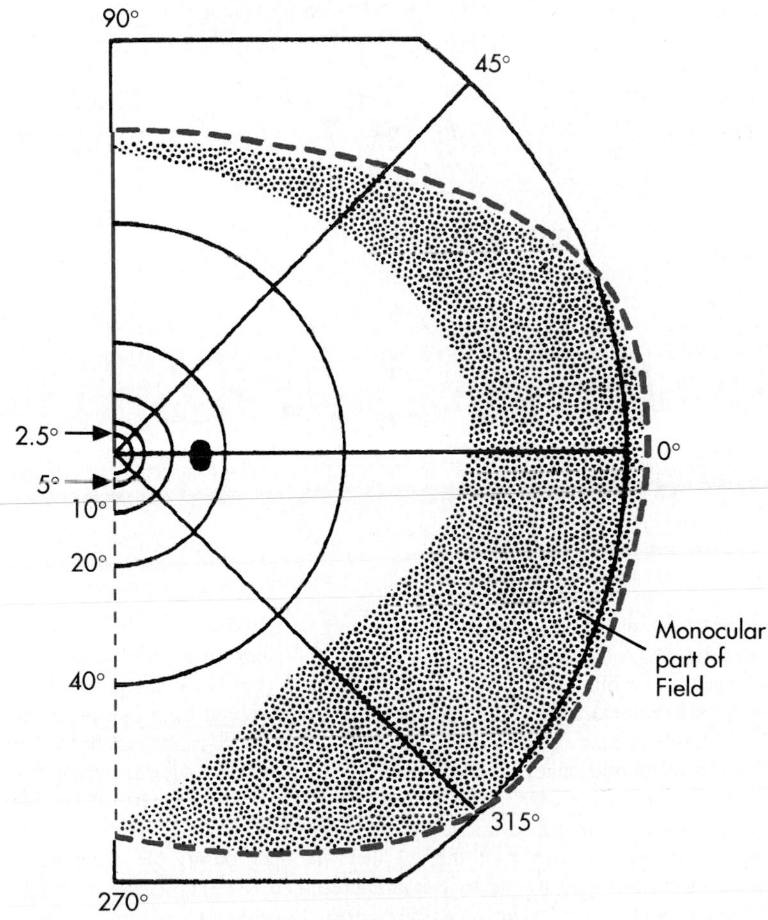


FIGURE 11-15, cont'd
For legend see opposite page.

A

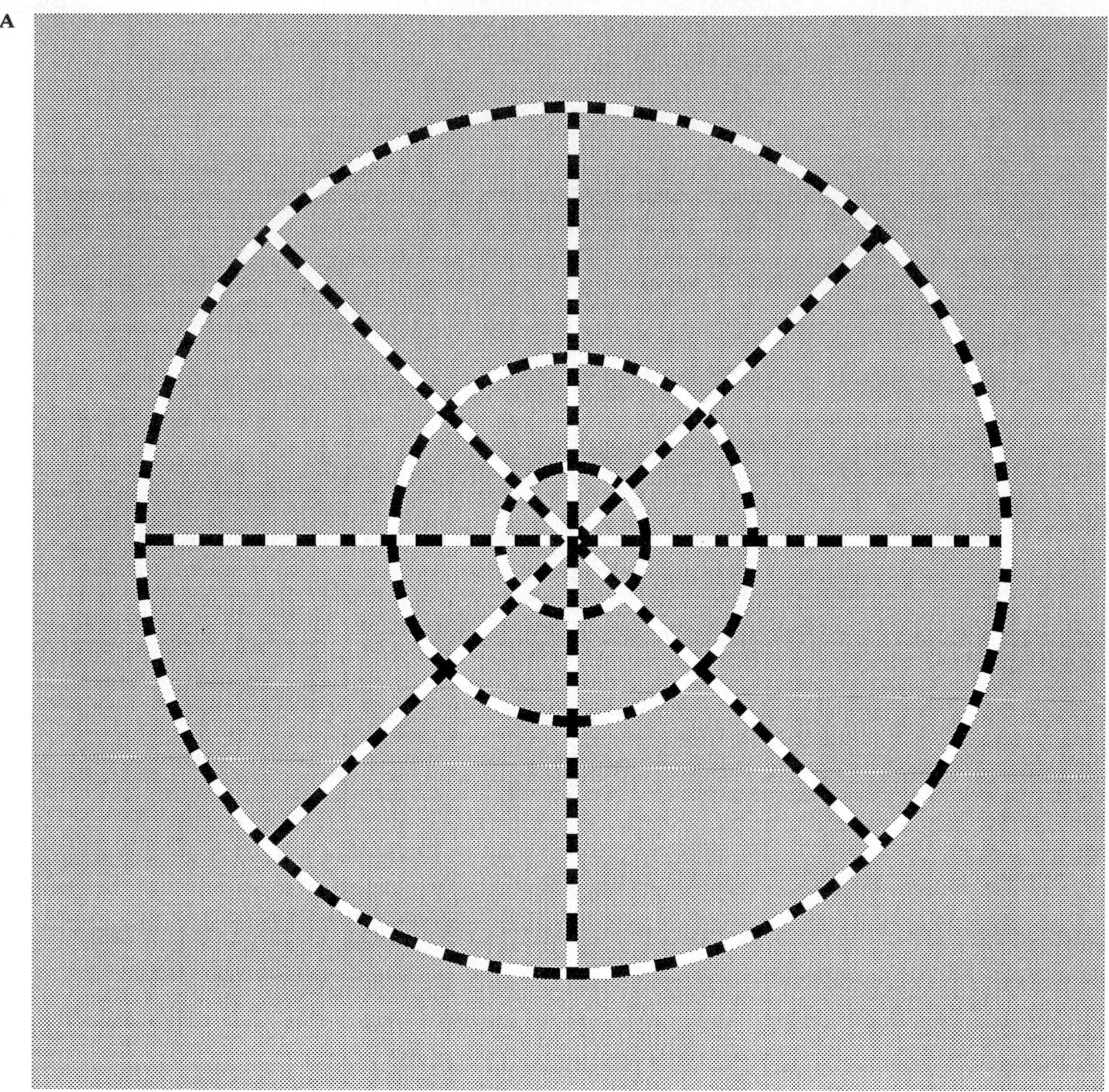

FIGURE 11-16

A remarkable, direct demonstration of the precise mapping of the visual field in the visual cortex of a monkey. The stimulus **(A)** was an array of dashed rings and lines on a gray background; during the experiment, the black and white segments reversed in contrast (the black segments turned white, and vice versa) at a freguency of 3 Hz. While watching the stimulus with one eye open the animal was injected with $^{14}C$-2-deoxyglucose, a radioactive analog of glucose that is taken up by active neurons and phosphorylated into a metabolite that cannot leave the cell. Subsequent autoradiography of a tangential section through the left visual cortex revealed a distorted but precise map **(B)** of the right half of the stimulus; each dark area corresponds to a small group of neurons that receive input from a particular small area of the visual field, primarily via the eye that was open during the experiment. The overall change in shape of the visual field by the time it is represented in striate cortex is diagrammed in **C**. (Adapted from Tootell RBH et al., *J Neurosci* 8:1531, 1988. Courtesy of Dr. Roger Tootell, Department of Neurobiology, Harvard Medical School.)

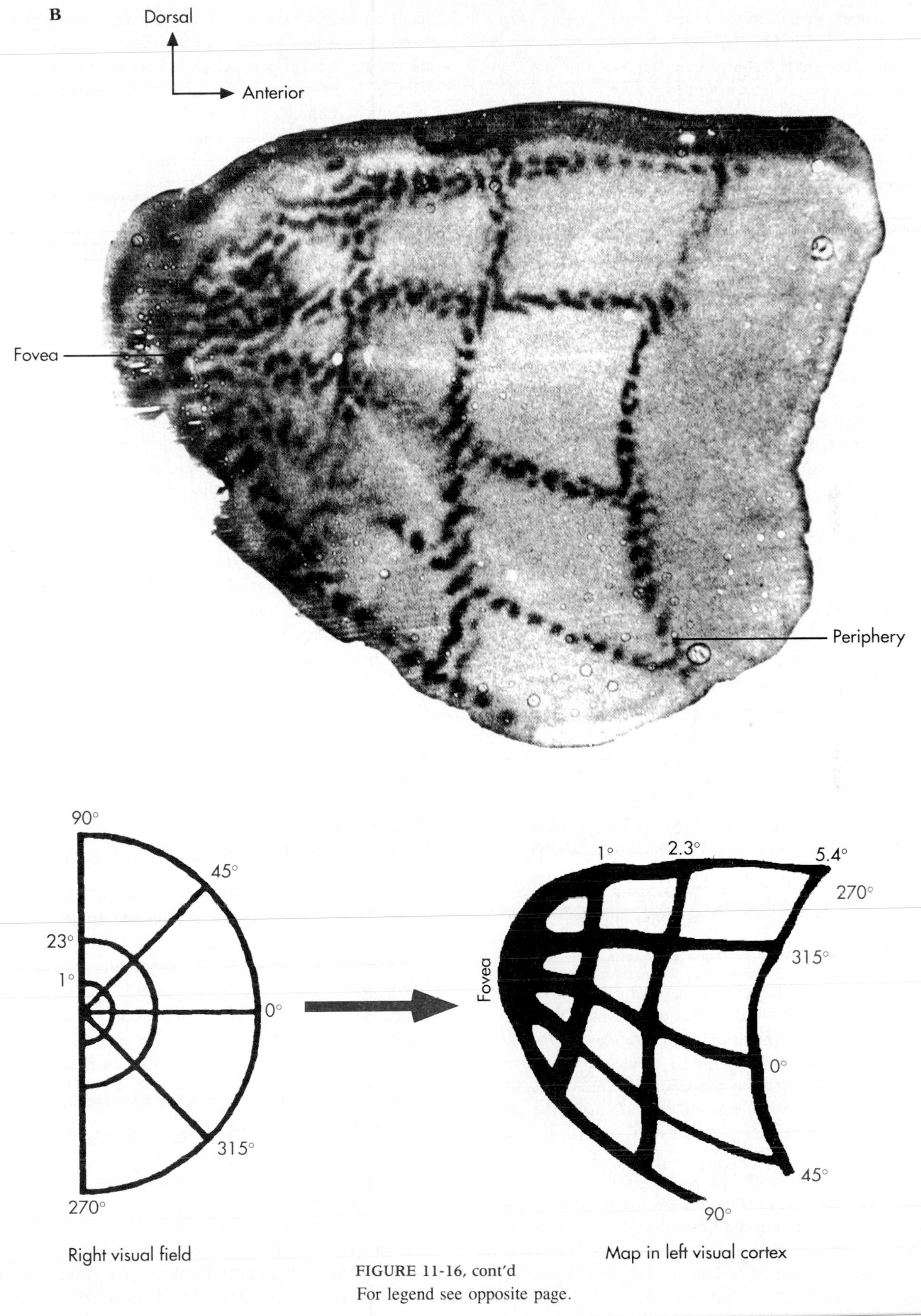


FIGURE 11-16, cont'd
For legend see opposite page.

Hence primary visual cortex is also called *striate cortex.*

The striate cortex parallels the calcarine sulcus and extends for a very short distance onto the posterior surface of the occipital lobe. It is surrounded by *area 18,* which in turn is surrounded by *area 19,* the two together comprising almost all the rest of the occipital lobe. Areas 18 and 19 are commonly referred to as the *visual association cortex* and are heavily interconnected with area 17. The parvocellular and magnocellular systems, as described later in this chapter, follow separate though interrelated routes through areas 17, 18, and 19.

### Superior colliculus

The common vertebrate plan of central visual connections includes not only a projection from the retina to the lateral geniculate nucleus (or its equivalent), but also a projection to the superior colliculus (or its equivalent). In lower vertebrates the collicular (or tectal) pathway is the more important, but in primates it is much less so. Nevertheless, the major inputs to the primate superior colliculus are still visual: one arising in the retina and the second in the striate cortex. The retinal input consists of a substantial number of fibers in each optic tract that bypass the lateral geniculate nucleus, pass over the medial geniculate nucleus in a bundle called the *brachium of the superior colliculus* (or *superior brachium*) (Figure 10-8), and terminate retinotopically in the superior colliculus and in the nearby *pretectal area* (described later). A few of these fibers are collaterals of axons that also terminate in the lateral geniculate nucleus, but most arise from separate subpopulations of ganglion cells. The cortical input consists of cells in area 17 that project to the superior colliculus (again via its brachium) and end in a pattern that coincides with the retinotopic map in the colliculus.

In addition to visual inputs, the superior colliculus receives (1) somatosensory inputs (sometimes referred to as the *spinotectal* or *spinomesencephalic tract*), many of them collaterals of fibers in somatosensory pathways ascending to the thalamus; (2) auditory inputs, chiefly by way of projections from the inferior colliculus; and (3) additional inputs from other areas of the cortex.

Efferent connections of the superior colliculus include projections to the reticular formation, the inferior colliculus, and the cervical spinal cord (the *tectospinal tract*). Of interest with respect to the visual system, the superior colliculus also projects to the posterior thalamus, notably to the lateral geniculate nucleus and the pulvinar. The pulvinar, in turn, projects to cortical areas 18 and 19, the visual association cortex.

The function of the human superior colliculus is poorly understood. It is presumed to play a role in certain reflexes, such as orienting the head to visual (or other) stimuli, and in certain kinds of eye movements. However, no known clinical condition in humans can be attributed specifically to damage to the superior colliculus. On the other hand, monkeys have been shown, with careful training, to have considerable visual capacity after extensive lesions of the striate cortex, particularly when dealing with moving stimuli. In a few rare cases of selective damage to the striate cortex, humans too have been found to have residual visual capacities that are strange and paradoxical: for example, despite having no conscious awareness of visual stimuli in the "blind" portions of their visual fields, they may be able to point to such stimuli quite accurately. There are a number of alternatives for the anatomical basis for this residual visual capacity; an example is the pathway to areas 18 and 19 via the superior colliculus and pulvinar. The relative importance of the various possible pathways is poorly understood at present, as is the function of these paths in the intact nervous system.

### Retinohypothalamic fibers

Photic input is involved in many neuroendocrine functions, so one might expect that there would be projections from the retina to the hypothalamus. It has now been shown directly that such fibers exist in a variety of mammals (including primates like us); these fibers end in a small hypothalamic nucleus above the optic chiasm called the *suprachiasmatic nucleus*. Many of our physical functions wax and wane with a 24-hour rhythm (*circadian rhythm,* from the Latin words *circa* and *diem* meaning about a day). For example, our body temperature rises and falls about a degree, being highest late in the afternoon and lowest early in the morning, when we are normally asleep. Many other circadian rhythms are known, involving such things as hormone secretion, eating, drinking, alertness, and excretion of various electrolytes. If no information about day length is available (as in the case of an animal living in constant light or constant darkness), the cycles of these rhythms become a little longer than 24 hours. This implies that one or more "clocks" exist within our bodies, that left to their own devices these clocks have a period of slightly more than 24 hours, and that under normal circumstances information about day length *entrains* the clocks to a period of 24 hours. There is now considerable evidence that the suprachiasmatic nucleus of the hypothalamus is a "master clock" for the timing of many (but not all) circadian rhythms and that direct retinal input to the suprachiasmatic nucleus provides the information for entraining these rhythms to a 24-hour cycle.

## PROCESSING OF VISUAL INFORMATION

The visual system can be viewed as a series of synapses beginning in the outer plexiform layer and extending to and beyond the visual association cortex of areas 18 and 19. At each level a certain amount of information processing takes place, so cortical neurons respond best to stimuli that are quite different from those best able to stimulate individual rods and cones. A cell at any given level in the visual system is conventionally characterized by its *recep-*

*tive field,* which refers to that area of the retina in which changing conditions of illumination produce an alteration of the cell's activity. By extension, receptive fields can also be defined in terms of the particular part of the outside world whose image falls on this region of the retina. One initially surprising observation about the receptive fields of the bipolar cells and more proximal neurons is that the intensity of illumination is relatively unimportant in determining a cell's level of activity. Rather, the important parameter is the contrast between different areas of the receptive field. That is, the visual system is especially attuned to the detection of borders between light and dark areas.

Recordings from individual ganglion cells show that their receptive fields are composed of two concentric, roughly circular zones. Illumination of the central area (the *center*) causes either an increase or a decrease in the background firing rate, whereas illumination of the peripheral area (the *surround*) has the opposite effect. Simultaneous illumination of both center and surround causes relatively little change in firing rate, since the antagonistic effects of the two areas tend to cancel each other. Cells of the parvocellular and magnocellular systems differ from each other in the sizes of their receptive fields, their color sensitivity and some temporal aspects of their responses, but not in their basic center-surround organization. Thus even at the level of the ganglion cell, the contrast between two different areas of the receptive fields is of paramount importance.

The properties of the center of such receptive fields reflect the "straight-through" receptor-bipolar-ganglion cell path. The properties of the surround result at least partially from the influence of receptors in the surround on receptors in the center by way of horizontal cells. Thus the basic spatial organization of ganglion cell receptive fields occurs in the outer plexiform layer. Further lateral interactions in the inner plexiform layer, mediated by amacrine cells, are thought to modify such things as the temporal characteristics of the ganglion cell response. For example, some ganglion cells respond only transiently to a change in illumination, whereas others show a maintained change in discharge rate. Many lower vertebrates have much more complex ganglion cell receptive fields, and there is a corresponding increase in the thickness of the inner plexiform layer and a proliferation of amacrine cell synapses.

Receptive fields of cells in the lateral geniculate nucleus are generally similar to those of ganglion cells. The contrast detection mechanism is somewhat more efficient, so that uniform illumination causes less response than in the case of ganglion cells.

The receptive fields of cortical neurons are rather more complicated, and names such as "simple," "complex," and "hypercomplex" have been coined to describe these cells. Simple cells respond best either to a dark bar on a light background or to a light bar on a dark background; uniform illumination has essentially no effect. In addition, the bar must be oriented at a particular angle. It has been hypothesized that the receptive fields of simple cells result from the convergence of a large number of geniculate axons onto a single cortical neuron; if the receptive fields of these axons fell along a straight line, a bar-shaped receptive field with flanking antagonistic areas could result. Complex and hypercomplex cells respond best to edges, bars, and corners and have particular orientation and movement properties. Many of their properties, like those of the simple cells, could be explained by the convergence of simpler neurons onto a single cell.

This account of visual processing is obviously highly simplified. It is selective as well in that data dealing with color vision and binocular interactions have not been discussed. It is known, for example, that many cells in the primate visual system have wavelength-specific properties and that there are cortical neurons that are sensitive to the location of an object in three-dimensional space as well as to its size and shape. Aspects like color and depth are processed in parallel with form and movement. These various qualities begin to be sorted out in the division of the lateral geniculate into parvocellular and magnocellular layers. The sorting continues as a partially separate-partially interconnected sequence of projections of the parvocellular and magnocellular systems through areas 17, 18, and 19. While the details are incompletely understood, and the independence of the two systems is far from total, in general the parvocellular system (color, detailed form) projects to more ventral portions of areas 18 and 19 and the magnocellular system (location, movement) to more dorsal portions (Figure 11-17).

## PLASTICITY

The visual system has provided a unique opportunity to study the extent to which connections within the CNS are genetically determined and unchangeable and the extent to which they can be influenced by the environment.

Recordings from neurons in the visual cortex of newborn cats and monkeys never previously exposed to light reveal that the basic properties of these neurons are similar to those of adults. This indicates that the wiring pattern of the visual system is, to a great extent, genetically determined and does not depend on visual input for its formation.

If, however, one eye of a newborn animal is covered for the first few months of its life, that eye will be permanently blind (in a perceptual sense) when uncovered. At the same time, cortical neurons are found to respond only to stimulation of the eye that had not been covered. This appears to be primarily the result of the replacement of "idle" synapses by connections reflecting activity in the noncovered eye.

This effect of covering an eye is specific to the first few months of life, and no deficit results if it occurs later. Also

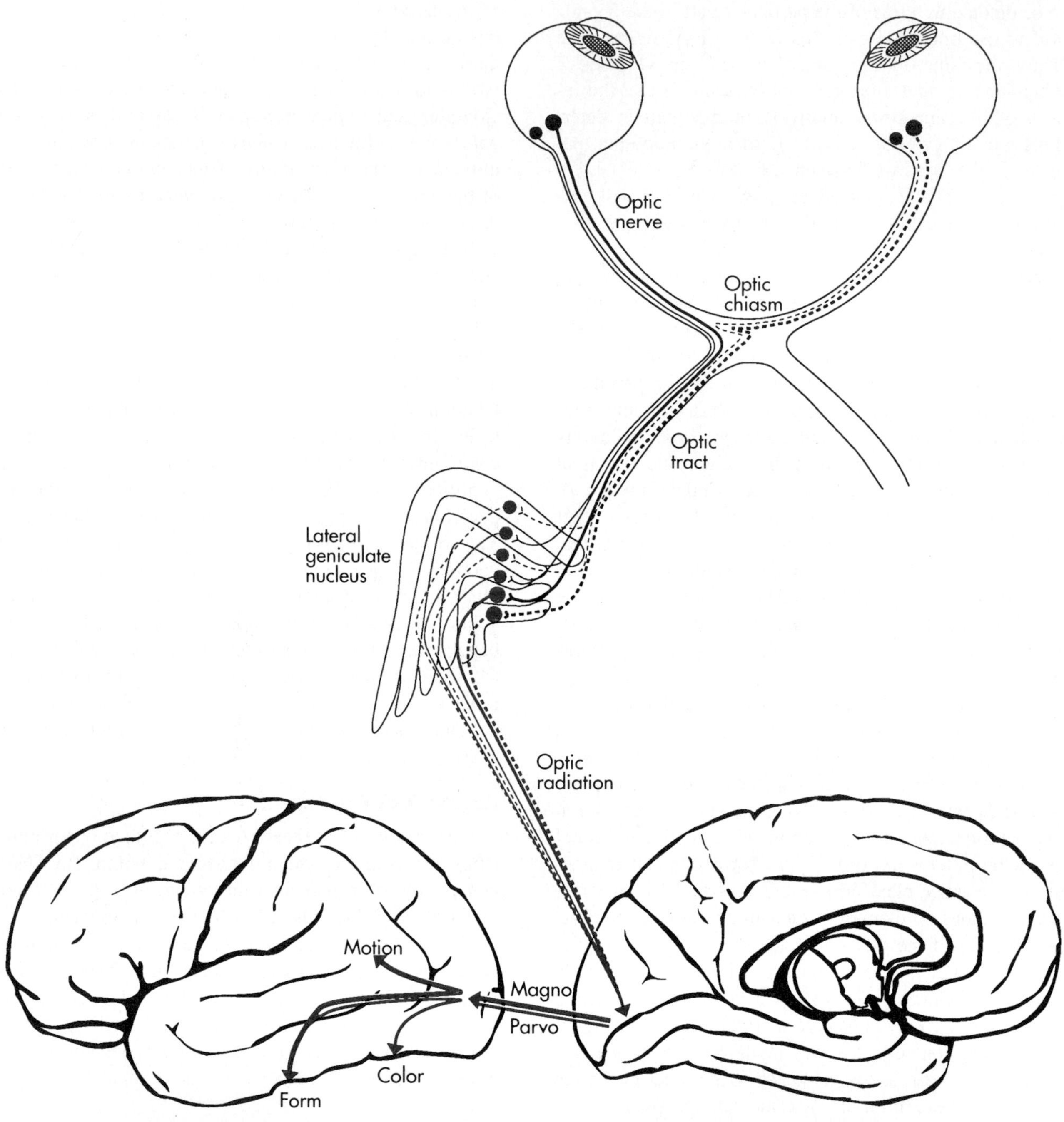


FIGURE 11-17
Schematic indication of the distribution of higher order visual processing among different cortical areas. The actual distribution system is far more complex than illustrated here; for example, dozens of separate visual areas, related to each other by literally hundreds of sets of interconnections, have been described in primate cortex. However, in a very general sense there is a superior stream of connections (dominated by the magnocellular system) concerned with the location and motion of objects and an inferior stream of connections (dominated by the parvocellular system) concerned with the form and color of objects.

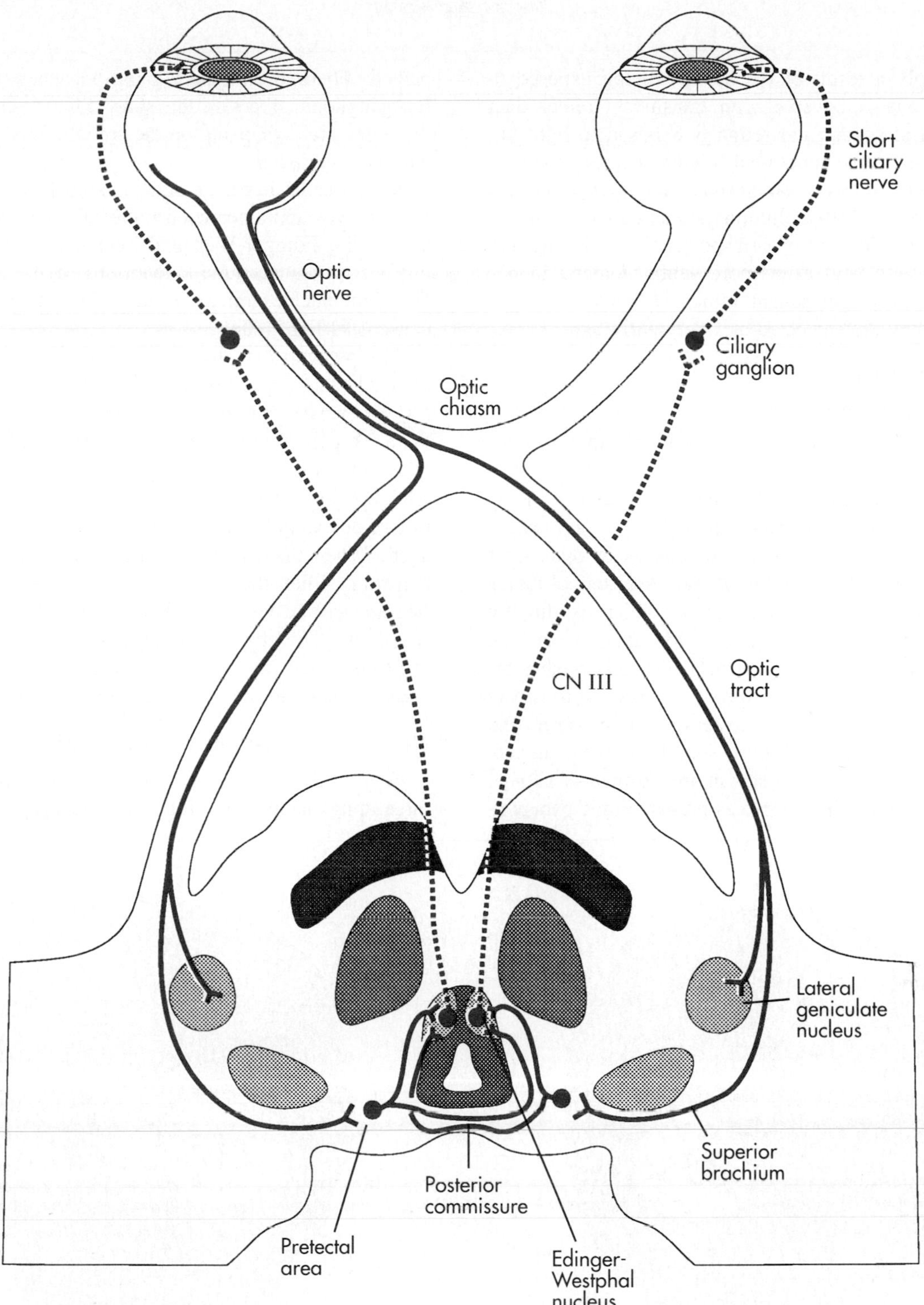


FIGURE 11-18
Pathway of the pupillary light reflex. For the sake of simplicity, crossing fibers from one pretectal area to the contralateral Edinger-Westphal nucleus are shown as passing only through the posterior commissure. In fact, some also cross ventral to the aqueduct.

Modified from Nolte J: Iris and pupil. In Records RE, editor: Physiology of the human eye and visual system, New York, 1979, Harper & Row.

it is not simply a result of the eye not being exposed to light. If the eye is covered with translucent rather than opaque material so that the retina is exposed to light but not patterns, the same functional blindness results. This is consistent with the fact that normal cortical neurons respond as poorly to diffuse illumination as they do to no illumination at all. This also corresponds to the finding that infantile cataracts (and even more subtle defects) in humans can result in permanent blindness (called *amblyopia*), unless they are corrected at a very early age.

## VISUAL REFLEXES

### Pupillary light reflex

Light directed into one eye causes both pupils to constrict. The response of the pupil of the illuminated eye is called the *direct pupillary light reflex,* whereas that of the other eye is called the *consensual pupillary light reflex*. The afferent limb of the reflex arc consists of optic tract axons that enter the brachium of the superior colliculus and terminate in the *pretectal area,* which is directly rostral to the superior colliculus at the junction between midbrain and diencephalon. Pretectal neurons project bilaterally to the Edinger-Westphal nucleus, with fibers crossing both through the posterior commissure and through the periaqueductal gray ventral to the aqueduct (Figure 11-18). Axons of cells in the Edinger-Westphal nucleus travel in the third nerve as preganglionic parasympathetic fibers to the ciliary ganglion, where they synapse. Postganglionic fibers in the short ciliary nerves complete the reflex arc, synapsing on the smooth muscle cells of the pupillary sphincter.

Since one optic tract contains axons from ganglion cells in both eyes and since each pretectal area projects bilaterally to the Edinger-Westphal nucleus, light directed into one eye causes the same amount of activity in the Edinger-Westphal nucleus on each side. This is the basis of the consensual light reflex.

The pathways of the pupillary light reflex are utilized clinically in a procedure known as the *swinging flashlight test* for damage to one retina or optic nerve (Figure 11-19). With the patient seated in a dimly lit room, a light source is quickly moved back and forth from one eye to the other, while the examiner observes the behavior of each pupil in turn. For example, assume the right optic nerve is damaged. When the left eye is illuminated, both pupils will constrict. When the right eye is illuminated, the light reflex arc will be less effectively activated, and both pupils will dilate. Therefore when the light is moved from the left eye to the right, the right pupil will be seen to dilate, indicating damage to the right retina or optic nerve.

### Near reflex (accommodation reflex)

When visual attention is directed to a nearby object, three things happen in a reflex manner: (1) *convergence* of

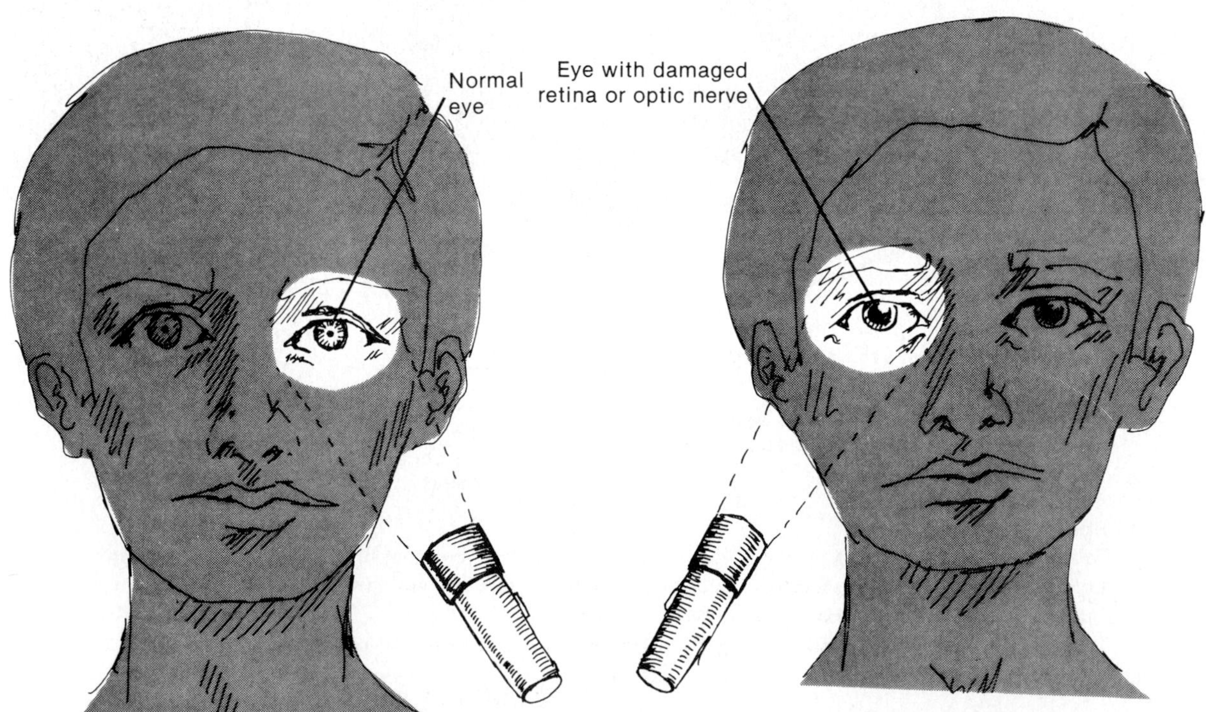


FIGURE 11-19
Swinging flashlight test with the results expected from an individual with a damaged right retina or optic nerve.

the two eyes, so the image of the object falls on both foveas; (2) contraction of the ciliary muscle and a resultant thickening of the lens *(accommodation),* so the image of the object is in focus on the retina; and (3) pupillary *constriction,* which improves the optical performance of the eye by reducing certain types of aberration and by increasing its depth of focus.

Unlike the pupillary light reflex, the *near reflex* requires the participation of the cerebral cortex. The pathway involved is poorly understood but is generally considered to follow the normal visual pathway to the striate cortex, project to the visual association cortex, and go from there to the superior colliculus and/or pretectal area (Figure 11-20). Impulses are then relayed to the oculomotor nucleus, stimulating medial rectus motor neurons and preganglionic motor neurons of the Edinger-Westphal nucleus.

Although the same preganglionic parasympathetic fibers are thought to mediate the pupillary constriction of both the light reflex and the near reflex, these two types of constriction can nevertheless be dissociated in certain pathological conditions. An *Argyll Robertson pupil* refers to a condition (usually bilateral and usually a manifestation of neurosyphilis) in which the pupil constricts during the near reflex but not in response to light. The site of the lesion involved is not known with certainty, but it is often assumed to be in that portion of the pretectal area subserving the light reflex.

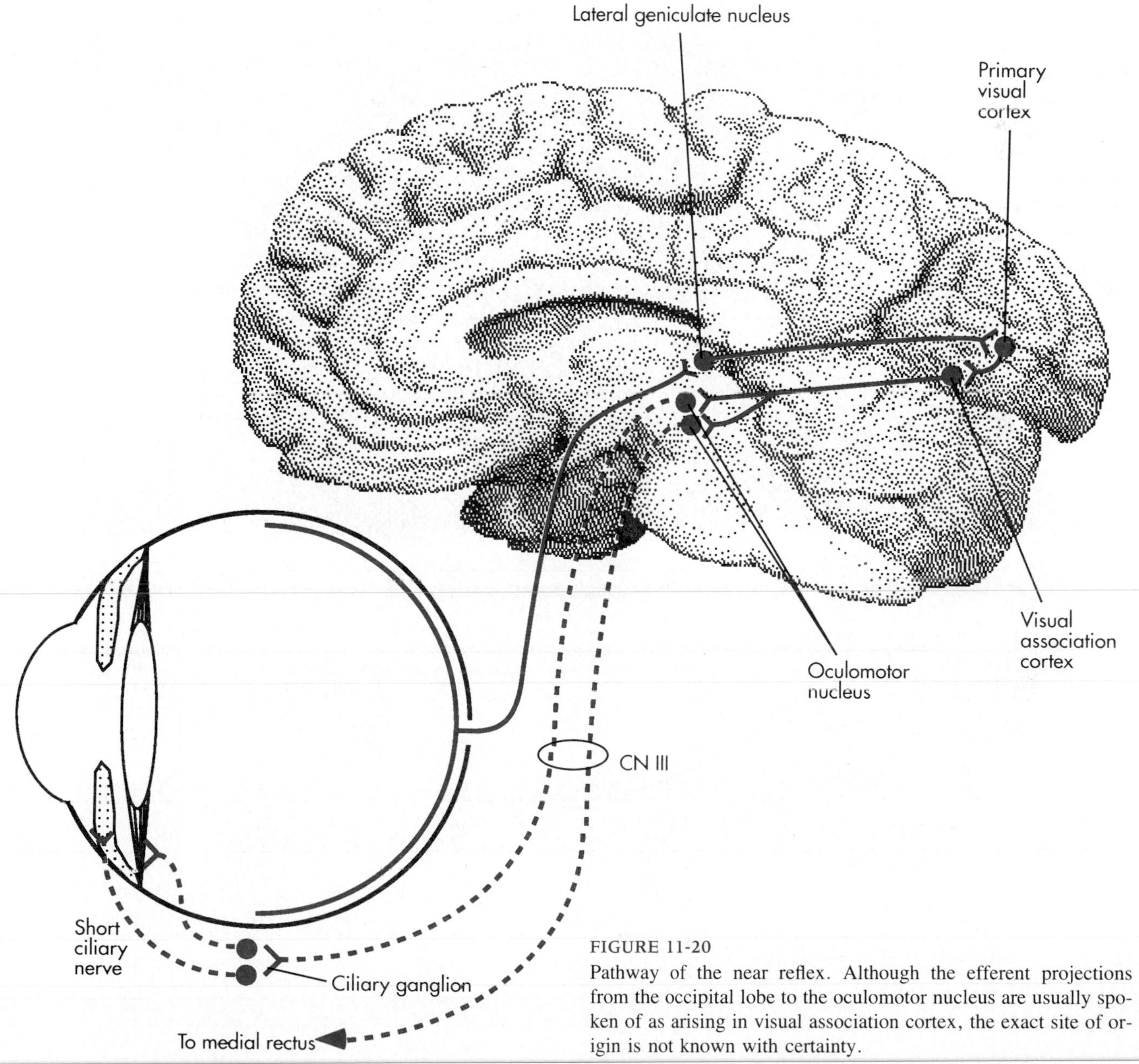


FIGURE 11-20
Pathway of the near reflex. Although the efferent projections from the occipital lobe to the oculomotor nucleus are usually spoken of as arising in visual association cortex, the exact site of origin is not known with certainty.

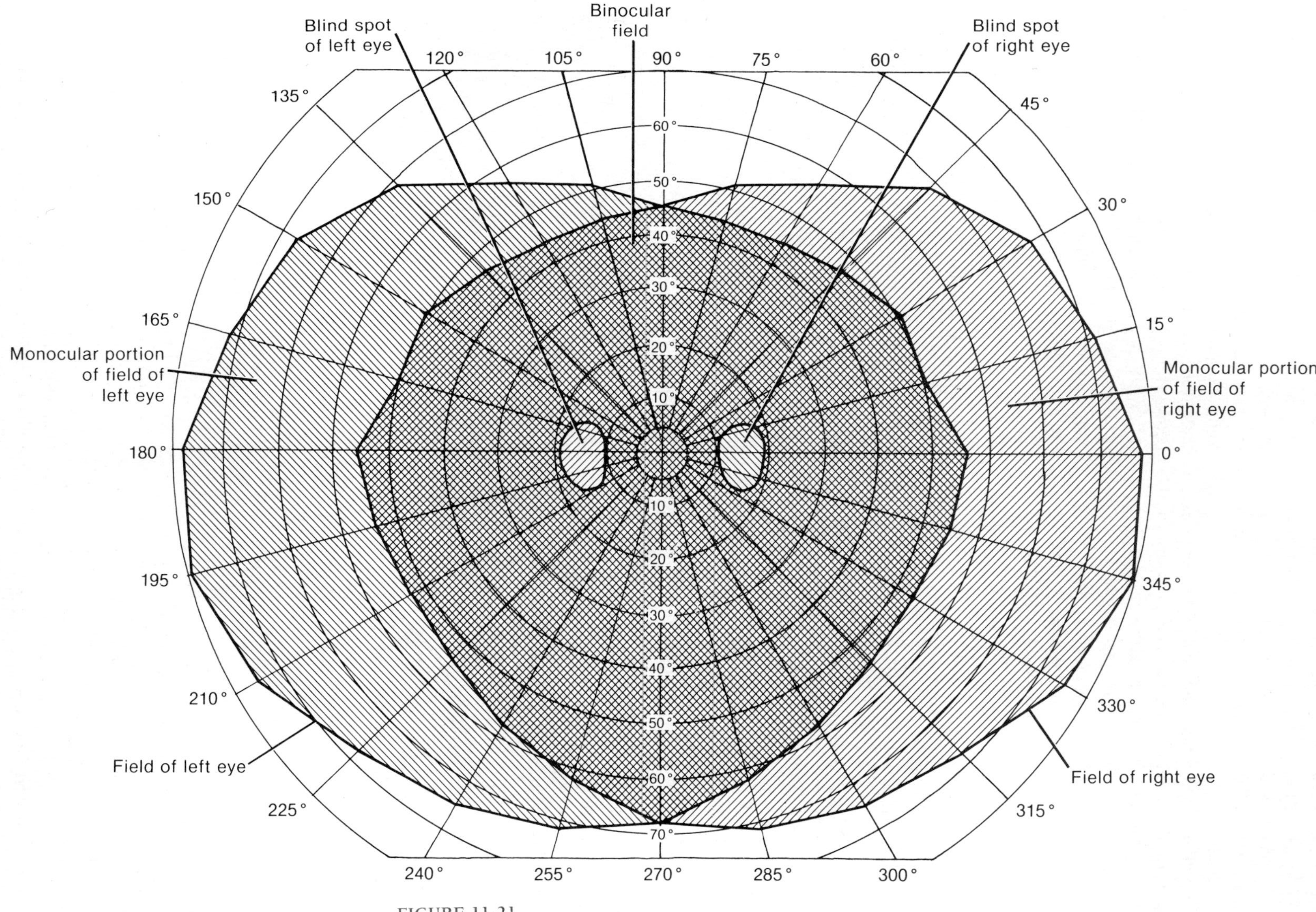


FIGURE 11-21
Normal visual fields for the two eyes, superimposed on each other.
Courtesy of Dr. Bruce Wilson and Marilyn Haner, Denver General Hospital.

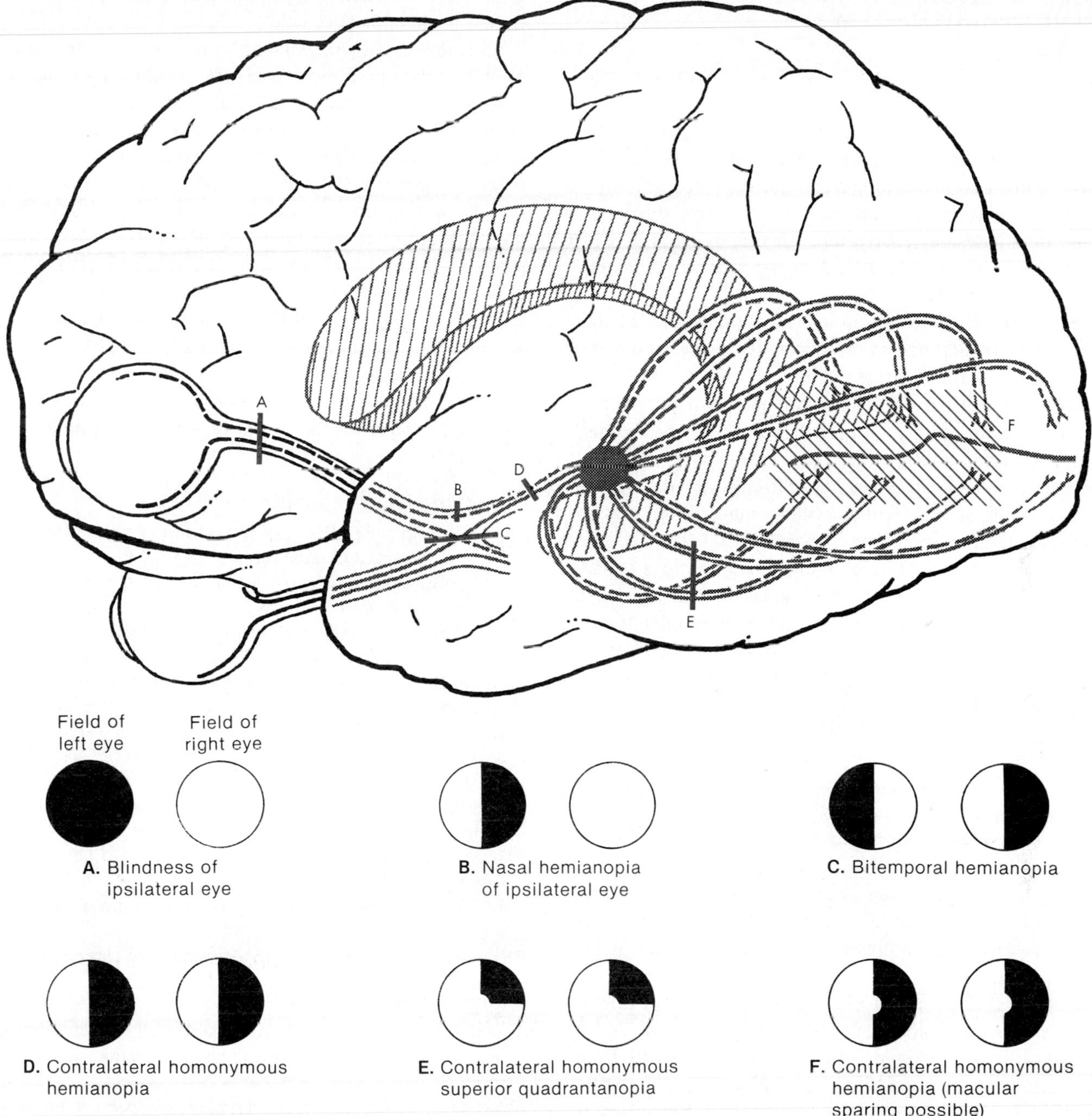


FIGURE 11-22
Visual field deficits caused by lesions at various points along the visual pathway. **A,** Destruction of one optic nerve causes blindness of the eye in which that nerve arises. **B,** Damage to one side of the optic chiasm destroys the noncrossing fibers from the ipsilateral eye; these fibers arise in the temporal retina, so a nasal hemianopia of the ipsilateral eye results. **C,** Pressure on the middle of the optic chiasm, typically from a pituitary tumor, destroys the crossing fibers from both eyes, causing a bitemporal hemianopia (one type of heteronymous hemianopia). **D,** Destruction of one optic tract causes contralateral homonymous hemianopia. **E,** Damage to one temporal lobe could destroy part of the optic radiation, specifically the fibers representing the contralateral superior quadrant of each visual field; since the optic radiation is rather spread out at this point, some fibers are likely to be spared (for example, in this case the macular fibers remain intact). **F,** Massive damage to one occipital lobe (such as might be caused by occlusion of one posterior cerebral artery) causes contralateral homonymous hemianopia; the macular representation is quite large, and some of it is likely to survive, resulting in macular sparing.

## SOME FUNCTIONAL ASPECTS OF THE VISUAL SYSTEM

### Visual deficits

Visual fields are tested by moving a small object in from the periphery until the patient, with one eye covered, reports seeing it. By repeating this for many different directions of approach, a chart of the visual field can be made (Figure 11-21). Each eye can normally see a surprising 90 degrees from the visual axis in a temporal direction, but the field is less extensive in other directions. The area of overlap of the two visual fields is the area in which binocular vision is possible.

Deficits resulting from damage to various parts of the visual pathway are named according to certain conventions. Most important, visual defects are always named according to the visual field loss and not according to the area of the retina that is nonfunctional. Since the retinal image is inverted and reversed, damage to temporal areas of the retina would cause nasal field losses, and damage to superior areas of the retina would cause inferior field losses. The combining form "-anopia" (or "-anopsia") is used to denote loss of one or more quadrants of a visual field; *hemianopia* would refer to loss of half of the visual field, *quadrantanopia* to loss of one quarter of a visual field. Finally the term *homonymous* denotes a condition in which the visual field losses are similar for both eyes, and *heteronymous* denotes a condition in which the two eyes have nonoverlapping field losses.

Using this terminology, it is possible to name the deficits resulting from damage at most locations in the visual pathway (Figure 11-22); some of the names are quite spectacular. A lesion of one optic nerve causes blindness of that eye. Damage in the central region of the optic chiasm, affecting the crossing fibers, causes a heteronymous hemianopia (or in this case, a *bitemporal hemianopia*). This can result from midline pressure exerted by a tumor of the pituitary, which lies close to the chiasm (compare Figure 2-16). Lateral pressure on one side of the chiasm, affecting the noncrossing fibers on that side, would cause an ipsilateral *nasal hemianopia*. This occasionally results from an aneurysm of the internal carotid artery, which lies adjacent to the chiasm (see Figure 5-2). In the rare event of aneurysms of both internal carotid arteries, a *binasal hemianopia* could result. Destruction of one optic tract would interrupt all the fibers carrying information from the contralateral visual fields, causing a contralateral *homonymous hemianopia*.

Damage to the optic radiation is rarely extensive enough to cause complete hemianopia, and roughly quadrantic deficits are more often the result. For example, a large destructive lesion of the left temporal lobe, interrupting the fibers of Meyer's loop (which represent inferior retinal quadrants), would produce a *right homonymous superior quadrantanopia*. Lesions in either optic radiation or visual cortex leave the pupillary light reflex undisturbed, as would be predicted from the anatomical pathways involved in this reflex.

In cases of massive damage to the visual cortex of one occipital lobe (as, for example, after occlusion of one posterior cerebral artery), a contralateral homonymous hemianopia would be the expected result. In fact, it is frequently observed clinically that vision is preserved over much of the fovea. This phenomenon is called *macular* (or *foveal*) *sparing*, and its existence, extent, and basis have been a topic of debate for many years. Part of its origin probably lies in the disproportionately large representation of the fovea in the striate cortex; even very large cortical lesions may leave part of the foveal region undamaged. In addition, the distributions of the middle and posterior cerebral arteries overlap near the occipital pole. Therefore even total occlusion of the posterior cerebral artery allows for supply of part of the foveal region by the middle cerebral artery.

## ADDITIONAL READINGS


Altman J, Carpenter MB: Fiber projections of the superior colliculus in the cat, *J Comp Neurol* 116:157, 1961.

Bender MB, Bodis-Wollner I: Visual dysfunction in optic tract lesions, *Ann Neurol* 3:187, 1978. *Clinical observations of nonidentical visual losses in the two eyes, or of selective deficits of only some visual functions, following optic tract damage.*

Brouwer B, Zeeman WPC: The projection of the retina in the primary optic neuron in monkeys, *Brain* 49:1, 1926. *A description of the retinotopic organization of the optic nerve, chiasm, and tract, and of the pattern of termination of the optic tract in the lateral geniculate nucleus.*

Clarke S, Miklossy J: Occipital cortex in man: organization of callosal connections, related myelo- and cytoarchitecture, and putative boundaries of functional visual areas, *J Comp Neurol* 298:188, 1990.

Curcio CA et al: Human photoreceptor topography, *J Comp Neurol* 292:497, 1990.

Denny-Brown D, Chambers RA: Physiological aspects of visual perception. I. Functional aspects of visual cortex, *Arch Neurol* 33:219, 1976.

Denny-Brown D, Fischer EG: Physiological aspects of visual perception. II. The subcortical visual direction of behavior, *Arch Neurol* 33:228, 1976.

Dowling JE: *The retina: an approachable part of the brain,* Cambridge, 1987, The Belknap Press of Harvard University Press.

Holmes G: The organization of the visual cortex in man, *Proc R Soc Lond* B132:348, 1945.

Horton JC, Hoyt WF: The representation of the visual field in human striate cortex. A revision of the classic Holmes map, *Arch Ophthalmol* 109:816, 1991.

Hoyt WF, Luis O: The primate chiasm, *Arch Ophthalmol* 70:69, 1963.

Hubel DH, Wiesel TN: Functional architecture of macaque monkey visual cortex, *Proc R Soc Lond* B198:1, 1977. *A detailed discussion of the elegant experiments on the primate visual system done by these two investigators over the previous 20 years.*

Humphrey NK, Weiskrantz L: Vision in monkeys after removal of the striate cortex, *Nature* 215:595, 1967.

Ishikawa S, Sakiya H, Kondo Y: The center for controlling the near reflex in the midbrain of the monkey: a double labelling study, *Brain Res* 519:217, 1990.

Jampel RS: Representation of the near-response on the cerebral cortex of the macaque, *Am J Ophthalmol* 48:573, 1959.

Kafka MS: Central nervous system control of mammalian circadian rhythms, *Fed Proc* 42:2782, 1982. *The introduction to a series of articles on this topic.*

Kupfer C: The projection of the macula in the lateral geniculate nucleus in man, *Am J Ophthalmoml* 54:597, 1962.

Livingstone MS et al: Physiological and anatomical evidence for a magnocellular defect in developmental dyslexia, *Proc Nat Acad Sci* 88:7943, 1991. *Recent evidence that an abnormality in the visual channel specialized for the analysis of rapidly changing stimuli could underlie dyslexia.*

Livingstone M, Hubel D: Segregation of form, color, movement, and depth: anatomy, physiology, and perception, *Science* 240:740, 1988. *An intriguing summary pointing out some striking correlations between the basic properties of visual system neurons and the ways in which we perceive things visually.*

Lowenstein O, Loewenfeld IE: *The pupil.* In Davson H, editor: *The eye.* Vol. 3. *Muscular mechanisms,* New York, 1969, Academic Press.

Magoun HW et al: The afferent path of the pupillary light reflex in the monkey, *Brain* 59:234, 1936.

McNaughton PA: Light response of vertebrate photoreceptors, *Physiol Rev* 70:847, 1990.

Mohler CW, Wurtz RH: Role of striate cortex and superior colliculus in visual guidance of saccadic eye movements in monkeys, *J Neurophysiol* 40:74, 1977.

Moore RY: Retinohypothalamic projection in mammals: a comparative study, *Brain Res* 49:403, 1973.

Nguyen-Legros J: Fine structure of the pigment epithelium in the vertebrate retina, *Int Rev Cytol* (Suppl.) 7:287, 1978.

Nordby K: *Vision in a complete achromat: a personal account.* In Hess RF, Sharpe LT, Nordby K, editors: *Night vision: basic, clinical and applied aspects,* Cambridge, 1990, Cambridge University Press. *Rarely, someone is born with a complete absence of cones. As this personal description indicates, color blindness is only one of the consequences.*

Pearlman AL, Birch J, Meadows JC: Cerebral color blindness: an acquired defect in hue discrimination. *Ann Neurol* 5:253, 1979. *One example of the notion that the primary visual cortex and visual association cortex are not like a screen on which the retinal image is projected; rather, a number of different subareas deal selectively with different aspects of the visual world.*

Perry VH, Cowey A: Retinal ganglion cells that project to the superior colliculus and pretectum in the macaque monkey, *Neuroscience* 12:1125, 1984.

Pollack JG, Hickey TL: The distribution of retinocollicular axon terminals in rhesus monkey, *J Comp Neurol* 185:587, 1979.

Pugh EN Jr, Lamb TD: Cyclic GMP and calcium: the internal messengers of excitation and adaptation in vertebrate photoreceptors, *Vision Res* 30:1923, 1990.

Reese BE, Cowey A: Fibre organization of the monkey optic tract: I. Segregation of functionally distinct optic axons; II. Noncongruent representation of the two half-retinae, *J Comp Neurol* 295:385 and 401, 1990.

Rushton WAH: King Charles II and the blind spot, *Vision Res* 19:225, 1979.

Schneider GE: Two visual systems, *Science* 163:895, 1969. *Differential effects of collicular and cortical damage on a hamster's visual capabilities.*

Schwartz WJ, Gainer H: Suprachiasmatic nucleus: use of $^{14}$C-labeled deoxyglucose uptake as a functional marker, *Science* 197:1089, 1977.

Sherman SM, Koch C: The control of retinogeniculate transmission in the mammalian lateral geniculate nucleus, *Exp Brain Res* 63:1, 1986. *The lateral geniculate probably has an important role in regulating the access of visual information to the cerebral cortex.*

Sherman SM, Spear PD: Organization of visual pathways in normal and visually deprived cats, *Physiol Rev* 62:738, 1982.

Tootell RBH et al: Functional anatomy of macaque striate cortex. II. Retinotopic organization, *J Neurosci* 8:1531, 1988.

Wässle H, Boycott BB: Functional architecture of the mammalian retina, *Physiol Rev* 71:447, 1991.

Weiskrantz L et al: Visual capacity in the hemianopic field following a restricted cortical ablation, *Brain* 97:709, 1974. *Remarkable account of the visual capabilities remaining in one individual after known selective damage to his striate cortex.*

Wilson ME, Cragg BG: Projections from the lateral geniculate nucleus in the cat and monkey, *J Anat* 101:677, 1967.

Wong-Riley MTT: Connections between the pulvinar nucleus and the prestriate cortex in the squirrel monkey as revealed by peroxidase histochemistry and autoradiography, *Brain Res* 134:249, 1977.

Wray SH: *Neuro-ophthalmologic manifestations of pituitary and parasellar lesions.* In Keener EB, editor: *Clinical neurosurgery,* Baltimore, 1977, Williams & Wilkins.

Zeki S: A century of cerebral achromatopsia, *Brain* 113.1721, 1990.

Zeki S: Colour vision and functional specialisation in the visual cortex, *Disc Neurosci* 6(2):11, 1990.

Zihl J, von Cramon D, Mai N: Selective disturbance of movement vision after bilateral brain damage, *Brain* 106:313, 1983. *Another example of the apparent parcellation of visual cortical areas into regions dealing with particular aspects of a visual stimulus.*

# CHAPTER 12

## *Corticospinal and Corticobulbar Tracts*

Each of us has fewer than 1 million motor neurons with which to control muscles. Without them, we would be completely unable to communicate with the outside world. With them, however, we are capable of an enormous range of complex activities, from automatic and semiautomatic movements such as postural adjustments to the characteristically human movements involved in speaking and writing. The ways in which a wide variety of neural structures interact to make these activities possible is the topic of Chapters 12 to 14.

### LEVELS OF ORGANIZATION OF MOTOR SYSTEMS

Determinants of activity in motor neurons may be very broadly divided into three overlapping classes:

1. *Built-in patterns* of neural connections
2. *Descending pathways* that modulate the activity of motor neurons; these effects may be direct or they may be indirect by way of influences on built-in neural subsystems
3. *Higher centers* that influence the activity of descending pathways

#### Built-in patterns

The stretch reflex is an obvious and simple example of a built-in pattern of neural connections that controls, to some extent, the activity of motor neurons. Stretching a muscle stimulates its muscle spindles, whose afferent fibers end on motor neurons that in turn cause the muscle to contract (Figure 7-8). Other reflexes, such as the flexor reflex (Figures 7-10 and 7-12), are more complex and involve a number of muscles and spinal segments. Finally, there are networks of interneurons in the brainstem and spinal cord that can act as pattern generators for movements such as walking. While some of the same interneurons that are involved in reflexes may also be part of the circuitry of these *central programs* (as they are often called), these programs are more than simply a stringing together of reflexes, each one triggering the next. One indication is that the principal features of central programs can persist in the absence of afferent input. As an extreme example, the spinal cord of a lamprey (a primitive, jawless fish) can be kept alive in a dish for several days. Such a spinal cord, completely isolated from the rest of the lamprey, can exhibit in its ventral roots oscillating bursts of action potentials that in an intact animal would produce rhythmic, coordinated swimming movements.

#### Descending pathways

Several descending pathways with effects on somatic motor neurons have already been mentioned (Figure 7-20). The *vestibulospinal tracts* are important mediators of postural adjustments. The *corticospinal tract* classically has been considered the principal mediator of voluntary movement, although as discussed in this chapter, its real role is not so clear these days. The *reticulospinal tracts* and, to a lesser extent, the *rubrospinal tract* are the principal alternate routes for the mediation of voluntary movement. The rubrospinal tract originates in the red nucleus, crosses to the other side of the midbrain, descends in the lateral part of the brainstem tegmentum, and travels through the lateral funiculus of the spinal cord in company with the lateral corticospinal tract. The rubrospinal tract of humans is quite small, and the reticulospinal tracts are the major alternate route to the spinal cord. A *tectospinal tract* has also been described, descending from the superior colliculus through the contralateral anterior funiculus of cervical levels of the spinal cord. It is assumed to be important in reflex turning of the head in response to visual and perhaps other stimuli, but little is actually known of its function in humans.

## Higher centers

Even though corticospinal, rubrospinal, reticulospinal, and vestibulospinal fibers are able to influence motor neurons and their local connections, this still does not explain how a voluntary movement is made. At the present time we are able to say very little about the nature of the little person within the CNS who pulls the strings when we decide to move. We can, however, specify some of the structures and connections that must be involved in the sense that damage to these structures and connections results in defective movements. In addition to the portions of the CNS already mentioned, these structures include the basal ganglia, the cerebellum, and portions of the thalamus. The basal ganglia and the cerebellum are the subjects of Chapters 13 and 14, but the general way in which the various components of the motor system are interconnected is briefly discussed here.

In one sense, the components of the motor system are organized hierarchically, as though premotor areas of the cortex devise the plan for a movement and pass this information on to the motor cortex, which then issues commands to motor neurons either directly or indirectly by way of nuclei and interneurons of the brainstem and spinal cord (Figure 12-1, *A*). In another sense the components of the motor system are organized in parallel, much as in the case of sensory pathways; messages are conveyed to motor neurons not only from motor cortex but also from premotor areas themselves. The cerebellum and basal ganglia are involved in various aspects of planning and monitoring movements but have no outputs of their own to the spinal cord. Rather, they act primarily by affecting motor and premotor cortex (Figure 12-1, *B*).

This is an extremely simplified overview of the central motor apparatus and omits a number of important details. Some of these details are mentioned in this and the next two chapters, whereas others are beyond the scope of this

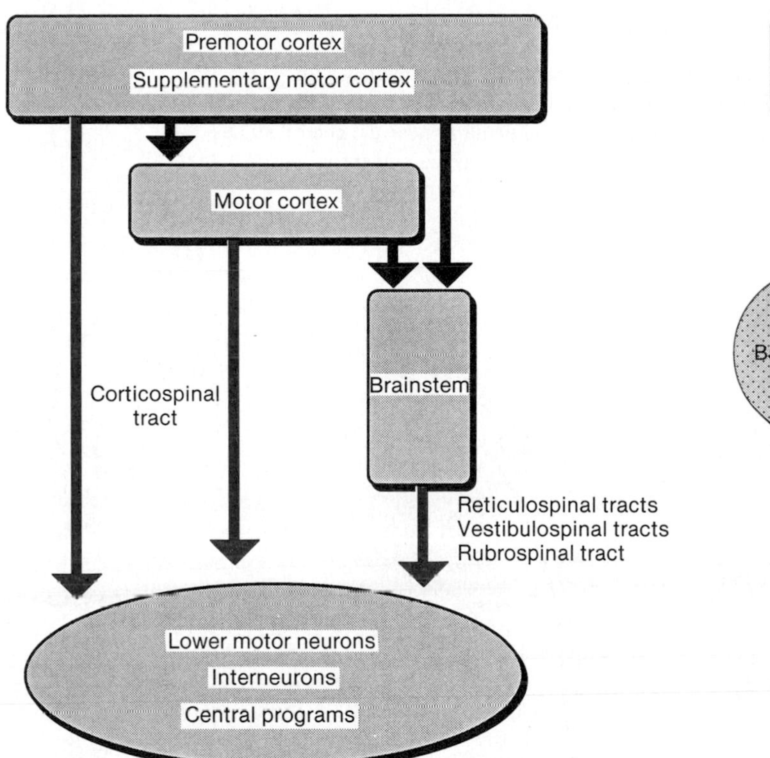


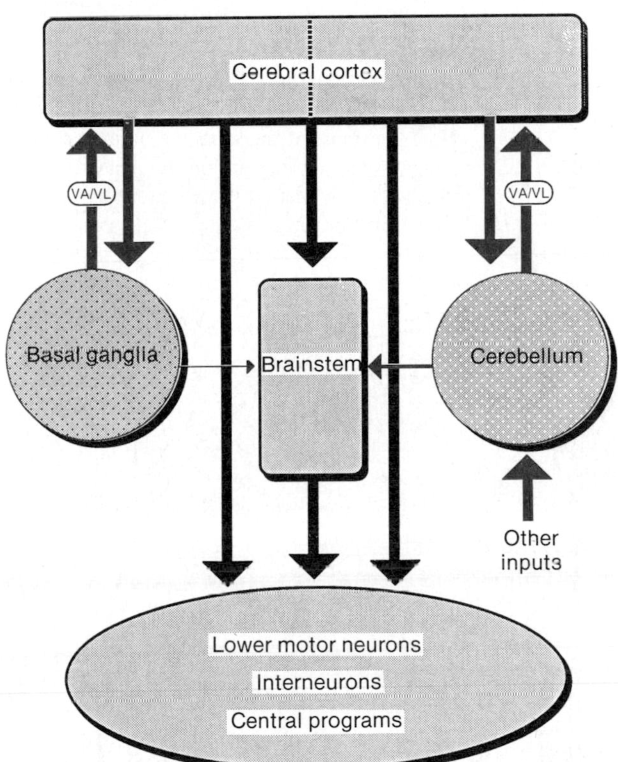


FIGURE 12-1
Overview of descending motor control pathways. **A,** Pathways that directly affect motor neurons and motor programs. The brainstem and the pool of lower motor neurons are indicated as separate entities in this schematic diagram, but some motor neurons and programs are, of course, located physically in the brainstem. **B,** The cerebellum and basal ganglia influence movement primarily by influencing the output from cerebral cortex to brainstem and spinal cord. (These connections are discussed in greater detail in Chapters 13 and 14.) Each acts to a great extent through different cortical areas, and each also has additional outputs to brainstem nuclei (minor for the basal ganglia, more substantial for the cerebellum). The basal ganglia receive inputs primarily from the cerebral cortex, as well as from other parts of the basal ganglia system. The cerebellum, in contrast, receives large quantities of sensory information from noncortical sources.

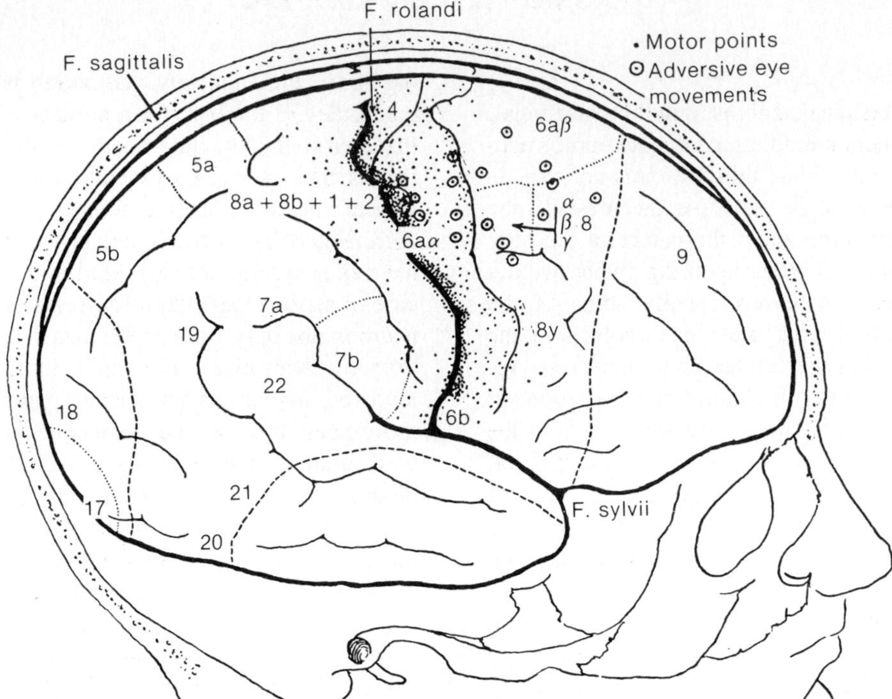


FIGURE 12-2
Composite diagram of the locations that yielded discrete movements when stimulated with a very weak electrical current in a series of conscious human patients during the course of neurosurgical procedures. Note that most of the sensitive points lie on the precentral gyrus, particularly near the central sulcus, but a significant number are on the postcentral gyrus and a few are anterior to the precentral gyrus.
From Penfield, W, Boldrey E: Brain 60:389, 1937.

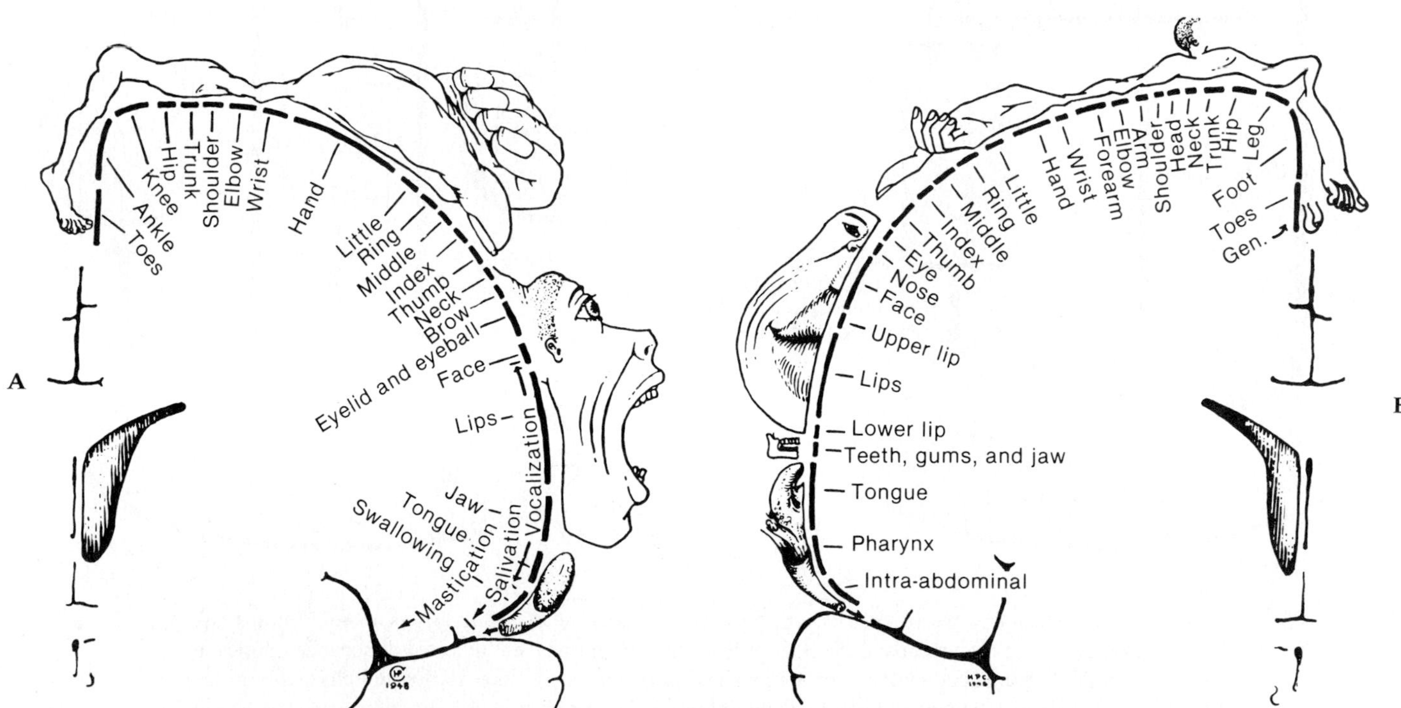


FIGURE 12-3
Somatotopic mappings in human motor **(A)** and somatosensory **(B)** cortex obtained by electrical stimulation of the surface of the brains of conscious patients undergoing neurosurgery. The size of a given part of the homunculus is roughly proportional to the size of the cortical area devoted to that body part.
From The cerebral cortex of man by W. Penfield and T. Rasmussen. Copyright © 1950 by Macmillan Publishing Co., Inc., renewed 1978 by T. Rasmussen.

book. For example, no mention has been made of the role of sensory input to this system. Such input is clearly involved, since we are easily able to make appropriate modifications in the walking program to accommodate an increased load such as a backpack or modifications in the running program to accommodate the sight of an impending brick wall. A variety of pathological conditions reflect motor deficits resulting from sensory losses. One example already cited is the ataxia resulting from damage to the posterior columns.

## CORTICOSPINAL TRACT

During the nineteenth century it was discovered that electrical stimulation of certain areas of the mammalian cerebral cortex causes movements of the contralateral side of the body. In humans the area with the lowest threshold for this effect lies in the precentral gyrus (Figure 12-2) and so has come to be called the *primary motor cortex*. Subsequent work showed that there is a distorted mapping of the body in the primary motor cortex, so stimulation of restricted cortical areas causes contraction of small groups of muscles or even single muscles. The somatotopic map (Figure 12-3) is distorted in such a way that the parts of the body capable of intricate movements (such as the fingers and lips) have disproportionately large representations. The *motor homunculus* (Latin for little person) is thus similar to the sensory homunculus in the somatosensory cortex of the postcentral gyrus, and this corresponds to (among other things) the notion that detailed sensory information is required for fine motor control.* There is a second map of the body in the *premotor cortex* directly anterior to primary motor cortex and a third in the *supplementary motor area,* located on the medial surface of the hemisphere just anterior to the representation of the foot in primary motor cortex (Figure 12-4). Movements can be elicited by electrically stimulating the premotor and supplementary motor areas, but more current is required than in the case of primary motor cortex. In addition, the movements are more complex. Stimulating the premotor cortex may cause turning of the trunk to the opposite side or

*Other species have maps distorted in different but appropriate ways. For example, nearly two thirds of the fibers leaving an elephant's motor cortex are bound for its facial motor nucleus, reflecting an elephant's fine control over trunk movements; only one third of the fibers reach the spinal cord.

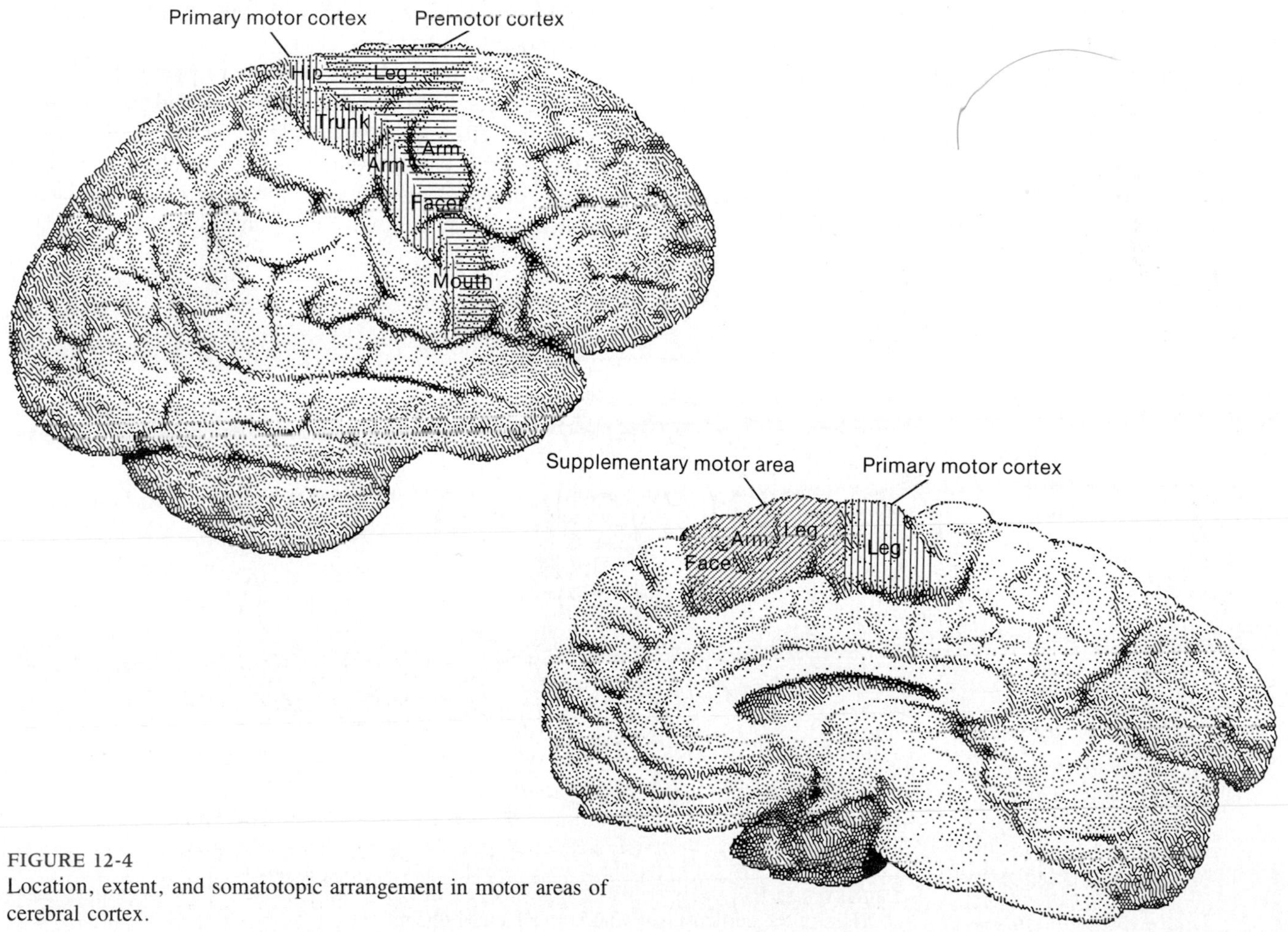


FIGURE 12-4
Location, extent, and somatotopic arrangement in motor areas of cerebral cortex.

movement of the entire contralateral arm. Stimulating the supplementary motor area can cause bilateral movements, vocalizations, or the arrest of speech.

It was also known in the previous century that the primary motor cortex contains giant pyramidal cells called *Betz cells,* whose axons descend to the spinal cord through the medullary pyramids; it was further known that cerebral lesions that destroy either the area containing motor cortex or the axons of the Betz cells as they pass through the posterior limb of the internal capsule cause contralateral spastic paralysis. Therefore it became accepted neurological thinking that the corticospinal tract (1) consists exclusively of large axons, (2) originates in the precentral gyrus, (3) proceeds exclusively to the spinal cord, (4) is necessary for voluntary movement, and (5) is a tract whose destruction results in spastic paralysis. However, it has gradually become apparent that this traditional description is incorrect in almost every way.

1. The large (up to 22 μm) axons of Betz cells are included in the corticospinal tract, but they account for only about 3% of the tract's 1 million fibers. The vast majority of corticospinal fibers are much smaller, in the 1 to 4 μm range. Whether the small fibers have a role different from that of the larger fibers is not known.

2. Betz cells reside specifically in primary motor cortex, but only about half of the corticospinal fibers originate in this cortical area. The remainder come from the premotor and supplementary motor areas and from the parietal lobe, particularly the somatosensory cortex of the postcentral gyrus (Figure 12-5). In view of this fact, many investigators now refer to the cortical complex on both sides of the central sulcus as the *sensorimotor cortex.*

3. Corticospinal fibers, as their name implies, end in the spinal cord. However, in their course from cortex to cord they give rise to large numbers of collaterals that end in a wide variety of locations, including the basal ganglia, the thalamus, the reticular formation, and various sensory nuclei such as the posterior column nuclei. Even within the spinal cord some end in the posterior horn, others end in the intermediate gray matter, and a minority end directly on alpha and gamma motor neurons.

These numerous connections make it seem unlikely that the corticospinal tract has a single, easily specified function. The projections to sensory nuclei, for example, might serve to compensate somehow for the altered afferent activity to be caused by an impending movement.

The corticospinal tract does, of course, have a major effect on motor neurons as well, both directly and indirectly by way of interneurons. In general, both alpha and gamma motor neurons are affected similarly. The utility of this *alpha-gamma coactivation* can be seen in Figure 6-8. If only the alpha motor neurons were activated, during the resulting contraction the muscle spindles would be "destretched" and hence inactive. Stretch reflexes thus would be inoperative and unable to help compensate for sudden changes in load during the movement. Activating the gamma motor neurons as well serves to maintain spindle sensitivity throughout the movement.

4. Studies in which both medullary pyramids of monkeys were carefully and selectively severed have demonstrated that after an initial period of flaccid paralysis, surprisingly little chronic motor deficit results from a total loss of corticospinal function. In moving about their cages, these animals are virtually indistinguishable from normal

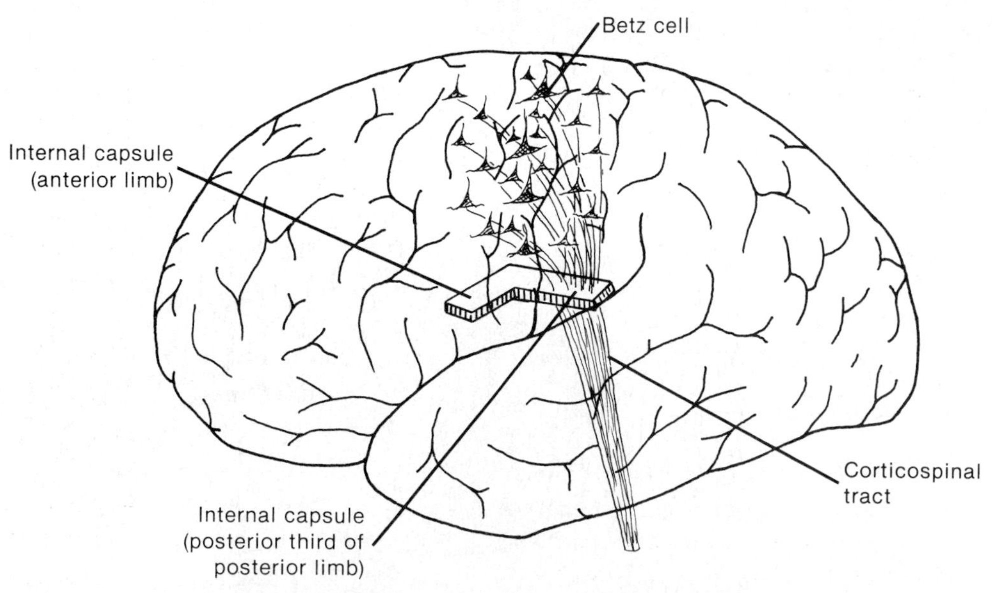


FIGURE 12-5
Origin of the corticospinal (and corticobulbar) fibers.

monkeys. The only behaviorally obvious deficit is a permanent inability to use their fingers individually as, for example, in picking up a small object between thumb and forefinger. This is a serious loss for creatures who use their hands as much and as skillfully as primates do, but nevertheless it falls far short of being a generalized weakness or paralysis of voluntary movements.

If lesions of medial portions of the medullary reticular formation are added to the corticospinal lesion, a severe and permanent disability of the axial muscles results. Conversely, if lesions of the lateral portions of the medullary reticular formation are added to the corticospinal lesion, a severe and permanent disability of independent use of the arms (including, of course, the fingers) results. Evidently the reticulospinal and/or rubrospinal tracts can compensate for the role normally played by the corticospinal tract in most aspects of voluntary movement.

Naturally occurring lesions in humans are never so neatly restricted as those in the monkeys just mentioned, and comparable cases of humans with selective damage to the pyramids are rare. However, there once was a neurosurgical procedure (whose rationale is explained in the next chapter) in which the corticospinal tract was cut in the cerebral peduncle. In these cases, the results were quite similar to those encountered with pyramid-sectioned monkeys, and relatively little chronic deficit resulted.

5. Spastic paralysis, commonly the result of a stroke involving the internal capsule, is characterized by (among other things) increased muscle tone and hyperactive reflexes. However, selective damage to the corticospinal tract, as in the experiments just referred to, causes little chronic change in tone or reflexes. The reason for the apparent discrepancy can be seen in Figure 12-1. Damage to a medullary pyramid affects a select group of fibers, the final portions of certain axons just before they reach the spinal cord. In contrast, damage to motor/premotor cortex or to the internal capsule affects not only corticospinal fibers but also projections from the cortex to the thalamus, basal ganglia, reticular formation, and other structures. Furthermore, even if it were possible to selectively damage only corticospinal fibers in the internal capsule, they would be affected before they gave off their many collaterals rather than after (as in the case of damage to the pyramid). Which part of this additional damage is responsible for the appearance of spasticity is not known with certainty, but the loss of certain projections from the premotor cortex to the reticular formation, and consequent reticulospinal dysfunction, is a likely cause.

## CORTICOBULBAR TRACT

Some corticospinal fibers, as we have seen, end directly on spinal motor neurons, whereas the rest end in the posterior horn, in the intermediate gray matter, or on interneurons of the anterior horn. Those not ending directly on motor neurons have a variety of effects, ranging from regulating the access of information to ascending pathways to affecting the activity of motor neurons via interneurons. In a similar manner, other fibers leave the cerebral cortex, descend through the internal capsule (immediately anterior to the corticospinal tract), and end in the brainstem on cells of sensory relay nuclei, of the reticular formation, and of motor nuclei of some cranial nerves. Strictly speaking, this entire collection of fibers is the *corticobulbar tract*.* However, in common usage the term "corticobulbar tract" is often used to refer selectively to those fibers that affect the motor neurons of cranial nerves (Figure 12-6). As in the spinal cord, some of these corticobulbar fibers end directly on motor neurons, but most act through interneurons of the reticular formation. The oculomotor, trochlear, and abducens nuclei receive no direct corticobulbar fibers; there are other peculiarities about the innervation of these nuclei, so they are treated separately in the next section. Thus the following discussion pertains to the trigeminal, facial, and hypoglossal motor nuclei, the nucleus ambiguus, and the spinal accessory nucleus.

In general, these nuclei receive a bilateral corticobulbar innervation. The fibers originate from the face portion of the motor cortex and from other areas of the frontal and parietal lobes as well. They accompany the corticospinal tract almost to the level of the nucleus they influence. Here they part company with the corticospinal tract and end in the appropriate motor nucleus on both sides or in the adjacent reticular formation. The major exception to this general pattern is in the case of the facial motor nucleus. As mentioned in Chapter 9, motor neurons to the lower facial muscles are innervated mainly by contralateral cortex, whereas those to upper facial muscles are bilaterally innervated. The result is that an individual with unilateral corticobulbar damage (as in a lesion of one cerebral peduncle) would be unable to smile or bare the teeth symmetrically or puff out the contralateral cheek; however, the ability to blink and wrinkle the forehead on both sides would remain. In addition, even though the hypoglossal and trigeminal motor nuclei and those neurons of the spinal accessory nucleus that innervate the trapezius receive some input from the cortex of both hemispheres, the input from the contralateral side predominates (to a degree that varies from one individual to another). Hence, after damage to the motor cortex, internal capsule, or cerebral peduncle on one side, there may be slight (and typically transient) weakness of the contralateral trapezius and masseter and the contralateral side of the tongue.

### Eye movements

Since maximum visual acuity is restricted to the fovea, it is important that the image of an object of interest fall on this part of the retina. Our eyes do a fairly remarkable job

*"Bulb" is an old term for the medulla or, by extension, for the entire brainstem.

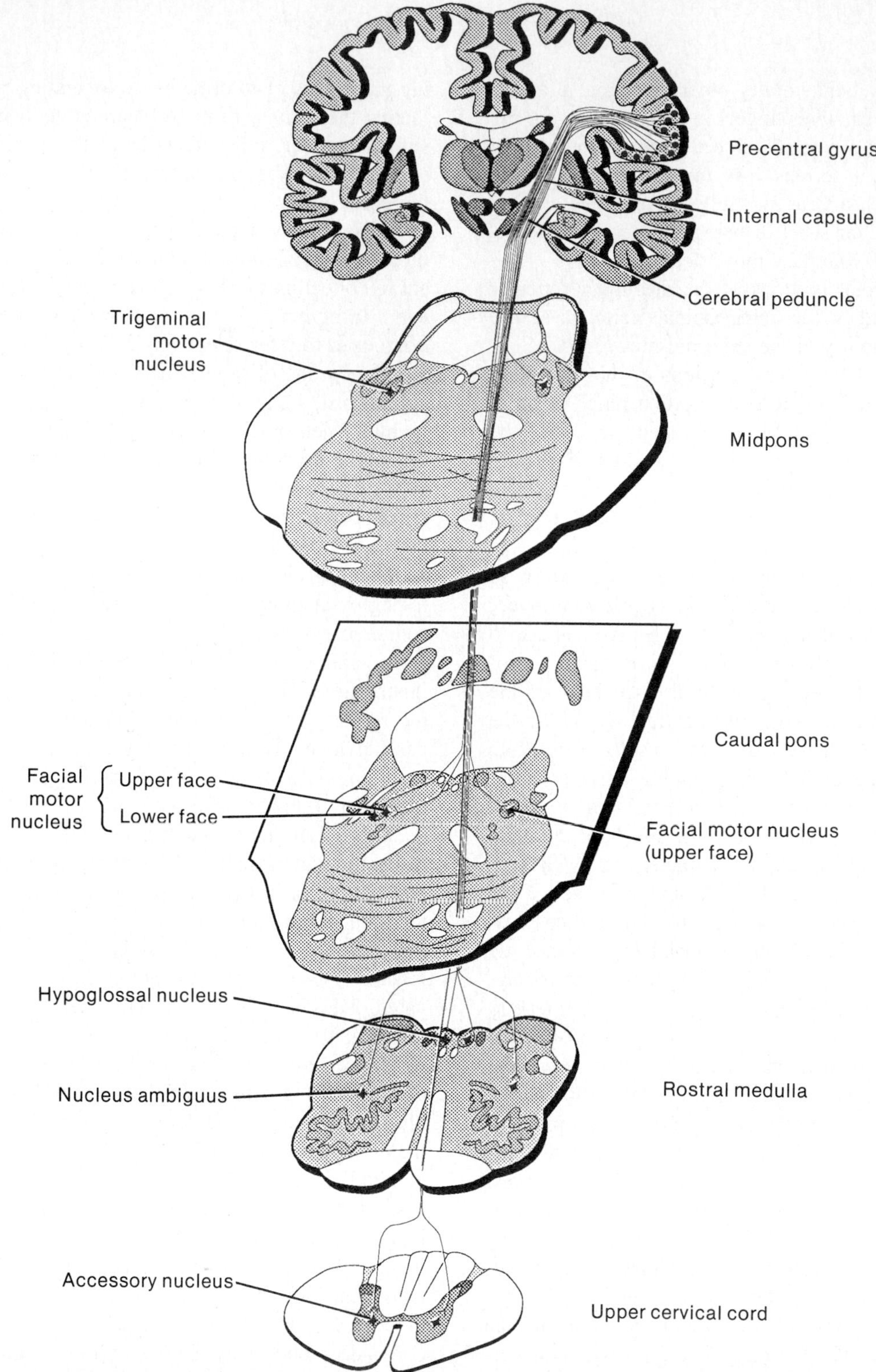


FIGURE 12-6
Corticobulbar pathway (except for cranial nerves III, IV, and VI). Three simplifications were used to keep the diagram manageable. First, corticobulbar fibers are shown ending directly on motor neurons, but most actually end on interneurons in the reticular formation. Second, corticobulbar fibers are shown with an equal bilateral distribution to the trigeminal, hypoglossal, and accessory nuclei. The trigeminal and hypoglossal nuclei and the trapezius motor neurons of the accessory nucleus often receive a preponderance of crossed fibers; sternocleidomastoid motor neurons of the accessory nucleus often receive a preponderance of uncrossed (actually, doubly crossed) fibers. Finally, all corticobulbar fibers are shown accompanying the corticospinal tract, whereas many actually leave this tract at various levels caudal to the cerebral peduncle and pursue a variety of aberrant courses through the brainstem.

of tracking (or moving to look at) various objects as the objects and/or we move about in three dimensional space. Throughout this process the two eyes stay aligned with each other to a high degree of accuracy. Two general types of movement are involved: (1) *vergence movements,* in which the two eyes move in opposite directions, as in the convergence that occurs when we look at a nearby object, and (2) *conjugate movements,* in which the two eyes move the same amount in the same direction, as in visually tracking an object that moves about at a fixed distance from us. Normally vergence and conjugate movements are smoothly integrated with one another so that images of the outside world fall on the two retinas in proper registration.

Little is known of the pathways involved in vergence movements. It is thought that the visual association cortex of the occipital lobe is important, along with projections from there to the midbrain (see Figure 11-20). The pathway ultimately influences the oculomotor nuclei (particularly the motor neurons to the two medial recti), which then converge the eyes. Consistent with this are the observations that damage to the midbrain and occasionally to the occipital lobes interferes with convergence, whereas damage to more caudal portions of the brainstem (including the MLF) does not.

Conjugate movements serve two general purposes—to move an object's image onto the fovea and then to keep it there. We use fast eye movements called *saccades* to redirect gaze so that an image falls on the fovea. These are brief, rapid movements of the kind we use to move our eyes voluntarily in any given direction and of the kind we use for the fast phase of nystagmus. We use two kinds of slower eye movements to keep an image on the fovea, corresponding to the fact that an image could move on the retina if we moved or if the object moved. The first of these is the vestibuloocular reflex, which compensates for head movements. Second, we use *smooth pursuit* movements to track a visual stimulus that is itself moving.* Smooth pursuit movements are also seen in the slow phase of optokinetic nystagmus (Figure 9-40).

A network of neural structures in both the brainstem and the cerebral hemispheres is involved in the initiation and coordination of conjugate eye movements. Basically it involves motor programs for these eye movements, located in the brainstem, together with cerebral centers that are able to trigger and modulate these brainstem mechanisms.

*It comes as a surprise to most that with the head stationary, we can only move our eyes smoothly when we are tracking a slowly moving object. This is easily demonstrated, however. Watch someone's eyes as he or she tries to move them slowly and smoothly while there is nothing to track, or concentrate on your own eyes while you try to do the same thing. In either case the result will be the same: a series of rapid, jerky movements. Some individuals can learn to have voluntary control of smooth tracking movements, but under normal circumstances and for most people, this is impossible.

### Brainstem mechanisms

The neural machinery for generating rapid horizontal movements is located in the medial reticular formation of the pons, near the abducens nucleus.* Signals from this region project to the abducens nucleus (see Figure 9-8), with each side of the brainstem directing movements to the ipsilateral side (Figure 12-7). The machinery for rapid vertical movements is located in the reticular formation of the rostral midbrain. Some recent experimental evidence and many years of clinical experience indicate that upward and downward movements are generated from slightly different locations. One of the common early effects of pineal tumors is paralysis of upward gaze (together with disturbances of convergence). Downward gaze is usually affected only later or when lesions are situated more deeply in the mesencephalic tegmentum. Both upward and downward gaze seem to be represented bilaterally in the midbrain, since unilateral lesions do not cause paralysis of vertical movements.

The neural mechanisms of the brainstem for smooth pursuit eye movements are not as well known as those for saccades. The vestibular nuclei and the flocculus of the cerebellum seem to be important for both horizontal and vertical slow movements (whether elicited by vestibular or visual stimuli), but other structures are involved as well.

### Cortical mechanisms

Stimulation of widespread cortical areas causes eye movements. Stimuli delivered to the occipital lobe or to a restricted area of the frontal lobe are particularly effective.

The *frontal eye field,* located in the posterior portion of the middle frontal gyrus just in front of the representation of the face in the premotor cortex (Figures 12-2 and 12-7), is involved in the initiation of rapid eye movements. Stimulation here causes horizontal or oblique conjugate movements to the contralateral side. Damage to the frontal eye field of one hemisphere causes inability to look voluntarily to the contralateral side. It can easily be shown, however, that the appropriate muscles are not paralyzed because the individual is able to visually track an object moving in any direction . Vertical eye movements are not impaired after a unilateral lesion, and even the deficit in horizontal movements is transitory, with recovery usually occurring in a matter of days. It is unclear how much of this recovery of function reflects other cortical areas working through the superior colliculus, and how much reflects increased activity of the contralateral frontal eye field.

The visual association cortex of the occipital lobe is considered to be involved in the initiation of pursuit and vergence movements. Posterior parts of the parietal and temporal lobes may be involved as well. Relatively little is actually known about these cortical mechanisms; occipital

*This particular portion of the reticular formation is now commonly referred to as the *paramedian pontine reticular formation,* or *PPRF*.

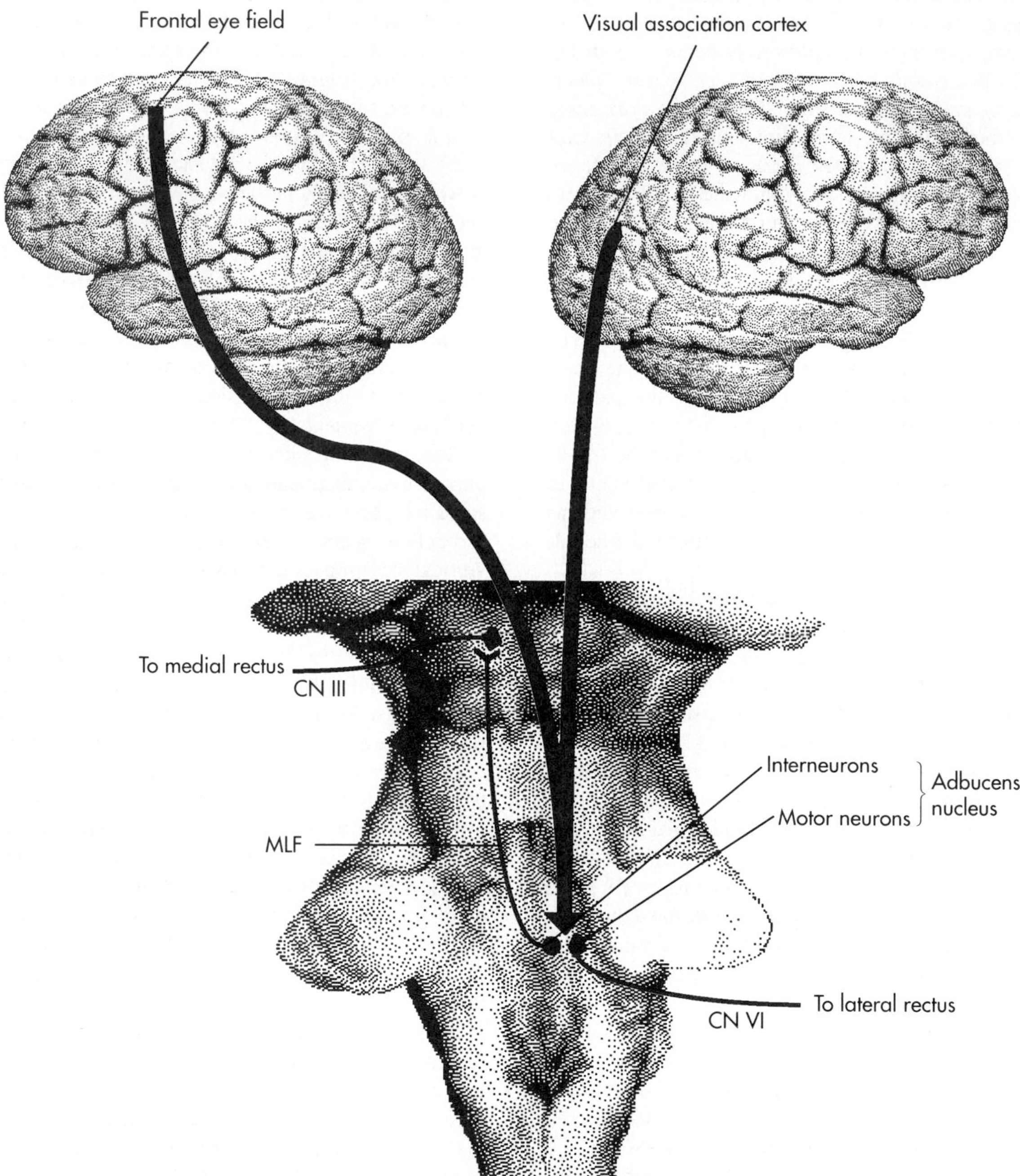


FIGURE 12-7
Cortical areas concerned with conjugate eye movements to the right; see text for details. The pathway for saccades originates in the frontal eye field. The pathway for smooth pursuit probably originates in the vicinity of the occipital-temporal-parietal junction. Both pathways descend through the internal capsule (the saccade pathway decussating in the caudal midbrain) and ultimately reach the right adbucens nucleus. Intermediate stops such as the pontine reticular formation or the flocculus are not shown.

damage typically causes visual deficits, so problems with eye movements may be difficult to evaluate. Movements in all directions may be represented in each hemisphere, since the deficits that persist are not pronounced. Somewhat surprisingly, unilateral damage causes more prominent, though usually transient, problems with slow movements to the *ipsilateral* side.

This localization of function seems to make good intuitive sense. The frontal eye field is adjacent to the motor cortex and could reasonably be expected to play a role in voluntary eye movements. Vergence, and particularly tracking, movements are associated with the perception of visual stimuli, so it would not be surprising if visual cortex and visual association cortex played a role in these eye movements.

## SOME FUNCTIONAL ASPECTS OF THE CORTICOSPINAL TRACT

The *pyramidal tract* received its name historically from the medullary pyramids and, like many other historically named neural structures, has now come to mean different things to different people. For some, it has the functional meaning of the combination of the corticospinal and corticobulbar tracts, with the emphasis on the fibers that more or less directly affect motor neurons. For others, it retains the historical-anatomical meaning and is the collection of fibers in the medullary pyramids. For still others, it means the collection of neurons whose destruction results in the clinically observed *pyramidal tract syndrome* (discussed shortly). People are sometimes misled into thinking that all three of these meanings refer to the same collection of fibers, but a major point of this chapter has been that they do not. For example, selective destruction of the medullary pyramids, though rare, is perverse enough not to cause the pyramidal tract syndrome. Also many corticospinal and corticobulbar fibers have no particular effect on motor neurons but instead modulate transmission through ascending pathways.

The pyramidal system (in the third sense, referring to fibers whose destruction causes spastic paralysis) is commonly considered in contrast to the *extrapyramidal* system. Strictly speaking, "extra-pyramidal" should mean everything except the pyramidal system (that is, at the very least, the cerebellum and basal ganglia). However, it is generally used with reference to the basal ganglia only. This pyramidal-versus-extrapyramidal terminology is rife with inconsistencies in logic and opportunities for confusion. For example (as Figure 12-1, *B,* indicates and the next chapter expands on), the principal route through which the basal ganglia are able to affect motor output is via the cerebral cortex and from there at least partially by way of corticospinal neurons. Also, as noted previously, collaterals of at least some corticospinal fibers project to the basal ganglia; should these collaterals be considered part of the pyramidal or extrapyramidal system? Since the two systems are so thoroughly intertwined, this pyramidal-versus-extrapyramidal terminology is being progressively abandoned. The change is happening slowly though, because the terms have been widely used for a long time and provide a convenient shorthand way to speak of two broad classes of motor disorders. As is seen in the next chapter, the effects of damage to the basal ganglia are quite distinct from the pyramidal tract syndrome.

### Spastic hemiplegia (pyramidal tract syndrome)

The most common cause of motor problems clinically attributed to the pyramidal system is a cerebrovascular accident involving the motor and premotor cortex or the posterior limb of the internal capsule. Immediately after the stroke a period of flaccid paralysis ensues, analogous to spinal shock. After a period of days to weeks, tone and reflexes return and increase, and the situation resolves into *spastic hemiplegia* or *hemiparesis.** Muscle tone is increased in a characteristic way, so that when a muscle is stretched rapidly (as by an examiner forcibly flexing the patient's leg), its resistance to further stretch increases greatly. (Slow stretch meets little resistance.) At some point this increased resistance suddenly melts away, and the limb collapses in flexion (or extension, if the arm is forcibly extended). This sudden collapse is called the *clasp-knife effect* and is usually attributed to inhibition of motor neurons by reflex connections of Golgi tendon organs (Figure 7-9); inhibitory effects of other muscle receptors are also likely to be important. The increased tone is especially pronounced in the flexors of the arm and fingers and in the extensors of the leg, leading to a typical hemiparetic stance and gait. Standard stretch reflexes such as the knee-jerk reflex are hyperactive. Sudden stretch of a muscle may lead to *clonus,* a rapid series of rhythmic contractions maintained for the duration of the stretch. This combination of hypertonia and hyperreflexia is spasticity. In addition, certain normal reflexes disappear and some abnormal reflexes appear. The best known of the latter is Babinski's sign. Interestingly, Babinski's sign is normally seen in human infants before the corticospinal tract is fully myelinated and functional and is also seen after selective damage to the corticospinal tract in the cerebral peduncle.

Some voluntary movement eventually returns, again in a characteristic pattern. Proximal muscles recover more than distal muscles, and movements of the fingers are the most severely and permanently affected. Skilled movements recover less than do coarser movements of entire limbs, suggesting that a major role of the corticospinal tract is to increase the speed and dexterity of movements

---

*Hemiplegia (from the Greek *-plegia* meaning stroke), strictly speaking, means total paralysis on one side. Since some voluntary movement returns after injury to the motor cortex or internal capsule, the condition is actually a hemiparesis (from the Greek *paresis* meaning slackening), indicating weakness or partial paralysis.

whose basic characteristics can be generated by other descending pathways.

### Premotor and supplementary motor areas

As indicated in Figure 12-1, both the premotor and supplementary motor areas give rise not only to corticospinal and corticoreticular fibers but also to projections to primary motor cortex. Thus some of the movements elicited by stimulating premotor and supplementary motor cortex arise via direct connections and others via primary motor cortex. For example, hand movements can no longer be produced by stimulation of the supplementary motor area after primary motor cortex has been removed, whereas trunk movements are unaffected. However, these two cortical areas are more than simply additional sources of motor command signals; recent evidence shows that they play distinctive roles in the control of movement.

The premotor cortex is selectively related to the cere-

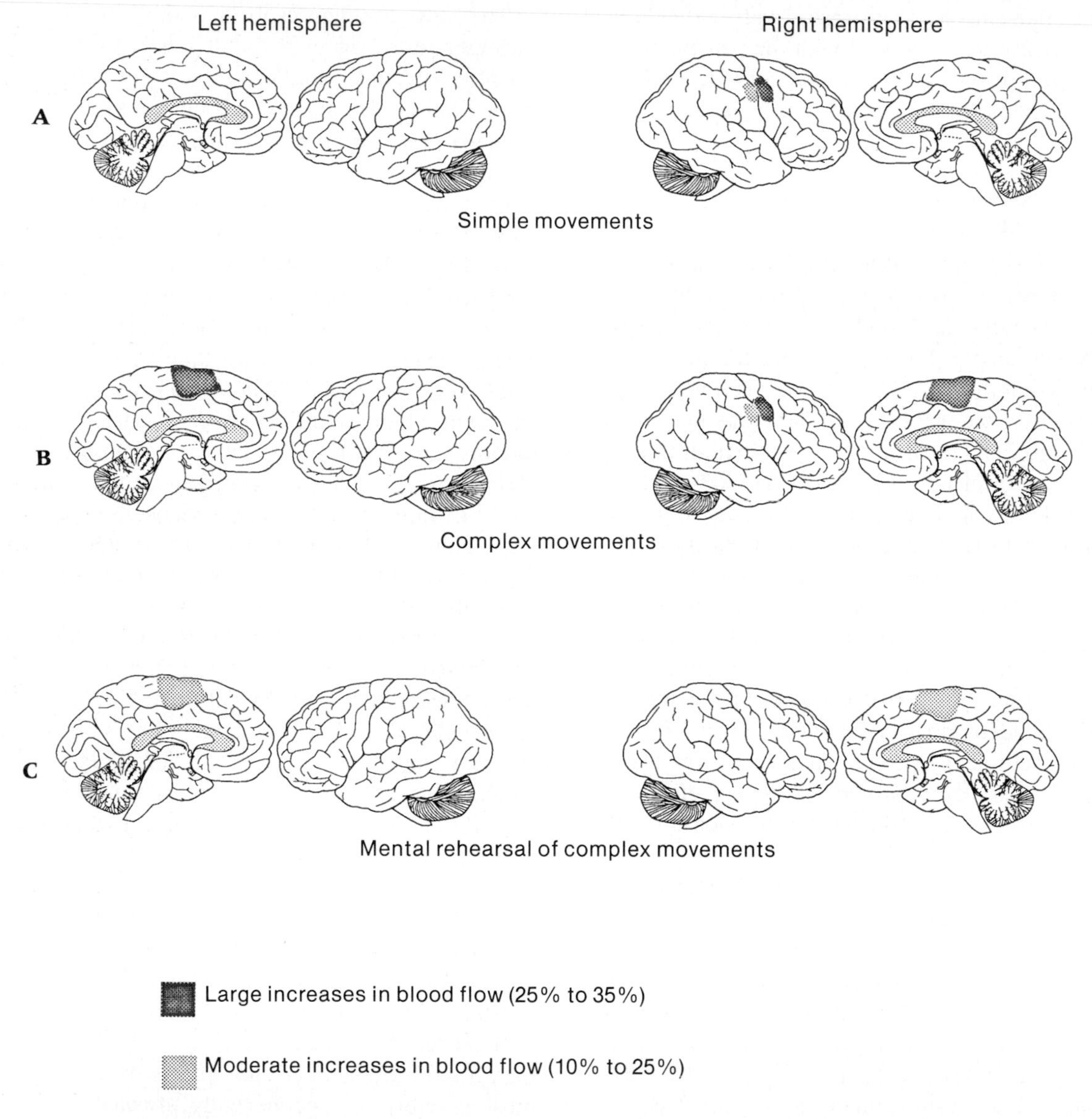


FIGURE 12-8
Changes in cerebral blood flow during real or imagined movements; in this illustration all movements involve the left hand. In **A,** the subject repeatedly flexes the left index finger, compressing a spring. Blood flow to primary motor cortex increases on the right; blood flow also increases in the corresponding part of the right postcentral gyrus, presumably because of the somatosensory input created by the repeated flexions. In **B** the subject rapidly touches each finger of the left hand to the left thumb; now blood flow also increases *bilaterally* in the supplementary motor area. In **C** the subject mentally rehearses the complex movement in **B** but does not actually perform it; blood flow increases only in the supplementary motor area (still bilaterally).
From the data of Roland PE et al: J Neurophysiol 43:118, 1980.

bellum and the supplementary motor area to the basal ganglia, as discussed further in the next two chapters. Such connections suggest that these cortical areas may have special roles in planning and preparing for movements. Studies of changes in regional cerebral blood flow have provided evidence consistent with this suggestion (Figure 12-8). Blood flow to the supplementary motor area and to the motor and premotor cortex increases when an individual performs a complex movement. However, if the individual merely rehearses the movement mentally but does not actually perform it, blood flow increases only in the supplementary motor area.

## ADDITIONAL READINGS


Balagura S, Katz RG: Undecussated innervation to the sternocleidomastoid muscle: a reinstatement, *Ann Neurol* 7:84, 1980.

Brinkman C: Supplementary motor area of the monkey's cerebral cortex: short- and long-term deficits after unilateral ablation and the effects of subsequent callosal section, *J Neurosci* 4:918, 1984.

Brinkman J, Kuypers HGJM: Cerebral control of contralateral and ipsilateral arm, hand and finger movements in the split-brain rhesus monkey, *Brain* 96:653, 1973. *Complex but interesting experiments whose results indicate that each cerebral hemisphere can exercise some control over the movements of both arms but not the fingers of both hands.*

Brodal, A: Self-observations and neuro-anatomical considerations after a stroke, *Brain* 96:675, 1973. *A fascinating account by an eminent neuroanatomist of a stroke suffered by him and the pattern of his recovery. Such an individual is able to provide information about motor control and other cerebral functions that is probably impossible to obtain in any other way.*

Brooks VB: *The neural basis of motor control,* New York, 1986, Oxford University Press.

Bucy P, Keplinger JE, Siqueira EB: Destruction of the "pyramidal tract" in man, *J Neurosurg* 21:385, 1964.

Cruccu G, Fornarelli M, Manfredi M: Impairment of masticatory function in hemiplegia, *Neurol* 38:301, 1988.

Davidoff RA: The pyramidal tract, *Neurol* 40:332, 1990.

Freund H-J: Premotor area and preparation of movement *Rev Neurol (Paris)* 146:543, 1990.

Gilman S, Lieberman JS, Marco LA: Spinal mechanisms underlying the effects of unilateral ablation of areas 4 and 6 in monkeys, *Brain* 97:49, 1974. *How are motor and premotor cortex related to the mechanism of spasticity?*

Goldberg G: Supplementary motor area structure and function: review and hypotheses, *Behav Brain Sci* 8:567, 1985.

Grillner S: Neurobiological bases of rhythmic motor acts in vertebrates, *Science* 228:143, 1985. *A brief review of central pattern generators.*

Grillner S, Wallén P: Central pattern generators for locomotion, with special reference to vertebrates, *Annu Rev Neurosci* 8:233, 1985.

Künzle H, Akert K: Efferent connections of cortical area 8 (frontal eye field) in *Macaca fascicularis:* a reinvestigation using the autoradiographic technique, *J Comp Neurol* 173:147, 1977.

Kuypers HGJM: Corticobulbar connexions to the pons and lower brain-stem in man, *Brain* 81:364, 1958.

Laplane D et al: Clinical consequences of corticectomies involving the supplementary motor area in man, *J Neurol Sci* 34:301, 1977.

Lawrence DG, Hopkins DA: The development of motor control in the rhesus monkey: evidence concerning the role of corticomotoneuronal connections, *Brain* 99:235, 1966.

Lawrence DG, Kuypers HGJM: The functional organization of the motor system in the monkey. I. The effects of bilateral pyramidal lesions. II. The effects of lesions of the descending brain-stem pathways, *Brain* 91:1 and 15, 1968. *Two classic papers on the chronic effects of selective corticospinal lesions in primates, including information about which other descending pathways are able to compensate for loss of the corticospinal tract.*

Leigh RJ, Zee DS: *The neurology of eye movements,* ed 2, Philadelphia, 1991, FA Davis.

Libet B: Unconscious cerebral initiative and the role of conscious will in voluntary action, *Behav Brain Sci* 8:529, 1985. *Under certain conditions, electrical changes related to voluntary movement appear to start in the brain* ***before*** *a person is aware of having decided to move. This paper and the commentaries that follow it discuss these experiments, their validity, and their philosophical implications.*

Luppino G et al: Multiple representations of body movements in mesial area 6 and the adjacent cingulate cortex: an intracortical microstimulation study in the macaque monkey, *J Comp Neurol* 311:463, 1991. *In additional to the supplementary motor area, the medial surface of the hemisphere contains two additional regions from which movements can be elicited.*

Lynch JC et al: Parietal lobe mechanisms for directed visual attention, *J Neurophysiol* 40:362, 1977.

Mastaglia FL, Knezevic W, Thompson PD: Weakness of head turning in hemiplegia: a quantitative study, *J Neurol Neurosurg Psychiatry* 49:195, 1986. *One sternocleidomastoid turns your head to the contralateral side. It would therefore make sense if the corticobulbar fibers to its motor neurons came from the ipsilateral cerebral hemisphere, and this is apparently the case.*

Morrow MJ, Sharpe JA: Cerebral hemispheric localization of smooth pursuit asymmetry, *Neurol* 40:284, 1990.

Mushiake H, Inase M, Tanji J: Neuronal activity in the primate premotor, supplementary, and precentral motor cortex during visually guided and internally determined sequential movements, *J Neurophysiol* 66:705, 1991. *Electrophysiological evidence that the supplementary motor area is more involved in movements repeated from memory, and premotor cortex more involved in movements that follow sensory cues.*

Nathan PW, Smith MC: The rubrospinal and central tegmental tracts in man, *Brain* 105:223, 1982.

Nathan PW, Smith MC, Deacon P: The corticospinal tracts in man. Course and location of fibres at different segmental levels, *Brain* 113:303, 1990.

Okano K, Tanji J: Neuronal activities in the primate motor fields of the agranular frontal cortex preceding visually triggered and self-paced movement, *Exp Brain Res* 66:155, 1987. *Description of a population of neurons in the supplementary motor area that change their firing rate many hundreds of milliseconds before a voluntary movement begins.*

Polit A, Bizzi E: Processes controlling arm movements in monkeys, *Science* 201:1235, 1978. *An article dealing with the motor abilities of a monkey receiving no afferent input from one arm.*

Ralston DD, Ralston HJ III: The terminations of corticospinal tract axons in the macaque monkey, *J Comp Neurol* 242:325, 1985.

Russell JR, DeMyer W: The quantitative cortical origin of pyramidal axons of *Macaca rhesus, Neurology* 11:96, 1961.

Schiller PH, True SD, Conway JL: Effects of frontal eye field and superior colliculus ablations on eye movements, *Science* 206:590, 1979.

Stein RB: Peripheral control of movement, *Physiol Rev* 54:215, 1974.

Talbott RE, Humphrey DR, editors: *Posture and movement,* New York, 1979, Raven Press.

Wiesendanger M: *The pyramidal tract: its structure and function.* In Towe AL, Luschei ES, editors: *Handbook of behavioral neurobiology.* Vol. 5. *Motor coordination,* New York, 1981, Plenum Press.

Wiesendanger M: Recent developments in studies of the supplementary motor area of primates, *Rev Physiol Biochem Pharmacol* 103:1, 1986.

Wise SP: The primate premotor cortex: past, present and preparatory, *Annu Rev Neurosci* 8:1, 1985.

# CHAPTER 13

## Basal Ganglia

In 1817 James Parkinson, an English country physician, published a brief monograph entitled *An Essay on the Shaking Palsy,* in which he described the symptoms of several individuals who had the disease that now bears his name. Parkinsonian patients, as described in more detail later in this chapter, are characterized by tremor, generally increased muscle tone, and difficulty in initiating voluntary movements (which are unusually slow once begun). Disorders of this sort, whose signs typically include involuntary movements and generalized alterations in muscle tone, have come to be associated with damage to the basal ganglia. They are often referred to as *extrapyramidal disorders,* although as explained in the previous chapter, such terminology can be somewhat misleading; for example, at least some of the involuntary movements are actually effected through the corticospinal tract.

### TERMINOLOGY

The term "basal ganglia" originally referred to all the masses of gray matter buried within the cerebrum and thus included the *putamen, caudate nucleus, globus pallidus, amygdala, claustrum,* and occasionally even the *thalamus* (Figures 13-1 and 13-2). However, it is now used to refer to those structures whose damage causes "extrapyramidal" syndromes. This list of structures includes at least one brainstem nucleus but excludes some nuclei buried within the cerebrum. Thus the amygdala, claustrum, and thalamus are no longer spoken of as basal ganglia, since the amygdala is part of the limbic system,* the claustrum has a largely unknown function, and the thalamus is part of a multitude of different pathways. Use of the term "basal ganglia" still varies, but most people mean the combination of caudate nucleus, putamen, globus pallidus, *subthalamic nucleus,* and *substantia nigra.*

Various names are applied to different combinations of members of the basal ganglia (Figure 13-3). The putamen and globus pallidus together comprise the *lenticular* or *lentiform nucleus* (from the Latin word for lentil). Bridges of gray matter growing across the internal capsule between the putamen and the caudate nucleus give this region a striped appearance in many planes of section, so the combination of the caudate and lenticular nuclei is called the *corpus striatum.* The caudate nucleus and putamen have a common embryological origin, identical histological appearances, and similar connections, so both together are called the *neostriatum,** or simply the *striatum.* Thus the striatum is a major subdivision of the corpus striatum.

These assorted names give rise to prefixes and suffixes that are used to describe fibers coming from or going to different members of the basal ganglia. "Strio-" and "-striate" are used for the striatum; thus *striopallidal* fibers go from the caudate nucleus or putamen to the globus pallidus, and *corticostriate* fibers go from the cerebral cortex to the caudate nucleus or putamen. The globus pallidus is also called the *pallidum,* so *pallidothalamic* fibers go from the globus pallidus to the thalamus. *Nigroreticular* fibers go from the substantia nigra to the reticular formation.

### TOPOGRAPHY

The lenticular nucleus is shaped somewhat like a wedge cut from a sphere (Figures 13-1 and 13-2). The putamen (from the Latin for husk), which is approximately coexten-

*Although, as discussed briefly in Chapter 16, there are connections between the limbic system and the basal ganglia, including projections from the amygdala to the striatum.

*"Neo-" refers to the fact that the neostriatum is generally considered to be a recent phylogenetic acquisition. Using similar terminology, the globus pallidus and the amygdala are occasionally referred to as the *paleostriatum* and the *archistriatum,* respectively.

Genu of corpus callosum
Head of caudate nucleus
Lateral ventricle (anterior horn)
Internal capsule (anterior limb)
Septum pellucidum
External capsule
Extreme capsule
Ventral tier nuclei
A
Claustrum
Putamen
Dorsomedial nucleus
Globus pallidus
Pulvinar
Tail of caudate nucleus

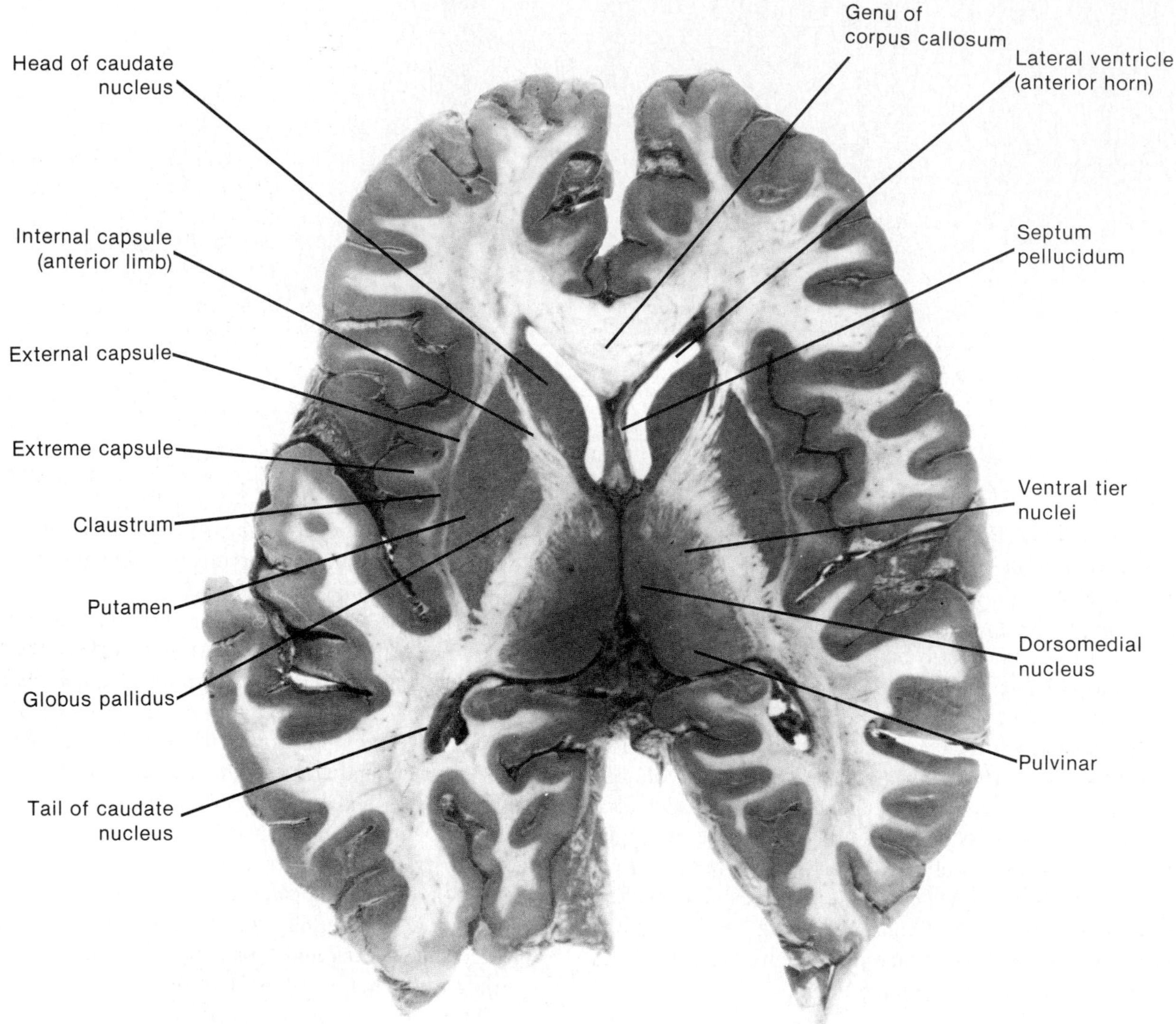

B

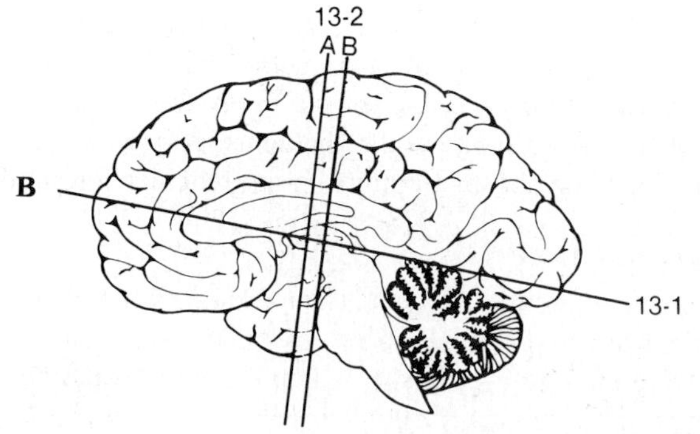


FIGURE 13-1
**A,** Basal ganglia and surrounding structures as seen in an approximately horizontal section. **B,** Planes of section for Figures 13-1 and 13-2.

---

FIGURE 13-2
Basal ganglia and surrounding structures as seen in coronal sections. (Shown on opposite page.)

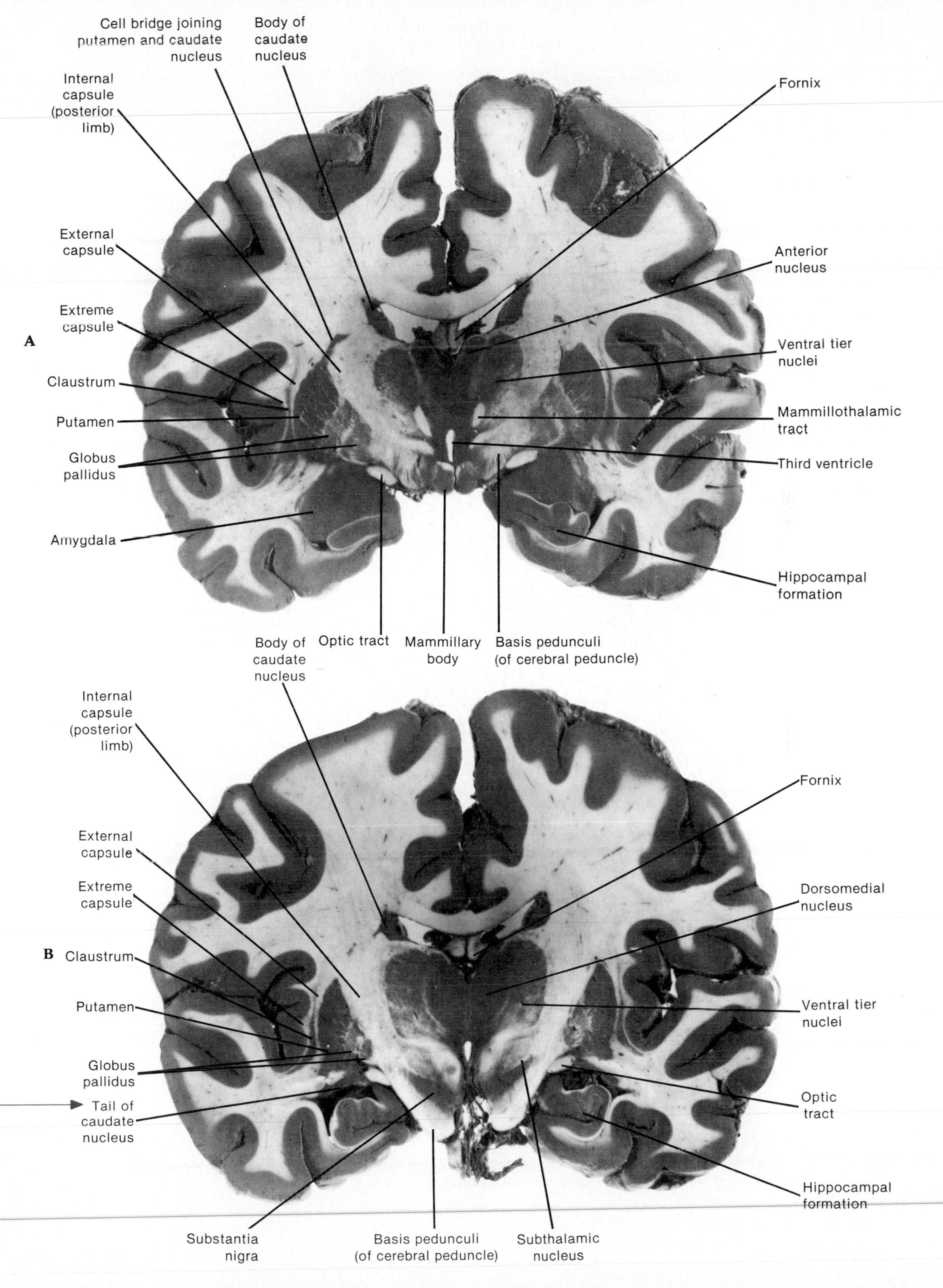
A
Cell bridge joining putamen and caudate nucleus
Body of caudate nucleus
Internal capsule (posterior limb)
Fornix
External capsule
Anterior nucleus
Extreme capsule
Ventral tier nuclei
Claustrum
Putamen
Mammillothalamic tract
Globus pallidus
Third ventricle
Amygdala
Hippocampal formation
Optic tract
Mammillary body
Basis pedunculi (of cerebral peduncle)
B
Body of caudate nucleus
Internal capsule (posterior limb)
Fornix
External capsule
Extreme capsule
Dorsomedial nucleus
Claustrum
Putamen
Ventral tier nuclei
Globus pallidus
Tail of caudate nucleus
Optic tract
Hippocampal formation
Substantia nigra
Basis pedunculi (of cerebral peduncle)
Subthalamic nucleus

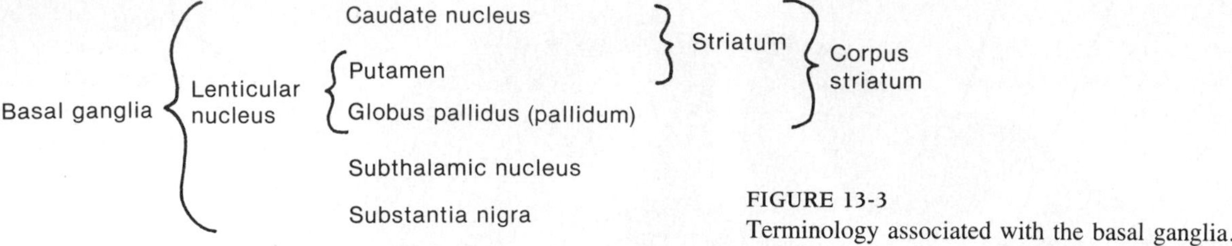


FIGURE 13-3
Terminology associated with the basal ganglia.

sive with the insula, forms the outermost portion of this wedge. It is separated from the more medial globus pallidus by a thin *lateral medullary lamina* of myelinated fibers. The globus pallidus is itself divided into *medial* and *lateral* (or *internal* and *external*) portions by a *medial medullary lamina*. In unstained sections through the lenticular nucleus, the globus pallidus has a distinctively pale appearance as a result of the large number of myelinated fibers that traverse it, terminate in it, and originate in it. (In myelin-stained sections like those shown in Figures 13-10 and 13-13, it is therefore relatively dark.)

The caudate nucleus starts out embryologically from the same mass of cells that gives rise to the putamen. In the course of development, the caudate nucleus remains in the wall of the lateral ventricle and grows around with it in a C-shaped course. The caudate nucleus of the adult has an enlarged *head* that bulges into the anterior horn, a *body* that forms the lateral wall of the body of the ventricle, and a slender *tail* that borders on the inferior horn (Figures 2-18 to 2-22, 13-1, 13-2, and 13-4). The caudate nucleus and putamen retain their embryological continuity just above the orbital surface of the frontal lobe, where the

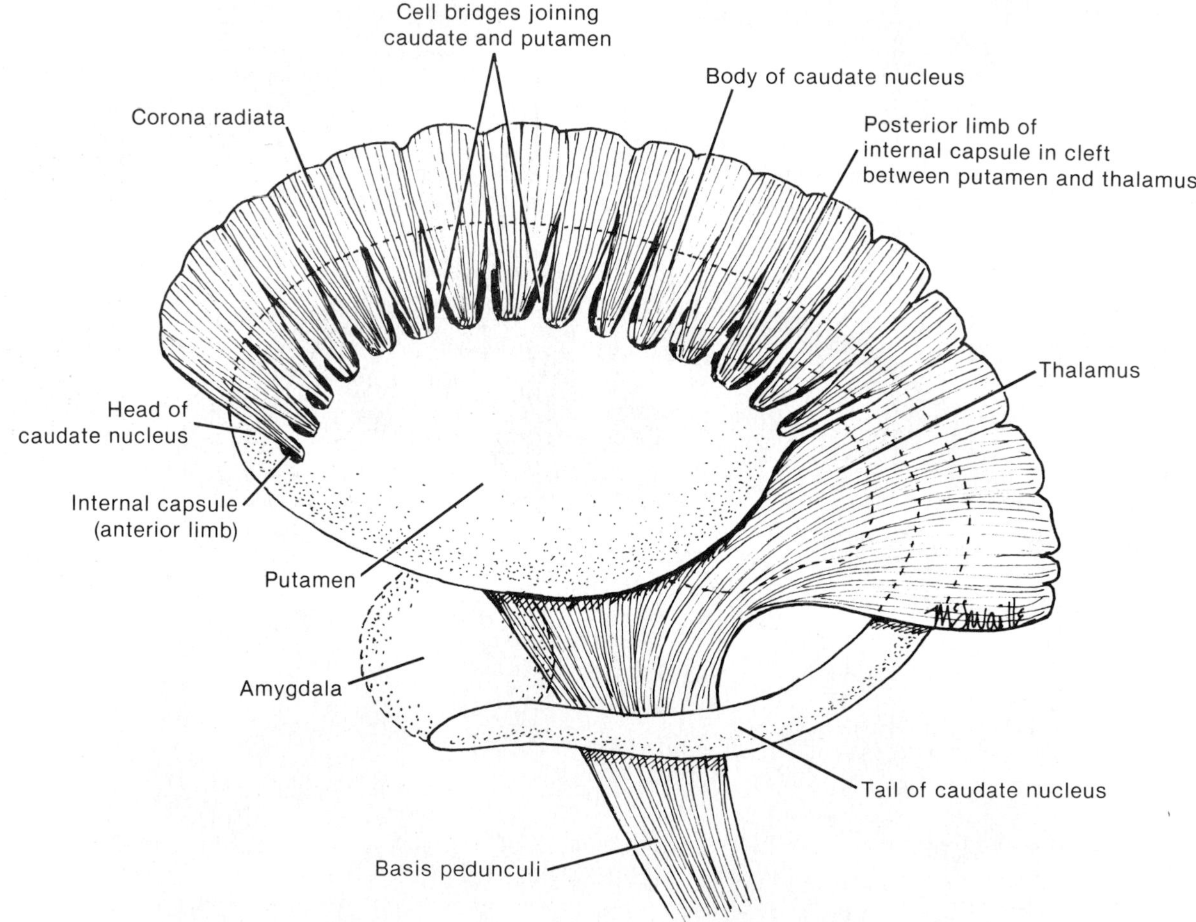


FIGURE 13-4
Schematic drawing of what the corpus striatum, amygdala, thalamus, and internal capsule would look like if they were all isolated from the rest of the brain.

head of the caudate appears to be continuous with the anterior part of the putamen. In the temporal lobe, the tail of the caudate nucleus is continuous with the amygdala, which in turn is continuous with the putamen (Figures 13-2 and 13-4), but these physical continuities are of no apparent functional significance.

## CONNECTIONS OF THE BASAL GANGLIA

The principal circuit of the basal ganglia is a loop that starts with projections from multiple cortical areas to the corpus striatum and then returns, by way of the thalamus, to one of these multiple cortical areas (Figure 13-5, *A*). There are multiple versions of this loop, all similar in principle but each utilizing different cortical areas and a distinctive portion of the corpus striatum. Each loop includes at least a portion of the frontal lobe among the cortical input areas, and each loop returns to a frontal area.

The major circuit through which the basal ganglia participate in the control of movement provides one example of such a loop (Figure 13-5, *B*). The corpus striatum forms by far the largest part of the basal ganglia, yet it has no way to affect motor neurons directly (see Figure 12-1). Thus the only way the corpus striatum can play a role in the control of movement is by somehow influencing one or more of the descending pathways mentioned in the previous chapter. It does so primarily by affecting the activity of motor areas of the cerebral cortex. Somatosensory and motor areas project to a portion of the striatum (mostly putamen), which in turn projects by way of the globus pallidus to the VL/VA; the circuit is completed by projections from the VL/VA back to the supplementary motor and premotor areas of the cortex. Other basal ganglia loops use their own distinctive portions of the striatum, globus pallidus, thalamus, and cerebral cortex.

Most of the remaining connections of the basal ganglia, described a little later in this chapter, fall into three categories: interconnections of the substantia nigra with the striatum (Figure 13-6, *A*), interconnections of the subthalamic nucleus with the globus pallidus (Figure 13-6, *B*), and interconnections of thalamic intralaminar nuclei with the corpus striatum. In the account that follows, only the best documented connections of the basal ganglia are de-

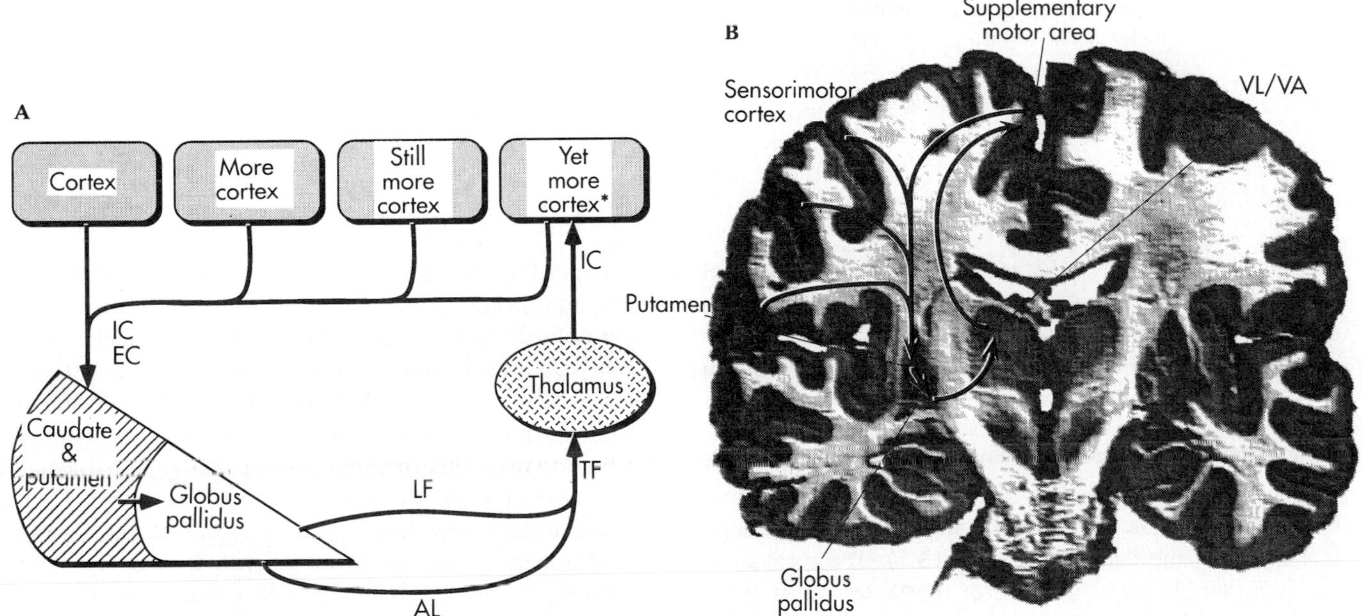


FIGURE 13-5
The principal circuit involving the basal ganglia. **A,** a schematic diagram showing the general elements of this circuit. The loop starts in multiple cortical areas and ends in one of these areas (*) in the frontal lobe. The bundles through which the fibers of this circuit travel are indicated by abbreviations: *AL,* ansa lenticularis; *EC,* external capsule; *IC,* internal capsule; *LF,* lenticular fasciculus; *TF,* thalamic fasciculus. Different parts of the striatum are related to different cortical areas. **B,** shows the principal circuit involving the basal ganglia, projected onto a coronal slice similar to that shown in Figure 13-2B. At this level, near the central sulcus, the circuit primarily involves sensory and motor cortex on either side of the central sulcus, the putamen, and the supplementary motor area. These connections are mostly uncrossed, but there is some bilaterality (not shown). Connections of the caudate nucleus are similar in principle but involve different cortical areas. See text for details.

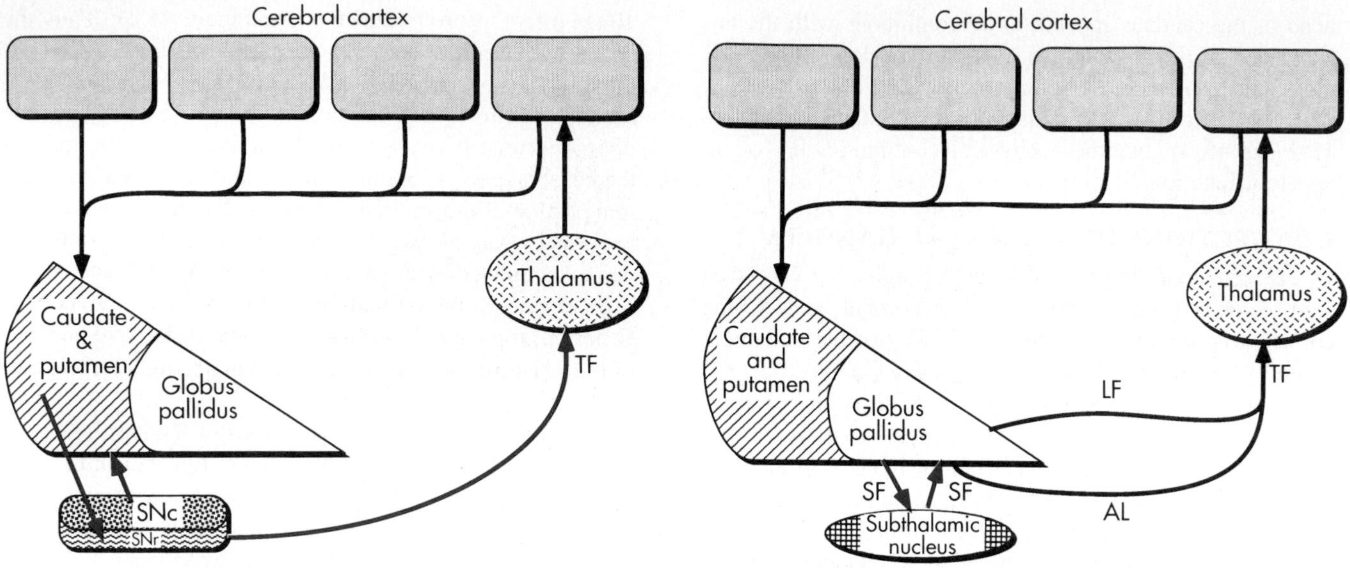


FIGURE 13-6
Two additional basal ganglia circuits of importance. **A,** The substantia nigra is interconnected with the striatum. As described further in the text, the pigmented, compact part of the substantia nigra (*SNc*) projects to the striatum; the striatum projects to the reticular part of the substantia nigra (*SNr*), which, like the globus pallidus, projects to the thalamus via the thalamic fasciculus (*TF*). **B,** The subthalamic nucleus is reciprocally connected with the globus pallidus. As described further in the text, this allows a degree of subthalamic control over pallidal output. Abbreviations for fiber bundles: *AL,* ansa lenticularis; *LF,* lenticular fasciculus; *SF,* subthalamic fasciculus; *TF,* thalamic fasciculus. A basal ganglia loop involving the centromedian and parafascicular nuclei of the thalamus is also prominent anatomically, but was omitted from these schematic diagrams because its functional significance is unclear.

scribed. Unfortunately, the precise function of most of these connections is unknown. However, there has been enough recent progress that we can not only consider the consequences of damage to some of these connections, but also begin to speculate about their normal functions.

## Striatum

The caudate nucleus and putamen receive inputs from the cerebral cortex, the substantia nigra, and the intralaminar nuclei of the thalamus (Figure 13-7). The cortical input is by far the most massive of the three. These fibers originate in all areas of the cortex, pass through the internal and external capsules, and end in a roughly topographical pattern in the striatum. The projection from the motor and somatosensory cortex thus goes mostly to the putamen. The caudate nucleus, as it curves around with the ventricular system, receives most of the projections from association areas; as the size and location of the head of the caudate might imply, the projection is particularly heavy from prefrontal cortex. Thus the basal ganglia are constantly informed about most aspects of cortical function. The substantia nigra projects to all areas of the striatum in a point-to-point fashion by way of very fine axons that use dopamine as their neurotransmitter. Destruction of this *nigrostriatal* pathway is the major factor causing Parkinson's disease. Finally, the intralaminar nuclei, especially the centromedian and parafascicular nuclei, project to the striatum. Many of these same fibers, as mentioned in Chapter 10, have collateral branches that end in the cerebral cortex. This *thalamostriate* pathway is particularly well developed in primates, but virtually nothing is known of its function. As described later in this chapter, various clinical findings can be associated with damage to different parts of the basal ganglia and their connections; however, there are no particular symptoms that we can ascribe to malfunction of the thalamus–corpus striatum–thalamus loop.

Striatal efferents collect into numerous bundles of myelinated fibers that converge on the globus pallidus. Most of them are *striopallidal* fibers; some terminate in the internal segment of the globe pallidus, others in the external segment. Still others pass through the globus pallidus and reach the substantia nigra.

The caudate nucleus and putamen are cytologically uniform, and it was thought for a time that they were functionally uniform as well. However, recent work has shown

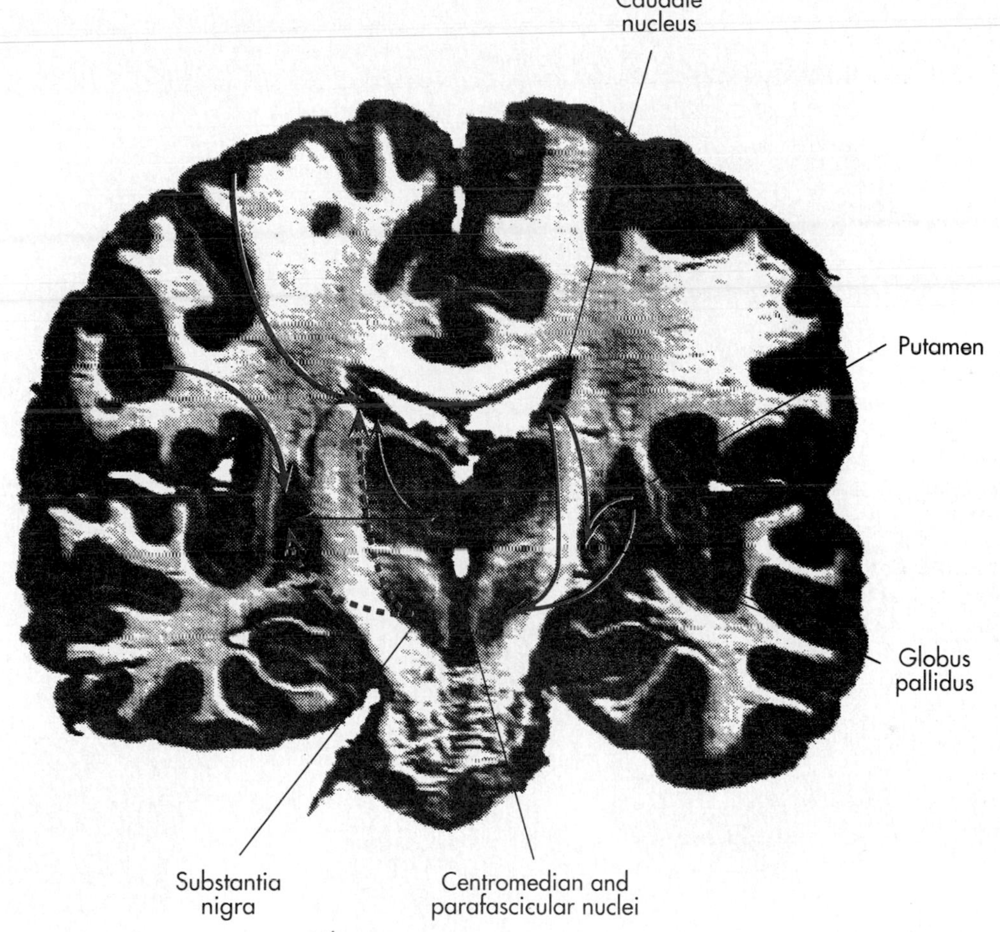


FIGURE 13-7
Connections of the striatum (putamen and caudate nucleus); afferents to the striatum on the left, efferents from the striatum on the right. The plane of section is the same as in Figure 13-6. Some anatomical liberties were taken in the labelling of this and similar figures in this chapter, since the centromedian nucleus and VL/VLA are not in the same coronal plane, and since most cortical afferents to the caudate nucleus actually arise anterior to this level.

that they are divided up into small modules according to types of connections and types of neurotransmitters (Figure 13-8). It seems likely that these various modules fit together in some as yet undefined way to form striatal functional units.

In addition, it now appears that the caudate nucleus and putamen have somewhat different functions. The putamen receives most of the inputs from motor and somatosensory areas of cortex and projects by way of the globus pallidus and thalamus to the premotor and supplementary motor areas. Corresponding to this, individual neurons in the putamen fire in conjunction with particular movements or positions, and stimulation of small areas of the putamen causes discrete movements. Thus the putamen is probably centrally involved in most of the motor functions of the basal ganglia. The caudate nucleus, in contrast, receives most of its inputs from association areas of cortex and projects by way of the globus pallidus and thalamus mostly to prefrontal areas. Few caudate neurons respond to movements or positions. Thus the caudate nucleus is involved more prominently in cognitive functions and less directly in movement.

Finally, it has become clear in recent years that the region of apparent continuity of the putamen and caudate nucleus should be recognized as a separate subdivision of the striatum. This subdivision, called the *ventral striatum**, has connections with the limbic system and is discussed briefly in Chapter 16.

## Globus pallidus

Afferents to both segments of the globus pallidus arise in the striatum and the subthalamic nucleus (Figure 13-9). As Figure 13-10 shows, the subthalamic nucleus is located

*The major component of the ventral striatum in human brains is the *nucleus accumbens*, which was named historically for its physical location. Its original name was *nucleus accumbens septi*—literally, "the nucleus leaning against the septum"—because the region of apparent fusion of the putamen and caudate nucleus appears to lean up against the base of the septum pellucidum (see Figure 16-5).

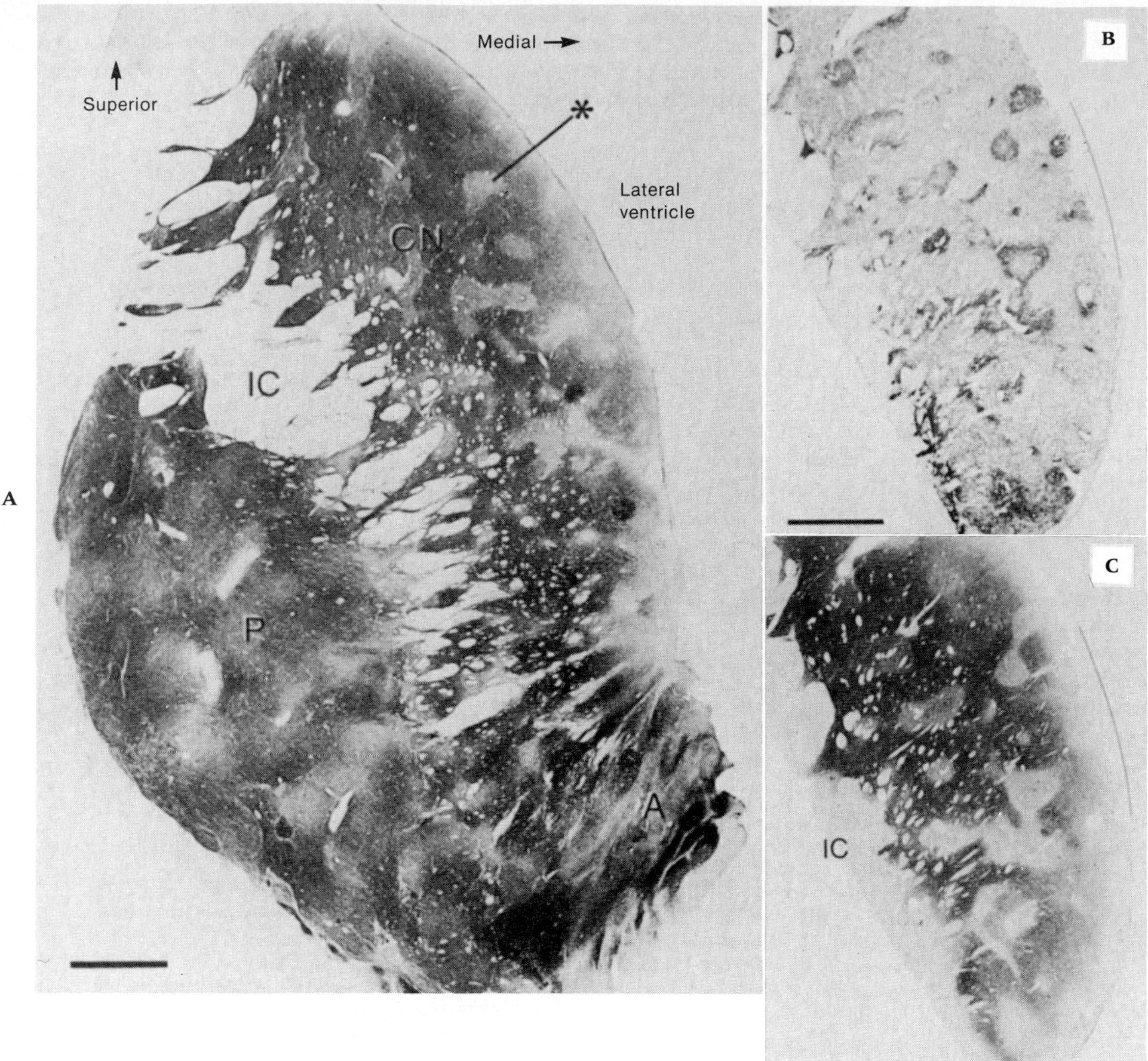


FIGURE 13-8
Chemical compartmentalization of the striatum. **A,** A coronal section through a human putamen (P) and caudate nucleus (CN), separated by the anterior limb of the internal capsule (IC). The area of fusion of the caudate and putamen is called nucleus accumbens (A) and, as described briefly in Chapter 16, has limbic connections. Histochemical staining for the enzyme acetylcholinesterase (AChE) was applied to the section, revealing that the striatum is made up of an AChE-rich background *(matrix)* with embedded AChE-poor regions (one indicated by an asterisk). The AChE-poor regions are about 300 to 600 μm wide and are often referred to as *striosomes*. Scale mark = 3 mm. Matrix and striosome regions have a number of other chemical differences. An example is shown in **B** and **C,** two adjacent coronal sections through the head of a human caudate nucleus. The section in **B** was stained immunocytochemically for enkephalin; the section in **C** was stained for AChE. High enkephalin levels are found precisely in the striosomes, especially around their peripheries. Scale mark = 3 mm.

From Graybiel AM: Neurochemically specified subsystems in the basal ganglia. In Functions of the basal ganglia, Ciba Foundation Symposium 107, London, 1984, Pitman.

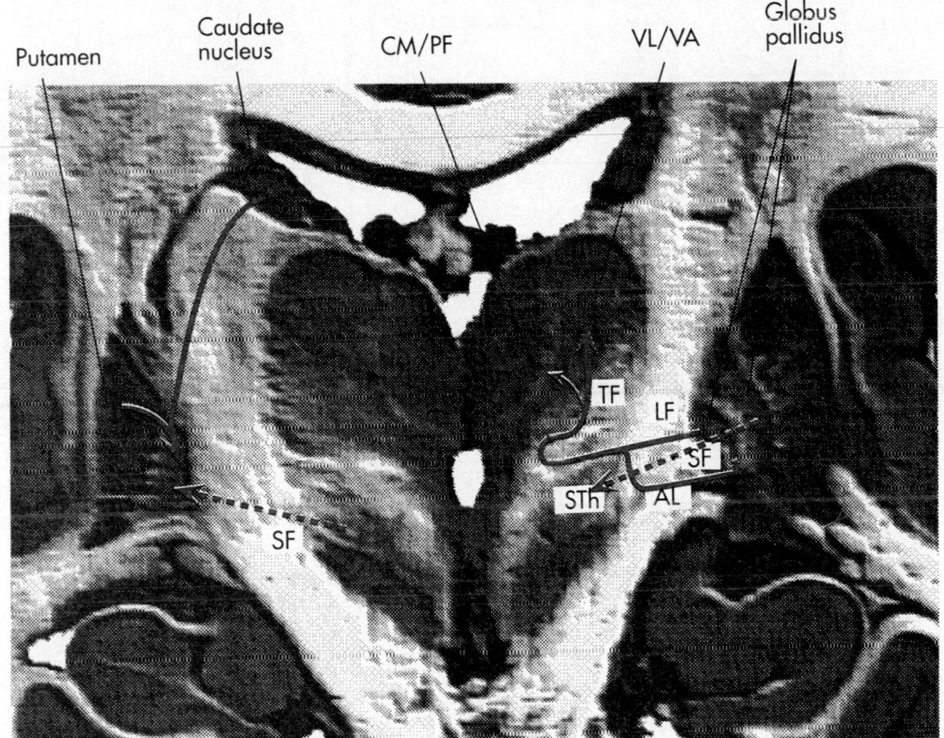


FIGURE 13-9
Connections of the globus pallidus; afferents to the globus pallidus on the left, efferents from the globus pallidus on the right. Plane of section as in Figure 13-6. Here again, the figure is drawn as though VL/VA and the centromedian nucleus were in the same coronal plane, when in fact the centromedian and parafascicular nuclei are mostly posterior to this level. *AL,* Ansa lenticularis; *CM/PF,* centromedian and parafascicular nuclei; *LF,* lenticular fasciculus; *SF,* subthalamic fasciculus; *STh,* subthalamic nucleus; *TF,* thalamic fasciculus.

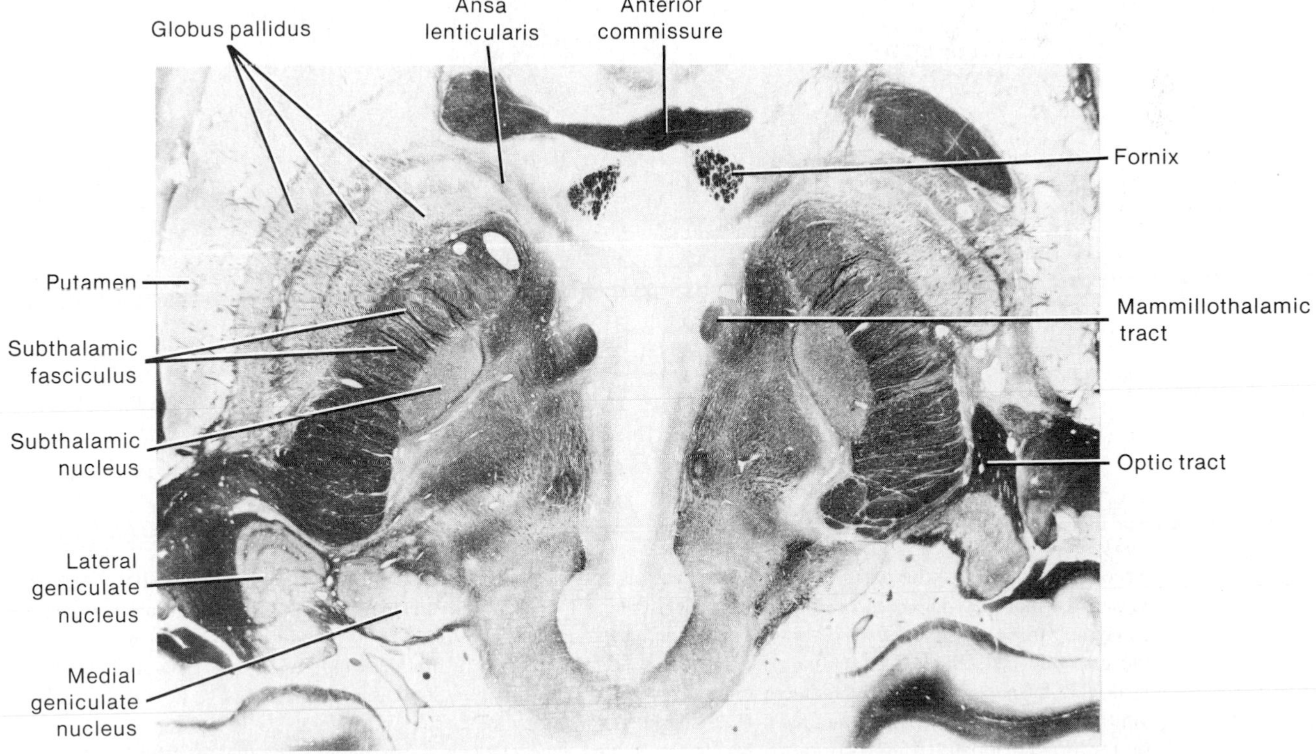


FIGURE 13-10
The subthalamic fasciculus as seen in a horizontal section (same section as Figure 11-12). Subthalamic fasciculus is a collective term for the small bundles of fibers that pass through the internal capsule interconnecting the subthalamic nucleus and the globus pallidus.

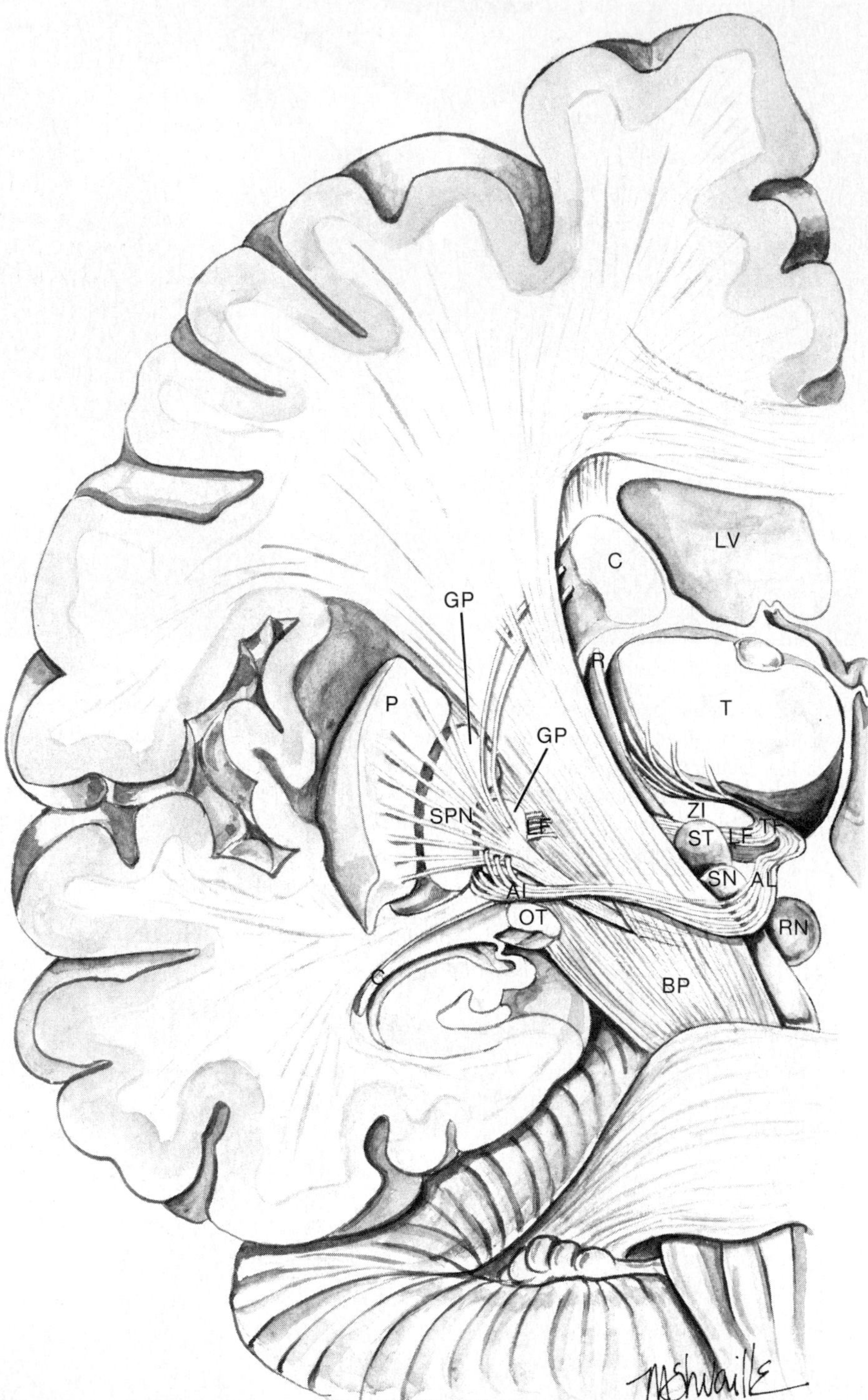


FIGURE 13-11

Schematic drawing of the paths of the ansa lenticularis and the lenticular fasciculus as seen in an anterior view of a partially dissected brain. The ansa lenticularis loops around the medial edge of the internal capsule, while the lenticular fasciculus passes through the internal capsule. The two bundles join to form the thalamic fasciculus. The subthalamic fasciculus is not indicated in this drawing. *AL,* Ansa lenticularis; *BP,* basis pedunculi; *C,* caudate nucleus; *GP,* globus pallidus; *LF,* lenticular fasciculus; *LV,* lateral ventricle; *OT,* optic tract; *P,* putamen; *R,* thalamic reticular nucleus; *RN,* red nucleus; *SN,* substantia nigra; *SPN,* striopallidal and strionigral fibers; *ST,* subthalamic nucleus; *T,* thalamus; *TF,* thalamic fasciculus; *ZI,* zona incerta.

Modified from Nieuwenhuys R et al: The human central nervous system, New York, 1978, Springer-Verlag.

right across the internal capsule from the globus pallidus. The small bundles of fibers that cross the internal capsule and interconnect these two nuclei are collectively called the *subthalamic fasciculus*.

Although the two segments of the globus pallidus have similar inputs, their efferents are separate and distinct (Figure 13-9). The external segment projects through the subthalamic fasciculus to the subthalamic nucleus. The internal pallidal segment projects mainly to the thalamus through two collections of fibers (Figure 13-11). One collection, the *lenticular fasciculus*, runs directly through the internal capsule and then passes medially as a sheet of fibers between the subthalamic nucleus and the zona incerta (Figure 13-12). At the medial edge of the zona incerta, the lenticular fasciculus makes a hairpin turn in a lateral and dorsal direction and enters the thalamus. The second collection loops around the medial edge of the internal capsule as the *ansa lenticularis* (the Latin word *ansa* means loop) (Figure 13-11 and 13-13); it joins the lenticular fasciculus in the *thalamic fasciculus**, which then enters the thalamus. The thalamic fasciculus terminates in a variety of thalamic nuclei. Fibers related to movement control end in the VL/VA, those related to the caudate nucleus and prefrontal cortex end in the dorsomedial nucleus and in part of the VA, and others end in the centromedian and parafascicular nuclei. The VL/VA and dorsomedial nuclei then project to frontal cortex, thus completing the principal circuit through the basal ganglia (Figure 13-5).

A few fibers leave the ansa lenticularis and lenticular fasciculus to end in the habenula, in the substantia nigra, and in a portion of the midbrain tegmentum that in turn projects to the reticular formation. However, their numbers are meager compared to the major outputs to the thalamus and subthalamic nucleus.

*This complex bundle also includes cerebellar output fibers described in the next chapter.

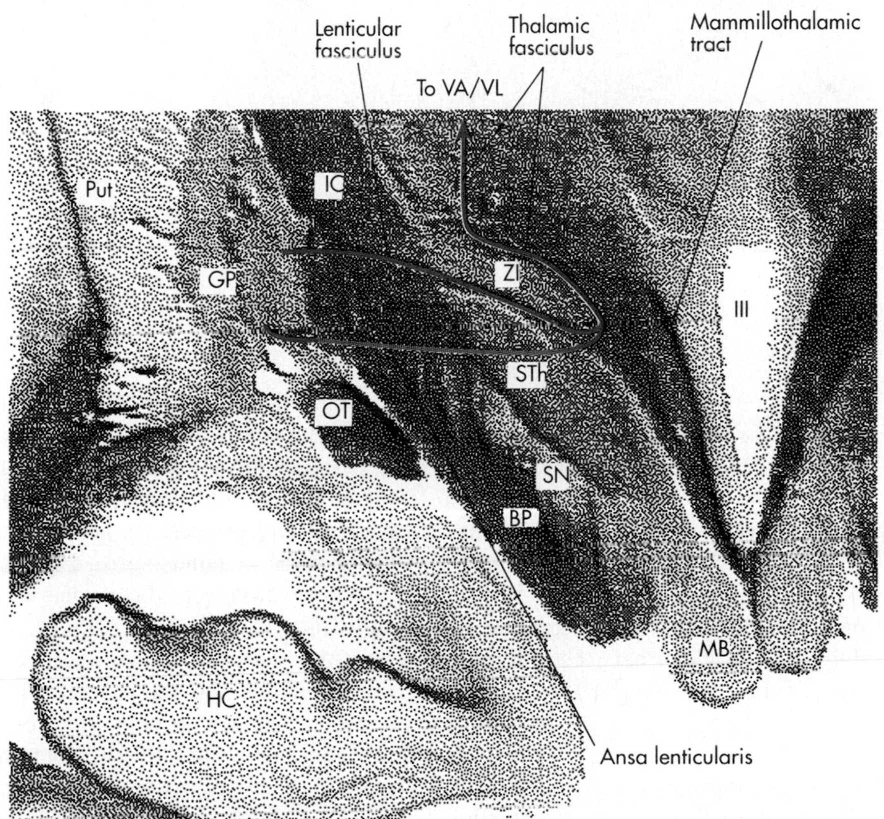


FIGURE 13-12
Output fibers from the globus pallidus seen in an enlarged portion of a coronal section similar to that shown in Figure 10-10. Most of the ansa lenticularis is shown as a shaded line, because these fibers loop around the medial edge of the internal capsule, out ot the plane of section; they then join the lenticular fasciculus to form the thalamic fasciculus. *BP*, Basis pedunculi (of cerebral peduncle); *GP*, globus pallidus; *HC*, hippocampal formation; *IC*, internal capsule (posterior limb); *III*, third ventricle; *MB*, mammillary body, *OT*, optic tract; *Put*, putamen; *SN*, substantia nigra; *STh*, subthalamic nucleus; *ZI*, zona incerta.

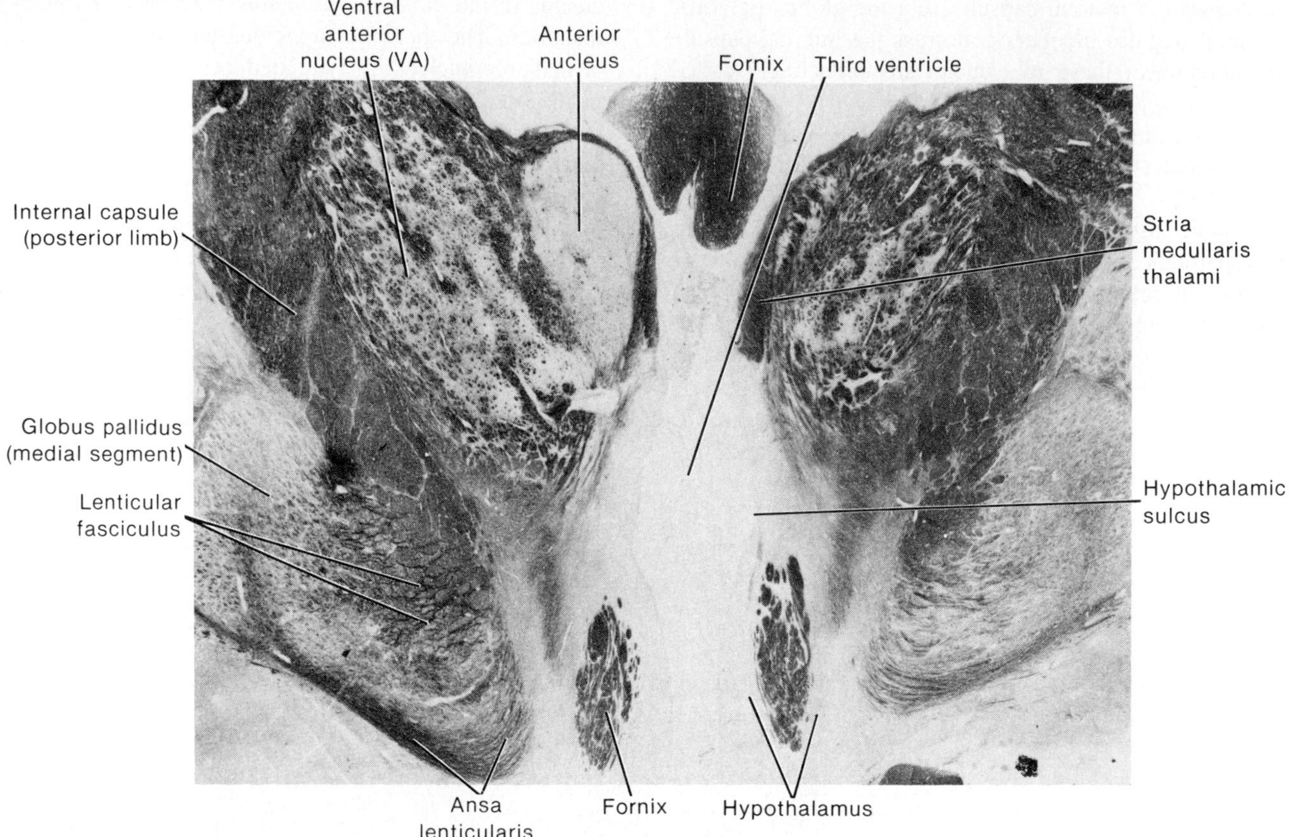


FIGURE 13-13
The ansa lenticularis seen in an enlarged portion of a coronal section similar to that shown in Figure 10-11.

## Subthalamic nucleus

The principal contacts of the subthalamic nucleus are simple and straightforward, consisting of interconnections with the globus pallidus, together with some efferent projections to the substantia nigra (Figure 13-14). These connections form the substrate of an indirect route through the basal ganglia (Figure 13-15) that plays a major role in determining the output of the globus pallidus. Alterations in the activity of the subthalamic nucleus have been implicated in several disorders of the basal ganglia (see Figure 13-17).

## Substantia nigra

The region referred to as the substantia nigra actually has two parts, a dorsal *compact part* containing closely packed, pigmented neurons and a *reticular part* nearer the cerebral peduncle containing more loosely packed neurons, most of which are nonpigmented.These correspond to two distinctly different ways in which the substantia nigra participates in the circuitry of the basal ganglia (Figures 13-6, *A* and 13-14).

The reticular part of the substantia nigra resembles in many respects a displaced portion of the globus pallidus. Like the globus pallidus, the reticular part of the substantia nigra receives inputs from the striatum and the subthalamic nucleus, and projects to the VL/VA and dorsomedial nucleus of the thalamus. It is in fact a more important route for information from the caudate nucleus to reach the thalamus than is the globus pallidus. In addition, projections from the reticular part of the substantia nigra to the superior colliculus and the reticular formation have been described. The connection with the superior colliculus is probably one route through which the basal ganglia participate in the control of eye movements.

The pigmented neurons of the compact part of the substantia nigra, which use dopamine as their neurotransmitter, project in a precisely organized topographic fashion to the caudate nucleus and putamen. These dopaminergic endings in the striatum ultimately modulate the output from the globus pallidus (Figure 13-17). Defects in this influence can result in movement disorders (putamen connections) and presumably in cognitive deficits as well (caudate connections).

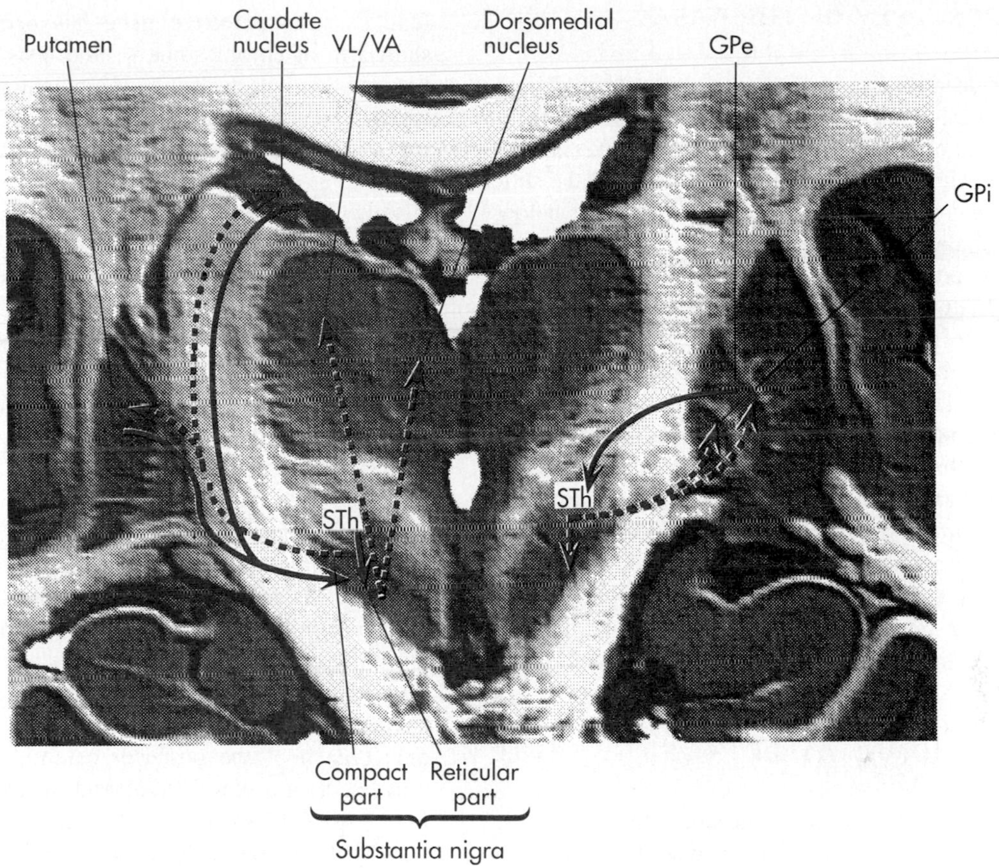


FIGURE 13-14
Connections of the substantia nigra and the subthalamic nucleus (*Sth*). Major afferents (solid) and efferents (dashed) of the substantia nigra are shown on the left. The substantia nigra has some additional connections that are not shown in this figure; see text for details. Major afferents (solid) and efferents (dashed) of the subthalamic nucleus are shown on the right. *GPe,* external segment of the globus pallidus; *GPi,* internal segment of the globus pallidus.

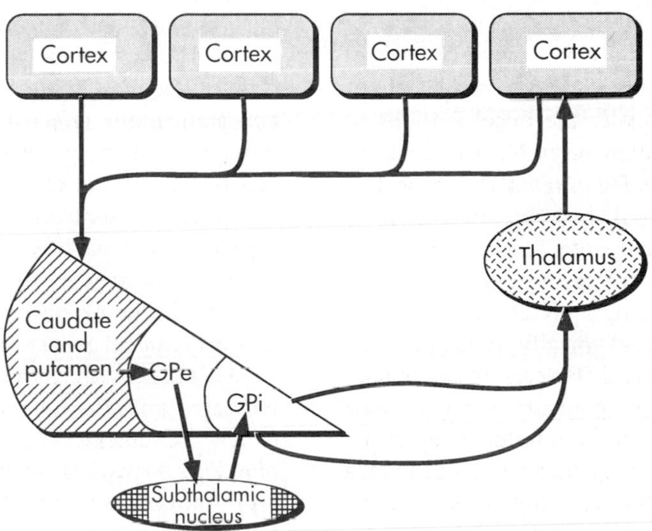


FIGURE 13-15
The subthalamic nucleus provides part of the substrate of an indirect route through the basal ganglia (compare to Figure 13-5, *A*).

## VASCULAR SUPPLY OF THE BASAL GANGLIA

Like other deep structures located superior to the circle of Willis, the basal ganglia receive their blood supply from small ganglionic or penetrating branches of arteries in and adjacent to the circle. One would therefore expect the substantia nigra and subthalamic nucleus, located just below the posterior thalamus (Figure 13-2, *B*) to be supplied by branches from posterior portions of the circle of Willis. The corpus striatum is mostly anterior to this level (Figure 13-1, *A*), and so its supply should come from more anterior portions of the circle. Hence the substantia nigra and subthalamic nucleus are mainly supplied by penetrating branches of the posterior cerebral and posterior communicating arteries, the striatum by penetrating branches of the middle cerebral artery (also referred to as lateral striate or lenticulostriate arteries), and the globus pallidus by the anterior choroidal artery. Branches of the anterior cerebral artery often help supply the striatum in the vicinity of nucleus accumbens; one of these may be a particularly large branch referred to as the *medial striate artery* (of Heubner).

## SOME FUNCTIONAL ASPECTS OF THE BASAL GANGLIA

Involuntary movements and disturbances of muscle tone figure prominently in the best known disorders involving the basal ganglia. The involuntary movements are customarily subdivided into tremors and states of *chorea, athetosis,* and *ballismus*. The disturbances of tone may be such that tone is increased in flexors and extensors generally (as in the rigidity of Parkinson's disease), or tone may be increased in only some muscles so that the patient's body is bent or twisted into an abnormal, relatively fixed posture. The latter condition is called *dystonia*. In still other cases, tone may be decreased.

Patients with chorea (from the Greek word for dance) exhibit a series of nearly continuous rapid movements of the face, tongue, or limbs (usually the distal portions of the limbs). The movements often resemble fragments of normal voluntary movements. *Huntington's disease* formerly called *Huntington's chorea)* is a hereditary disorder characterized by neuronal degeneration that is particularly severe in the striatum, especially in the caudate nucleus (Figure 13-16), and to a lesser extent affects neurons in the cerebral cortex and elsewhere. Typically symptoms first appear between the ages of 30 and 50 years as involuntary choreiform movements. The movements slowly become more pronounced, and this symptom is followed by or accompanied by gradually developing dementia. The chorea is presumably caused by striatal degeneration and the dementia by some combination of caudate and cortical degeneration. This is a particularly nasty disease, since it is inherited in a dominant fashion, but is usually not manifested until after individuals are old enough to have started families. The defective gene has been localized to the short arm of chromosome 4, and tests are now being developed that will determine if a potential victim is indeed a carrier. Hence, it will be possible to determine whether half of the children of an individual at risk are likely to be affected.

Athetosis (from the Greek word meaning without position) is characterized by slow, writhing movements, most pronounced in the hands and fingers so that a patient may be unable to keep the affected limb in a fixed position (hence the name "athetosis"). The responsible lesion seems to be in the striatum. All intermediate forms between chorea and athetosis are seen, and questionable cases are often referred to as *choreoathetosis*. No one knows why a particular lesion in the striatum should induce one state rather than the other.

*Hemiballismus* (ballismus comes from the Greek word meaning jumping about) is one of the most dramatic of the disorders of the basal ganglia. Its most prominent characteristic is wild flailing movements of one arm and leg. The responsible lesion is in the contralateral subthalamic nucleus. Hemiballismus is most often seen in older people, having been caused by a stroke involving a small ganglionic branch of the posterior cerebral artery. The reason movements are seen contralateral to the lesion is apparent from Figure 13-14: each subthalamic nucleus is related by way of the globus pallidus and the VL/VA to the ipsilateral motor cortex, which in turn is concerned with movements of the contralateral side of the body.

*Parkinsonism* is the most common and probably the best-known disease involving the basal ganglia. The symptoms are variable in relative severity and onset, but they usually include tremor, rigidity, and difficulty in moving. The tremor is a *resting tremor,* characteristically involving the hands in a "pill-rolling" movement; it diminishes during voluntary movement and increases during emotional stress. The *rigidity* is caused by increased tone in all muscles, although strength is nearly normal and reflexes are not particularly affected. The rigidity may be uniform throughout the range of movements imposed by an examiner (called *plastic* or *lead-pipe rigidity*), or it may be interrupted by a series of brief relaxations (called *cog-wheel rigidity*). Thus parkinsonian rigidity is quite distinct from spasticity: in spastic patients muscle tone is increased selectively in the extensors of the leg and the flexors of the arm and can be overcome in the clasp-knife reaction, and stretch reflexes are hyperactive. Finally, the difficulty in moving (*bradykinesia,* or slow movements; *hypokinesia,* or few movements) is shown by such things as decreased blinking, an expressionless face, and the absence of the arm movements normally associated with walking. Bradykinesia and hypokinesia are fundamental deficits; they are not simply the result of rigidity, since patients whose rigidity is not pronounced can nevertheless have great difficulty moving.

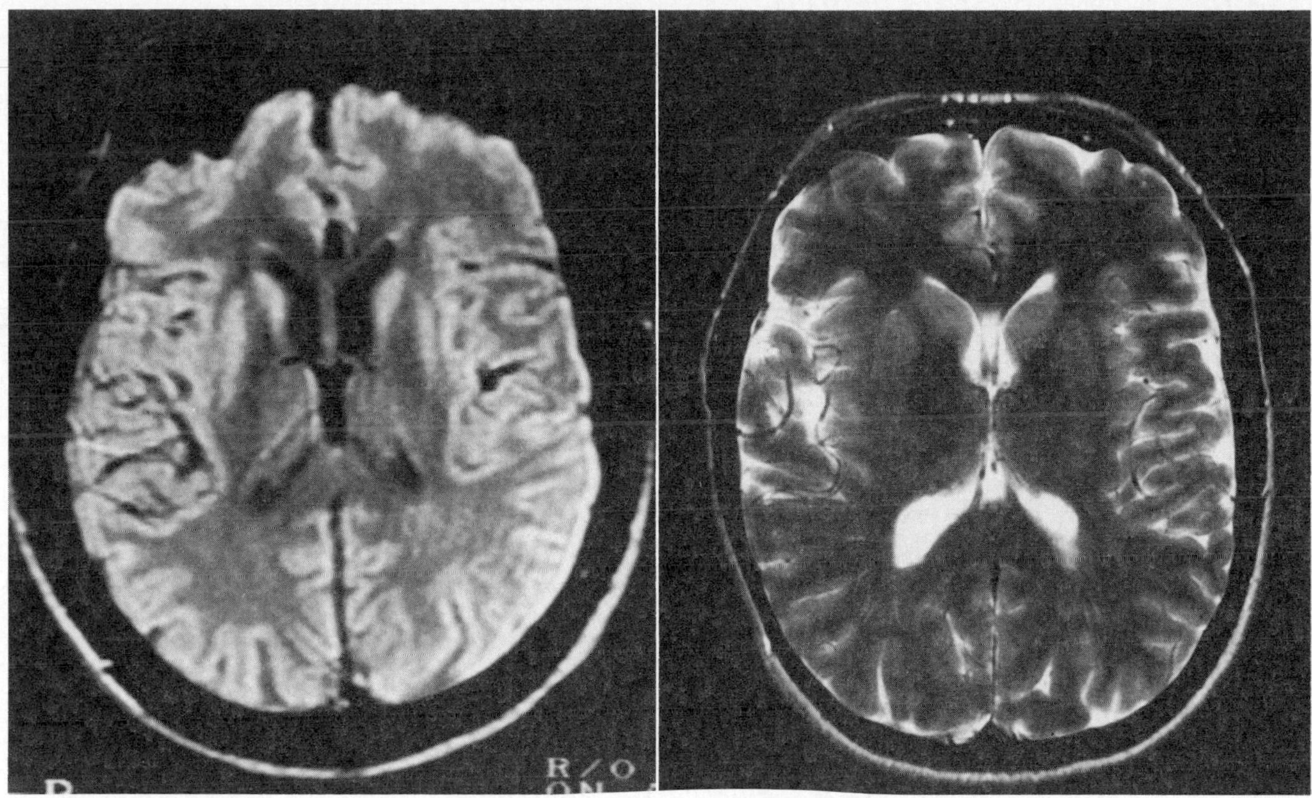


FIGURE 13-16
Horizontal MRIs of a patient with Huntington's disease (*A*) and of a normal individual (*B*, the same subject shown in Figures 4-15—4-17). Notice how much smaller the caudate nucleus and putamen are in *A*, and how the anterior horn of the lateral ventricle has expanded to take up the volume vacated by the caudate nucleus. *A*, courtesy of Dr. Erwin B. Montgomery, Jr., The University of Arizona College of Medicine. *B*, courtesy of Dr. Roger Bird, St. Joseph's Hospital, Phoenix, Arizona.

## Mechanism and treatment of disorders

Many disorders of the basal ganglia include striking positive signs (for example, tremor, rigidity, and ballistic movements), in which motor neurons are made to fire when they should not; they may also include negative signs as well (for example, hypokinesia), in which motor neurons cannot easily be made to fire by their owner. Recent advances in our knowledge of the anatomy and physiology of the basal ganglia now allow some tentative explanations of these clinical observations.

Each small portion of the internal segment of the globus pallidus has an inhibitory influence on the restricted portion of the thalamus to which it projects. Thalamocortical projections are excitatory. Hence changes in the activity of a small portion of the globus pallidus cause inverse changes in the activity of a corresponding small cortical area. Thus the basal ganglia may function by facilitating activity in some cortical areas and suppressing activity in others. One recent model proposes that the "direct" cortex → striatum → globus pallidus → thalamus → cortex loop facilitates selected cortical activity (Figure 13-17, *A*), while activity in the "indirect" loop involving the subthalamic nucleus suppresses other cortical activity (Figure 13-17, *B*). A further implication is that decreased activity of neurons in the subthalamic nucleus should cause disorders with many involuntary movements (hyperkinetic disorders), whereas increased activity of subthalamic neurons should cause hypokinetic disorders. Many of the clinical observations described earlier are consistent with this. The involuntary movements of hemiballismus result from direct damage to the contralateral subthalamic nucleus. In addition, degeneration of inhibitory striatal neurons, as in Huntington's disease, results in decreased subthalamic activity and the appearance of involuntary choreiform movements (Figure 13-17, *C*). Finally, removal of the dopaminergic input to the striatum, as in Parkinson's disease and its accompanying hypokinesia, results in increased subthalamic activity (Figure 13-17, *D*).

James Parkinson remarked in his original description on one patient whose tremors disappeared on one side after

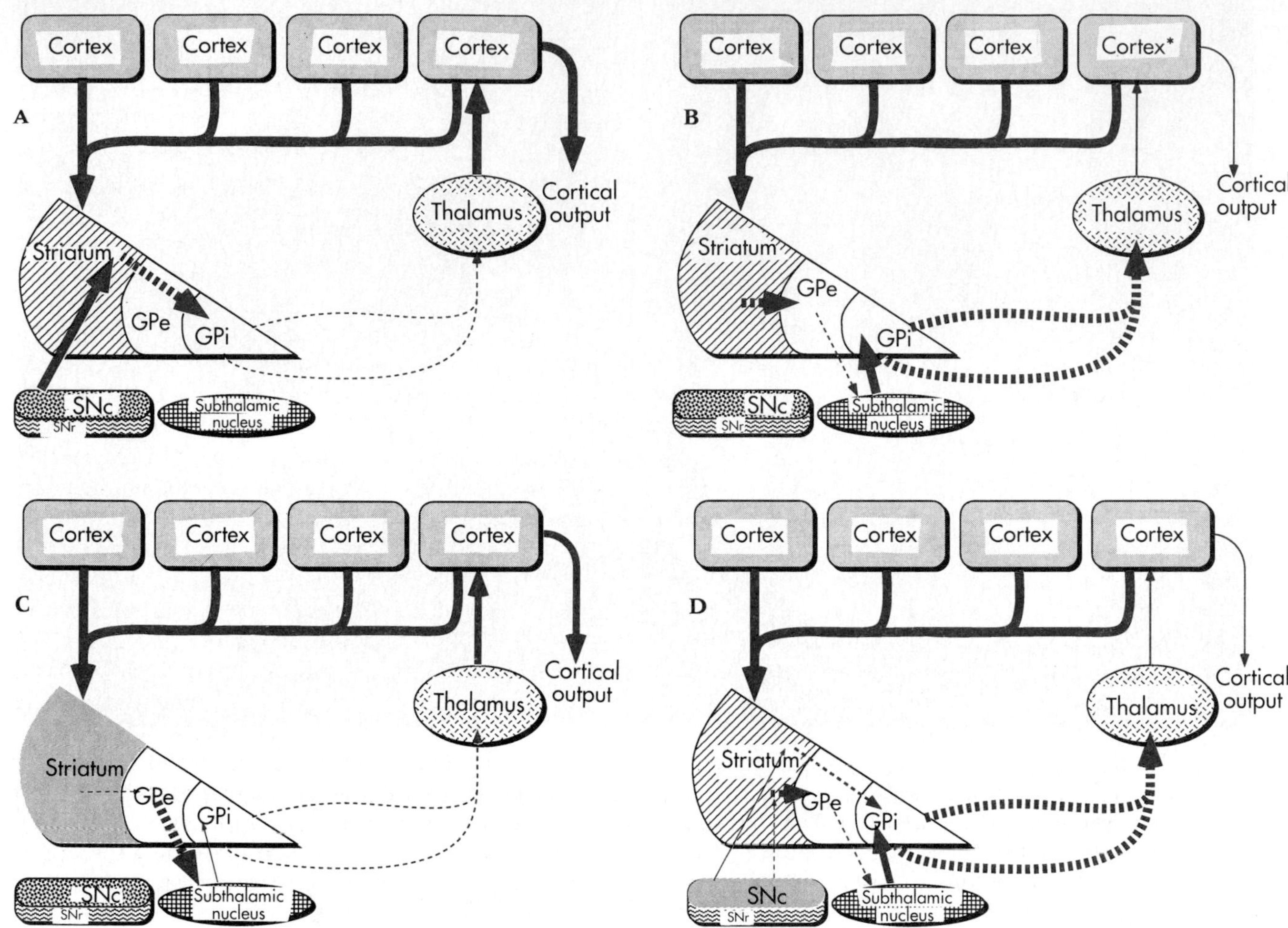


FIGURE 13-17

Some of the excitatory and inhibitory interactions in the basal ganglia, with an indication of how they may function together to affect cortical output in health and disease. This is by no means a complete depiction of all such interactions in the basal ganglia, but it does provide an illustration of how alteration of single elements could unbalance the entire system. Excitatory connections are solid, inhibitory connections are dashed, and the level of activity roughly indicated by the thickness of a line. **A,** The effect of the direct pathway through the basal ganglia in a normal individual. Cortical inputs and inputs from the compact part of the substantia nigra (*SNc*) have a net excitatory effect on striatal output neurons, which are inhibitory. Hence striatal output neurons decrease the output of the internal pallidal segment (*GPi*), which would otherwise inhibit the thalamus. This allows the thalamus to facilitate certain cortical outputs. **B,** The effect of the indirect pathway, utilizing the subthalamic nucleus, in a normal individual. In this case, diminished output from the external pallidal segment (*GPe*) leads indirectly to increased inhibition of the thalamus and to diminished output from another cortical area (*). Acting together, the direct and indirect pathways (**A** and **B**) could facilitate activity in some cortical areas while inhibiting activity in others. **C,** Loss of striatal projection neurons (as in Huntington's disease) would lead to decreased output from the internal pallidal segment via the indirect pathway. This could in turn lead to a failure to suppress some cortical outputs, which could manifest itself as involuntary movements. **D,** In Parkinson's disease loss of dopaminergic neurons from the compact part of the substantia nigra (*SNc*) causes decreased activity in the direct projections from the striatum to the internal pallidal segment. In addition, although not indicated in *B,* this nigral projection is thought to *inhibit* the striatal neurons in the indirect pathway; loss of this inhibition causes increased subthalamic activity. The combined effect of loss of these dopamine neurons would be inhibition of the thalamus, causing a diminished cortical output that could underlie bradykinesia and hypokinesia. Adapted from Bergman H et al. [*Science* 249:1436, 1990] and others.

suffering a stroke. This seems consistent with the idea that altered activity in the cortex → basal ganglia → cortex loop underlies these movement disorders, and it was reasoned some time ago that surgical intervention in some part of the loop might alleviate some symptoms. Since the globus pallidus affects motor areas of the cortex by way of the VL/VA complex, one logical site for surgical destruction might seem to be this part of the thalamus.

Somewhat astoundingly, this turns out to be effective. Stereotactic lesions in the VL/VA region (*thalamotomy;* the VL is the principal target) or in the internal segment of the globus pallidus are reasonably successful in relieving the tremor and rigidity of parkinsonism, the flailing movements of hemiballismus, and some (but not all) other involuntary movements and abnormalities of tone. In the case of hemiballismus, the excessive activity of the basal ganglia is apparently expressed primarily through the corticospinal tract. This tract has been sectioned in the cerebral peduncle in a few humans (on the side contralateral to the ballistic movements) for the relief of hemiballismus. The involuntary movements were permanently abolished and a transient flaccid paralysis ensued on the side contralateral to the surgery; however, as explained in the previous chapter, there were rather limited long-term deficits. Unfortunately, such surgery has less effect on negative signs such as hypokinesia, as though the role of the basal ganglia in facilitating selected patterns of movement cannot be replaced.

Considering the proximity of the VL/VA to the internal capsule and considering that thalamotomy does not relieve the negative signs, this surgery has always been a last resort, and other forms of treatment have long been sought. Postmortem examination of the brains of patients with parkinsonism indicated that damage is most consistently evident in the substantia nigra, reflecting degeneration of the pigmented nigral cells that normally manufacture dopamine and transport it to the striatum. It was therefore reasoned that if the dopamine could somehow be replaced, the symptoms might be ameliorated. Since dopamine does not cross the blood-brain barrier, it is necessary to administer *l*-dopa (levodopa), a precursor of dopamine that does cross the barrier.

While this form of therapy has been a great help for many patients, it also has a number of shortcomings. Therefore, other therapeutic approaches continue to be sought. One promising area of current research has been attempts to replace degenerated nigral cells. Since the central nervous system is largely isolated from the immune system, rejection of implanted tissue is not as great a concern as in other organs, and dopaminergic cells from human fetal midbrains have been successfully implanted into the striatum of a small number of parkinsonian patients. The extent to which such implants can mimic a patient's original substantia nigra, and the long-term efficacy of such treatment, are not yet known.

Additional avenues of research in basal ganglia disorders have been opened by the recent development of a primate model of Parkinson's disease. In the early 1980s several young individuals with what appeared to be severe Parkinson's disease were found to have injected themselves with a synthetic heroin analog contaminated with a compound called MPTP (1-methyl-4-phenyl-1,2,3,6-tetrahydropyridine). It was quickly found that MPTP is selectively toxic to dopaminergic neurons of the primate substantia nigra. This not only made certain types of controlled experiments more feasible, but also lent additional credence to the idea that some as yet unidentified environmental agent plays a major role in most cases of Parkinson's disease.

The basal ganglia have proved to be a treasure trove of chemically coded neural subsystems, as described in Chapter 17. The dopaminergic projection from the substantia nigra to the striatum is one example, but there are many others. The many common features of the various syndromes caused by damage to diverse parts of the basal ganglia give rise to the concept of these neural structures as forming a finely tuned system in which malfunction of any part can throw the whole system out of balance. The study of the balancing mechanisms in neurochemical terms is currently an active area of research. Thus a decrease in dopamine levels in the striatum causes parkinsonian symptoms. This can occur naturally (in Parkinson's disease) or as a side effect of drugs that act as dopamine antagonists (such as the phenothiazines used for psychiatric disorders). In contrast, increased levels of dopamine in the striatum, as in parkinsonian patients who receive too much *l*-dopa, can cause choreiform and athetoid movements as though the system were now tilted in the opposite direction. Great interest has been generated by the discovery that striatal synthesis of the transmitter γ-aminobutyric acid (GABA) is decreased in patients with Huntington's disease. A number of other transmitters in the basal ganglia are known or suspected, but their study is still at an early stage.

## ADDITIONAL READINGS


Alexander L: The vascular supply of the striopallidum, *Res Publ Assoc Res Nerv Ment Dis* 21:77, 1942.

Alexander GE, DeLong MR: Microstimulation of the primate neostriatum. II. Somatotopic organization of striatal microexcitable zones and their relation to neuronal response properties, *J Neurophysiol* 53:1417, 1985.

Alexander GE, DeLong MR, Strick PL: Parallel organization of functionally segregated circuits linking basal ganglia and cortex, *Ann Rev Neurosci* 9:357, 1986.

Alheid GF, Heimer L, Switzer RC III: Basal ganglia. In Paxinos G, editor: *The human nervous system,* San Diego, 1990, Academic Press.

Bergman H, Wichmann T, DeLong MR: Reversal of experimental parkinsonism by lesions of the subthalamic nucleus, *Science* 249:1436, 1990. *Recent work emphasizing the critical role of the subthalamic nucleus in the movement abnormalities seen in multiple basal ganglia disorders, including Parkinson's disease.*

Carpenter MB: Athetosis and the basal ganglia: review of the literature and study of forty-two cases, *Arch Neurol Psychiatry* 63:875, 1950.

Dick JPR et al: Simple and complex movements in a patient with infarction of the supplementary motor area, *Movement Disorders* 1:255, 1986. *Clinical evidence bearing on the relationship between the putamen and the supplementary motor area.*

Flowers K: Some frequency response characteristics of parkinsonism on pursuit tracking, *Brain* 101:19, 1978.

Flowers K: Lack of prediction in the motor behavior of parkinsonism, *Brain* 101:35, 1978.

Gage FH, Fisher LJ: Intracerebral grafting: a tool for the neurobiologist, *Neuron* 6:1, 1991.

Goldman PS, Nauta WJH: An intricately patterned prefrontocaudate projection in the rhesus monkey, *J Comp Neurol* 171:369, 1977. *Early results indicating that the traditional view of the striatum as a uniformly organized structure is an oversimplification.*

Goldman-Rakic PS, Selemon LD: New frontiers in basal ganglia research, *Trends Neurosci* 13:241, 1990.

Graybiel AM: Neurochemically defined subsystems in the basal ganglia. In *Functions of the basal ganglia,* Ciba Foundation Symposium, vol. 107, London, 1984, Pitman Medical Publishing Co, Ltd.

Graybiel AM, Baughman RW, Eckenstein F: Cholinergic neuropil of the striatum observes striosomal boundaries, *Nature* 323:625, 1986.

Graybiel AM, Ragsdale CW, Jr: Histochemically distinct compartments in the striatum of human, monkey, and cat demonstrated by acetylthiocholinesterase staining, *Proc Natl Acad Sci* 75:5723, 1978. *Additional results, complementary to those of Goldman and Nauta, indicating that the striatum is a jigsaw puzzle in terms of both connections and neurotransmitters.*

Hallett M, Shahani BT, Young RR: Analysis of stereotyped voluntary movements at the elbow in patients with Parkinson's disease, *J Neurol Neurosurg Psychiatry* 40:1129, 1977.

Hopkins DA, Niesser LW: Substantia nigra projections to the reticular formation, superior colliculus and central gray in the rat, cat and monkey, *Neurosci Lett* 2:253, 1976.

Hore J, Meyer-Lohmann J, Brooks VB: Basal ganglia cooling disables learned arm movements of monkeys in the absence of visual guidance, *Science* 195:584, 1977. *Some exciting work bearing on the possible role of the basal ganglia in the formulation of voluntary movements.*

Kemp JM, Powell TPS: The connexions of the striatum and globus pallidus: synthesis and speculation, *Philos Trans R Soc Lond* B262:441, 1971.

Kopin IJ, Markey SP: MPTP toxicity: implications for research in Parkinson's disease, *Ann Rev Neurosci* 11:81, 1988.

Langston JW et al: Chronic parkinsonism in humans due to a product of meperidine-analog synthesis, *Science* 219:979, 1983. *One of the original descriptions of MPTP-induced parkinsonism.*

Laplane D et al: Clinical consequences of corticectomies involving the supplementary motor area in man, *J Neurol Sci* 34:301, 1977.

Lindvall O et al: Grafts of fetal dopamine neurons survive and improve motor function in Parkinson's disease, *Science* 247:574, 1990.

Martin JP: *The basal ganglia and posture,* Tunbridge Wells, U.K., 1967, Pitman Medical Publishing.

Mendez MF, Adams NL, Lewandowski KS: Neurobehavioral changes associated with caudate lesions, *Neurol* 39:349, 1989.

Molina-Negro P: Surgery for abnormal movements. In Rasmussen T, Marino R, editors: *Functional neurosurgery,* New York, 1979, Raven Press.

Richfield EK, Twyman R, Berent S: Neurological syndrome following bilateral damage to the head of the caudate nuclei, *Ann Neurol* 22:768, 1987.

Rinne JO et al: Dementia in Parkinson's disease is related to neuronal loss in the medial substantia nigra, *Ann Neurol* 26:47, 1989. *Additional evidence about the role of the basal ganglia in cognitive functions—the medial part of the substantia nigra is preferentially connected to the caudate nucleus.*

Sadikot AF, Parent A, Franois C: The centre médian and parafascicular thalamic nuclei project respectively to the sensorimotor and associative-limbic striatal territories in the squirrel monkey, *Brain Res* 510:161, 1990.

Sandler M, Feuerstein C, Scatton B: *Neurotransmitter interactions in the basal ganglia,* New York, 1987, Raven Press.

Schell GF, Strick PL: The origin of thalamic inputs to the arcuate premotor and supplementary motor areas, *J Neurosci* 4:539, 1984. *An influential paper pointing out that the cerebellum and basal ganglia have separate projections to the thalamus and influence separate areas of the cortex.*

Selemon LD, Goldman-Rakic PS: Longitudinal topography and interdigitation of corticostriatal projections in the rhesus monkey, *J Neurosci* 5:776, 1985.

Smith Y, Parent A: Differential connections of caudate nucleus and putamen in the squirrel monkey *(Saimiri sciureus), Neuroscience* 18:347, 1986.

Smith Y, Hazrati L-N, Parent A: Efferent projections of the subthalamic nucleus in the squirrel monkey as studied by the PHA-L anterograde tracing method, *J Comp Neurol* 294:306, 1990.

Spokes EGS: Neurochemical alterations in Huntington's chorea: a study of post-mortem brain tissue, *Brain* 103:179, 1980.

Tetrud JW, Langston JW: The effect of deprenyl (Selegiline) on the natural history of Parkinson's disease, *Science* 245:519, 1989. *An important recent advance in the treatment of Parkinson's disease—a pharmacological strategy, suggested by studies of the mechanism of MPTP toxicity, that may slow the degenerative process in the substantia nigra.*

Weiner WJ, Lang AE: *Movement disorders: a comprehensive survey,* Mount Kisco, NY, 1989, Futura Publishing.

Whittier JR: Ballism and the subthalamic nucleus (nucleus hypothalamicus; corpus Luysi): review of the literature and study of thirty cases, *Arch Neurol Psychiatry* 58:672, 1947.

# CHAPTER 14

# Cerebellum

Cerebellum literally means "little brain," and in a real sense it is. This semidetached mass of neural tissue covers most of the posterior surface of the brainstem, anchored there by three pairs of fiber bundles called *cerebellar peduncles*. Sensory inputs of virtually every description find their way to the uniquely structured cortex of the cerebellum, which in turn projects (via a set of *deep cerebellar nuclei*) to various sites in the brainstem and thalamus. Although the cerebellum is extensively concerned with the processing of sensory information, and although it has few ways to influence motor neurons directly, it is considered part of the motor system because cerebellar damage results in abnormalities of equilibrium, of muscle tone and postural control, and of coordination of voluntary movements.

## GENERAL PLAN OF THE CEREBELLUM

### Gross anatomy

The outside of the cerebellum has a banded appearance, as though its surface were folded like an accordion (Figures 14-1 to 14-5). This folding is a successful device for increasing the cerebellar surface area; if the cortex could be drawn out into a flat sheet, it would be over 1 meter long (Figure 14-6). Deep fissures, most easily seen in sagittal sections (Figure 14-5), indent the cerebellar surface. Smaller fissures indent the walls of these deep fissures, with the result that the entire cerebellar surface is made up of cortical ridges called *folia,** most of which are transversely oriented. Beneath the cortex is a mass of white matter, the *medullary center* of the cerebellum, which is composed of fibers going to or coming from the cerebellar cortex.

* The white matter of the cerebellum has a tree-like appearance in sagittal sections (Figure 14-5), and so was named *arbor vitae* ("tree of life") by early anatomists. In a continuation of the tree analogy, each of the cortical folds on the surface of the arbor vitae is called a folium (Latin for leaf, as in foliage).

The first fissure to appear during development is the *posterolateral fissure,* which separates the *flocculonodular lobe* from the *corpus cerebelli*. In humans, the corpus cerebelli is by far the larger of the two, and the posterolateral fissure is so deep that the *flocculus* of each side is almost pinched off from the rest of the cerebellum (Figures 14-4 and 14-5). The *primary fissure,* a prominent landmark in midsagittal sections of the cerebellum, subdivides the corpus cerebelli into *anterior* and *posterior lobes* (Figures 14-1 and 14-5).

The cerebellum may also be subdivided into longitudinal zones, perpendicular to the fissures, which cut across the anterior, posterior, and flocculonodular lobes (Figure 14-7, *A*). The most medial zone, straddling the midline, is the *vermis* (from the Latin for worm). On either side of the vermis is a large *cerebellar hemisphere*. Each hemisphere is subdivided into a medial longitudinal strip adjacent to the vermis, called the *intermediate* or *paravermal zone,* and a larger, more lateral portion. The vermis is fairly clearly set off from the hemispheres on the inferior surface of the cerebellum (Figure 14-3), but other longitudinal lines of separation are not very obvious from the outside (for example, Figure 14-1). The demarcation into longitudinal zones is based on function and on patterns of connections, as is described shortly. Cerebellar cortex has the same structure everywhere and is smoothly continuous from one hemisphere across the midline to the other. The fissures that carve the cerebellum into *lobules* and folia are also continuous across the midline, so each transverse wedge of cerebellum has a vermal portion and a more lateral portion. Thus the *nodulus* is the vermal portion of the flocculonodular lobe and continues laterally into the flocculus. An assortment of exotic names is applied to the lobules and the vermal areas of the corpus cerebelli (Figure 14-7, *B*), and a Roman numeral system is used as well for

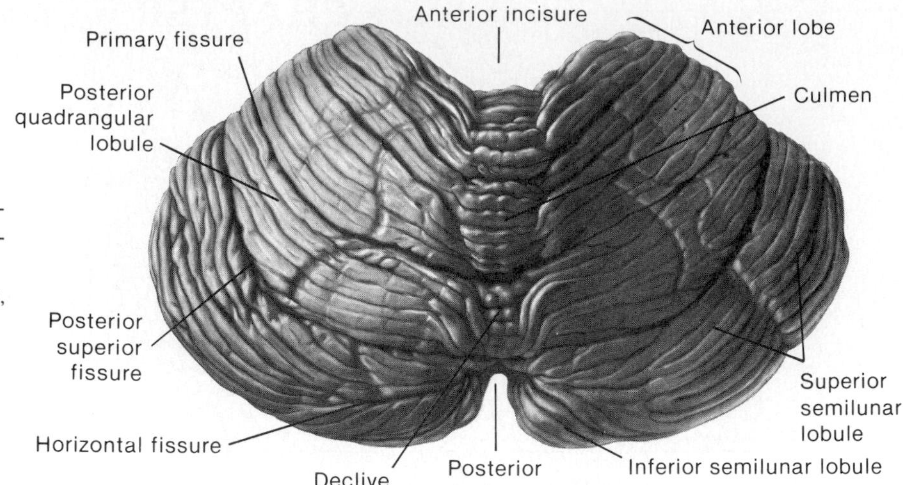


FIGURE 14-1
Superior surface of the cerebellum (the surface normally covered by the tentorium cerebelli).
From Mettler FA: Neuroanatomy, ed. 2, St. Louis, 1948, Mosby-Year Book.

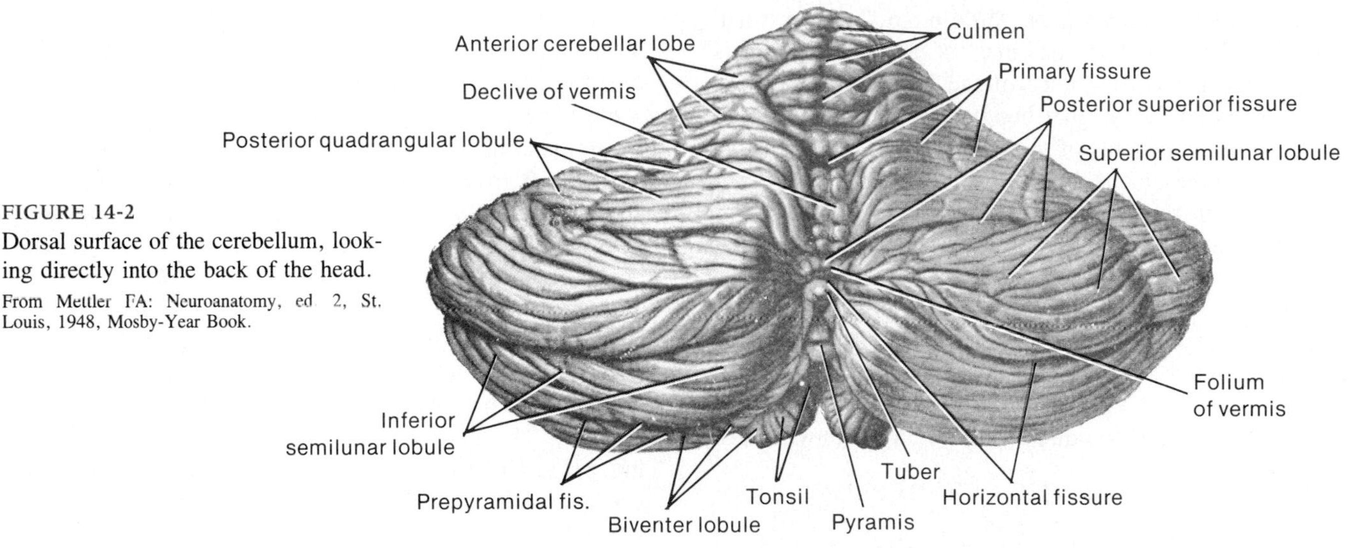


FIGURE 14-2
Dorsal surface of the cerebellum, looking directly into the back of the head.
From Mettler FA: Neuroanatomy, ed. 2, St. Louis, 1948, Mosby-Year Book.

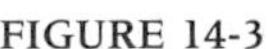
FIGURE 14-3
Cerebellum seen from behind and below, as though one were sighting up the spinal cord.
From Mettler FA: Neuroanatomy, ed. 2, St. Louis, 1948, Mosby-Year Book.

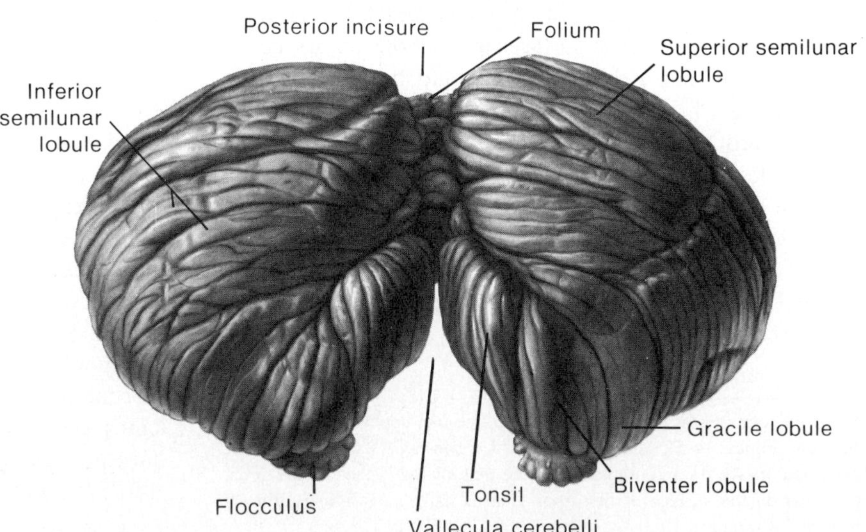

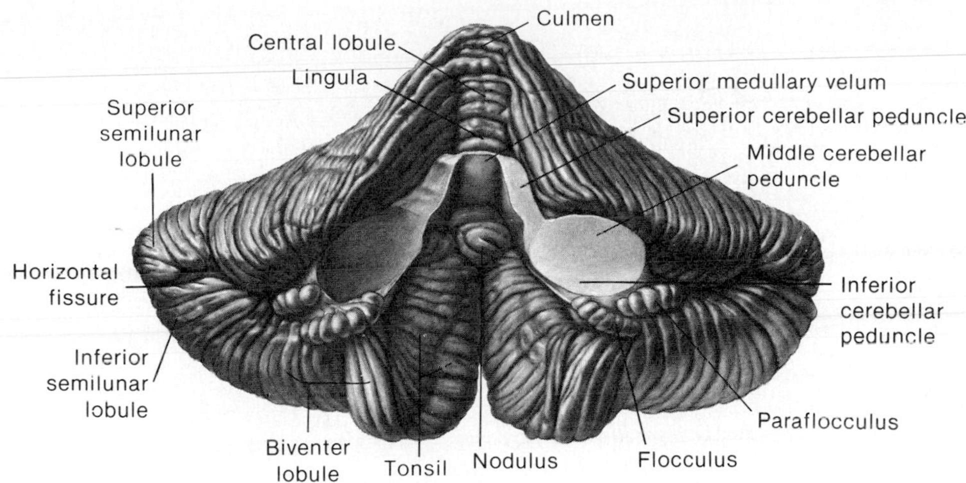


FIGURE 14-4
Ventral surface of a cerebellum that had been removed from the brainstem by severing the cerebellar peduncles. The view is as if one were looking up from the floor of the fourth ventricle toward its roof, looking directly at someone who is observing Figure 14-2.
From Mettler FA: Neuroanatomy, ed. 2, St. Louis, 1948, Mosby-Year Book.

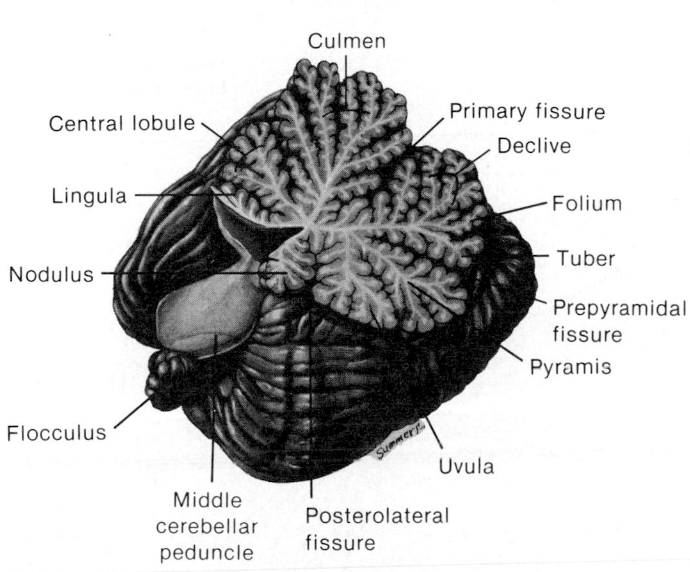


FIGURE 14-5
Medial surface of a hemisected cerebellum, demonstrating the depth of many of the cerebellar fissures and the way in which the fissures divide the vermis into a number of lobules. The same fissures continue laterally and divide up the cerebellar hemispheres.
From Mettler, FA: Neuroanatomy, ed. 2, St. Louis, 1948, Mosby-Year Book.

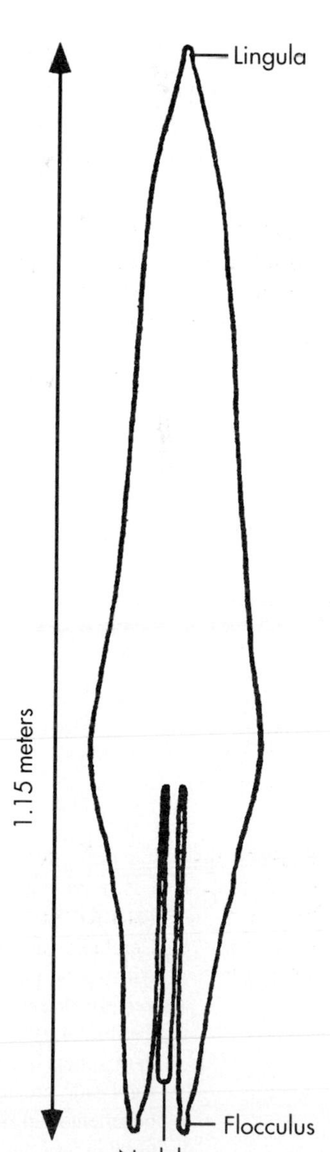


FIGURE 14-6
What the human cerebellar cortex would look like if it could be peeled off the surface of the cerebellum and laid out as a flat sheet.
Redrawn from Braitenberg V, Atwood RP: *J Comp Neurol* 109:1, 1958.

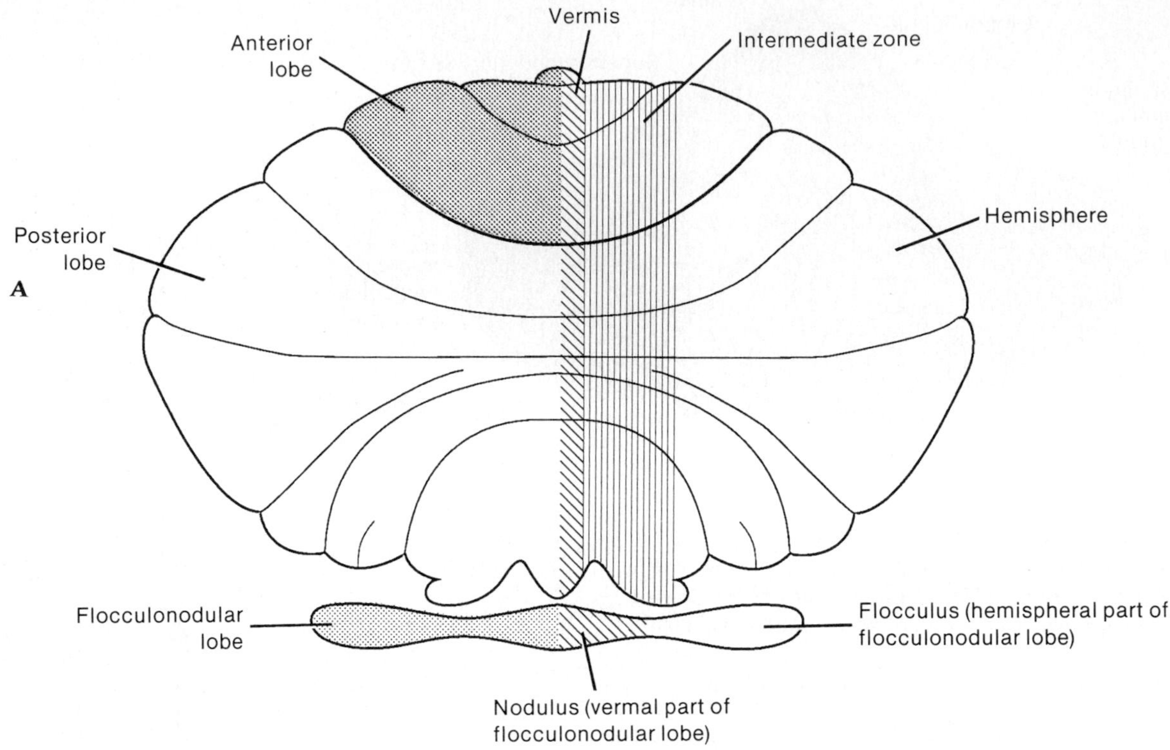


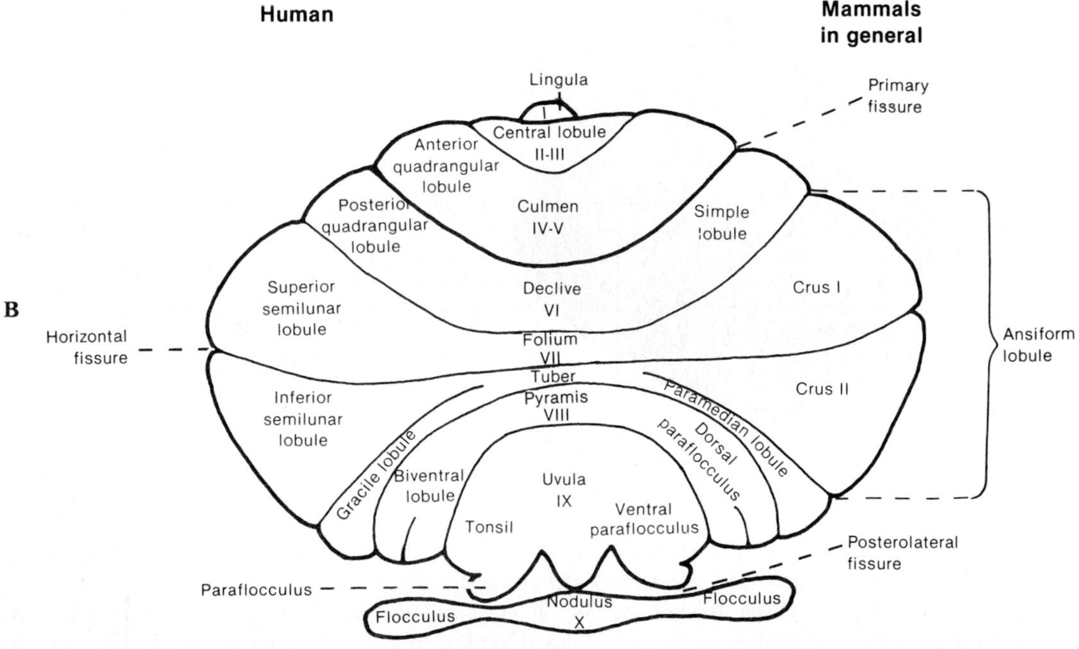


FIGURE 14-7
Cerebellar terminology on a schematic cerebellum projected as though the cerebellum were flattened out with its vermis now in one plane (compare with Figures 14-1 to 14-5). **A,** General division into transversely oriented lobes (on the left side of the diagram) and into longitudinal zones (on the right). **B,** Terminology for the various subdivisions of the vermis (including Roman numerals) and lobules of the hemispheres. On the left side of the diagram are terms classically used for the human cerebellum. On the right side are terms from comparative anatomy used more frequently in describing the cerebella of experimental animals.

Modified from Larsell O: Anatomy of the nervous system, ed. 2, New York, 1951, Appleton-Century-Crofts.

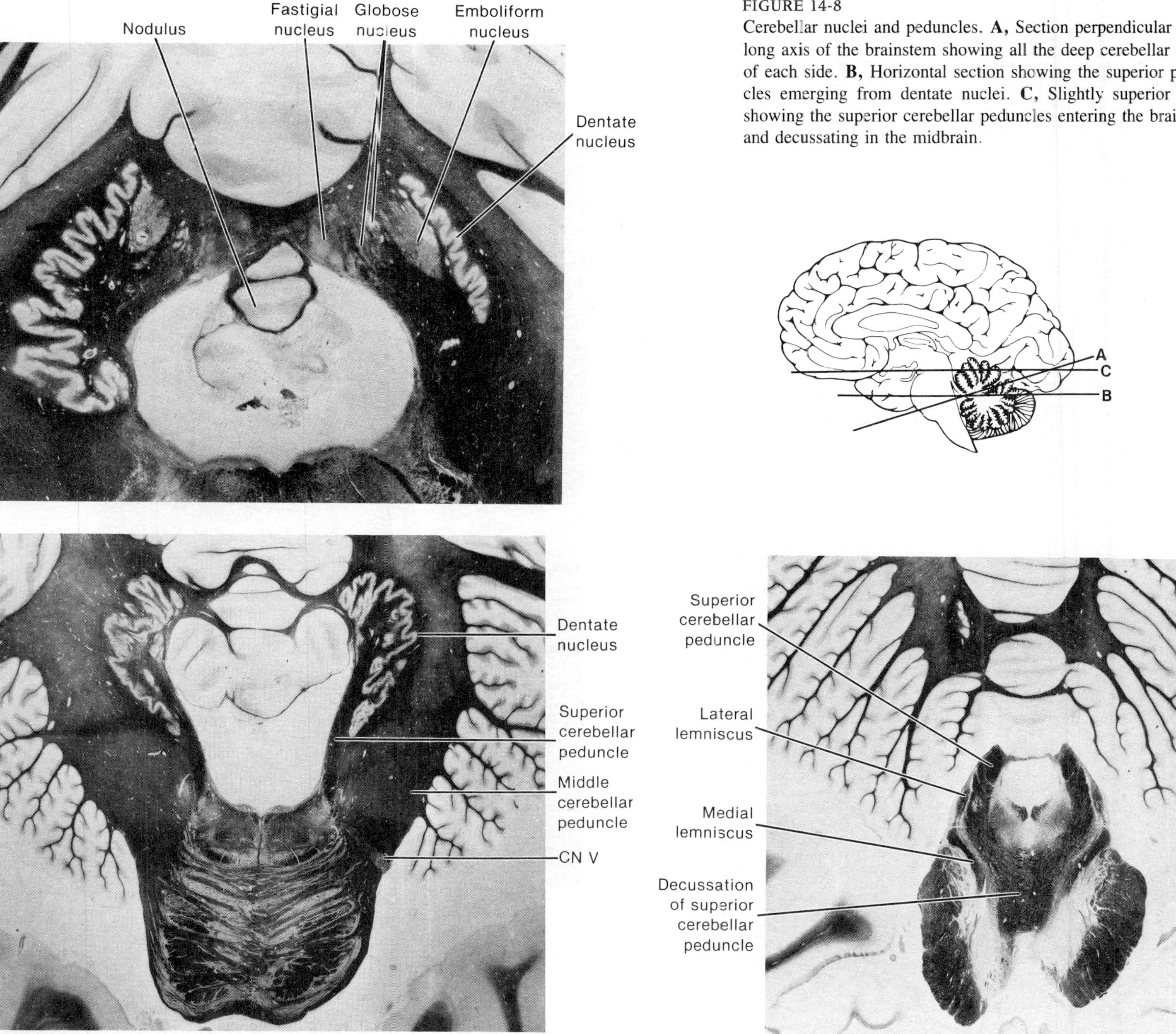


FIGURE 14-8
Cerebellar nuclei and peduncles. **A,** Section perpendicular to the long axis of the brainstem showing all the deep cerebellar nuclei of each side. **B,** Horizontal section showing the superior peduncles emerging from dentate nuclei. **C,** Slightly superior to **B,** showing the superior cerebellar peduncles entering the brainstem and decussating in the midbrain.

the vermis, but for the most part these names and numbers are of limited utility in clinical settings. The *tonsils* are the hemispheral portions just across the posterolateral fissure from the flocculi; appropriately enough, their vermal continuation is the *uvula*.

The cerebellum is attached to the brainstem by three substantial peduncles on each side. The *inferior cerebellar peduncle* (or *restiform body**) (Figures 8-8 and 8-9) is composed mainly of afferents to the cerebellum from the spinal cord and brainstem. The *middle cerebellar peduncle* (or *brachium pontis,* Figure 8-10) is the largest of the three. It is composed virtually exclusively of afferents to the cerebellum from the *pontine nuclei* of the contralateral side. The *superior cerebellar peduncle* (or *brachium conjunctivum,*† Figures 8-11 to 8-14 and 14-8) contains the major efferent pathways from the cerebellum.

*There is a bit of a logical inconsistency in using the terms *inferior cerebellar peduncle* and *restiform body* interchangeably. The *juxtarestiform body,* carrying vestibular traffic to and from the cerebellum, is also part of the inferior cerebellar peduncle. In common usage, the logical inconsistency is often ignored.

†A similar logical inconsistency exists in using the terms *superior cerebellar peduncle* and *brachium conjunctivum* synonymously. Brachium conjunctivum refers specifically to the large mass of cerebellar efferents bound mostly for the red nucleus and thalamus, whereas the total superior cerebellar peduncle also includes a few cerebellar afferents such as those of the anterior spinocerebellar tract.

A series of *deep cerebellar nuclei* is buried in the medullary center of each side of the cerebellum (Figures 14-8 and 14-9). The most lateral is the *dentate nucleus,* a crumpled sheet of cells that looks strikingly like the inferior olivary nucleus. Most of the fibers in the superior cerebellar peduncle originate from the dentate nucleus and emerge from its medially facing mouth, or *hilus*. Medial to the dentate nucleus are the *emboliform nucleus* and the *globose nucleus*. In most nonhuman cerebella, the equivalent cells form a single nuclear mass called the *interposed nucleus* (or *nucleus interpositus*), and so even in human neuroanatomy the term *interposed nucleus* is often used for the combination of the emboliform and globose nuclei. Finally, the most medial of the deep cerebellar nuclei is the *fastigial nucleus*.

## Cerebellar cortex

The cortex of the cerebellum has a uniform and fairly simple three-layered structure (Figure 14-10). The most superficial layer is the *molecular layer,* consisting mainly of the axons and dendrites of various cerebellar neurons. Deep to the molecular layer is a single layer of large neurons called *Purkinje cells*. Finally, adjacent to the medullary center is the *granular layer,* composed mainly of small *granule cells* arranged in a stratum many cells thick.

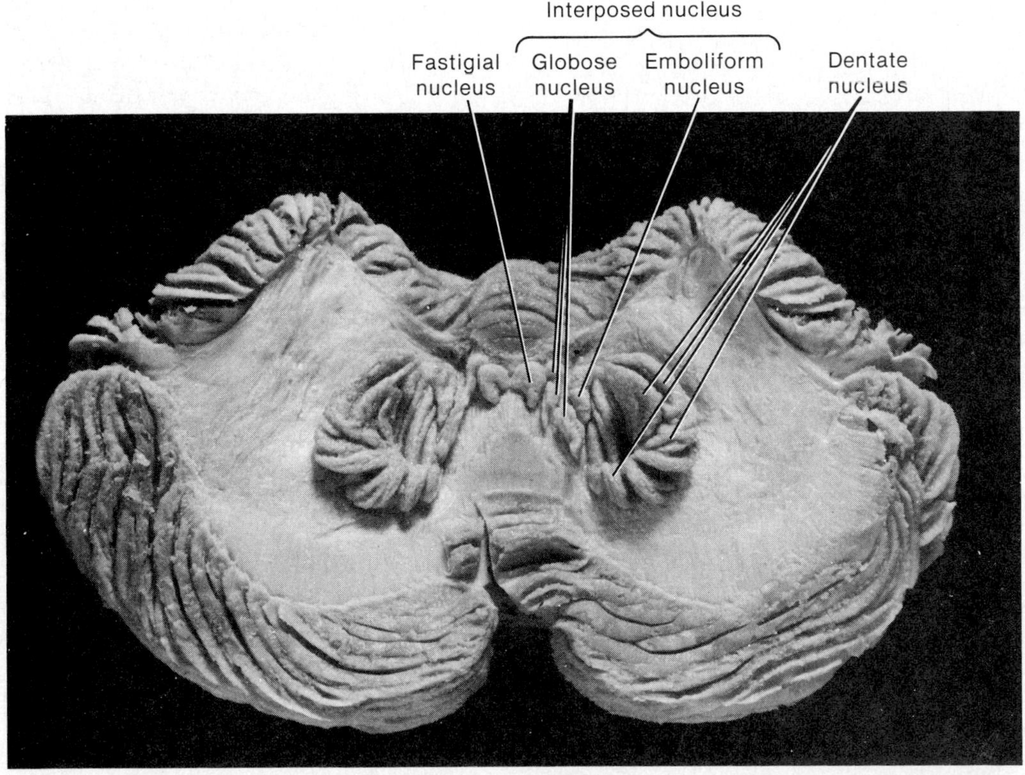


FIGURE 14-9
A beautiful dissection demonstrating the deep nuclei of a human cerebellum. From Gluhbegovic N: *J Anat* 137:396, 1983.
Courtesy of Dr. N. Gluhbegovic, University of Utrecht.

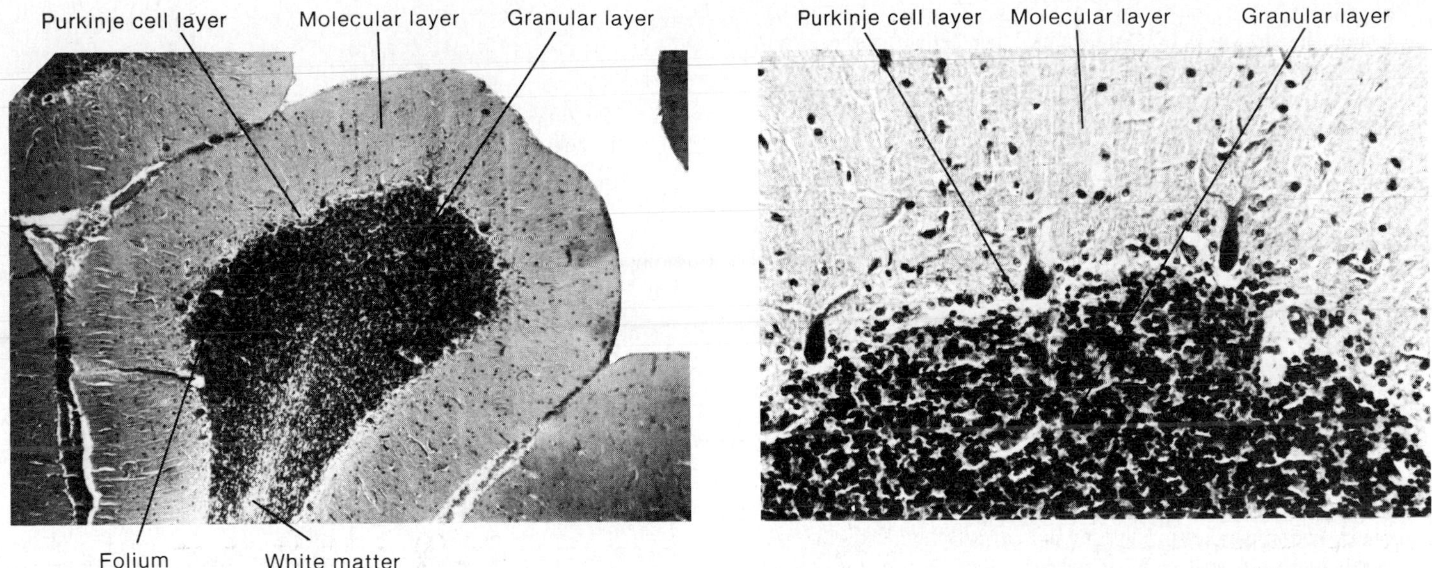


FIGURE 14-10
Low-power and high-power micrographs of the cerebellar cortex showing its three layers. From Willis WD, Jr and Grossman RG: Medical neurobiology, ed 3, St. Louis, 1981, Mosby Year-Book, Inc.

The molecular and granular layers also contain characteristic types of interneurons (Figure 14-11), but the fundamental circuitry of the cerebellar cortex can be described in terms of Purkinje cells, granule cells, and the afferents to the cortex (Figures 14-11 and 14-13, *A*).

Purkinje cells are the only neurons whose axons leave the cortex. They are, in addition, among the most anatomically distinctive neurons to be found in the nervous system. Each Purkinje cell has an intricate, extensive dendritic tree that is flattened out in a plane perpendicular to the long axis of the folium in which it resides (Figure 14-11). Each granule cell sends its axon into the molecular layer, where it bifurcates to form a fine, unmyelinated *parallel fiber* that extends for about 5 mm along the long axis of the folium. In its course, each parallel fiber passes through and synapses on the dendritic trees of a succession of Purkinje cells (as many as 500 of them). Each of us is estimated to have an incredible $10^{10}$ or more granule cells, and each of our 15 million Purkinje cells receives synapses from perhaps $10^5$ of them.

There are two sets of afferent fibers to the cerebellar cortex: *climbing fibers* and *mossy fibers*. A single climbing fiber ends directly on each Purkinje cell, winding around the proximal portions of its dendrites like ivy climbing a trellis (Figure 14-12). All of these climbing fibers arise in the contralateral inferior olivary nucleus. By elimination, then, all the rest of the afferents to the cerebellar cortex are mossy fibers. Mossy fibers end on the dendrites of granule cells, so this is an indirect route to the Purkinje cells (mossy fiber → granule cell → parallel fiber → Purkinje cell).

## Deep nuclei

Although Purkinje cell axons are the only route out of the cerebellar cortex, few of them leave the cerebellum itself. Rather, they project to the deep nuclei, which in turn give rise to the cerebellar output. However, it has become clear in recent years that the deep nuclei are not just simple relay stations; they have a more intricate relationship with the cerebellar cortex than had been realized previously (Figure 14-14). For example, climbing fibers and some mossy fibers send collateral branches to the deep nuclei. Nuclear cells are thus in a position to sample many of the same inputs the cortex receives and to compare the original inputs to the results of cortical computations on them. Furthermore, in addition to giving rise to axons that leave the cerebellum, the deep nuclei project back to the same areas of cerebellar cortex from which they receive Purkinje axons. The functional implications of these recently discovered connections are unknown, but they make it less surprising that the consequences of cerebellar damage are much more severe and long-lasting when the deep nuclei are included in the lesion.

## Functional divisions

The cerebellum is involved in equilibrium, in muscle tone and postural control, and in the coordination of voluntary movements; thus it would seem reasonable for it to receive vestibular, spinal, and cerebral cortical inputs. This is indeed the case, and even though the cerebellar cortex has the same anatomical appearance everywhere, different areas are concerned with particular functions. The flocculonodular lobe and part of the uvula receive ves-

FIGURE 14-11
Composite drawings of Golgi-stained cerebellar neurons, from sections cut in three nearly orthogonal planes. *A,* A transverse section cut perpendicular to the long axis of a folium, showing mossy fibers, climbing fibers, and the major neuronal cell types of the cerebellar cortex. The elements of the principal circuit through the cerebellar cortex (see Figure 14-13, *A*) can be seen clearly. Other cell types in the cerebellar cortex: *Basket cells,* whose dendrites spread out in the molecular layer and whose axons branch to enclose the cell bodies of a series of Purkinje cells; *stellate cells,* whose axons and dendrites all ramify in the molecular layer; and *Golgi cells,* whose dendrites spread out in the molecular layer and whose axons end on granule cell dendrites. *B,* A section parallel to the long axis of a folium, cut at an oblique angle so that it passes through the molecular layer on the right and the Purkinje cell layer on the left. This view demonstrates how the parallel fibers and the flattened dendritic trees of Purkinje cells are oriented perpendicular to each other. *C,* Another section parallel to the long axis of a folium, this time perpendicular to its surface to demonstrate the layers of the cerebellar cortex.

(Inset in *A* from Mettler FA: *Neuroanatomy,* ed. 2, St. Louis, 1948, Mosby-Year Book. All other parts redrawn from Ramón y Cajal S: *Histologie du système nerveux de l'homme et des vertébres,* Paris, 1909-1911, Norbert Maloine.

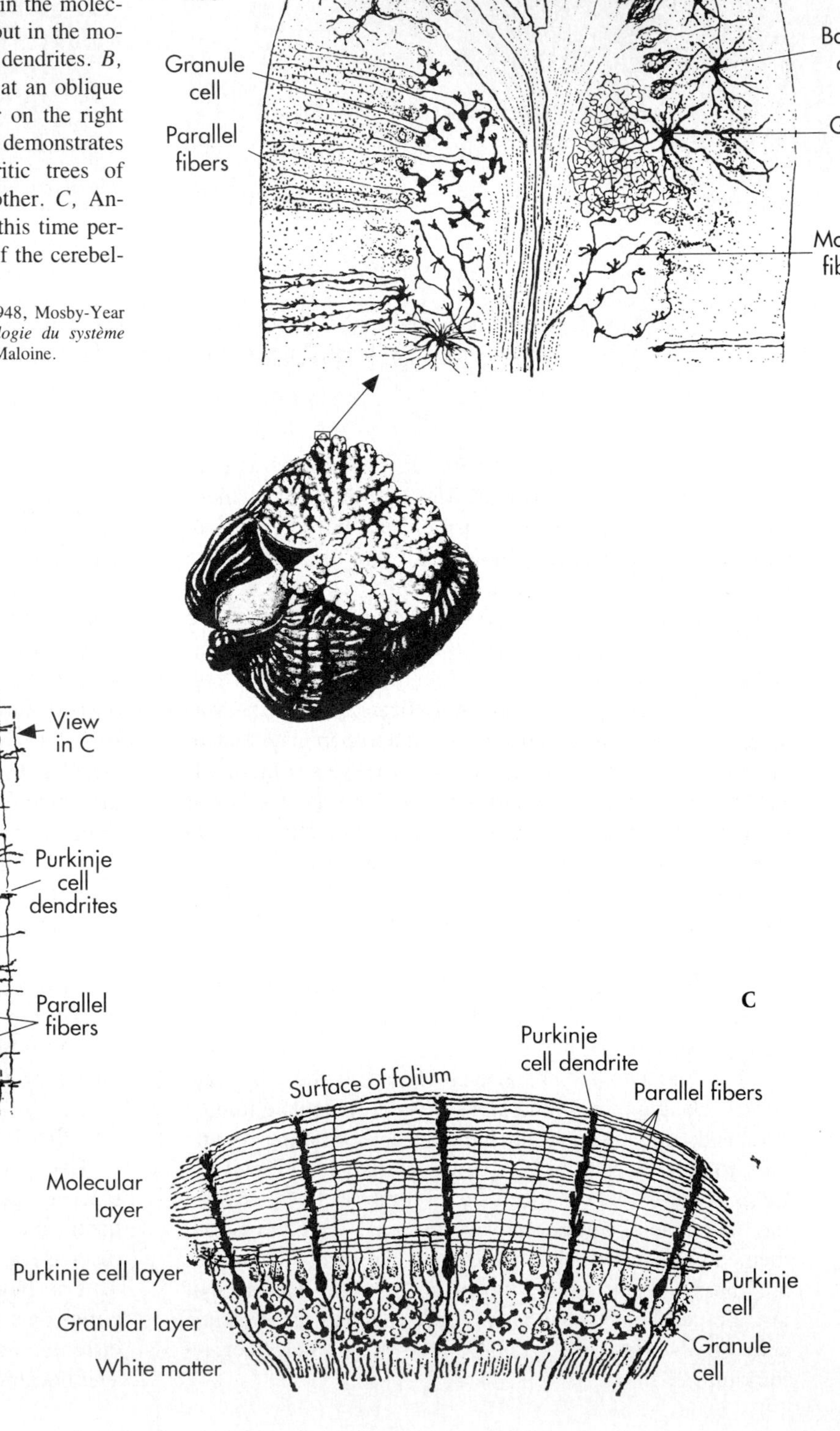

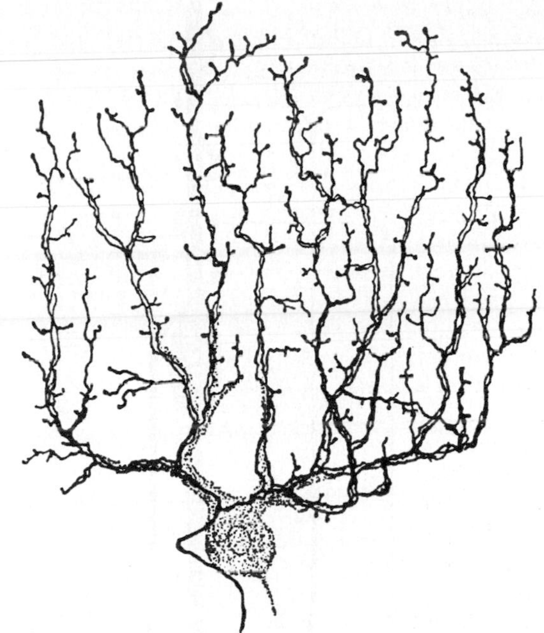

FIGURE 14-12
A drawing of a Golgi-stained climbing fiber, demonstrating the origin of its name as it climbs up the dendritic tree of a Purkinje cell (shown in color).

Redrawn from Ramón y Cajal S: *Histologie du système nerveux de l'homme et des vertebres,* Paris, 1909-1911, Norbert Maloine.

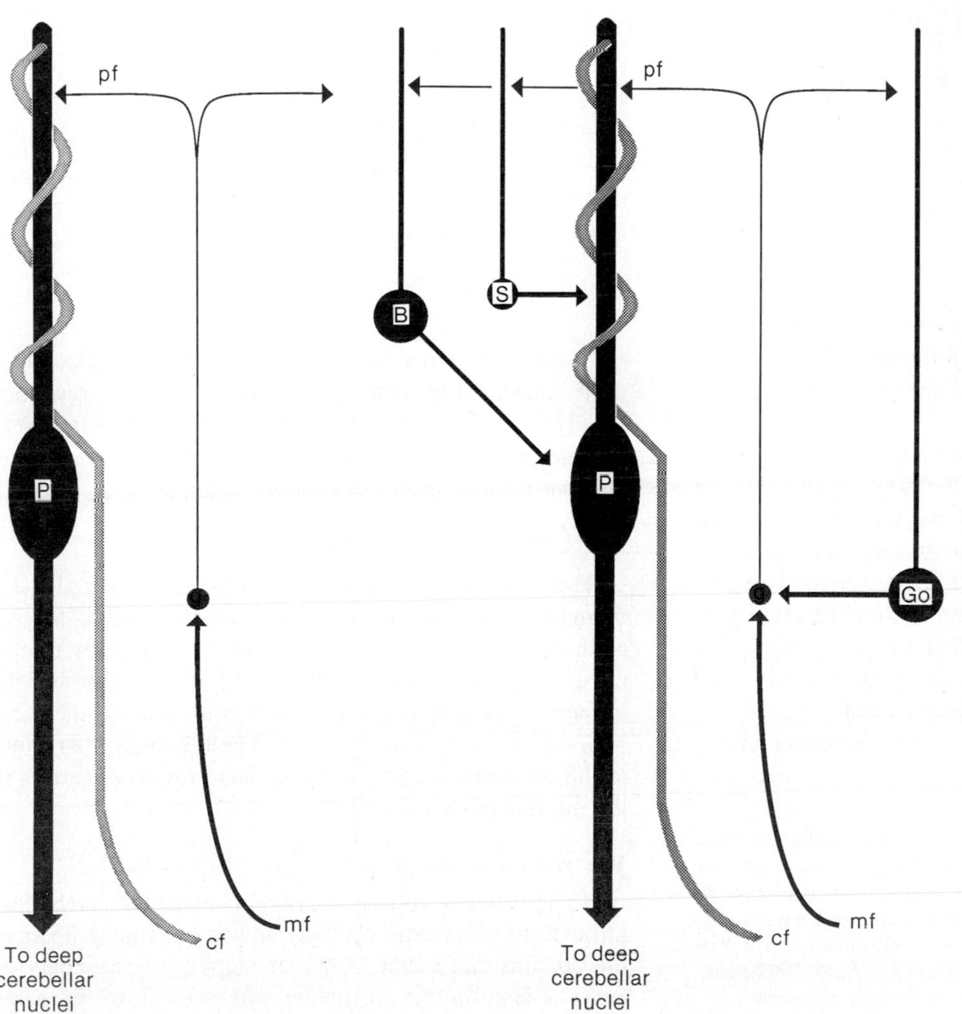


FIGURE 14-13
**A,** Schematic diagram of the principal circuit through the cerebellar cortex. Inhibitory connections are shown in black, excitatory in color. **B,** Major interconnections in cerebellar cortex; inhibitory connections shown in black, excitatory in color. One striking thing about the cerebellar cortex is the large amount of inhibition used in processing there: The mossy fiber *(mf)*-granule cell *(g)* inputs and the climbing fiber *(cf)* inputs are excitatory, but everything else is inhibitory. Golgi cells *(Go)* make inhibitory feedback connections onto granule cells. Basket cells *(B)* and stellate cells *(S)* make inhibitory synapses on the cell bodies and dendrites, respectively, of Purkinje cells *(P)*. Finally, all synapses of Purkinje cells, as far as we know, are inhibitory.

Modified from Thach WT: Brain Res 40:89, 1972.

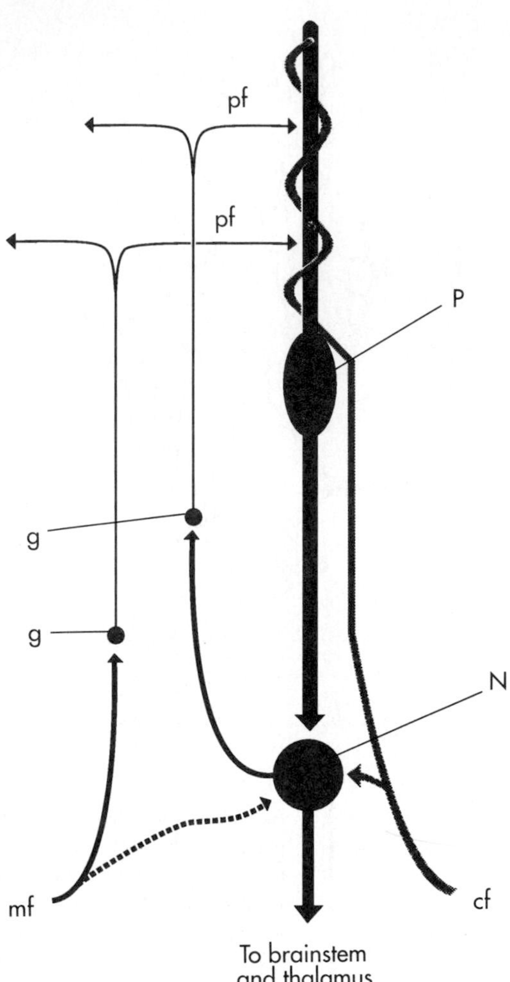


FIGURE 14-14
Schematic diagram of general interconnections of cerebellar cortex and deep cerebellar nuclei. Climbing fibers (*cf*) and some mossy fibers (*mf*) send collaterals to cells of deep nuclei (*N*) before continuing to cerebellar cortex, where climbing fibers end directly on Purkinje cells (*P*) and mossy fibers influence Purkinje cells indirectly through granule cell (*g*)–parallel fiber (*pf*) pathway. Purinje cells in turn end on cells of deep nuclei, and deep nuclei send mossy fibers to cortex as well as massive numbers of fibers to extracerebellar sites in the brainstem and thalamus.
Modified from Thach, W.T.: Brain Res, 40:89, 1972.

tibular inputs, and so this area is referred to as the *vestibulocerebellum*. Most of the vermal and paravermal regions (except for the nodulus and uvula) receive spinal inputs and so are called the *spinocerebellum*. Projections from the cerebral cortex (via relays in the pontine nuclei) form the single major input to lateral parts of the cerebellar hemispheres, so the lateral hemispheres are sometimes referred to as the *cerebrocerebellum* or the *neocerebellum*.* There is a certain amount of overlap of these functional divisions in terms of connections. For example, the spinocerebellum receives afferents from pontine nuclei, and parts of it receive vestibular afferents as well.

Different areas of the cerebellar cortex are preferentially related not only to particular inputs but also to particular deep nuclei. The dentate nucleus receives projections mainly from the lateral parts of the cerebellar hemispheres, the interposed nucleus from the paravermal cortex, and the fastigial nucleus from the vermis (Figure 14-18).

*Many authors use the terms *archicerebellum, paleocerebellum,* and *neocerebellum* synonymously with *vestibulocerebellum, spinocerebellum,* and *cerebrocerebellum* in reference to what is thought to be the phylogenetic sequence of development of these different cerebellar areas. Unfortunately, different authors use these terms in slightly different ways. Vestibulocerebellum, spinocerebellum, and neocerebellum, as defined here, seem to be the most common usage of the terminology at present.

## CEREBELLAR INPUTS

The cerebellar cortex receives some of its complement of mossy fibers from the deep cerebellar nuclei; the remaining mossy fibers carry information from three principal extracerebellar sources (Figure 14-15): (1) the vestibular nerve and nuclei, (2) the spinal cord, and (3) the cerebral cortex (via pontine nuclei). The climbing fiber input to the cerebellar cortex, as mentioned previously, arises in the inferior olivary nucleus.

### Vestibular system

Some primary vestibular afferents enter the cerebellum through the juxtarestiform body and end as mossy fibers in the nodulus and uvula. A larger number of secondary fibers, arising in the vestibular nuclei, follow the same

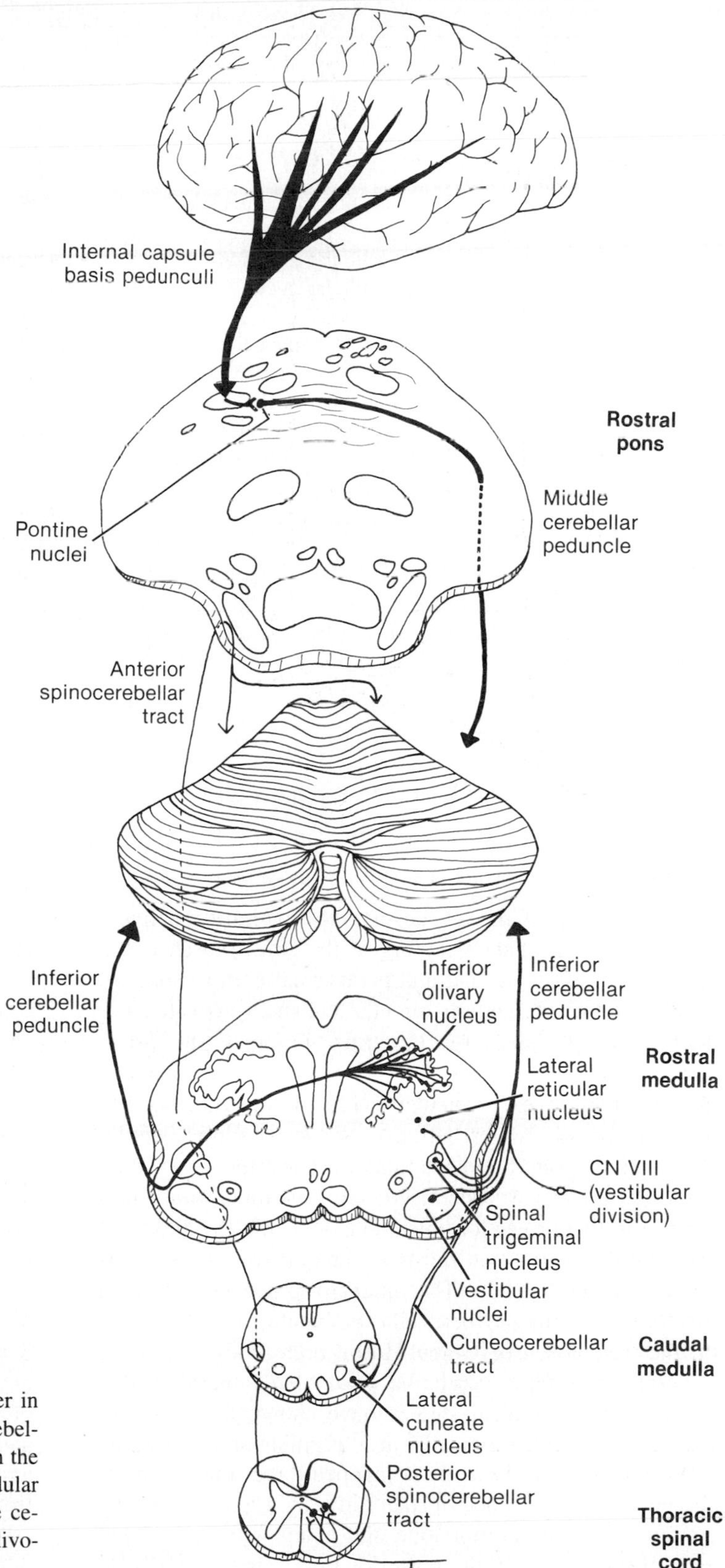


FIGURE 14-15
Principal inputs to the cerebellar cortex. As explained further in the text, spinocerebellar, cuneocerebellar, and trigeminocerebellar fibers end in the vermis and intermediate zone; fibers from the vestibular nerve and nuclei end mainly in the flocculonodular lobe; pontocerebellar fibers, conveying information from the cerebral cortex, end throughout the cerebellar cortex, as do olivocerebellar fibers.

**TABLE 9** *Inputs to cerebellar cortex**

| Tract | Origin | Termination | Peduncle |
|---|---|---|---|
| Anterior spinocerebellar | Contralateral spinal cord | Vermis and intermediate zone, mostly ipsilateral to origin (recrosses in cerebellum) | Superior |
| Posterior spinocerebellar | Clarke's nucleus | Vermis and intermediate zone, mostly ipsilateral | Inferior |
| Cuneocerebellar | Lateral cuneate nucleus | Vermis and intermediate zone, mostly ipsilateral | Inferior |
| Vestibulocerebellar‡ | Vestibular ganglion | Ipsilateral nodulus and uvula | Inferior (juxtarestiform body) |
| Vestibulocerebellar§ | Vestibular nuclei | Flocculus, modulus, and vermis, bilaterally | Inferior (juxtarestiform body) |
| Reticulocerebellar | Lateral, paramedian, and tegmental reticular nuclei | Mainly vermis and intermediate zone, mostly ipsilateral | Inferior |
| Trigeminocerebellar | Spinal and main sensory nuclei of trigeminal nerve | Vermis and intermediate zone, mostly ipsilateral | Inferior |
| Olivocerebellar | Inferior olivary and accessory olivary nuclei | All contralateral areas | Inferior |
| Pontocerebellar | Pontine nuclei | All contralateral areas except the flocculonodular lobe; some to ipsilateral vermis | Middle |

*Inputs from deep cerebellar nuclei not included.
‡Primary afferents.
§Second order fibers.

course to the flocculonodular lobe and most of the vermis, bilaterally.

## Spinal cord

A great deal of somatosensory information (principally from various mechanoreceptors of the skin, muscles, and joints) reaches the vermal and paravermal cortex. Some of it reaches the cerebellum directly via the spinocerebellar tracts and the cuneocerebellar tract (Figure 7-18). Some arrives indirectly by way of the reticular formation (remember that several reticular nuclei of the medulla and pons project to the cerebellum). Not surprisingly, similar information from the head also reaches the cerebellum from the trigeminal system. All the trigeminal nuclei participate in this projection to some extent, but the bulk of it arises in the rostral two thirds of the spinal nucleus (interpolar and oral nuclei). The anterior spinocerebellar tract travels in the superior cerebellar peduncle, but all the rest of the somatosensory input from both body and head traverses the inferior cerebellar peduncle (Table 8).

Electrophysiological studies have shown that this projection ends somatotopically in a peculiar and interesting way. Each part of the body is mapped three times onto the cerebellar cortex, once ipsilaterally in a pattern mostly contained in the anterior lobe and again with some bilateral representation in the posterior lobe (Figure 14-17). In each of the three somatotopic maps, the head is nearest the primary fissure and the trunk is adjacent to the midline.

## Cerebral cortex

You may recall that the basis pedunculi of the cerebral peduncle is considerably larger than the medullary pyramid. One basis pedunculi contains about 21 million fibers, of which only about 1 million continue on into the ipsilateral pyramid. Some of the remaining 20 million fibers are bound for the reticular formation or for the motor nuclei of cranial nerves, but the vast majority end in ipsilateral pontine nuclei. The pontine nuclei of one side contain about 12 million cells that project through the middle cerebellar peduncle to virtually all parts of the cerebellar cortex.* Almost all of these fibers cross the midline in the basal pons and end on the contralateral side of the cerebellum; indeed the pathway is usually treated as entirely crossed. However, a few fibers (particularly some of those destined for the vermis) end ipsilaterally.

The corticopontocerebellar pathway is therefore a mammoth one, dwarfing the corticospinal tract by comparison. Several areas of the cerebral cortex project to the pontine nuclei (Figure 14-16), but contributions from the vicinity of the central sulcus predominate (that is, from the motor and premotor cortex and from somatosensory cortex and adjacent parts of the parietal lobe). There are projections from other parts of the cortex, such as auditory, visual and association areas, but these are not as heavy as the others

*The nodulus receives no pontocerebellar fibers and the flocculus receives only a few.

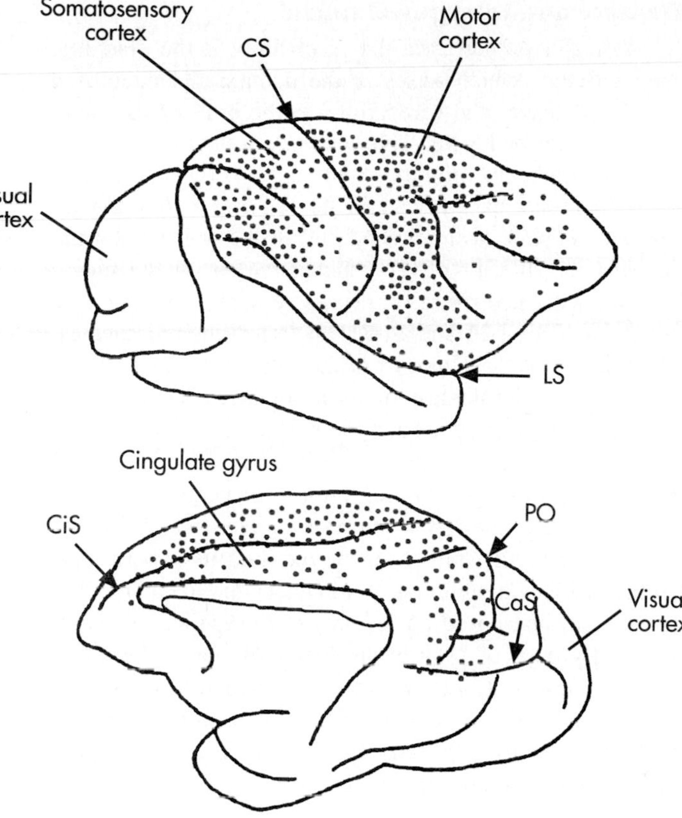


FIGURE 14-16
Distribution of labeled neurons in the cerebral cortex of a monkey after a tracer substance was injected into the basal pons and transported back to the cells that project to the pons. Most of the labeled neurons are in or near motor and somatosensory cortex, but there are also a significant number in limbic (e.g., cingulate) and association (e.g., prefrontal, temporal) areas. Abbreviations: CaS, calcarine sulcus; CiS, cingulate sulcus; CS, central sulcus; PO, parietooccipital sulcus.

Redrawn from Glickstein M et al: *J Comp Neurol* 235:343, 1985.

just mentioned. The vermis and intermediate zone preferentially receive their cortical input from the motor cortex of the precentral gyrus, and the pathway is somatotopically organized so that the pontocerebellar fibers end in the same pattern as do those carrying information from the spinal cord (Figure 14-17). The lateral parts of the cerebellar hemispheres, in contrast, receive most of their cortical input from premotor, somatosensory, and association areas of the cerebral cortex.

### Inferior olivary nucleus

The inferior olivary nucleus (actually a complex of a *principal* and two *accessory* olivary nuclei) is unique among structures providing afferents to the cerebellum. All olivary efferents emerge medially, enter the contralateral inferior cerebellar peduncle, and blanket the entire contralateral cerebellar cortex with climbing fibers.

The information these climbing fibers convey comes from diverse sources, including the spinal cord, the red nucleus, the cerebral cortex, and the cerebellum itself. Fibers from the ipsilateral red nucleus, forming the bulk of the central tegmental tract, are the numerically most important olivary input. Spinal inputs, all crossed, reach the inferior olivary complex both directly (via *spinoolivary fibers*) and indirectly (through relays in the posterior column nuclei). A few fibers from the cerebral cortex of both sides, mostly from motor cortex, also reach the olive. Finally, there is a topographically highly organized projection from the contralateral dentate and interposed nuclei to the inferior olivary complex (Figure 14-19).

A structure with these sorts of connections would be expected to play an important role in cerebellar function. This appears to be the case, since selective destruction of the inferior olive in experimental animals has acute effects similar to those of destruction of the entire contralateral half of the cerebellum (described shortly). However, selec-

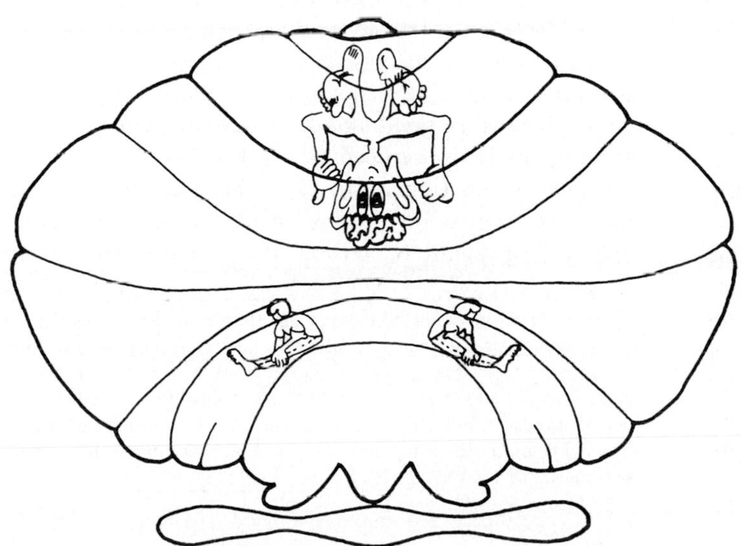

FIGURE 14-17
Arrangement of visual, auditory, and somatosensory inputs to the cerebellar cortex. Such maps have never actually been determined physiologically for the human cerebellum. Rather, they are inferred from data such as those of Snider (1950) for monkeys. The mapping is not nearly as precise as in the sensory and motor areas of the cerebral cortex, and is actually much more fragmented than portrayed here. The large eyes and ears of the upper homunculus are meant to indicate that this is the region that receives auditory and visual inputs.

tive olivary destruction is exceedingly rare in human pathology. Damage in this part of the brainstem is likely to affect the nearby pyramid or inferior cerebellar peduncle as well, and it becomes difficult to sort out those symptoms for which olivary damage is responsible.

### Other inputs

Electrophysiological studies have also shown that responses to visual and auditory stimuli can be recorded from the vermis, approximately midway along its length (Figure 14-17). The anatomical routes by which this information reaches the cerebellum are not known with certainty, but there are likely to be at least two routes. The auditory and visual areas of the cerebral cortex can influence the cerebellum by way of the standard corticopontocerebellar pathway. In addition, fibers from the superior and inferior colliculi convey visual and auditory information, respectively, to the cerebellum by way of relays in pontine nuclei. Visual information also reaches the flocculus, where it is used in the control of eye movements.

## CEREBELLAR OUTPUTS

The output of the cerebellar cortex is entirely in the form of the axons of Purkinje cells. Some of these, arising in the flocculonodular lobe and in parts of the vermis of both anterior and posterior lobes as well, leave the cerebellum via the juxtarestiform body and end in the vestibular nuclei. This then provides the only reasonably direct access the cerebellar cortex has to motor neurons of the spinal cord (via the vestibulospinal tracts); all other Purkinje axons end in the deep cerebellar nuclei. They do so in an orderly medial-to-lateral way; the vermis projects to the fastigial nucleus, the paravermal or intermediate zone projects to the interposed nucleus, and the lateral hemisphere projects to the dentate nucleus (Figure 14-18).

The output connections of the fastigial nucleus are distinctive, whereas those of the dentate and interposed nuclei are similar to each other. In addition to the connections described in the next three sections, all the deep nuclei project back to the cerebellar cortex.

### Fastigial nucleus

The fastigial output is directed primarily to the brainstem, ending in the vestibular nuclei of both sides and in the reticular formation, mainly contralaterally (Figure 14-19). Fibers that end ipsilaterally go right out through the juxtarestiform body. Those bound for contralateral targets cross the midline within the cerebellum, loop over the superior cerebellar peduncle as the *uncinate fasciculus* (or *hook bundle*), and descend through the contralateral juxtarestiform body. A few fibers also project to the contralateral VL/VA complex of the thalamus and to the contralateral cervical spinal cord.

### Dentate and interposed nuclei

The major output from the cerebellum is the brachium conjunctivum, which arises in the dentate and interposed nuclei and leaves the cerebellum as the bulk of the superior cerebellar peduncle. This peduncle joins the brainstem in the rostral pons (Figures 8-11 and 14-8); at this level some fibers turn caudally as the *descending limb of the superior cerebellar peduncle* and end in the reticular formation and the inferior olivary nucleus. Most of the fibers, however, continue rostrally, decussate in the midbrain (see Figures 8-13 to 8-15 and 14-8), and reach the red nucleus, where many of the fibers from the interposed nucleus and a minority of the dentate fibers terminate. The remaining fibers pass through or around the red nucleus, join the thalamic fasciculus, and end in the VL/VA complex of the thalamus. The projections of these two cerebellar nuclei therefore differ mainly in emphasis. The interposed nucleus preferentially influences the red nucleus, whereas the dentate nucleus preferentially influences the thalamus. The dentate and interposed nuclei project to separate but interdigitated groups of cells in the thalamus. From these thalamic cells, dentate information is conveyed to motor and premotor cortex, whereas information from the interposed nucleus is conveyed selectively to the limb areas of motor cortex (Figure 14-20 and 14-21).

## SOME FUNCTIONAL ASPECTS OF THE CEREBELLUM

The cerebellum is a great delight for anatomists and physiologists because of its uniform, precisely organized cortex and its well worked out connections. It is also something of an embarrassment because in the final analysis we do not understand much about how it works. However, characteristic motor disorders and no significant sensory deficit* follow cerebellar damage. Based on the nature of these motor disabilities (detailed in the next section) and on the anatomy and physiology of different parts of the cerebellum, a few general comments about function can be made.

The lateral hemispheres form the largest part of the human cerebellum. The major neural circuit in which they are involved is the great loop from several areas of the cerebral cortex to the cerebellum and back to the motor and premotor cortex (Figure 14-20). This circuitry suggests that the cerebellar hemispheres could be involved somehow in the planning of movements, acting by influencing

*"I have, however, examined every modality of sensation in many cases [of cerebellar damage] but have never found disturbances of any form ...No matter how irregular the movements may be, or how far the affected limb deviates from the point to which it should be moved, the patient always has a full and accurate recognition of its position in space." (From Holmes G: The symptoms of acute cerebellar injuries due to gunshot injuries, *Brain* 40:461, 1917.)

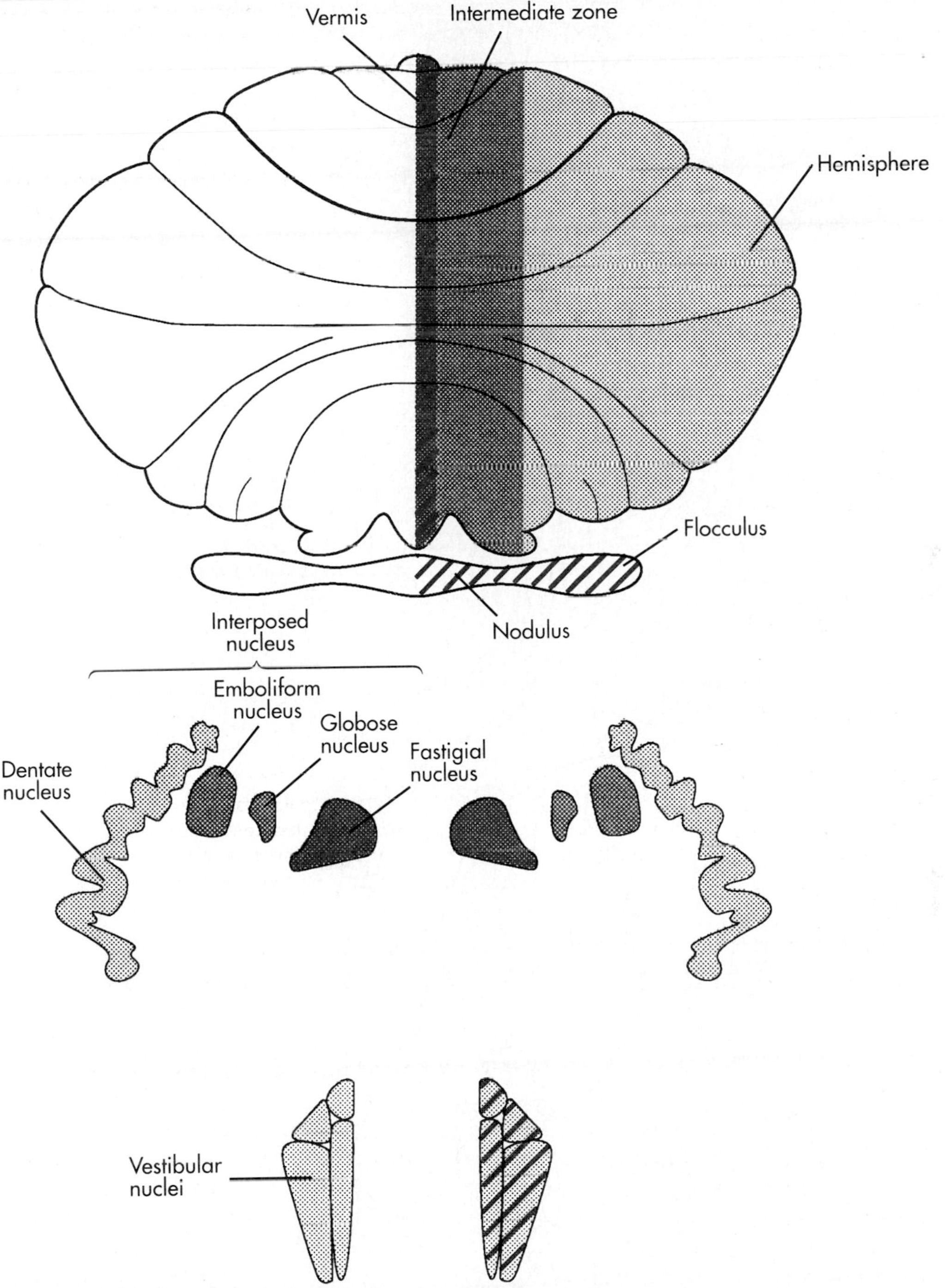


FIGURE 14-18
Projections from cerebellar cortex to deep cerebellar nuclei and vestibular nuclei. The cortex is generally divided into three longitudinal zones that project in a medial-to-lateral sequence to the fastigial, interposed, and dentate nuclei. Superimposed on this is a projection from the vermis and flocculonodular lobe directly to the vestibular nuclei.

Modified from Jansen J, Brodal A: Das Kleinhirn. In Möllendorff: Handbuch der mikroskopischen Anatomie des Menschen IV/8, Heidelberg, 1958, Springer-Verlag.

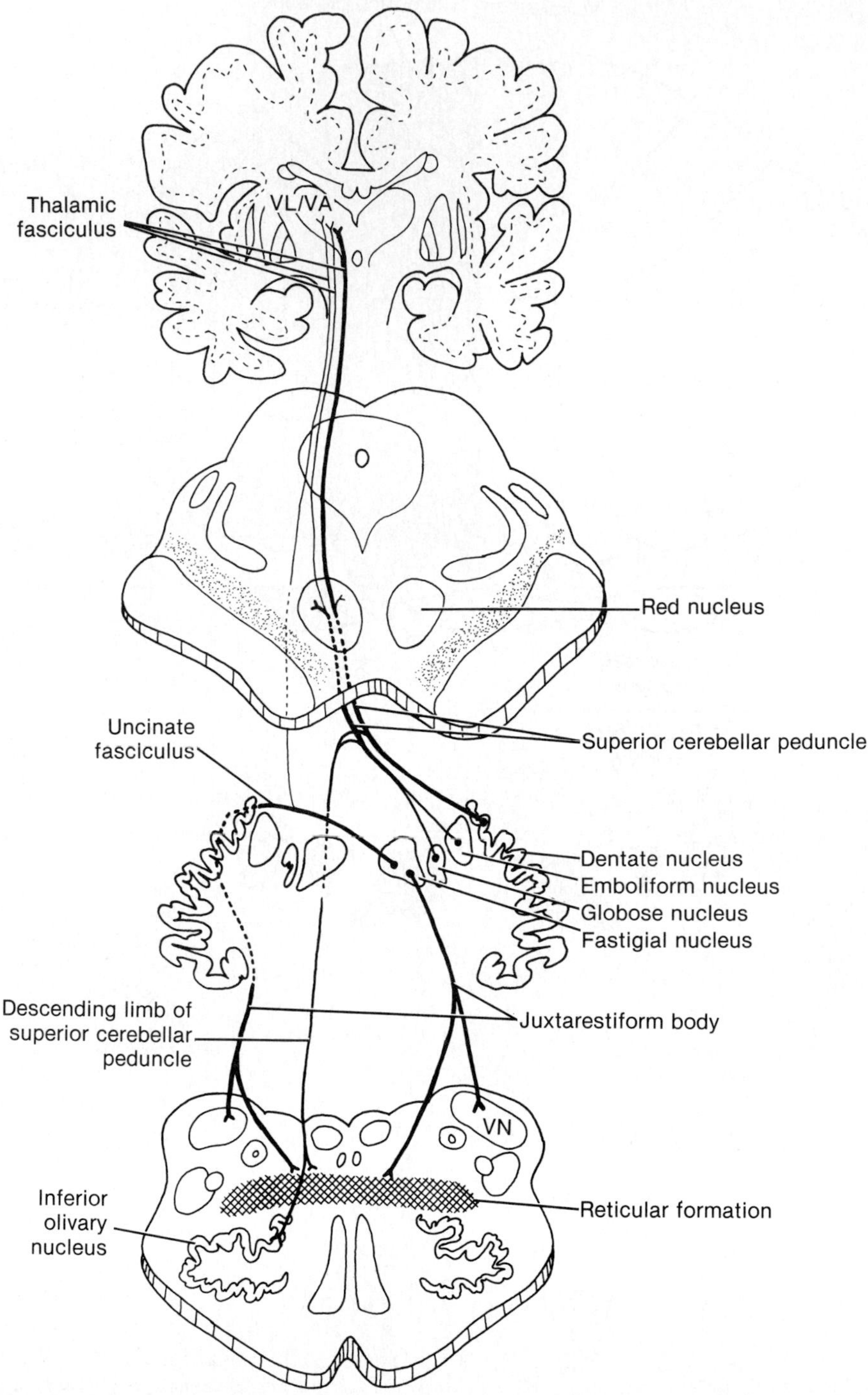


FIGURE 14-19

Principal efferent connections of the deep cerebellar nuclei. The fastigial nucleus projects bilaterally to the vestibular nuclei and the reticular formation; a few fibers reach the contralateral VL/VA complex. The interposed nucleus (globose + emboliform) projects heavily to the red nucleus and less heavily to the VL/VA complex; the dentate nucleus does just the opposite. Both the interposed and dentate nuclei also send fibers to the contralateral inferior olivary complex and reticular formation.

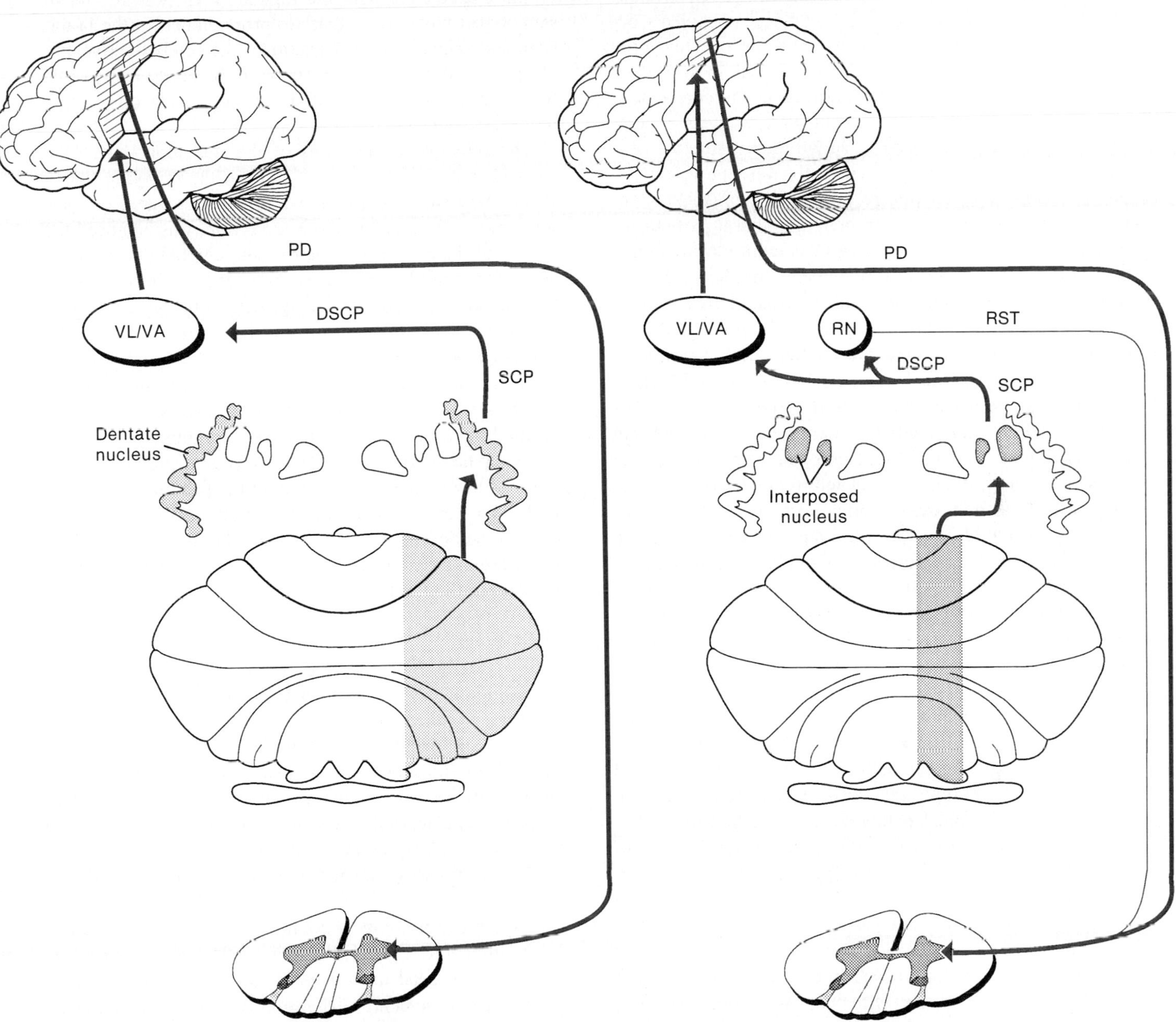


FIGURE 14-20
The principal output circuit through which the cerebellar hemispheres influence movement. The hemispheres receive input via the pontine nuclei from widespread areas of cerebral cortex (not shown) and then, via the dentate nucleus, superior cerebellar peduncle *(SCP),* and VL/VA, influence the output of motor and premotor cortex. Notice that this cerebellar output crosses the midline in the decussation of the superior cerebellar peduncles *(DSCP)* and that the output from motor and premotor cortex recrosses the midline in the pyramidal decussation *(PD)*. The result is that one cerebellar hemisphere affects the ipsilateral side of the spinal cord and brainstem.

FIGURE 14-21
The principal output circuits through which the intermediate zone of cerebellar cortex influences movement. While similar in many respects to hemispheral circuitry, in this case only the limb areas of motor cortex are affected; premotor cortex is not involved. However, the red nucleus *(RN)* and rubrospinal tract *(RST)* are also called into play. Here again there are compensating decussations; cerebellar output fibers cross in the decussation of the superior cerebellar peduncles *(DCSP)* and rubrospinal fibers cross on their way to the spinal cord. The few fastigial fibers that reach VL/VA behave in a similar manner, but their information is relayed to the trunk area of motor cortex.

the output of motor cortex. Consistent with this notion, it has been found that most neurons in the dentate nucleus change their firing rates before voluntary movements occur, and indeed many of them change firing rates even before activity in motor cortex changes. (This is not to say that voluntary movements are initiated in the cerebellum, since in anticipation of a movement, various areas of cerebral association cortex become active long before the dentate nucleus does.) Thus the currently most prevalent hypothesis about the function of the lateral hemisphere-dentate nucleus portion of the cerebellum is that it participates in the planning and programming of voluntary movements, particularly learned, skillful movements that become more rapid, precise, and automatic with practice. This is consistent with the clinical observation that although a great deal of compensation may take place after cerebellar injury, deficits in skilled learned movements (for example, piano playing) may be permanent. Note that the connections between cerebral and cerebellar hemispheres are entirely crossed (Figure 14-20). This means that, for example, the left side of the cerebellum is related to motor cortex on the right. Since the right motor cortex controls the left side of the body, it would be expected (and is observed) that the symptoms of unilateral cerebellar damage are found on the ipsilateral side of the body.

The major inputs to the intermediate or paravermal cortex are superimposed, somatotopically arranged projections from the motor cortex and spinal cord (Figure 14-17). The major output of this part of the cerebellum is via the interposed nucleus to the red nucleus and also back to the motor cortex (through the VL/VA, Figure 14-21). Thus the intermediate cerebellum can influence spinal cord motor neurons through the corticospinal tract and also through the rubrospinal pathway. This has led to the hypothesis that the intermediate zone of the cerebellum compares the commands emanating from motor cortex (it receives this information via pontine nuclei) with the actual position and velocity of the moving part (it receives this information via spinocerebellar and similar tracts), and then, by way of the interposed nucleus, issues correcting signals. This is consistent with the observation that most neurons of the interposed nucleus have firing rates related to voluntary movements, but unlike those of dentate neurons, their rates tend to change *during* rather than before movement. Note that here again a given side of the cerebellum winds up affecting ipsilateral motor neurons (for example, left side of cerebellum → right red nucleus → left side of spinal cord).

The vermis includes the representation of the trunk conveyed by the spinocerebellar tracts. Its major outputs reach the vestibular nuclei and the reticular formation both through the fastigial nucleus and through direct projections to the vestibular nuclei. The vestibulospinal and reticulospinal tracts then influence spinal motor neurons. Since this part of the cerebellum has so little effect on more rostral levels of the CNS, it seems reasonable that it should be most concerned with the regulation of posture and of stereotyped movements that are programmed in the brainstem and spinal cord. For example, the cerebellum-vestibulospinal pathway has been shown to be partly responsible for rhythmic modulation of the basic pattern of walking movements generated in the spinal cord.

The principal connections of the flocculonodular lobe are with the vestibular nerve and nuclei, implying that it should have something to do with the maintenance of equilibrium. As discussed in the next section, this is indeed the case, and damage to this part of the cerebellum causes a general disequilibrium and vertigo (one of the few situations in which cerebellar damage causes perceptual changes), as though some controls had been removed from the vestibular nuclei. In addition, the flocculus seems to have a special role in the coordination of slow eye movements, which is not surprising in view of the involvement of the vestibular nuclei in eye movements. Deciding how to track a moving target visually is not as easy as it sounds, since a target's image moves across the retina if the target moves, if the eyes move, or if the head moves. Some Purkinje cells in the flocculus receive all three kinds of information, make the appropriate computations, and reflect true target velocity in their output.

### Motor learning

We usually think of learning in terms of facts and concepts, although we also learn in terms of becoming more skillful in various kinds of movements. A common example is agility with hands and feet in playing a piano; another is the skillful shots in handball that can be developed over time. Evidence is accumulating that the cerebellum may play a special role in motor learning (Figure 14-22), and two well-studied examples are described in this section.

The vestibuloocular reflex was mentioned briefly in Chapter 9. This reflex occurs during head movement when the eyes move the same amount as the head but in the opposite direction. That is, the gain of the reflex is one: every degree of head movement elicits a degree of compensating eye movement. The result is that the direction of gaze stays constant, and the visual world remains stable. The basic circuitry of the reflex is a simple three-neuron chain. The afferent limb is formed by vestibular primary afferents. These synapse on cells of the vestibular nuclei, which in turn project to the motor neurons of extraocular muscles. If the optics of the eye were to change (e.g., if a person started to wear glasses), a reflex gain of one might no longer be appropriate, and it has been found that the vestibuloocular reflex arc is remarkably adaptable to changes in visual input. As an extreme example, if an experimental animal or a person wears reversing prisms, so that eye or head movement in one direction causes apparent movement in the opposite direction, an unaltered vestibuloocular reflex would be counterproductive. However,

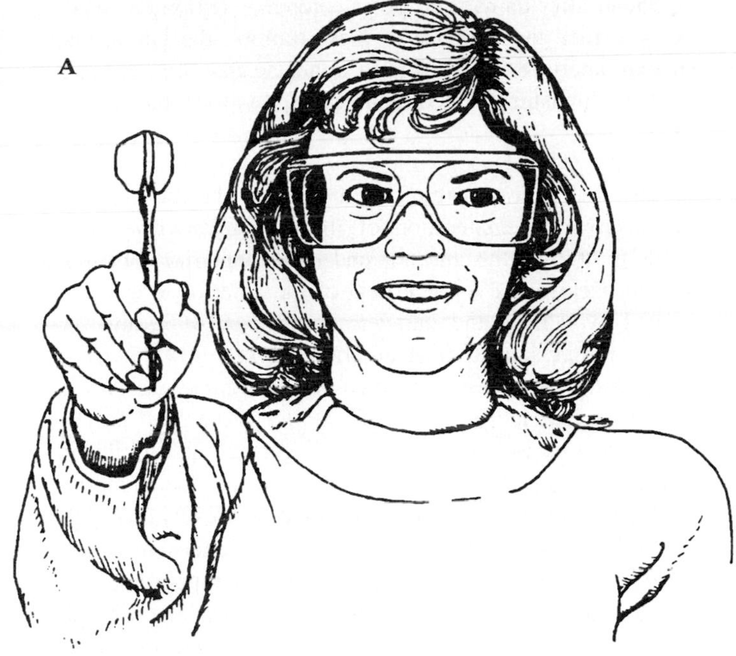

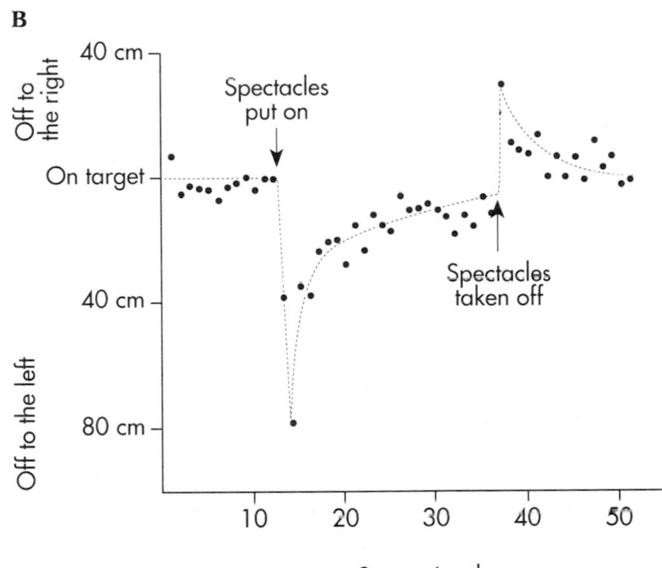


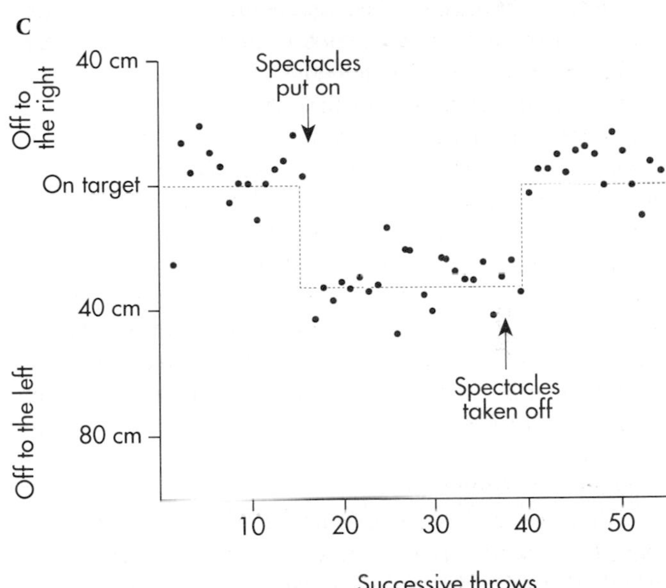


FIGURE 14-22
An example of the possible involvement of the cerebellum in motor learning, in this case learning to alter dart-throwing technique while wearing prisms that displace images to one side. *A,* The experimental arrangement. The subject is wearing spectacles containing prisms that bend the path of light 15° to the right. The effects of the prisms can be seen by the apparent displacement of the part of her face behind the spectacles and by the deviation of her eyes 15° to her left; she is actually looking directly at you, but must deviate her eyes to compensate for the prisms. *B,* The effects of prism spectacles on the dart-throwing ability of a normal subject. When the spectacles are first put on, the subject's throws become wide to the left. After a little practice the throws become reasonably accurate again, and at this point the thrower would look like the subject in *A,* with gaze deviated to one side but the dart aimed straight ahead. When the spectacles are removed, throws deviate to the right but then quickly become accurate again. *C,* The effects of prism spectacles on the dart-throwing ability of a patient with degenerative disease of the inferior olivary nuclei. In this case there is no compensation for the prism spectacles, and throws are wide to the left for as long as the spectacles are worn.

Adapted from Thach WT, Goodkin HP, Keating JG: The cerebellum and the adaptive coordination of movement, *Ann Rev Neurosci* 15:403, 1992.

if the prisms are worn continuously, the gain of the reflex slowly changes until by the end of a day or so it actually reverses direction. When the prisms are removed, the gain of the reflex slowly reverts to its usual state. Removal of the flocculus, or removal of a particular area of the inferior olivary nucleus, prevents these adaptive changes in the gain of the vestibuloocular reflex.

Some forms of conditioned responses, at least in experimental animals, have also been shown to depend on the cerebellum. The best-studied example is a conditioned eyeblink response. A puff of air directed at a rabbit's cornea elicits a reflex blink. If the puff of air is regularly preceded by a sound, then after a while the sound by itself elicits the same blink. Removal of a particular small area of the interposed nucleus abolishes the conditioned response of the ipsilateral eye, even though the reflex response to the air puff, as well as the conditioned response of the contralateral eye, is unaffected. Lesions of the inferior olivary nucleus prevent acquisition of the conditioned response by the contralateral eye of an unconditioned animal. If the response was acquired before the olivary lesion, it slowly fades after the lesion, as though the inferior olivary nucleus is required to establish and sustain the conditioned response.

The exact locations of the modifiable synapses underlying these long-term changes are not yet known with certainty. However, it seems possible that similar changes may underlie the acquisition of skilled, voluntary movements in general.

### Higher functions

Despite the fact that most corticopontine neurons reside in motor or somatosensory cortex, there are also many in limbic and association areas (Figure 14-16). This is consistent with scattered clinical reports that cerebellar damage or malformation can be associated with a variety of cognitive or behavioral disturbances. Just as the basal ganglia had traditionally been associated primarily with movement and are now thought to have broader functions, so too is the possible role of the cerebellum in nonmotor functions receiving increasing attention. It has recently been suggested that connections between the lateral cerebellum and association cortex may be involved in cognition, and that connections between the medial cerebellum and limbic cortex (as well as cerebellum-hypothalamus interconnections) may play a role in affective and autonomic functions.

### Clinical observations

Despite the fact that the cerebellum is clearly divided into longitudinal vermal-intermediate-hemispheric zones, syndromes referable to individual zones are rarely seen clinically. To destroy only the intermediate zone on one side, for example, a lesion would need to extend from the superior surface of the cerebellum near the midbrain to the inferior surface of the cerebellum overlying the medulla. The lesion would also need to extend into the depths of the cerebellar fissures. It is extremely unlikely that this could happen without damaging other parts of the cerebellum and possibly parts of the brainstem. As a result, what is typically seen clinically are problems referable to the flocculonodular lobe or to one or both sides of the corpus cerebelli as a whole.

#### *Flocculonodular lobe*

The nodulus sits on the roof of the caudal part of the fourth ventricle. Tumors called *medulloblastomas* occasionally arise in the roof of the ventricle, usually in young children, and are the most common cause of damage to the flocculonodular lobe. Affected individuals have a general loss of equilibrium—they sway from side to side when standing, walk with a staggering, wide-based gait, and tend to fall over. The basic mechanisms used in moving the limbs are unaffected, so that when the trunk is supported (for example, when lying in bed), movements of the arms and legs are normal. In contrast to the findings after damage to the cerebellar hemispheres, there is no tremor, and both reflexes and muscle tone remain normal. A variety of eye movement difficulties may also be seen, such as problems with pursuit eye movements, with maintaining eccentric gaze, or with making accurate voluntary eye movements. However, eye movement disorders may be found after damage to other cerebellar regions as well. As a further consequence of these tumors, the lateral and median apertures of the fourth ventricle may be squeezed shut, with ensuing noncommunicating hydrocephalus.

#### *Corpus cerebelli*

The malnutrition often accompanying chronic alcoholism causes a degeneration of the cerebellar cortex that tends to start at the anterior end of the anterior lobe and spread backwards. A great deal of the anterior lobe is occupied by vermis and paravermis (Figure 14-7), and the legs are represented most anteriorly (Figure 14-17). The result is a syndrome (called the *anterior lobe syndrome)* in which the legs are primarily affected, and the most prominent symptom is a broad-based, staggering gait, similar in many ways to that seen after damage to the flocculonodular lobe. In the anterior lobe syndrome, however, there is a general incoordination or *ataxia* (Greek for lack of order) of leg movements, even when the trunk is supported.

Most of the cerebellum is made up of the lateral hemisphere, and with a few exceptions like the one just mentioned, this is the region most heavily damaged in lesions of the corpus cerebelli. The result is called the *neocerebellar syndrome,* which is characterized by a variable combination of changes in muscle tone, reflexes, and the coordination of voluntary movements, all ipsilateral to the side of the lesion.

Widespread decreases in muscle tone *(hypotonia)* may follow small lesions, so that the limbs offer little resistance

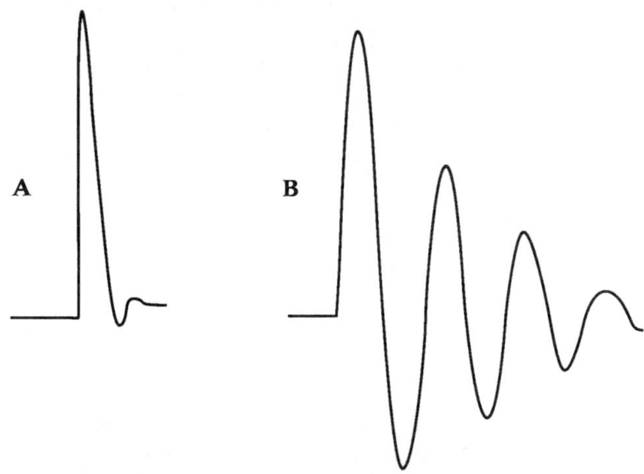


FIGURE 14-23
Reflex changes accompanying cerebellar damage. *A,* Tracing of limb movement during a knee-jerk reflex in a normal subject. Note that the brief reflex limb movement is followed by a small secondary movement that dies out quickly; even the small secondary movement is frequently missing in normal subjects. *B,* Tracing of a knee-jerk reflex of the right leg in a patient who had sustained right-sided cerebellar damage eight years previously. Note the poorly damped oscillation following the reflex response. Redrawn from Holmes G: *Brain* 40:461, 1917.

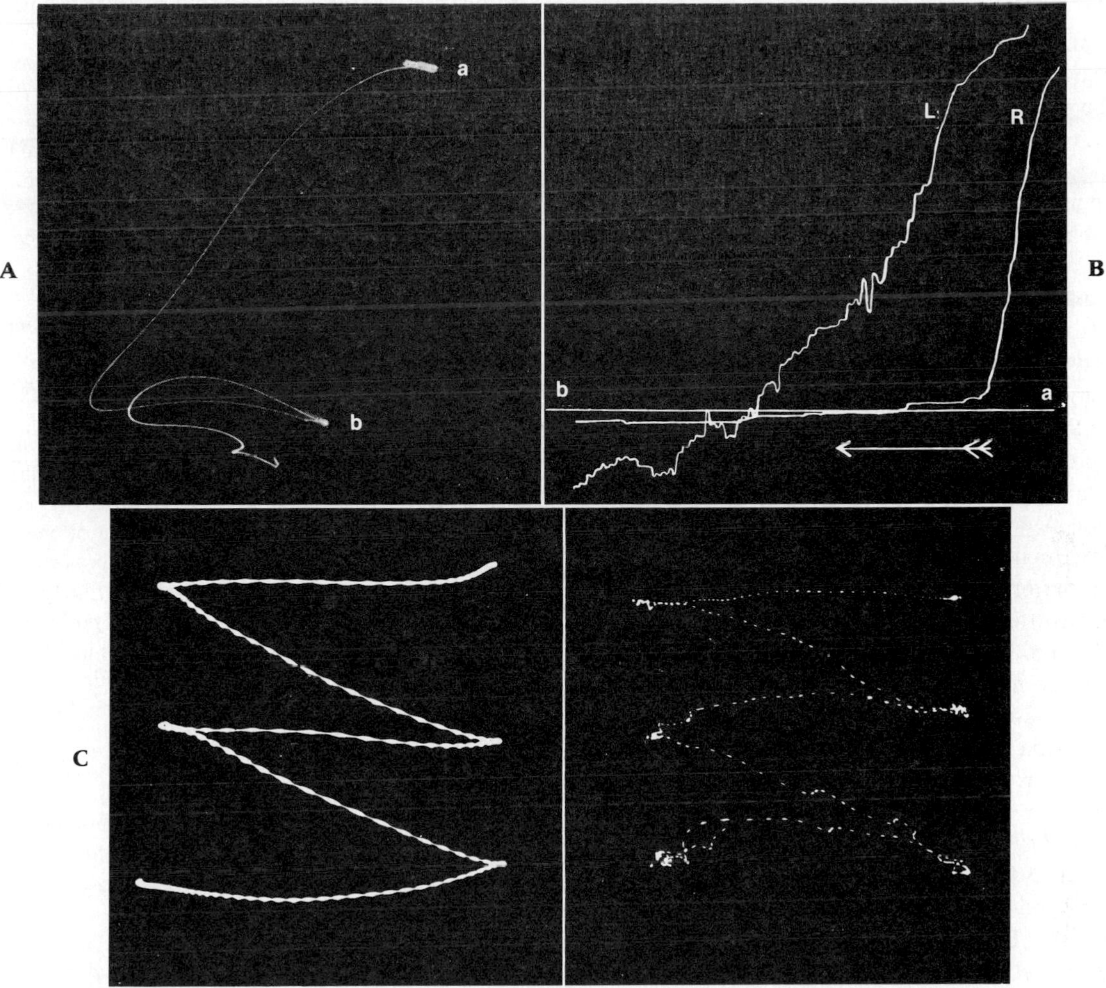


FIGURE 14-24

Movements made by patients with cerebellar lesions (all involving one or both hemispheres), recorded by the simple but ingenious technique of photographing a light bulb attached to the patient's finger (A and C) or by recording the movement on a revolving drum. **A,** A patient attempts to touch his nose (at *b*) with the tip of his finger, starting from point *a* above his head; the movement has two distinct parts to it instead of being a smooth, continuous sweep (decomposition of movement), and the patient misjudges the range (dysmetria), striking his nose and then making irregular corrective movements. **B,** A patient with left-sided cerebellar damage attempts to stretch two similar springs and then keep them stretched to the level of the line *ab;* time progresses from right to left in this record. The normal right arm *(R)* moves promptly and appropriately, but the left arm *(L)* starts slowly, moves slowly, makes many small corrective movements, overshoots the line *ab,* and is then unable to maintain a constant stretch. **C,** A patient with right-sided cerebellar damage moves each hand back and forth between a series of small targets; the light attached to his fingertip was flashing at a constant rate, so the separation between bright spots is a measure of finger velocity. The left hand (on left) performs smoothly and accurately, but the right hand (on right) moves at varying speeds and has particular difficulty stopping and changing direction.

From Holmes G: The cerebellum of man, Brain 62:1, 1939.

to passive movement and muscles feel abnormally soft and flaccid. Stretch reflexes are often reduced *(hyporeflexia)*, and as a result of the hypotonia a limb may swing back and forth after a reflex contraction (*pendular reflexes*, Figure 14-23).

Most prominent, however, is a lack of coordination of voluntary movements. This is caused by a fundamental deficit in the timing of movements and the regulation of their rates. As shown in Figure 14-24, voluntary movements take longer than usual to initiate, and there are problems in stopping them or changing their direction. This is manifest in a number of different ways: patients are likely to overshoot or undershoot targets *(dysmetria)*; corrective movements when the patient nears a target have the appearance of a tremor *(intention tremor)*; and rapid alternating movements, such as repeatedly pronating and supinating the forearm, may be especially difficult *(adiadochokinesia)*. Note that the intention tremor of cerebellar disease is quite different from the resting tremor seen in disorders of the basal ganglia, partly because it is seen during voluntary movements and partly because it is not so rhythmic or regular. When complex movements involving more than one joint are performed, the timing of different parts may be defective in different ways, leading to *decomposition of movement* (Figure 14-24, *A*). The complex movements used in speaking may be affected in this way, in which case the normal flow and rhythm of speech is disrupted; successive syllables may emerge slowly and separated from each other *(scanning speech)*.

In view of current notions of the function of the cerebellar hemispheres in the preprogramming of skilled voluntary movements, it is important to note again that the neocerebellar syndrome is not accompanied by any sensory deficits. The British neurologist Gordon Holmes described a patient who had incurred damage to his right cerebellar hemisphere and who said, "The movements of my left arm are done subconsciously, but I have to think out each movement of the right arm. I come to a dead stop in turning and have to think before I start again."

## ADDITIONAL READINGS


Aas J-E: Subcortical projections to the pontine nuclei in the cat, *J Comp Neurol* 282:331, 1989.

Amerenco P: The spectrum of cerebellar infarctions, *Neurol* 41:973, 1991.

Amici R, Avanzini G, Pacini L: *Cerebellar tumors, clinical analysis and physiopathologic correlations,* Munich, 1976, S. Karger.

Angevine JB, Jr, Mancall EL, Yakovlev PI: *The human cerebellum: an atlas of gross topography in serial sections.* Boston, 1961, Little, Brown & Co. *A review of various systems of cerebellar nomenclature and terminology together with a collection of beautiful sections cut in several different planes.*

Armstrong DM: The mammalian cerebellum and its contribution to movement control, *Int Rev Physiol* 17:239, 1978. *An extensive, physiologically oriented review.*

Asanuma C, Thach WT, Jones EG: Distribution of cerebellar terminations and their relation to other afferent terminations in the ventral lateral thalamic region of the monkey, *Brain Res Rev* 5:237, 1983.

Bloedel JR, Dichgans J, Precht W: *Cerebellar functions,* Berlin, 1985, Springer-Verlag.

Brecha N, Karten HJ: Accessory optic projections upon oculomotor nuclei and vestibulocerebellum, *Science* 203:913, 1979. *A recently unravelled route by which visual information used in guiding eye movements reaches the cerebellum.*

Brodal P: The cerebropontocerebellar pathway: salient features of its organization, *Exp Brain Res* Suppl. 6:108, 1982.

Carpenter MB, Batton RR III: Connections of the fastigial nucleus in the cat and monkey, *Exp Brain Res Suppl* 6:250, 1982.

Chan-Palay V: *Cerebellar dentate nucleus: organization, cytology, and transmitters,* New York, 1977, Springer-Verlag, Inc.

Courville J, de Montigny C, Lamarre Y: *The inferior olivary nucleus,* New York, 1980, Raven Press.

Demer JL, Robinson DA: Effects of reversible lesions and stimulation of olivocerebellar system on vestibuloocular reflex plasticity, *J Neurophysiol* 47:1084, 1982.

Dietrichs E, Walberg F: Cerebellar nuclear afferents—where do they originate? A reevaluation of the projections from some lower brain stem nuclei, *Anat Embryol* 177:165, 1987.

Dow RS, Moruzzi G: *The physiology and pathology of the cerebellum,* Minneapolis, 1958, University of Minnesota Press.

Flumerfelt BA, Otabe S, Courville J: Distinct projections to the red nucleus from the dentate and interposed nuclei in the monkey, *Brain Res* 50:408, 1973.

Gilman S, Bloedel JR, Lechtenberg R: *Disorders of the cerebellum,* Philadelphia, 1981, F.A. Davis Co.

Glickstein M, May JG III, Mercier BE: Corticopontine projection in the macaque: the distribution of labelled cortical cells after large injections of horseradish peroxidase in the pontine nuclei, *J Comp Neurol* 235:343, 1985.

Glickstein M, Yeo C: The cerebellum and motor learning, *J Cog Neurosci* 2:69, 1990. *A brief but enjoyable review of the history of theories about cerebellar function, and of recent evidence that it is important for motor learning.*

Grant G, Xu Q: Routes of entry into the cerebellum of spinocerebellar axons from the lower part of the spinal cord. An experimental study in the cat, *Exp Brain Res* 72:543, 1988.

Gould BB, Graybiel AM: Afferents to the cerebellar cortex in the cat: evidence for an intrinsic pathway leading from the deep nuclei to the cortex, *Brain Res* 110:601, 1976.

Haines DE, May PJ, Dietrichs E: Neuronal connections between the cerebellar nuclei and hypothalamus in *Macaca fascicularis, J Comp Neurol* 299:106, 1990.

Harvey RJ, Napper RMA: Quantitative studies on the mammalian cerebellum, *Prog Neurobiol* 36:437, 1991.

Holmes G: The cerebellum of man, *Brain* 62:1, 1939. *Still the all-time great description of the neocerebellar syndrome in man and the source of the striking illustrations used in Figure 14-24.*

Ikeda M: Projections from the spinal and the principal sensory nuclei of the trigeminal nerve to the cerebellar cortex in the cat, as studied by retrograde transport of horseradish peroxidase, *J Comp Neurol* 184:57, 1979.

Ito M: *The cerebellum and neural control,* New York, 1984, Raven Press.

Kalil K: Projections of the cerebellar and dorsal column nuclei upon the inferior olive in the rhesus monkey: an autoradiographic study, *J Comp Neurol* 188:43, 1979.

Keele SW, Ivry R: Does the cerebellum provide a common computation for diverse tasks? A timing hypothesis, *Ann NY Acad Sci* 608:179, 1990. *A broad hypothesis, proposing that the cerebellum comes into play whenever there is a need for accurate computations involving time—whether for timing movements or for judging durations or velocities.*

Langer T et al.: Afferents to the flocculus of the cerebellum in the rhesus macaque as revealed by retrograde transport of horseradish peroxidase, *J Comp Neurol* 235:1, 1985.

Langer T et al.: Floccular efferents in the rhesus macaque as revealed by autoradiography and horseradish peroxidase, *J Comp Neurol* 235:26, 1985.

Larsell O, Jansen J: *The comparative anatomy and histology of the cerebellum: the human cerebellum, cerebellar connections, and the cerebellar cortex,* Minneapolis, 1972, University of Minnesota Press.

Lechtenberg R, Gilman S: Speech disorders in cerebellar disease, *Ann Neurol* 3:285, 1978. *Cerebellar speech disorders are often considered to be caused by damage to the vermis, but this report presents an alternative view.*

Massion J, Rispal-Padel L: Spatial organization of the cerebello-thalamo-cortical pathway, *Brain Res* 40:61, 1972.

McCormick DA, Steinmetz JE, Thompson RF: Lesions of the inferior olivary complex cause extinction of the classically conditioned eyeblink response, *Brain Res* 359:120, 1985.

Mercier BE, Legg CR, Glickstein M: Basal ganglia and cerebellum receive different somatonsensory information, *Proc Nat Acad Sci* 87:4388, 1990.

Meyer-Lohmann J, Hore J, Brooks VB: Cerebellar participation in generation of prompt arm movements, *J Neurophysiol* 40:1038, 1977. *What happens to voluntary movements when one dentate nucleus is temporarily disabled.*

Miles FA, Fuller JH: Visual tracking and the primate flocculus, *Science* 189:1000, 1975.

Murphy MG, O'Leary JL: Neurological deficit in cats with lesions of the olivocerebellar system, *Arch Neurol* 24:145, 1971.

Orlovsky GN: Activity of vestibulospinal neurons during locomotion, *Brain Res* 46:85, 1972. *The activity is rhythmically modulated, and the modulation disappears after cerebellar lesions.*

Palay SL, Chan-Palay V: *Cerebellar cortex: cytology and organization,* New York, 1974, Springer-Verlag, Inc. *A beautiful book, full of Golgi-stained cells and electron micrographs.*

Payne JN: The cerebellar nucleo-cortical projection in the rat studied by the retrograde fluorescent double-labelling method, *Brain Res* 271:141, 1983.

Ritchie L: Effects of cerebellar lesions on saccadic eye movements, *J Neurophysiol* 39:1246, 1976.

Sanes JN, Dimitrov B, Hallet M: Motor learning in patients with cerebellar dysfunction, *Brain* 113:103, 1990.

Schmahmann JD: An emerging concept. The cerebellar contribution to higher function, *Arch Neurol* 48:1178, 1991.

Shepherd GM: *The synaptic organization of the brain,* ed. 3, New York, 1990, Oxford University Press. *A nice, readable book about a number of areas of the CNS; Chapter 7 covers the cerebellum.*

Snider RS: Recent contributions to the anatomy and physiology of the cerebellum, *Arch Neurol Psychiatry* 64:196, 1950. *A summary of the electrophysiologically determined mapping of the cerebral cortex and the body surface onto the cerebellar cortex.*

Soechting JF et al: Changes in a motor pattern following cerebellar and olivary lesions in the squirrel monkey, *Brain Res* 105:21, 1976.

Stein JF: Role of the cerebellum in the visual guidance of movement, *Nature* 323:217, 1986.

Thach WT: Goodkin HP, Keating JG: The cerebellum and the adaptive control of movement, *Ann Rev Neurosci* 15:403, 1992.

Thach WT, Timing of activity in cerebellar dentate nucleus and cerebral motor cortex during prompt volitional movement, *Brain Res* 88:233, 1975.

Thompson RF: The neurobiology of learning and memory, *Science* 233:941, 1986. *A recent review by one of the principal investigators of the role of the cerebellum in classical conditioning.*

Tolbert DL, Bantli H, Bloedel JR: Organizational features of the cat and monkey cerebellar nucleocortical projection, *J Comp Neurol* 182:39, 1978.

Victor M, Adams RD, Mancall EL: A restricted form of cerebellar cortical degeneration occurring in alcoholic patients, *Arch Neurol* 1:578, 1959.

Westheimer G, Blair SM: Oculomotor defects in cerebellectomized monkeys, *Invest Ophthalmol* 12:618, 1973.

CHAPTER

# 15

# *Cerebral Cortex*

The cerebral cortex is a sheet of neurons and their interconnections, about 2.5 sq ft in area, that plates the corrugated surface of the cerebral hemispheres in a layer just a few millimeters thick. This thin layer of gray matter is estimated to contain about 30 billion neurons, interconnected by 100,000 km of axons and dendrites. Figures 15-1, 15-2, and 15-3 show the gross topography of this cortical covering.

One of the more striking changes that has occurred in the course of the evolution of brains in vertebrate animals is the tremendous increase in the relative size of the cerebral hemispheres and the even greater increase in the area of cerebral cortex on their surfaces. One inference drawn from this fact (and one abundantly supported by clinical evidence) is that the cerebral cortex has a great deal to do with the abilities and activities we think of as reaching their highest level of development in humans (or in some cases as existing uniquely in humans). Obvious examples are language and abstract thinking. This is, of course, not the only function of the cerebral cortex; basic aspects of perception, movement, and adaptive response to the outside world also depend on it.

## HISTOLOGY

### Terminology

The cerebral cortex does not have the same structure everywhere. Almost all the cortex that can be seen from the outside of the brain is of a type called *neocortex,* "neo" referring to the common notion that it first appeared fairly late in vertebrate evolution (some neocortex, or at least its functional equivalent, actually seems to be present in all vertebrates, but mammals have much more than other vertebrates do). Neocortex accounts for more than 90% of our total cortical area. The remainder is made up of *paleocortex* and *archicortex,* named in reference to their possibly more ancient origins. Paleocortex covers some restricted parts of the base of the telencephalon (Figure 15-4), and archicortex comprises the hippocampal formation.

All neocortical areas go through a period during development in which they have a six-layered structure. As discussed shortly, this layered appearance persists in only some areas of the adult brain, but in view of its uniform early development, the neocortex is also referred to as *homogenetic cortex* or *isocortex*. In contrast, paleocortex and archicortex never go through such a six-layered stage and are referred to collectively as *heterogenetic cortex* or *allocortex* (from the Greek word *allo* meaning other). The hippocampal formation is a component of the limbic system, and the paleocortex, which develops in conjunction with the olfactory system, is closely interconnected with limbic structures. Both therefore are considered in Chapter 16, and the remainder of this chapter deals with the neocortex.

### Cell types

The two principal neuronal cell types in the neocortex are *stellate* (or *granule) cells* and *pyramidal cells*. Stellate cells come in a wide assortment of shapes, but they are typically small (in the range of less than 10 μm) multipolar neurons; their short axons do not leave the cortex. Pyramidal cells are named for their shape (Figure 15-5): a long *apical dendrite* leaves the top of each pyramidal cell and ascends vertically toward the cortical surface, and a series of *basal dendrites* emerges from nearer the base of the cell and spreads out horizontally. Pyramidal cells range in size from 10μm in diameter all the way up to the 70 to 100 μm giant pyramidal cells *(Betz cells)* of the motor cortex, which are among the largest neurons in the CNS. Most or all pyramidal cells have long axons that leave the cortex to reach either other cortical areas or various subcortical sites. Therefore stellate cells are the principal in-

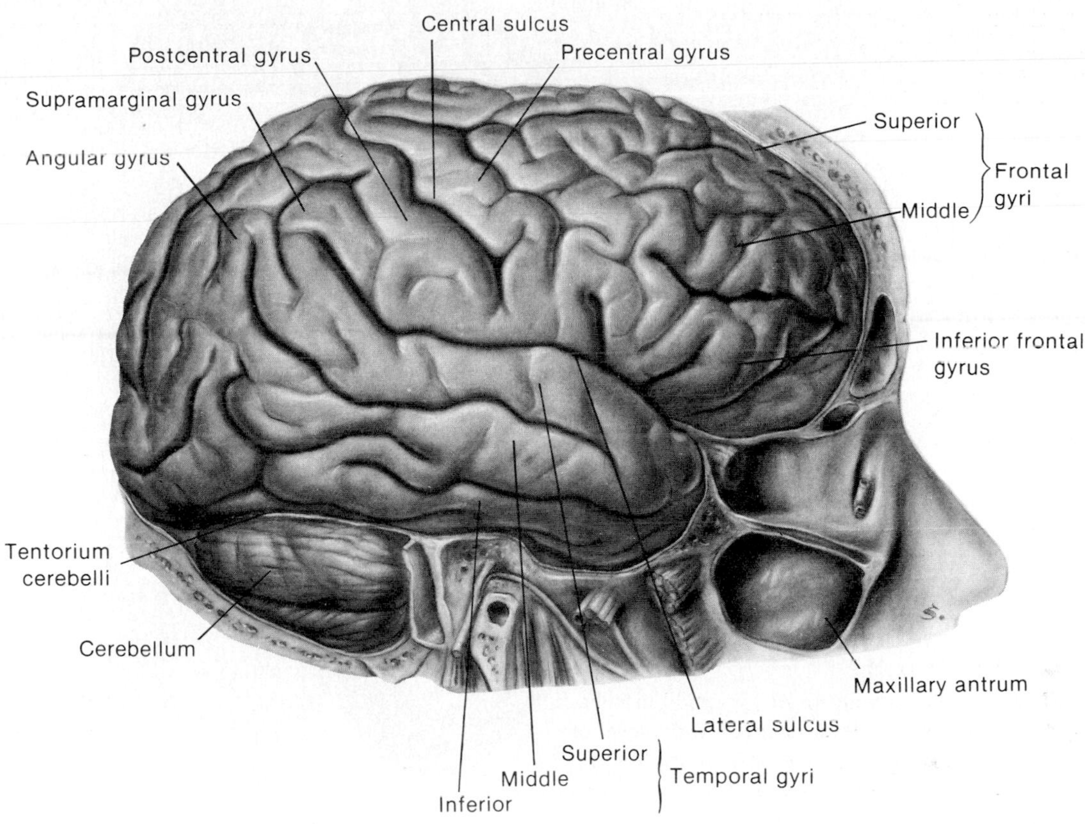


FIGURE 15-1
Lateral surface of the cerebral hemisphere with the major gyri indicated.
From Mettler FA: *Neuroanatomy*, ed 2, St. Louis, 1948, Mosby-Year Book.

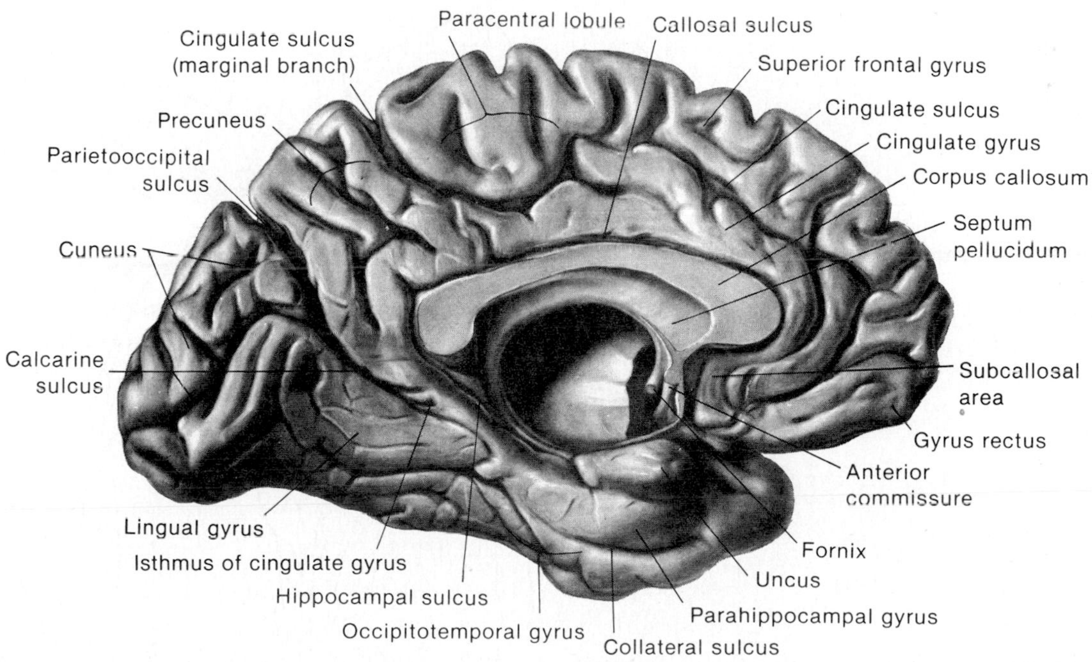


FIGURE 15-2
Medial surface of the cerebral hemisphere after the brainstem, cerebellum, and diencephalon have been removed; major gyri and other features are indicated.
From Mettler FA: *Neuroanatomy*, ed 2, St. Louis, 1948, Mosby-Year Book.

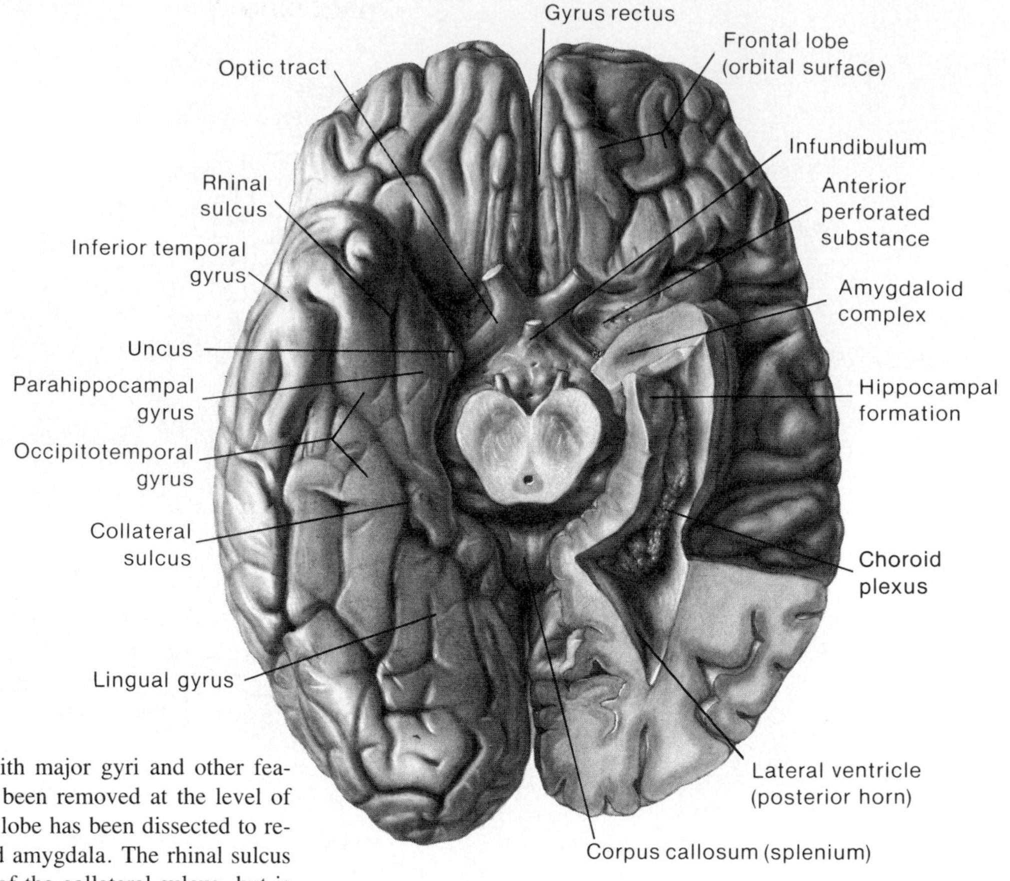


**FIGURE 15-3**

Inferior surface of the cerebrum with major gyri and other features indicated. The brainstem has been removed at the level of the midbrain, and the left temporal lobe has been dissected to reveal the hippocampal formation and amygdala. The rhinal sulcus looks like an anterior continuation of the collateral sulcus, but is actually a separate landmark.

From Mettler FA: *Neuroanatomy,* ed. 2, St. Louis, 1948, Mosby-Year Book.

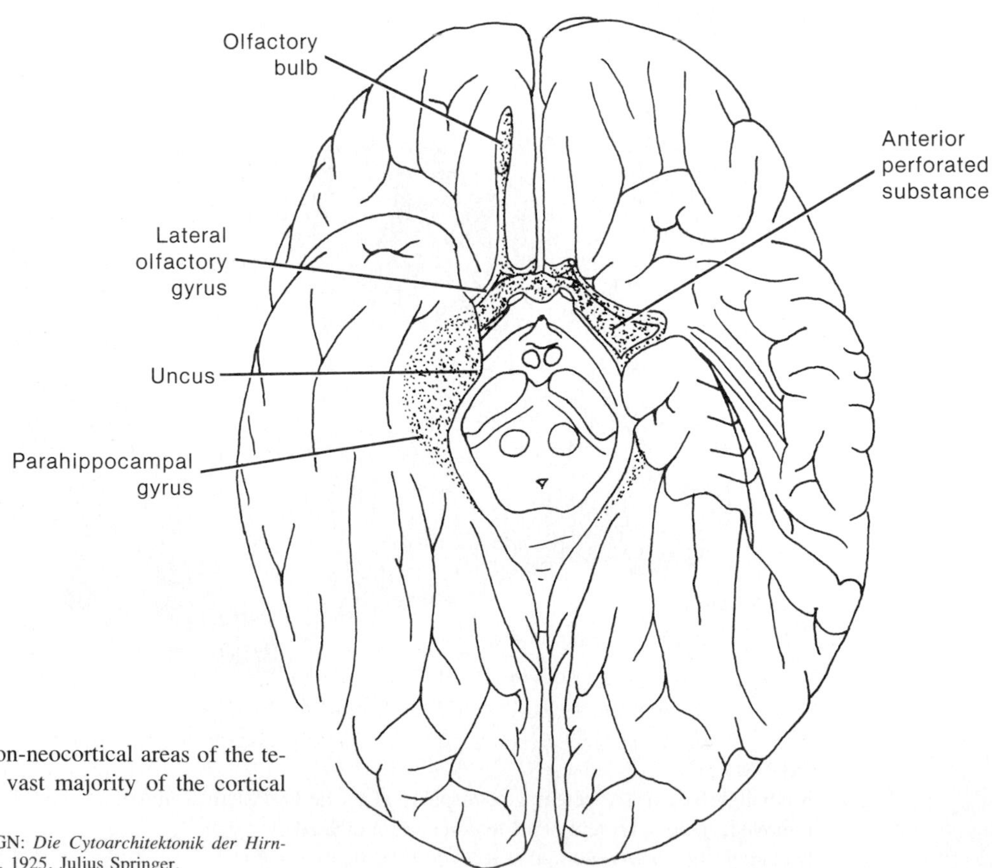


**FIGURE 15-4**

Inferior surface of the brain, with non-neocortical areas of the telencephalon stippled. Note that the vast majority of the cortical surface is neocortex.

Modified from Von Economo C, Koskinas GN: *Die Cytoarchitektonik der Hirnrinde des erwachsenen Menschen,* Heidelberg, 1925, Julius Springer.

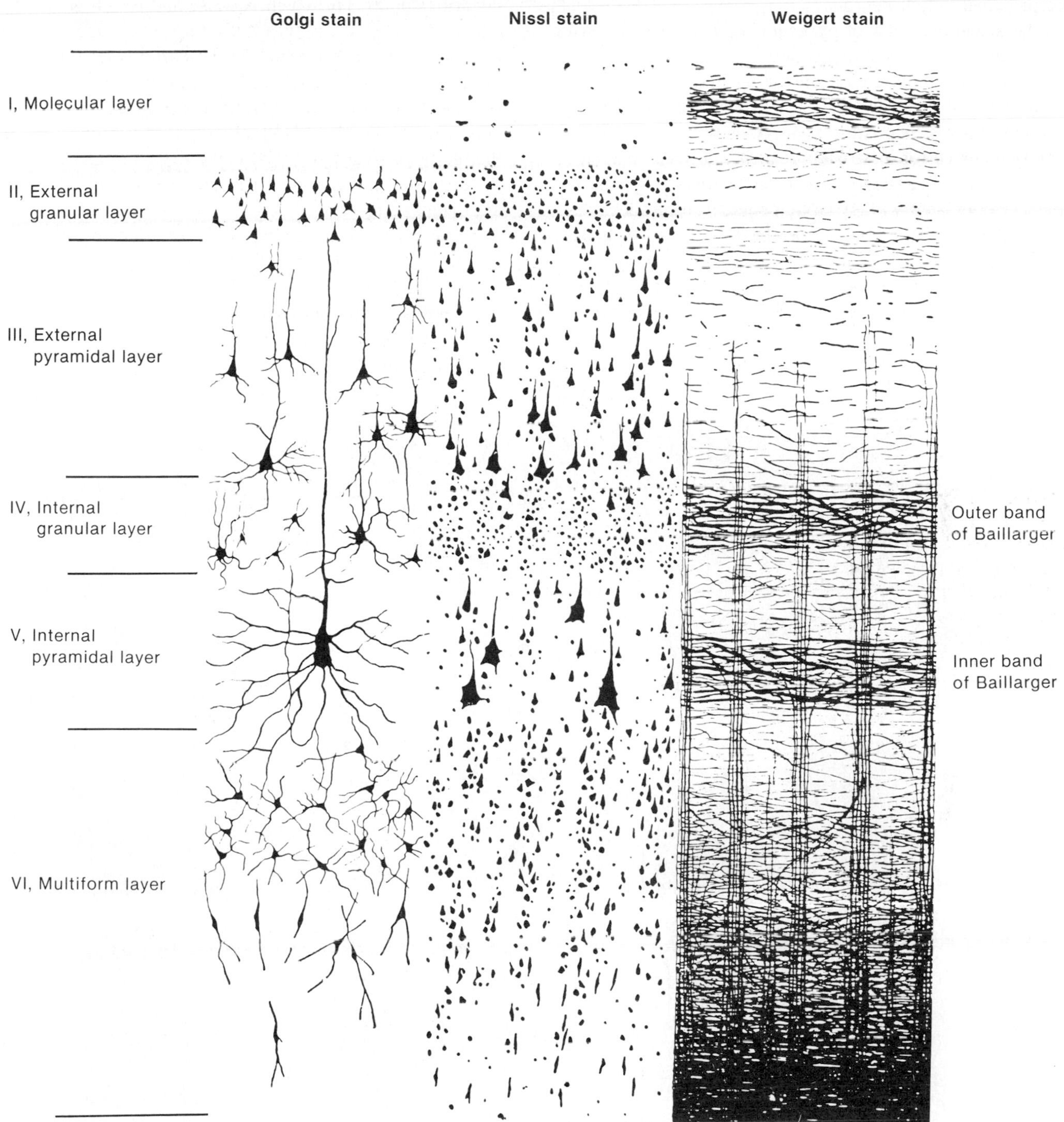


FIGURE 15-5
Cross section of neocortex stained by three different methods; the six cortical layers are indicated. The Golgi stain reveals the shapes of the arborizations of cortical neurons by completely staining a small percentage of them. The Nissl method stains the cell bodies of all neurons, showing their shapes and packing densities. The Weigert method stains myelin, revealing the horizontally oriented bands of Baillarger as well as vertically oriented collections of cortical afferents and efferents.

From Ranson SW, Clark SL: The anatomy of the nervous system, ed 10, Philadelphia, 1959, WB Saunders Co.

terneurons of the neocortex, whereas pyramidal cells are the principal output neurons.

The apical dendrites of pyramidal cells are studded with numerous small projections called *dendritic spines*. These spines are the preferential site of synaptic contacts onto pyramidal cell dendrites and have been the source of considerable interest and some mystery as well. They are not merely a device for increasing dendritic surface area, since the portions of a dendrite located between spines are sparsely populated with synaptic contacts. It has been suggested that dendritic spines may be the sites of synapses that are selectively modified as a result of learning, since small changes in the geometry of a spine could cause relatively large changes in its electrical properties and therefore in the efficacy of that synapse. Certain cases of mental retardation are accompanied by faulty development of dendritic spines, but which is cause and which is effect (if either) is not known. Certainly, however, the most remarkable change that occurs in the cortex after birth is the tremendous expansion of the dendritic trees of its neurons (Figure 15-6) and a parallel increase in the numbers of dendritic spines. It should be noted that spines are not unique to cortical pyramidal cells; they are also found on the dendrites of some other neurons, such as Purkinje cells and many striatal neurons.

Other neocortical cell types (in addition to the stellate and pyramidal cells) include *horizontal cells* (or *cells of Cajal), fusiform cells,* and *cells of Martinotti*. Horizontal cells ramify within the most superficial cortical layer; they are prominent during development, but most disappear af-

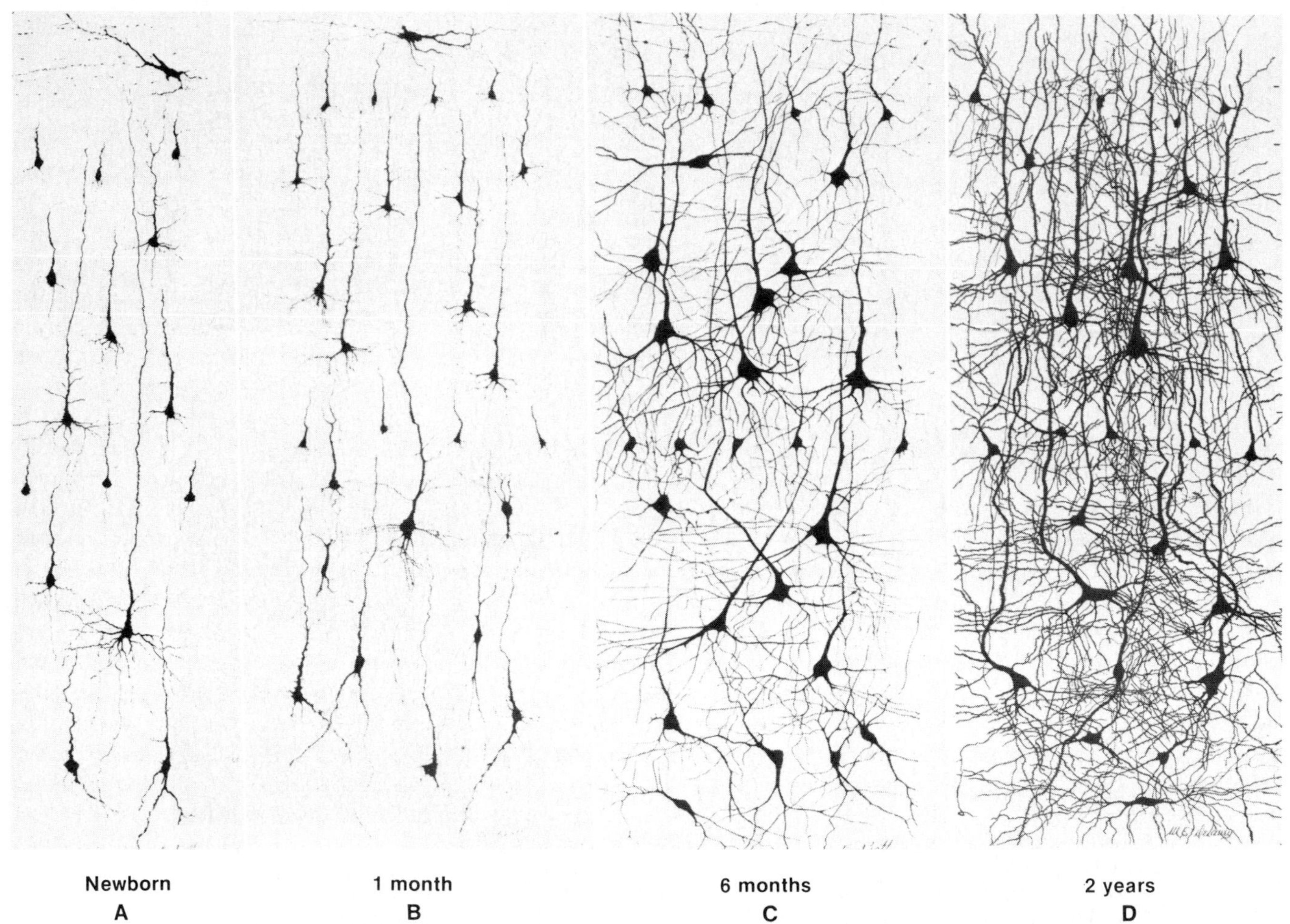


FIGURE 15-6
Golgi-stained sections of human cerebral cortex taken from equivalent areas of the anterior portion of the middle frontal gyrus at different ages. Note that although the packing density of cortical neurons does not appear to change, there is a tremendous increase in the complexity of dendritic arborizations with increasing age.

From Conel JL: *The postnatal development of the human cerebral cortex,* Cambridge, Mass., Harvard University Press. **A,** Vol. I, 1939; **B,** vol. II, 1941; **C,** vol. IV, 1951; **D,** vol. VI, 1959. Reprinted by permission.

ter birth. Fusiform cells are found in the deepest cortical layer; they are spindle shaped, with a tuft of dendrites emerging from each end of the spindle (Figure 15-5), but otherwise are similar to pyramidal cells and have an axon that leaves the cortex. Cells of Martinotti are found in all cortical layers, most abundantly in the deepest layers, and are unusual in having axons that ascend toward the surface.

### Cortical layers

The cells of the neocortex are arranged in a series of six layers, more apparent in some areas than in others. Most superficial is a cell-poor *molecular layer,* and deepest is the *polymorphic* (or *multiform) layer,* which is populated largely by fusiform cells. In between these two are four layers alternately populated mostly by stellate cells or mostly by pyramidal cells. The layers are commonly designated by Roman numerals and by names, as indicated in Figure 15-5.

Myelin staining reveals vertically oriented bundles of cortical afferents and efferents as well as horizontal bands through which these fibers and intracortical axons spread (Figure 15-5). Two particularly prominent horizontal bands are contained in layers IV and V and are called, respectively, the *outer* and *inner bands of Baillarger.*

The six neocortical cell layers are not equally prominent everywhere. Areas that give rise to many long axons (for example, the motor cortex) would be expected to have numerous large pyramidal cells, and this is indeed the case (Figure 15-7). In these areas, stellate cells appear minor by comparison, and layers II through V are dominated by pyramidal cells to the extent that individual layers are no longer obvious. Because of the apparent lack of stellate (granule) cells, such cortex is called *agranular*. In contrast, primary sensory areas project mainly to adjacent cortical areas and do not give rise to many long axons. They have a corresponding dearth of large pyramidal cells; here too, layers II through V look like one continuous layer, but in this case they are dominated by small stellate and pyramidal cells (Figure 15-7). Such cortex is therefore called *granular cortex* or *koniocortex* (from the Greek word *konia* meaning dust, referring to the numerous tiny cells). There is a continuum of structural types ranging between thick (4.5 mm) agranular cortex and thin (1.5 mm) granular cortex (Figure 15-7). The intermediate kinds, in which the six neocortical layers can be seen, are called *homotypical* cortices (as opposed to granular and agranular cortices, which are collectively called *heterotypical).*

The differences among cortical areas are to some extent more apparent than real. Beneath a square millimeter of any area of mammalian cortex, whether from a mouse or a human, lies approximately the same number of neurons (roughly 100,000). The only exception is the binocular portion of the primary visual cortex of primates, where the neurons are packed about 2.5 times as densely. About two thirds of the neurons in all cortical areas are pyramidal cells. Hence two thirds of the neurons in granular cortex are very small pyramidal cells. Different cortical areas have different appearances and functions because of the relative sizes of the cell types, the complexities of their dendritic trees, and the patterns of their connections. This fundamental similarity of all cortical areas is one aspect of the notion, discussed a little later in this chapter, that the cerebral cortex may be a large array of small repeated functional units.

### Cortical connections

Afferents to the cortex can come from only two general places: other cortical areas or subcortical sites. Afferents from other cortical sites, which are discussed at various points in this chapter, may arise in the same hemisphere *(association fibers)* or in the contralateral hemisphere *(commissural fibers).* The single major subcortical source of afferents is the thalamus, and its pattern of projections is described in Chapter 10. Other subcortical sites, such as the locus ceruleus and other chemically coded nuclei, also provide some afferents to the cortex (Chapter 17).

These various types of incoming fibers ramify within the cortex in different patterns (Figure 15-8). For example, specific thalamic afferents end in a dense arborization located primarily in layer IV*; fibers from other thalamic nuclei and from other cortical areas ascend vertically and terminate diffusely along their course in distinctive patterns (for example, those from association nuclei end mostly in layer I, those from intralaminar nuclei in layer VI, and those from other cortical areas in layers II and III).

Efferents from the cortex, like afferents to it, must be connected either with other cortical areas or with subcortical sites. Efferents to subcortical sites have been mentioned in various places throughout this book. Most of them descend through the internal capsule along a pathway that (for some) continues through the cerebral peduncle, the basal part of the pons, and the medullary pyramids, finally reaching the spinal cord. Along this pathway many other structures are contacted, including (but by no means limited to) the caudate nucleus and putamen, the thalamus, the superior colliculus, the red nucleus, the reticular formation, motor neurons of cranial and spinal nerves, and various sensory nuclei of the brainstem and spinal cord. Some corticostriate fibers travel through the external capsule. Just as afferents to the cortex have a distinctive laminar pattern of termination, so do efferents from the cortex

---

*Since the line of Gennari in the striate cortex represents a particularly large outer band of Baillarger and is located in layer IV, it is often assumed that it represents the massive projection from the lateral geniculate nucleus to the striate cortex. However, cutting all the afferents to the striate cortex does not cause the line of Gennari to disappear. Hence it is thought to be a collection of intracortical axons, although the details of its structure and function are unknown.

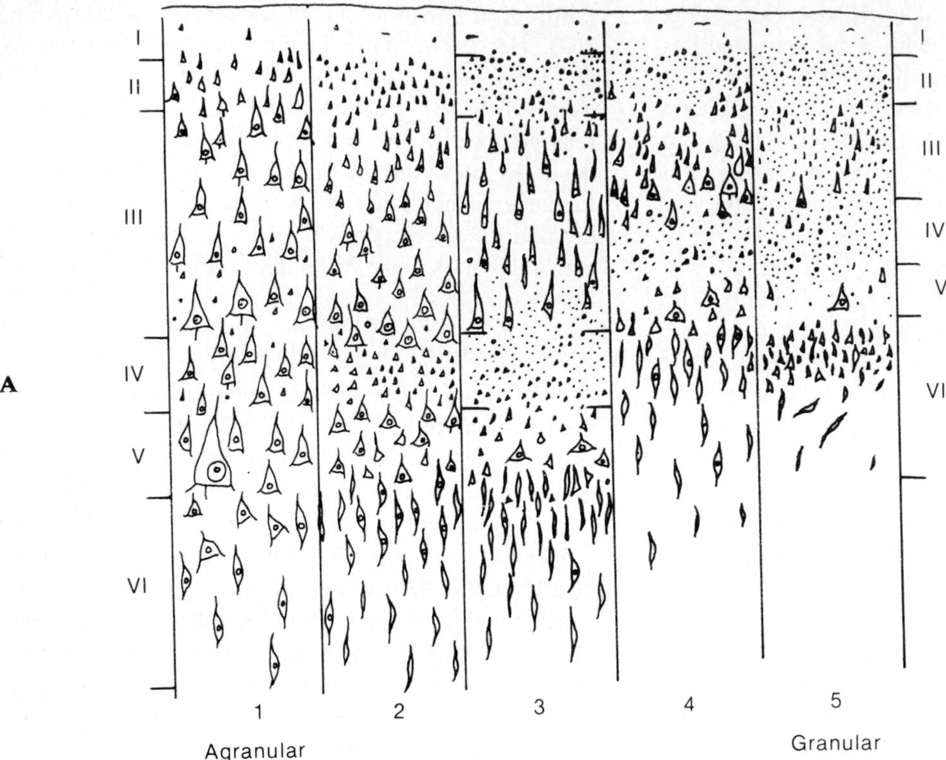


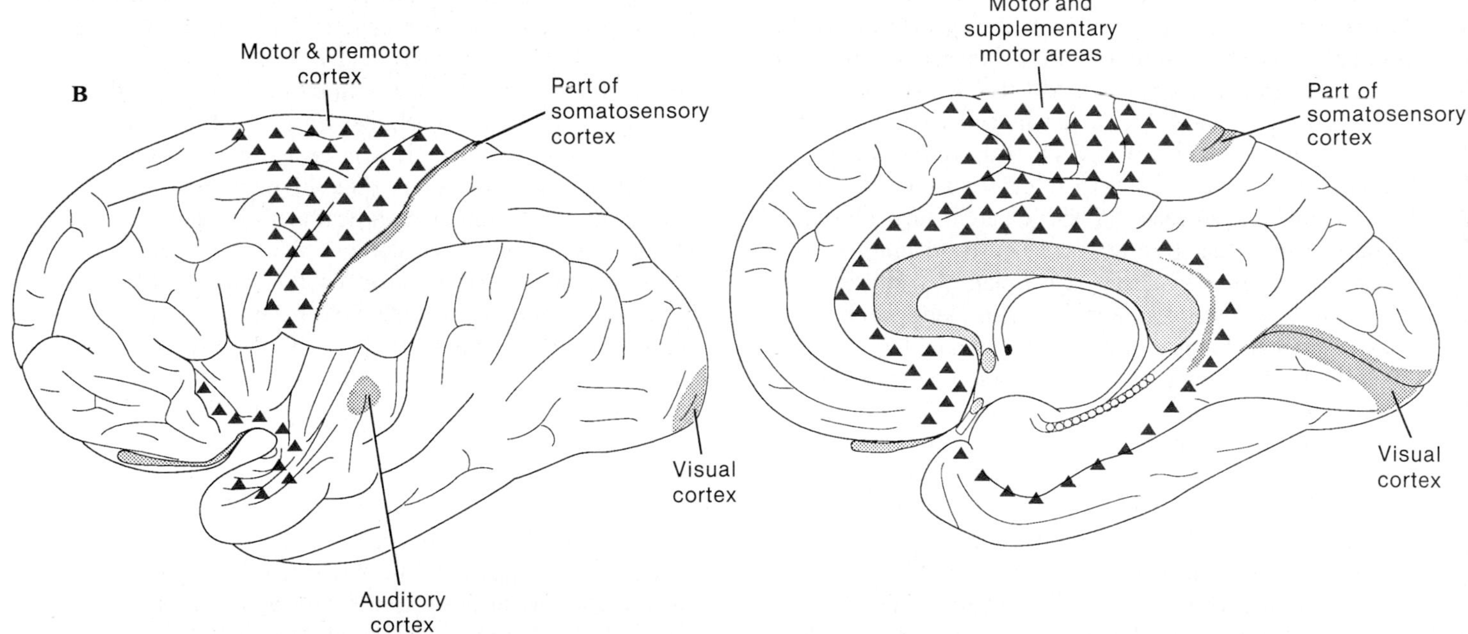


FIGURE 15-7

**A,** Different types of neocortex. At the two extremes are the heterotypical cortices: agranular cortex dominated by large pyramidal cells and granular cortex (koniocortex) dominated by small cells. Areas with intermediate structures in which six layers can be discerned are homotypical and were divided into three types by von Economo: 2, frontal type; 3, parietal type; 4, polar type; **B,** Distribution of heterotypical cortex. The lateral view, on the left, is drawn as though the lateral sulcus had been pried open, exposing the insula. Agranular cortex is found primarily in motor areas, granular cortex primarily in sensory areas (compare to Figure 15-15).

Modified from Von Economo C: *The cytoarchitectonics of the human cerebral cortex,* Oxford, 1929, Oxford University Press.

have a laminar pattern of origin. Although there is substantial overlap, layer III is the major source of corticocortical fibers, layer V of corticostriate fibers and fibers to the brainstem and spinal cord, and layer VI of corticothalamic fibers.

Most efferents to the cortex of the contralateral hemisphere pass through the corpus callosum, as described later in this chapter (Figure 15-20). Those interconnecting parts of the temporal lobes (particularly the middle and inferior temporal gyri) traverse the anterior commissure. Efferents to ipsilateral cortical areas come in all lengths, from very short ones that never leave the cortex to U-shaped fibers that dip under one sulcus to reach the next gyrus and longer association fibers that travel to a different lobe. The longer fibers collect into reasonably well-defined bundles (Figure 15-9) that can be found by gross dissection (Figure 15-10). The most prominent of these association bundles are the *superior longitudinal fasciculus,* the *superior* and *inferior occipitofrontal fasciculi,* and the *cingulum.* The superior longitudinal fasciculus (also called the *arcuate fasciculus)* sweeps along in a great arc above the insula from the frontal lobe to posterior portions of the hemisphere, where it fans out among the parietal, occipital, and temporal lobes. The superior occipitofrontal fasciculus, as its name implies, runs between the frontal and occipital lobes parallel to the corpus callosum for much of its course. Within the hemisphere, the superior occipitofrontal fasciculus is located between the corpus callosum and the caudate nucleus, and so it is also called the *subcallosal bundle.* The inferior occipitofrontal fasciculus passes below the insula from the frontal lobe through the temporal lobe and back to the occipital lobe. Its fibers fan out at both ends of the fasciculus, and those that hook around the margin of the lateral sulcus to interconnect the orbital cortex and anterior temporal cortex are often considered separately as the *uncinate fasciculus* (from the Latin *uncus*

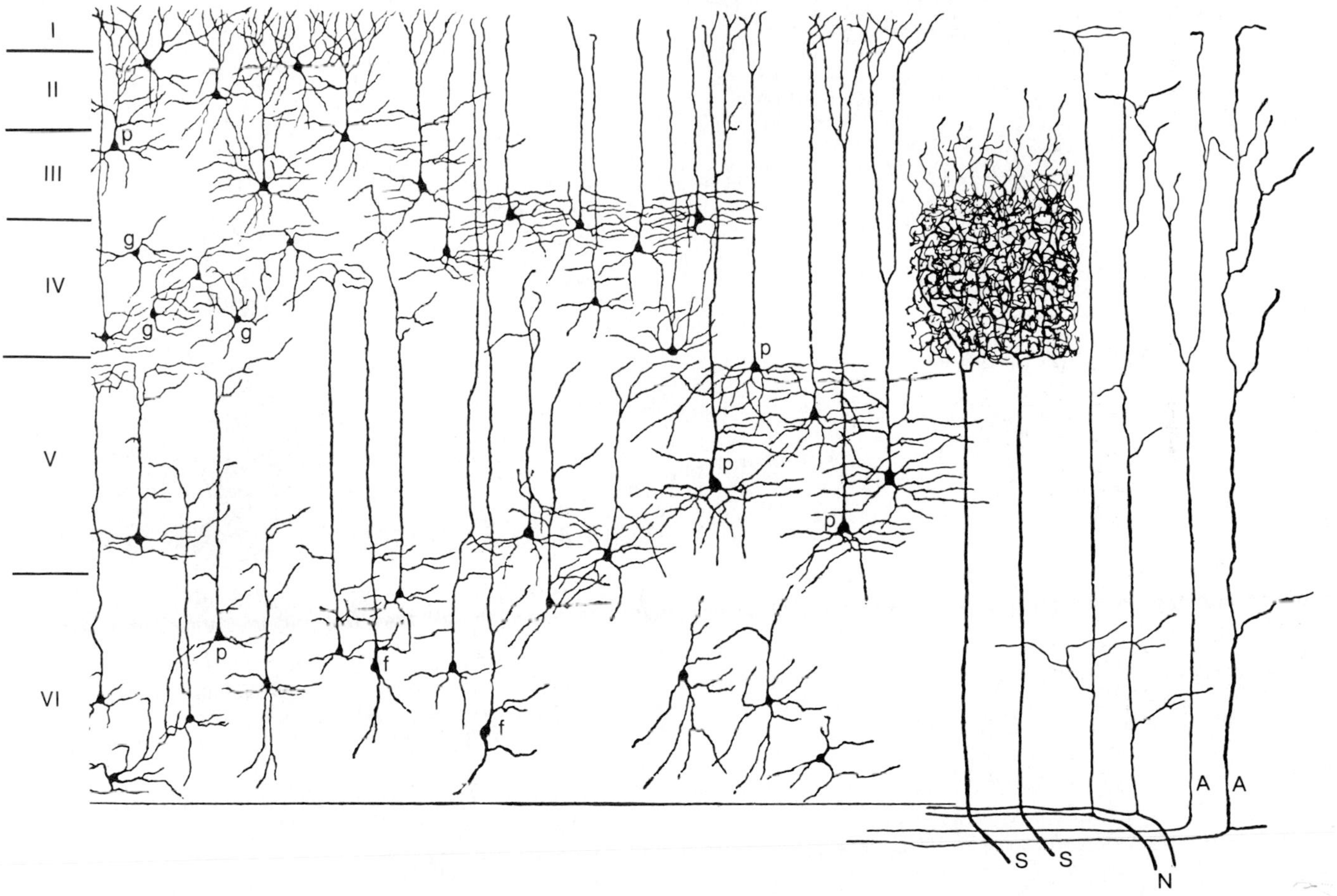


FIGURE 15-8
Types of cortical neurons as seen in Golgi-stained cerebral cortex from a mouse; main types of cortical afferents shown on the right. Cells: f, fusiform cells; *g,* granule (stellate) cells; *p,* pyramidal cells. Afferents: *A,* association fibers from other cortical areas; *N,* fibers from nonspecific thalamic nuclei; *S,* fibers from specific thalamic nuclei. Note the strongly vertical orientation of many cortical elements.

From Lorente de Nó R: Cerebral cortex: architecture, intracortical connections, motor projections. In Fulton JF: *Physiology of the nervous system,* ed 3, Oxford, 1949, Oxford University Press.

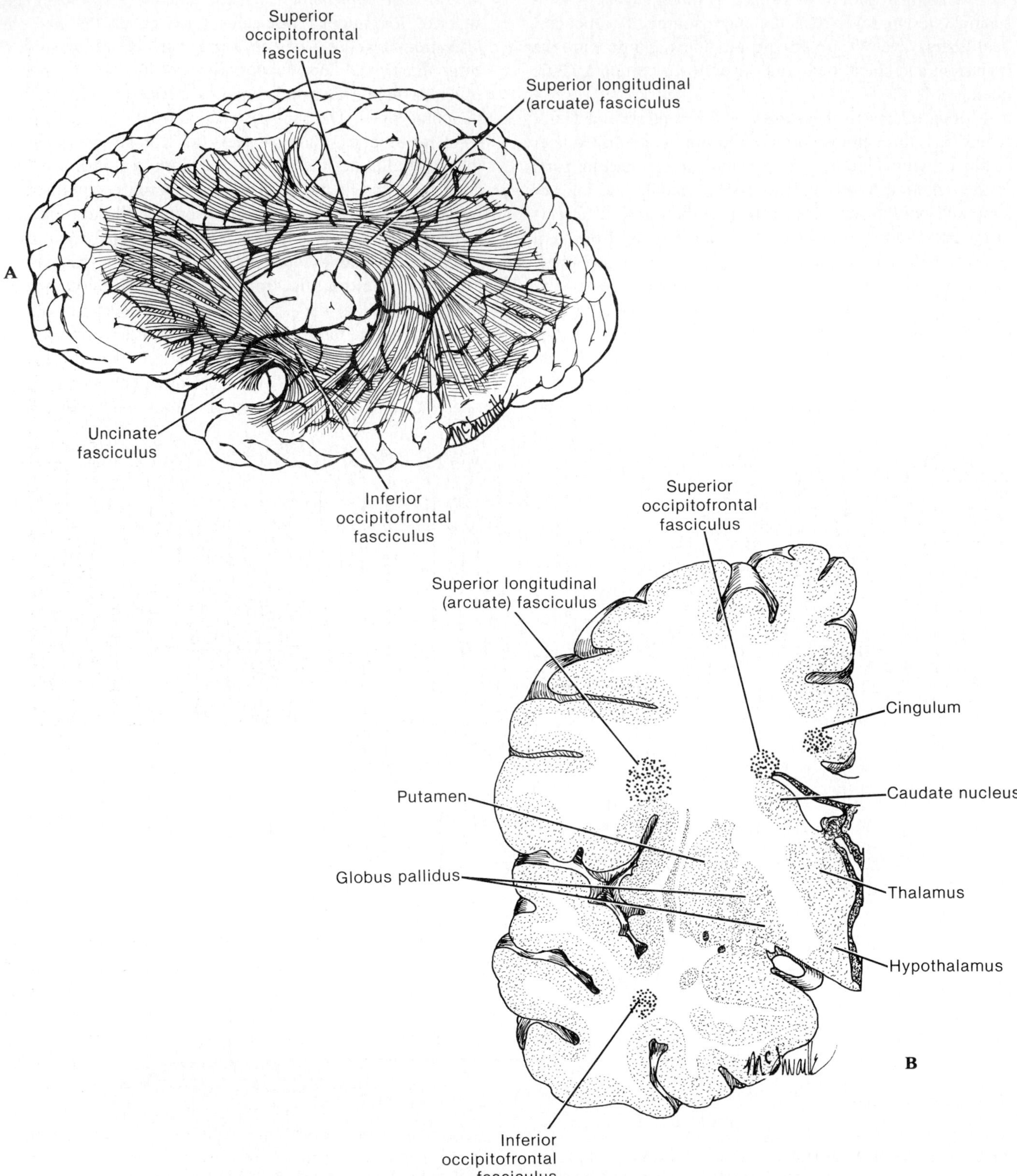


FIGURE 15-9
Long association bundles interconnecting cortical areas. **A,** Major bundles projected onto a lateral view of a cerebral hemisphere. **B,** Position of association bundles in a coronal section through one cerebral hemisphere.

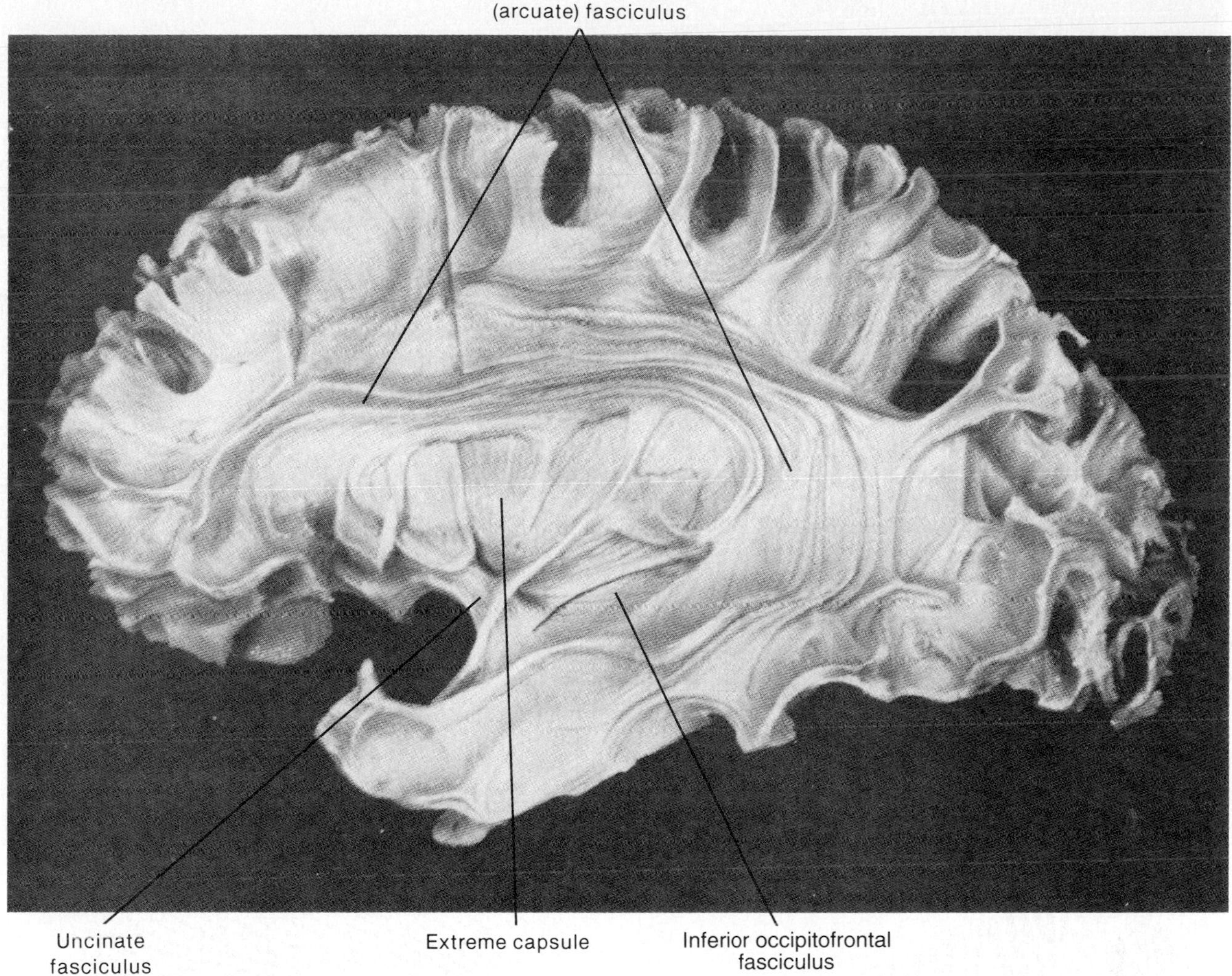


FIGURE 15-10
Some long association bundles as seen in a partially dissected left cerebral hemisphere.
From Ludwig E, Klingler J: *Atlas cerebri humani,* Boston, 1956, Little, Brown & Co.

meaning hook). Finally, the cingulum courses within the cingulate gyrus and continues around within the parahippocampal gyrus to nearly complete a circle. None of these association bundles should be thought of as discrete, point-to-point pathways from one place to another; rather, fibers enter and leave them all along their courses.

## Cortical columns

In spite of the fact that the cortex is horizontally laminated, one gets the strong impression that there is also a vertical organization ("vertical" meaning perpendicular to the surface). Apical dendrites of pyramidal cells have vertical courses, as do afferents to the cortex and the axons of some intracortical cells (Figure 15-8); even the cell bodies of cortical neurons often look as though they are arranged in vertical columns (Figure 15-5). Physiological studies and newer types of anatomical studies have shown that this is not just an illusion. If an electrode is slowly advanced through the somatosensory cortex along a path perpendicular to the cortical surface, all the cells encountered are found to respond with about the same latency to the same type of stimulus delivered to about the same region of the body. Similarly all the cells along a vertical path through the visual cortex respond best to bars or edges with the same orientation in about the same part of the visual field; if the electrode is moved over 50 μm or so, cells with a different preferred stimulus orientation are encountered. Furthermore, each cell along such a vertical path responds better to stimulation of one eye than to stimulation of the other eye; cells in a nearby vertical region may have not only a different preferred stimulus orientation but also a different preferred eye. The picture that has emerged is of

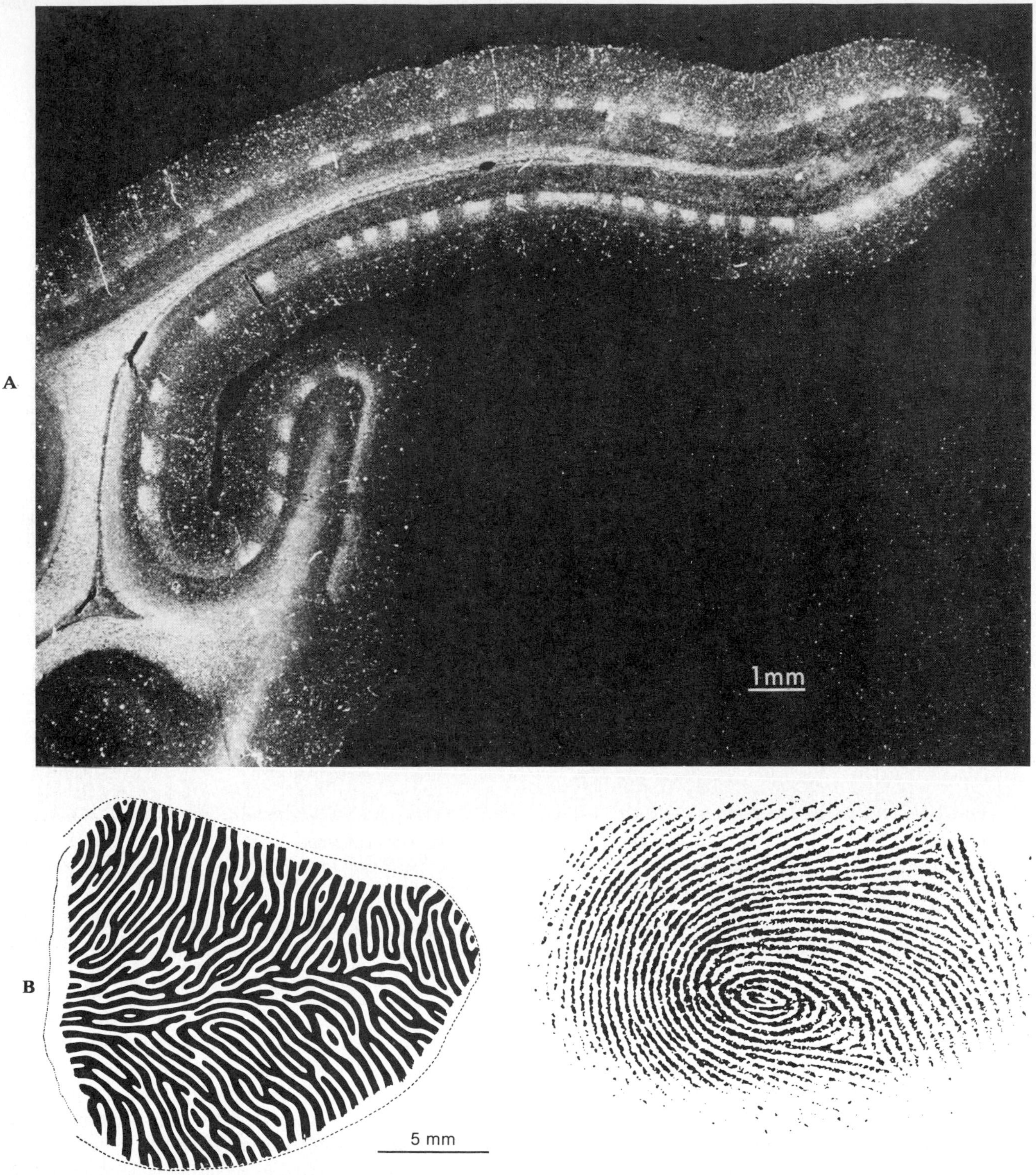

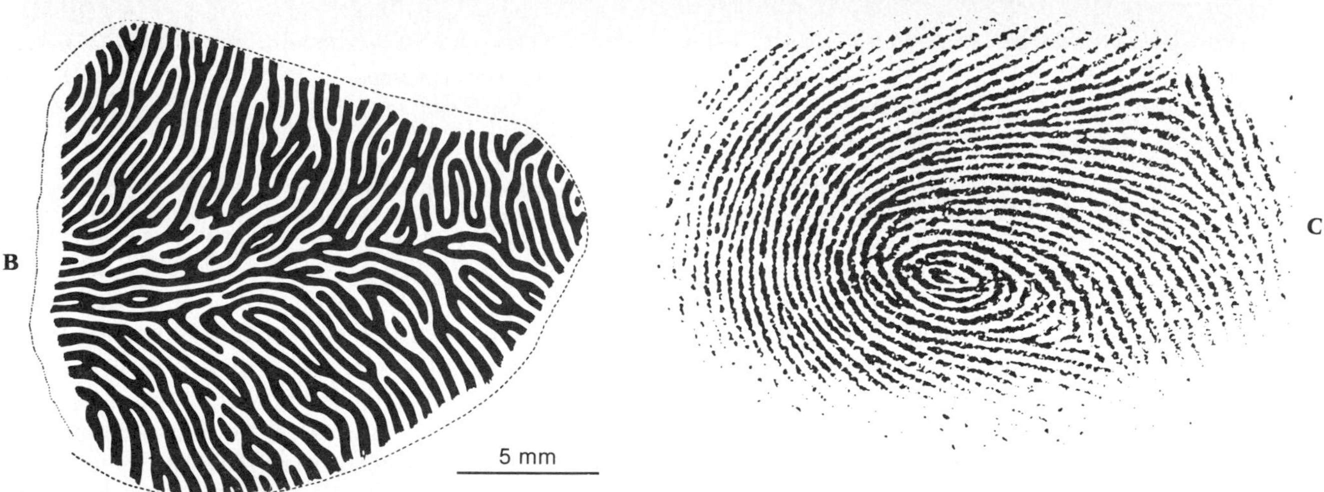


FIGURE 15-11

Cortical columns in the visual cortex of rhesus monkeys. **A,** Autoradiograph of a section through the visual cortex of a monkey whose ipsilateral eye had been injected with a radioactive amino acid 2 weeks before sectioning. The amino acid was taken up by the ganglion cells of that eye, transported to the lateral geniculate nucleus (presumably after being packaged into proteins), taken up by geniculate cells, and then transported to the visual cortex. Ocular dominance columns for the injected eye show up as light areas in layer IV (where the optic radiation terminates) in this autoradiograph seen with dark-field optics; the interspersed dark areas are ocular dominance columns for the contralateral eye. **B,** Reconstruction of the ocular dominance columns (seen as though one were looking down on the cortical surface) showing that the columns are really more or less parallel slabs. **C,** Fingerprint of a human index finger to the same scale as **B.**

From Hubel DH, Wiesel TN: Functional architecture of macaque monkey visual cortex, *Proc R Soc Lond B198:* 1, 1977. Courtesy of Dr. David Hubel. By permission of the Controller of Her Britannic Majesty's Stationery Office.

the organization of the cortex into vertical slabs or columns, each 50 to 500 μm wide, in which some parameter (for example, stimulus orientation) is constant for all cells. Vertical slabs of different types (for example, stimulus orientation or ocular dominance) may intersect one another in patterns that are still largely unknown.

This kind of columnar organization probably reflects a general strategy used in the construction of neocortex. For most areas this is currently impossible to test physiologically because we cannot define the "best" stimulus for the cells in most parts of the cortex. However, some of the new anatomical tracing techniques make it possible to visualize the columns (Figure 15-11), and there are indications that columnar organization is widespread. For example, it has now been shown that in at least some cortical areas, afferents from the thalamus, from other ipsilateral cortical areas, and from contralateral cortical areas each end in vertical slabs separated by slabs that do not receive that particular kind of input.

## LOCALIZATION OF FUNCTION

Just as there has been a long controversy about whether the nature of a stimulus is signalled by the type of peripheral receptor that is activated or by the pattern of activity in many receptors, so too there has been a controversy about localization of function in the cerebral cortex. At one extreme have been those who maintain (in a kind of phrenology moved inward) that particular patches of cortex are the unique sites of particular functions. At the other extreme have been those who maintain that large areas of cortex form uniform fields in which functions are not localized and that complex activities depend on the amount of such cortex that is intact, not on the particular areas. As is often the case, the truth appears to lie somewhere in between. Consider the "simple" visual examination of an object, for example. This involves analysis of its size, shape, color, movement, and position in space; correlation of that object with objects seen in the past; cross-correlation of the appearance of the object with its sound, smell, and other properties; and decision making about whether, for instance, to run away or to grab it. Not surprisingly, large expanses of cortex are involved in even simple activities like this, and performance of complex tasks can be impaired by damage to widely separated cortical areas. Nevertheless, many years of clinical experience have shown that reasonably predictable deficits are found after damage at various cerebral sites. This could mean that a given function actually is localized in a particular area, that the area performs one crucial step in the function, or that the area facilitates the activity of one or more other structures. Whichever is the case, the consistent association of some deficits with certain areas of damage provides a useful diagnostic tool, and we often speak as though functions are localized to specific cortical areas.

### Anatomical maps

Seeing that various cortical areas are structurally distinct from one another in fairly obvious ways (for example, granular versus agranular cortex), a number of anatomists have sought to map the cortex in terms of these differences and often of considerably more subtle differences. One mapping system whose terminology has come into widespread use is that devised by Brodmann (Figure 15-12), who divided the cortex of each hemisphere into 52 areas. The boundaries between many of these areas are not precise, as they often grade into each other by degrees. In addition, as noted previously, the correlation of functions with specific anatomical areas is not nearly as precise as once was hoped. Nevertheless, many of the numbers proposed by Brodmann are commonly used for reference purposes (Table 10).

### Cortical areas

The neocortex of each cerebral hemisphere is traditionally considered as made up of *primary sensory areas* (receiving inputs from thalamic relay nuclei), a *primary motor area* (giving rise to the pyramidal tract), *association areas,* and *limbic areas.* In this view the somatosensory cortex occupies the postcentral gyrus, the visual cortex the banks of the calcarine sulcus, the auditory cortex a small part of the superior temporal gyrus, and the motor cortex the precentral gyrus. These areas are characterized by a topographical organization in which the body surface, the outside world, or the range of audible frequencies is mapped onto the cortical surface (see Figures 11-15 and 12-3). The maps are distorted so that highly discriminating or finely controlled items have a disproportionately large representation (for example, the fovea in the visual cortex or the fingers in the motor and somatosensory cortex).

These primary areas come to occupy relatively less and less of the cortical surface over the course of mammalian evolution (Figure 15-13), and most of the human neocortex is of the association variety. Association cortex in turn is commonly divided into two broad types. The area adjacent to a primary area is typically a *unimodal association area,* devoted to an elaboration of the business of that primary area. Thus areas 18 and 19, which surround the primary visual cortex, are part of the *visual association cortex.* Similarly the superior parietal lobule, much of the superior temporal gyrus, and the premotor cortex are involved in somatosensory, auditory, and motor functions, respectively. This still leaves the inferior parietal lobule and large portions of the frontal and temporal lobes. Neurons in these areas typically respond to multiple sensory modalities and may change their response properties under different circumstances. For example, a neuron in the inferior parietal lobule might respond to a visual stimulus but *only* if it was something interesting, like a cue or a piece of food. These *multimodal* or *heteromodal association ar-*

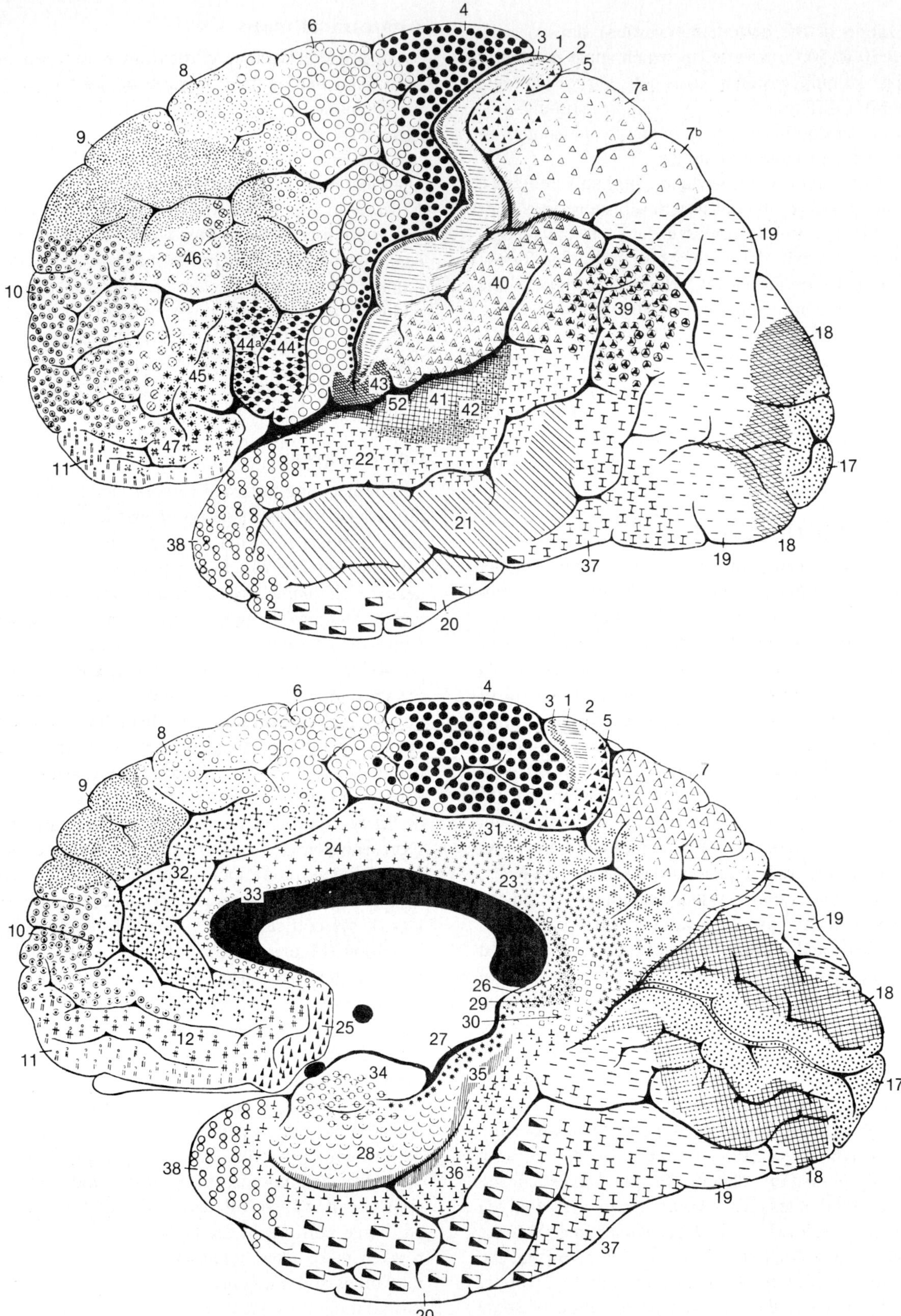


FIGURE 15-12
Brodmann's anatomically defined areas of the human cerebral cortex.

From Von Economo G, Koskinas GN: *Die cytoarchitektonik der Hirnrinde des erwachsenen Menschen,* Heidelberg, 1925, Julius Springer.

**TABLE 10** *Selected Brodmann's areas*

| Lobe | Number | Location | Other names |
|---|---|---|---|
| Frontal | 4 | Precentral gyrus, paracentral lobule | Primary motor area |
| | 6 | Superior and middle frontal gyri, precentral gyrus | Premotor area, supplementary motor area |
| | 8 | Superior and middle frontal gyri | Inferior portion = frontal eye field |
| | 44,45 | Opercular and triangular parts of inferior frontal gyrus | Broca's area |
| Parietal | 3,1,2 | Postcentral gyrus, paracentral lobule | Primary somatosensory area; S1 |
| | 5,7 | Superior parietal lobule | Somatosensory association area |
| | 39 | Inferior parietal lobule | Angular gyrus |
| | 40 | Inferior parietal lobule | Supramarginal gyrus |
| Occipital | 17 | Banks of calcarine sulcus | Primary visual area; V1 |
| | 18,19 | Surrounding 17 | Visual association area; V2, V3, V4, V5 |
| Temporal | 41 | Superior temporal gyrus | Primary auditory area; A1 |
| | 42* | Superior temporal gyrus | Auditory association area; A2 |
| | 22 | Superior temporal gyrus | Auditory association area; posterior portion = Wernicke's area |

*Considered part of the primary auditory cortex by many authors.

*eas* are therefore thought to be concerned somehow with high-level intellectual functions.

Although there is a great deal of validity to this broad view of cortical organization, it is also clear that it is a considerable oversimplification in some respects. For one thing, the distinction between primary areas and association areas is not nearly so clear as the traditional formulation implies. One example given in an earlier chapter is the finding that the pyramidal tract originates not just from the classical primary motor cortex but also from other areas, including the somatosensory cortex. As another example, we now know there are *several* separate, distinct, and topographically arranged representations of motor and sensory functions in the cortex. In addition, the concepts that primary sensory areas receive all the input (which is then acted on in some more complex fashion by the association cortex) and that motor activity is formulated in association areas and then funnels down to the primary motor area for expression are certainly not completely correct. Monkeys (and humans as well) with extensive damage to the precentral or postcentral gyrus are not rendered unable to move or to perceive tactile stimuli. They are impaired in these capacities, but the fact that they suffer only a partial disability indicates that other cortical areas play a role as well and that these other areas can function independently of the primary areas, at least to some extent (Figure 15-14).* The details of the ways in which different areas of the cor-

*The extent to which this applies varies in different association areas and in different species. In primates, for example, some portions of the visual and somatosensory association cortex absolutely depend on the primary areas for their continued function while other portions do not.

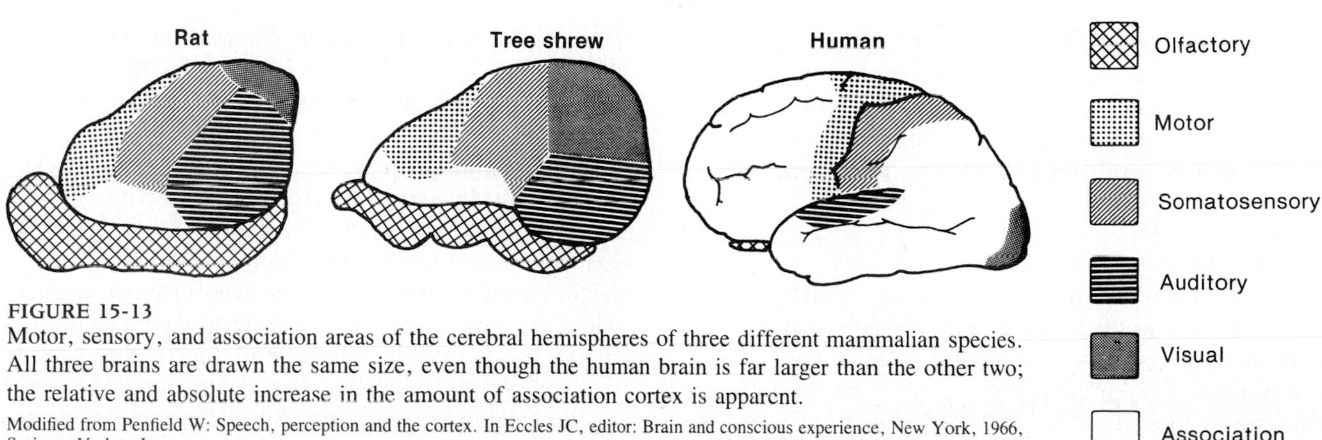


FIGURE 15-13
Motor, sensory, and association areas of the cerebral hemispheres of three different mammalian species. All three brains are drawn the same size, even though the human brain is far larger than the other two; the relative and absolute increase in the amount of association cortex is apparent.

Modified from Penfield W: Speech, perception and the cortex. In Eccles JC, editor: Brain and conscious experience, New York, 1966, Springer-Verlag, Inc.

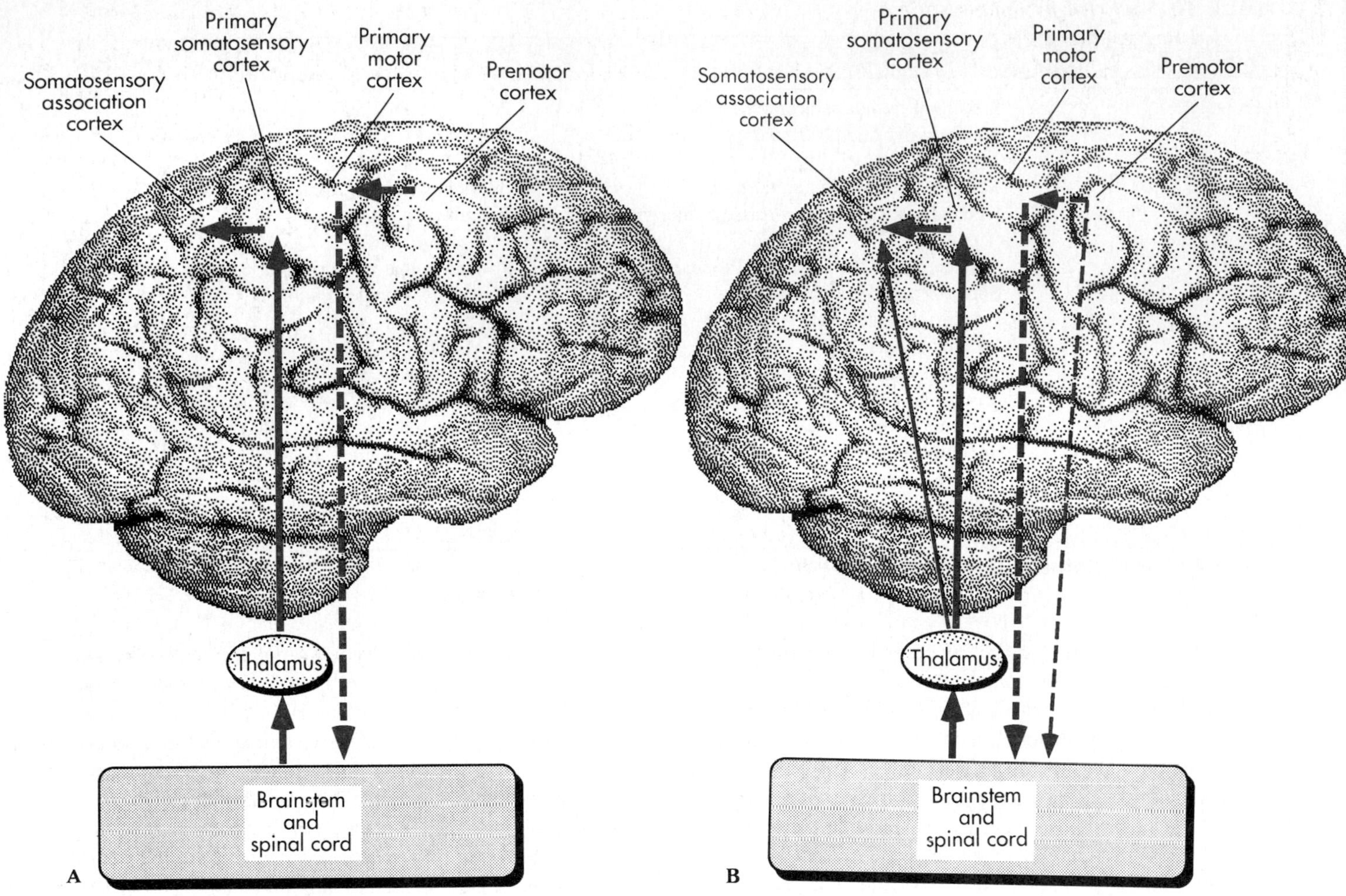


FIGURE 15-14
Cortical connections in sensory and motor systems. The somatosensory system is used as an example in this illustration, but the same principles apply to other sensory systems. **A,** Traditional serial-processing formulation. In this view, all sensory inflow from the thalamus ends in the primary sensory cortex, which then processes the information and passes it on to association areas. Similarly, all motor outflow originates in the primary motor cortex, which receives its inputs from motor association areas like the premotor area. **B,** Current formulation, in which there is a combination of serial and parallel processing. Sensory inflow from the thalamus is distributed to both primary and association areas. Similarly, motor outflow originates in both primary motor and motor association areas. In both cases, the primary area is of major importance, but association areas have some connections in parallel.

tex and other parts of the CNS cooperate to produce something like a simple voluntary movement or a simple visual perception are still largely mysterious. The best we can do at present is specify some known cortical connections and the consequences of damage to some cortical areas.

## Sensory areas

### *Somatosensory cortex*

Somatosensory information traveling rostrally in the medial lemniscus and in the spinothalamic and trigeminothalamic tracts relays in the VPL/VPM of the thalamus and projects through the posterior limb of the internal capsule mainly to areas 3, 1, and 2. These are three long, parallel strips of cortex that together occupy almost the entire postcentral gyrus; most of area 3 is in the posterior wall of the central sulcus. These areas are not only structurally distinct from one another, but they also differ slightly in their connections; in fact, the body surface is mapped separately in each area in terms of different types of sensory input. Cells in area 3 mostly reflect activity of slowly adapting cutaneous receptors, those of area 1 rapidly adapting cutaneous receptors, and those of area 2 deep receptors such as those of joints. The result is a map in which the progression from tongue to contralateral toe is spread out along an inferior-superior line (Figure 12-3) and in which sensory modalities are spread out along a much shorter anterior-posterior line. Since this is the most prominent (but not the only) area concerned with somatic sensation, it is often referred to as the *first somatosensory area,* or *S1*. Another parallel strip of cortex (area 3a), located in the depths of the central sulcus between areas 3 and 4, should probably be included in S1, since it receives information from muscle receptors. The fact that none of area 3a is exposed at the surface of the brain contributed to the long-held (but erroneous) notion that muscle receptors have no cortical representation and do not contribute to conscious experience.

A *second somatosensory area (S2)* has also been described; it receives its inputs not only from S1, but also to a lesser extent directly from the VPL/VPM. It occupies part of the parietal operculum, and much of it is buried in the lateral sulcus, possibly extending onto the insula (Figure 15-15). S2 is also somatotopically organized but in an order that is the reverse of that in S1; that is, the face areas of both maps are adjacent to one another, and the rest of the S2 map extends into the lateral sulcus. The cells in S2 tend to have bilateral receptive fields so that touching either of two symmetrically placed sites activates them.

Stimulation of the postcentral gyrus in conscious humans produces sensations usually described as tingling or numbness in a contralateral part of the body whose location is related in an orderly way to the site stimulated (Figure 12-3). The sensations generally do not resemble those caused by natural stimuli like bending a hair or touching the skin, presumably because electrical stimulation of the cortex is a poor imitation of the pattern of activity set up by natural stimuli. Interestingly, sensations of pain can rarely be elicited from the postcentral gyrus, and the way in which pain is represented in the cerebral cortex continues to be something of a mystery. Large lesions affecting all of the postcentral cortex cause a considerable impairment of the finer aspects of somatic sensation (such as judging the exact location or intensity of a stimulus) and a serious deficit in the sense of position and movement of the affected parts, but such damage does not abolish tactile sensation or sensation of pain. Indeed, on the few occasions when removal of the postcentral cortex was tried as a treatment for intractable pain, the patient's pain was usually relieved only partially and briefly, and this was often followed by a hyperpathic state reminiscent of thalamic pain. On the other hand, small lesions affecting only the part of the postcentral gyrus adjacent to the central sulcus cause localized losses of pain and temperature sensation in the somatotopically appropriate part of the body on the

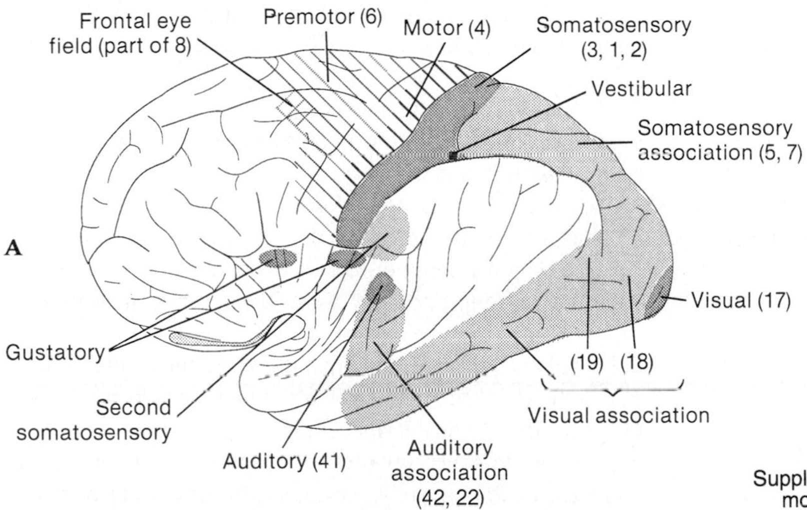


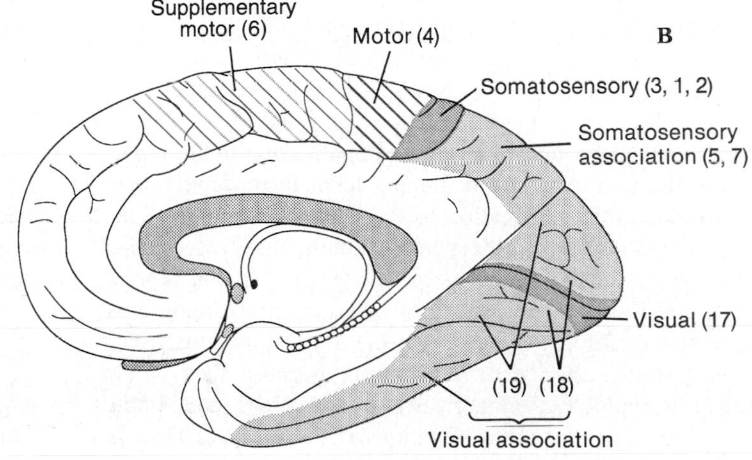


FIGURE 15-15
Summary diagram of some functional areas of the cerebral cortex. The lateral view, as in Figure 15-7, is drawn as though the lateral sulcus had been pried open, exposing the insula. Visual association cortex is particularly extensive in primate brains, occupying not only most of the occipital lobe but also much of the temporal lobe. Many of these various functional areas are associated with one of Brodmann's anatomically defined areas, although sometimes the correspondence is only approximate; commonly used Brodmann numbers are indicated in parentheses. The probable location of primary vestibular cortex is indicated by a filled square.

contralateral side. Corresponding to this clinical observation, neurons specifically responsive to painful stimuli have been found in the somatosensory cortex of monkeys at about the junction between areas 3 and 1. However, processing of pain information is not the exclusive province of S1. Pain-sensitive neurons have also been found in S2, and there have been clinical reports of loss of pain in humans following damage to S2. The relative roles of S1 and S2 (and possibly other cortical areas as well) in pain perception, and the reasons why large cortical lesions should cause a hyperpathic state, are not yet clear.

### *Visual cortex*

The retinotopic projection from the lateral geniculate nucleus to the banks of the calcarine sulcus, conveying information about the contralateral visual field, was described in Chapter 11. This primary visual cortex (called the *striate cortex)* corresponds to area 17 of Brodmann's map. Peripheral parts of the visual field are represented anteriorly, the fovea has a disproportionately large representation located posteriorly, and the vertical meridian is represented along the upper and lower borders of area 17 (Figure 11-15). Although area 17 looks fairly small on maps such as that in Figure 15-12, it really occupies a substantial amount of the cortical surface and appears small only because most of it forms the walls of the deep calcarine sulcus.

A two-part visual association cortex occupies the rest of the occipital lobe. Area 18 surrounds area 17 and is itself surrounded by area 19. This association cortex receives its visual information both from area 17 and via the superior colliculus-pulvinar pathway. Areas 18 and 19 are themselves complex mosaics of smaller, retinotopically organized areas, one interested in the movements of objects, another in the colors of objects, and still others in other properties. Additional visual association areas occupy much of the temporal lobe (Figure 15-15), reflecting the importance of vision for primates.

The relative roles of primary visual cortex and visual association cortex in human vision are poorly understood. It seems safe to say that the primary area is extremely important, since its destruction results in a total or near-total loss of conscious awareness of visual stimuli. A simplified view of its function, then, would be that the primary visual cortex does some initial processing on inputs from the lateral geniculate nucleus (for example, combining inputs from the two eyes and beginning to analyze depth), then distributes this information to the various subareas of the visual association cortex where motion, color, and other parameters are analyzed more elaborately. If this is true, bilateral lesions of the visual association cortex could conceivably disrupt single aspects of visual function. (Such cases would also be extremely rare because they would need to involve symmetrically placed areas and would need to spare the optic radiations.) A few cases have in fact been reported in which bilateral damage to the inferior surfaces of the occipital lobes caused color-blindness or in which more lateral damage near the occipital-temporal junction caused motion-blindness.

### *Auditory cortex*

The superior surface of the temporal lobe forms one wall of the lateral sulcus. Two *transverse temporal gyri* cross the posterior part of this surface and form Brodmann's areas 41 and 42. Area 41 is granular cortex (like areas 3 and 17) and receives most of the auditory radiation from the medial geniculate nucleus via the sublenticular part of the internal capsule; thus it serves as the *primary auditory cortex,* or *A1* (Figure 15-16). Just as the body is mapped onto the postcentral gyrus *(somatotopy)* and the retina is mapped onto striate cortex *(retinotopy),* so the spectrum of audible frequencies is mapped onto area 41 *(tonotopy).* Area 42 is adjacent to area 41 and receives auditory information both from area 41 and from the medial geniculate nucleus. This is analogous to the arrangement found in the second somatosensory area (S2), so area 42 is often referred to as A2.* The cortex surrounding area 41 in monkeys includes at least four different subareas, each with its own tonotopic map. The same is assumed to be true for humans, but the exact details of the arrangement of these multiple maps with respect to area 42 are not known. Area 42 is itself flanked by area 22, which forms much of the superior temporal gyrus and is called the *auditory association cortex.*

At levels rostral to the cochlear nuclei, both ears are represented in the auditory pathway of each side of the brain, although the contralateral ear predominates (Chapter 9). As a result, even total destruction of the auditory cortex has relatively little effect. An individual with such damage may have some difficulty localizing sounds on the contralateral side and may have some subtle hearing loss that is greater for the contralateral ear, but the deficits are not nearly comparable in magnitude to those that follow unilateral damage to the somatosensory or visual cortex. On the other hand, if the auditory association cortex of area 22 is damaged in the dominant hemisphere, severe language problems may ensue, as discussed later in this chapter.

### *Other sensory areas*

Gustatory information, relayed from the VPM through the posterior limb of the internal capsule, apparently reaches the parietal operculum and part of the anterior insula. These seem like logical places for gustatory cortex, since part is adjacent to the representation of the tongue in

*Terminology for area 42 varies among authors. Since it receives direct projections from the medial geniculate nucleus, some include it in the primary auditory cortex. Since it receives projections from area 41, others refer to it as part of the auditory association cortex.

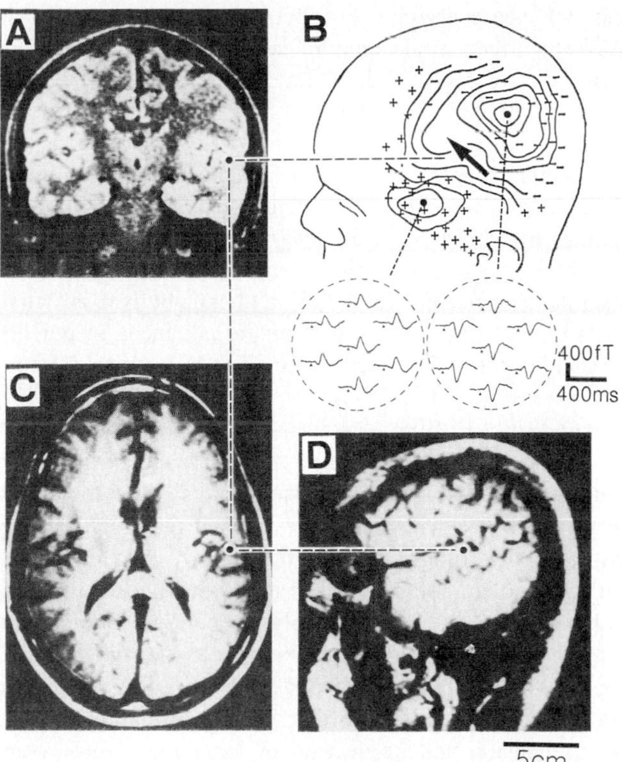


FIGURE 15-16
A striking demonstration of the location of auditory cortex on the superior surface of the superior temporal gyrus in a living human. The current flows associated with nerve impulses are accompanied by fluctuating external magnetic fields. The fields and their fluctuations are tiny, but the changes can be measured using extremely sensitive recording instruments based on special detectors called superconducting quantum interference devices *(SQUIDs)*. Magnetic field changes can then be mapped out using a technique called *magnetoencephalography*. In the study shown here, 1 kHz tone bursts 400 ms in duration were presented to the right ear and the resulting magnetic field changes were mapped out over the left hemisphere *(B)*; some of the actual magnetic field-change recordings are shown in the circular insets. The calculated source of these field changes was then mapped as a dot onto coronal, horizontal and sagittal magnetic resonance images of the same individual (*A*, *C*, and *D*, respectively). From Yamamoto T et al., *Proc Natl Acad Sci USA* 85:8732, 1988. Courtesy of Dr. R. Llinás, New York University Medical Center.

the somatosensory cortex and part is adjacent to an olfactory area (see Chapter 16); however, these probable gustatory areas are rarely exposed during surgical procedures, so little direct information is available about them for humans. A few cases have been reported in which stimulation of the parietal operculum or nearby insula caused sensations of taste or in which seizures originating in this vicinity were preceded by an aura that included sensations of taste.

The vestibular area was long thought to be located in the superior temporal gyrus near the auditory cortex, since stimulation of this region sometimes produces a sensation of movement or dizziness. However, more recent work on monkeys has shown that the most direct cortical projection from the vestibular nerve is to the parietal lobe adjacent to the representation of the head in the primary somatosensory cortex. The most likely location in humans (determined by extrapolation from monkeys and not by direct observation) is in the walls of the intraparietal sulcus near its junction with the postcentral sulcus (Figure 15-15). The feelings of dizziness elicited by stimulation of the superior temporal gyrus may indicate that there is a secondary vestibular area in the temporal lobe.

The olfactory system is unique in that it does not relay in the thalamus and that the primary olfactory cortex is paleocortical rather than neocortical. Since it is closely connected with elements of the limbic system, the olfactory cortex is discussed separately in the next chapter.

### Motor areas

Just as the somatosensory, visual, and auditory systems have multiple representations in the cortex, so too are there several areas from which movements can be elicited. The *primary motor cortex* corresponds to Brodmann's area 4, occupying a tapering strip in the precentral gyrus. Area 4 is agranular, the thickest cortex in the brain, containing a preponderance of large pyramidal cells including the giant pyramidal cells (Betz cells). In the midnineteenth century, before the motor cortex had been explored electrically, the British neurologist Hughlings Jackson predicted the pattern in which movements are mapped on the precentral gyrus, based on his careful observation of patients with epileptic foci in this area. He noted that such patients typically had seizures that started as a twitching in one part of the body and then spread to other regions on the same side in a sequence that was similar from one patient to another. This sequence corresponds to the now-familiar homunculus for the motor cortex, which is generally parallel to the homunculus found in the somatosensory cortex (Figure 12-3). As might be expected from the distortions of the motor homunculus, Jackson also observed that these seizures were more likely to begin as twitchings of the fingers or lips. Such attacks are still referred to as *jacksonian seizures* and the spread of motor activity as a *jacksonian march*. Stimulation of area 4 in conscious humans causes discrete movements involving one muscle or a small group of muscles (such as flexion of a single finger joint), which the patient is unable to prevent.* The movements are always contralateral to the side stimulated except in movements of the palate, the pharynx, the masseter, and often the tongue (but not the face), where the movements are bilateral; this

*However, the patient has no sensation of *willing* the movement.

corresponds nicely to the partly crossed-partly uncrossed corticobulbar projection (Figure 12-6).

Several cortical areas in addition to area 4 give rise to corticospinal fibers and to other cortical efferents that participate in motor control (Figure 12-5). Among them is area 6, which is also agranular cortex similar to area 4 except that it lacks Betz cells. Movements can be elicited by stimulating area 6 (the *premotor area),* but the threshold is slightly higher than in the case of area 4, the movements are slower, and they are more likely to involve larger groups of muscles. Corticospinal fibers also arise in the somatosensory cortex of the postcentral gyrus, and movements can be elicited from this region too, according to a pattern identical to the somatosensory homunculus. Finally, there is a *supplementary motor area* on the medial surface of the hemisphere; it is located anterior to the representation of the foot in the primary motor cortex, in the medial extension of area 6 (Figure 15-15). Stimulation of the supplementary motor area causes movements that are usually described as the assumption of postures and may involve muscles on both sides of the body. For example, there might be a turning of the head and trunk to the contralateral side, accompanied by raising the contralateral arm.

The multiple representation of movements in the cerebral cortex, with a primary area and several other nearby areas, is strikingly similar to the situation with sensory systems. In this case, too, the primary motor area seems to be the most important in terms of the deficits that follow its destruction. Lesions of area 4 cause an initial contralateral flaccid paralysis, which resolves fairly quickly into hemiparesis accompanied by mild spasticity. The paresis is worse for more distal muscles, and its effects are seen most when fine, skilled movements (such as individual finger movements) are attempted. There is disagreement as to the degree of spasticity (or whether there is any at all) following damage that is entirely restricted to area 4, but the spasticity is certainly slight compared to that seen in cases of more widespread cortical damage or of lesions of the internal capsule. Selective damage to area 6 or to the supplementary motor cortex does not produce paralysis or reflex changes, but if such damage accompanies destruction of the primary motor area, full-blown spastic hemiparesis results.

## Higher functions

Humans use language, create visual art and music, and otherwise behave in ways totally or nearly totally beyond the capacities of nonhuman species. Such behavior therefore can be studied only in humans, in contrast to our ability to obtain useful information about basic aspects of motor and sensory systems from experimental animals. Until the recent advent of techniques like PET scanning (Plates 11 and 12) this obviously constrained us to examining the effects of naturally occurring lesions of the brain or the effects of neurosurgical procedures, neither of which is likely to affect single anatomical areas in isolation. Our knowledge of higher mental functions is therefore largely based on clinical case studies, often on small numbers of patients with extremely rare lesions; as a result, it is not very satisfactory from a strictly scientific point of view. Nevertheless, as in the case of motor and sensory cortex, damage to certain cortical areas results in predictable deficits. PET scanning and related techniques, which can demonstrate changes in blood flow and metabolism in active areas of the brain, promise dramatic advances in our understanding of higher cortical function in the near future.

### *Cerebral dominance*

All the functions discussed thus far have been related equally to both cerebral hemispheres, so that the hemisphere in which a lesion occurs makes a difference only insofar as determining the side of the body on which a deficit is found. In contrast, it has long been known that language deficits are far more likely to occur after damage to the left hemisphere than after damage to the right. Thus it appears that language tends to be lateralized in the human brain, and the hemisphere that is more important for the comprehension and production of language is now commonly called the *dominant hemisphere*. Its mate is of course called the *nondominant hemisphere,* although this is rather chauvinistic terminology, since (as will be seen) the so-called nondominant hemisphere is quite superior in some things.

Nearly all right-handed people (more than 95%) have dominant left hemispheres. Left-handed people are more likely than right-handers to have dominant right hemispheres or to have some language representation in each hemisphere, but still the majority of left-handers are left-dominant. Thus the side that is dominant is correlated to some extent with handedness, but regardless of whether an individual is left-handed or right-handed, the left hemisphere is more likely to be dominant.

Brains, on casual inspection, look bilaterally symmetrical, but searches for an anatomical basis for the lateralization of language have revealed that a variety of asymmetries actually exist. As discussed in the next section, certain cortical areas abutting the lateral sulcus are important for linguistic functions, and so the consistent asymmetries found in the vicinity of the lateral sulcus are of great interest in this regard. The part of the superior surface of the superior temporal gyrus located posterior to the primary auditory cortex is called the *planum temporale* and is, on the average, considerably larger on the left than on the right. Since the lateral border of the planum temporale forms part of the lower bank of the lateral sulcus, it stands to reason that the lateral sulcus should extend farther posteriorly on the left than on the right. This too has been found to be the case (Figure 15-17). These asymmetries are present before birth, which seems to indicate that left-

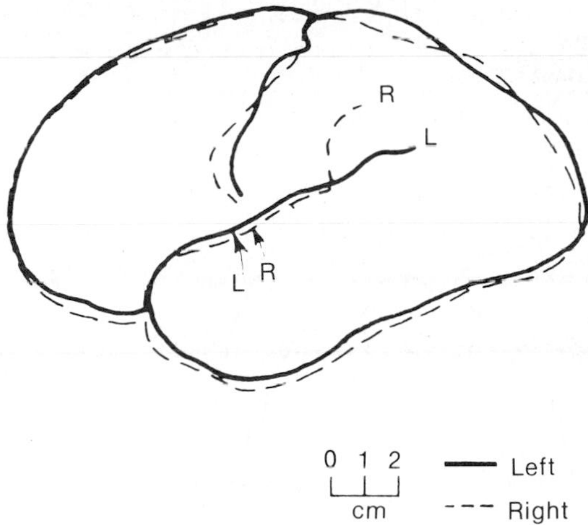


FIGURE 15-17
Typical asymmetry of the two lateral sulci of a single human brain. Both hemispheres were photographed, then one of the photographs was reversed and superimposed on the other. Notice that the left lateral sulcus *(L)* extends farther posteriorly than does the right *(R)*, corresponding to the fact that the planum temporale is usually larger on the left.
From Rubens AB, Mahowald MW, Hutton JT: *Neurology* 26:620, 1976.

hemisphere dominance for language is, at least in part, genetically determined. (This assumes, of course, that the connections of the planum temporale are as predetermined as its size.)

### *Language areas*

Stimulation of the part of motor cortex where the mouth is represented causes an inability to speak and at the same time produces involuntary grunts, cries, or other forms of vocalization. This is similar to what happens when any other part of the motor cortex is stimulated: there is a discrete movement during which the patient is powerless to use those muscles for anything else. However, there are two areas whose stimulation on the dominant side causes the patient to cease speaking but not to do something else with the vocal muscles; more strikingly, stimulation of these areas can cause the patient to make linguistic errors or be unable to find appropriate words. The first of these two areas occupies the opercular and triangular parts of the inferior frontal gyrus and is called *Broca's area*. The second area occupies the posterior part of the superior temporal gyrus and much of the inferior parietal lobule. This posterior part of the superior temporal gyrus is called *Wernicke's area;* some authors extend the meaning of the term to include the inferior parietal lobule as well.

Inability to use language is called *aphasia* and can be divided into two broad types. The first type is associated with damage to Broca's area (Figure 15-18). Broca's aphasics produce few words, either written or spoken, and have great difficulty producing them. They tend to leave out all but the most meaningful words in a sentence and to speak or write in a telegraphic manner. In marked contrast to their difficulties in producing language, Broca's aphasics have relatively little difficulty comprehending it. Broca's aphasia is also called *nonfluent, motor,* or *expressive aphasia*. The second type of aphasia is associated with damage to Wernicke's area (Figure 15-19). Wernicke's aphasics are able to produce written and spoken words, but the words or the sequences in which they are used are defective in their linguistic content. There may be substitutions of one word for another *(paraphasia),* insertion of new and meaningless words *(neologisms),* or stringing together of words and phrases in an order that conveys little or no meaning *(jargon aphasia)*. All of this suggests that such patients have difficulty comprehending whether their own speech makes sense, and indeed Wernicke's aphasics (in contrast to Broca's aphasics) are deficient in the comprehension of language generally. Because in this condition language can be produced but not understood, Wernicke's aphasia is also called *fluent, sensory,* or *receptive aphasia*.

These two broad types of aphasia are consistent with the notions that Broca's area contains the motor programs for the generation of language and Wernicke's area contains the mechanisms for the formulation of language. Destruction of Broca's area would then deprive the motor cortex of the instructions needed to generate language, but the muscles involved would be normal in other activities; comprehension of language would be relatively unaffected. Destruction of Wernicke's area would leave Broca's area unchecked so that words could be produced without regard for their meaning. This implies that there must be neural projections from Wernicke's area to Broca's area that would most likely travel in the superior longitudinal fasciculus (Figure 15-9). It could be predicted that selective destruction of these fibers would also leave Broca's area unchecked and would result in fluent aphasia. Such cases have been reported (with lesions at the predicted site), in which the patient speaks like a Wernicke's aphasic but has intact comprehension, since Wernicke's area itself is undamaged. This syndrome is called *conduction aphasia*. Destruction of the angular gyrus in the dominant hemisphere causes a type of fluent aphasia in which one major deficit is an inability to name objects *(anomic aphasia)*. This has been used to argue that the angular gyrus performs associations between objects and the symbols (such as words) for objects. According to this model, then, the sequence of cerebral events that occurs during the verbal description of a seen object is as follows: visual information reaches the occipital lobe, is processed in various ways in areas 17, 18, and 19, and is projected to the dominant angular gyrus, which associates words with the object and its attributes; the words (or their cerebral representations) are transferred to Wernicke's area, which assembles them into sentences and activates the appropriate mo-

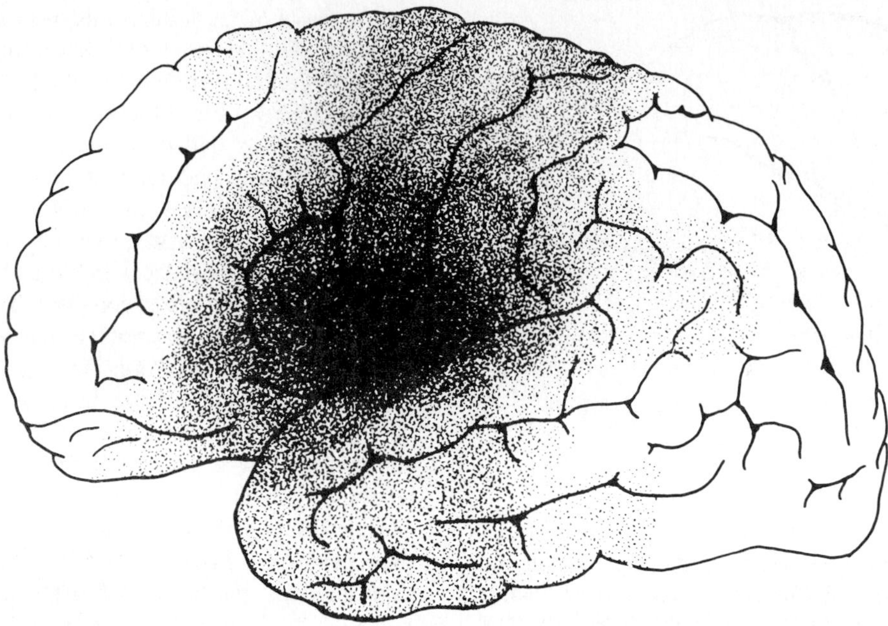

FIGURE 15-18
Site of damage causing Broca's aphasia. The areas infarcted in 14 patients, all diagnosed as suffering from Broca's aphasia, were determined by radioisotope brain scan. All 14 lesions were then superimposed, indicating a focus of damage in the posterior part of the left inferior frontal gyrus.
From Kertesz A, Lesk D, McCabe P: *Arch Neurol* 34:590, © 1977, American Medical Association.

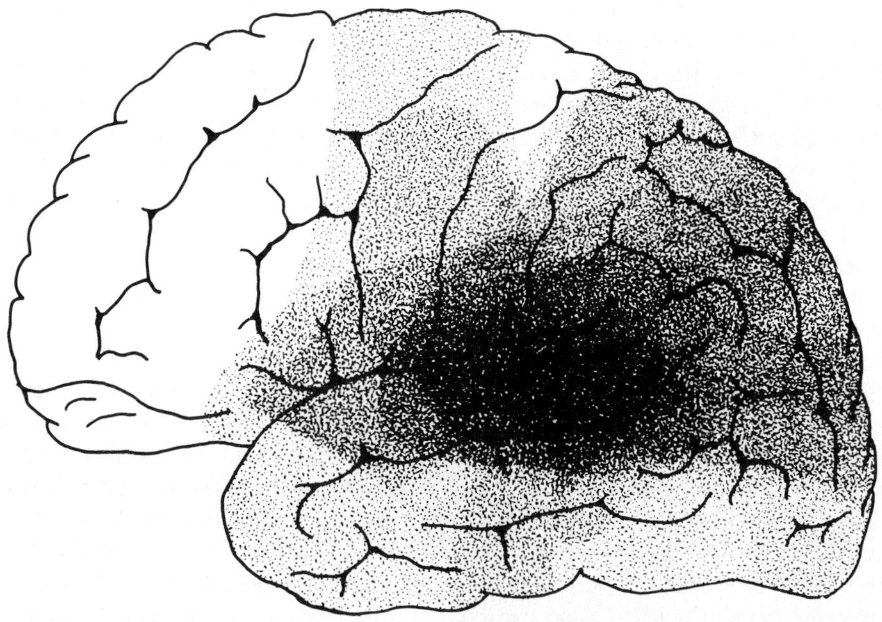

FIGURE 15-19
Site of damage causing Wernicke's aphasia. The areas infarcted in 13 patients, all diagnosed as suffering from Wernicke's aphasia, were determined by radioisotope brain scan. All 13 lesions were then superimposed, indicating a focus of damage in the posterior part of the left superior temporal gyrus.
From Kertesz A, Lesk D, McCabe P: Arch Neurol 34:590, © 1977, American Medical Association.

tor programs in Broca's area; these programs in turn activate the motor cortex.

As appealingly simple as such a model is (and as successful as it is in explaining a variety of aphasic disorders), it is certainly an oversimplification, and many investigators would violently disagree with it. For one thing, it requires an extraordinary degree of localization of very complex functions to specific small areas. For another, the types of aphasia just described are really abstractions, since they are never seen in pure form. This is partly because naturally occurring lesions are not neatly restricted to one of these areas* and partly because aphasias may not exist in pure form. For example, Broca's aphasics typically have a comprehension deficit for grammatically complex statements; comprehension is only spared relative to the severe deficit in production of language. Nevertheless, it is consistently found that within the cortical areas important for language, more anterior lesions result in greater deficits in production of language, and more posterior lesions result in greater deficits in comprehension.

Communication by language involves more than just selecting words and then assembling them according to grammatical rules. Most of the emotional content and part of the linguistic content as well is conveyed by varying emphases. This is true of language generally but especially of spoken language. For example, depending on how they were said, the words "Jack is here" could be a statement of fact or a question; they could convey a feeling of happiness or dread. The rhythmic and more or less musical aspects of speech are called *prosody*. There is clinical evidence that the right hemisphere plays a special role in producing and comprehending the affective aspects of the prosody of speech. The right hemisphere system for generating and comprehending prosody is apparently organized in a fashion analogous to the left hemisphere system for producing and comprehending language. That is, the right inferior frontal gyrus is involved in *producing* prosody and the right posterior temporoparietal region in *comprehending* it. One of the first such patients described was a school teacher with right frontal damage who had begun to have difficulty controlling her students because she was unable to convey feelings of anger or authority by voice or gesture (even though the feelings were there). She had *motor aprosodia*. Patients with more posterior lesions on the right may have *sensory aprosodia* and have difficulty comprehending the emotional content of the speech or gestures of others.

### Parietal lobe syndromes

Neurons in the primary somatosensory or visual cortices respond to easily defined and fairly simple stimuli like the onset of a light touch at a particular site on the back of the contralateral hand or a bar of light oriented at a specific angle and located in a particular part of the contralateral visual field. However, many of the neurons in the parietal association cortex (areas 5 and 7) of a monkey respond to considerably more complicated stimuli. Some respond to movement of the monkey's hand toward some desirable object (for example, a piece of food) but not at all to stretch of the muscles or rotation of the joints involved in the movement. Others respond only when the monkey visually fixates an object of interest and then continue to respond as the monkey tracks the object (if it moves). Removal of areas 5 and 7 causes a neglect of the contralateral half of the body; even though the tactile threshold is unchanged, the limbs on that side are used little, and reaching with them is inaccurate.

The consequences of large lesions of the right parietal lobe in humans are similar to those seen in monkeys but more complex.* Such a patient has difficulty with spatial orientation to everything on the left and may completely ignore the halves of objects to the left as well as the left half of his own body. Such a lesion is rarely confined to the parietal lobe and is often accompanied by hemiparesis and a hemisensory loss. The patient may deny that anything is wrong with the affected limbs and may even deny that they belong to him! In some cases there is a general deficit in spatial orientation that shows up as a difficulty in following maps or in finding locations even in familiar surroundings. Contralateral neglect sometimes, but much less frequently, follows left parietal damage. This may be partly (but not entirely) a result of the fact that left parietal lesions are likely to encroach on Wernicke's area and cause much more prominent aphasic disturbances.

Other deficits that may accompany damage to parietal occipital-temporal association cortex include peculiar disabilities called *agnosias* and *apraxias*. Agnosia (from the Greek word for lack of knowledge) means the inability to recognize objects when using a given sense, even though that sense is basically intact. A person with visual agnosia, for example, would be unable to recognize common objects by sight, even though the visual fields were perfectly intact and even though the ability to recognize the same objects using other senses (such as hearing or touch) might be intact. Apraxia (from the Greek word for lack of action) means an inability to perform an action, even though the muscles required are perfectly sound and able to perform the same action in a different context. An apraxic patient might be unable to touch her nose with her index finger when asked to imitate the examiner's movement, but would be quite capable of doing so spontaneously if her nose itched. There are a multitude of subcategories of ag-

*Full-blown Broca's ophasia, for example, is apparently always associated with damage not just to Broca's area but also to adjacent cortical areas, to the underlying white matter, and to the head of the caudate nucleus. Focal damage restricted to Broca's area causes a relatively mild and short-lived problem with language production.

*In this discussion of parietal lobe syndromes, some types of symptoms are related to right-sided damage and others to left-sided damage. It is assumed (but in general not proven) that these sides correspond in a given patient to the sides nondominant and dominant for language, respectively. Certainly this is true in the large majority of patients.

nosias and apraxias and numerous theories about whether some types are based on language deficits, spatial disorientation, or other more basic problems. Some (but not all) agnosias tend to be associated with bilateral damage. Apraxia often accompanies certain forms of aphasia, but it can result from a lesion on either side. The exact nature of the apraxia depends on the side and area damaged, and some forms of apraxia can also follow premotor damage.

### *Prefrontal cortex*

The parts of each frontal lobe anterior to areas 4, 6, and 8 do not cause movements when stimulated and are called *prefrontal cortex*. This part of the brain expanded dramatically during mammalian evolution (Figure 15-13) and now occupies the inside of the distinctive high forehead of humans. An early clue to the role of the prefrontal cortex in human behavior was provided by an unfortunate accident in the nineteenth century. In 1848, Phineas T. Gage, the foreman of a railroad construction crew, was setting a charge of explosives with a 13-pound, 3½-foot iron tamping rod (Figure 15-20). The charge exploded and blew the tamping iron through the front of his head, destroying a good deal of his prefrontal cortex. Remarkably, he survived the accident and regained his physical health in a few weeks. However, his personality changed dramatically. Before the accident, he was hard working, responsible, clever, and thoroughly respectable. After the accident, he seemed to have lost most of his industriousness and his awareness of social responsibilities.* He wandered aimlessly from job to job, exhibiting himself and his tamping iron in various carnivals, and was tactless and impulsive in his behavior, not particularly concerned about his future or the consequences of his actions.

*"The equilibrium or balance, so to speak, between his intellectual faculties and animal propensities, seems to have been destroyed. He is fitful, irreverent, indulging at times in the grossest profanity (which was not previously his custom), manifesting but little deference for his fellows, impatient of restraint or advice when it conflicts with his desires, at times pertinaciously obstinate, yet capricious and vacillating, devising many plans of future operation, which are no sooner arranged than they are abandoned. . . .In this regard his mind was radically changed, so decidedly that his friends and acquaintances said that he was 'no longer Gage.' " (Harlow HM: Recovery from the passage of an iron bar through the head, Mass Med Soc Publ 2:327, 1868.)

A

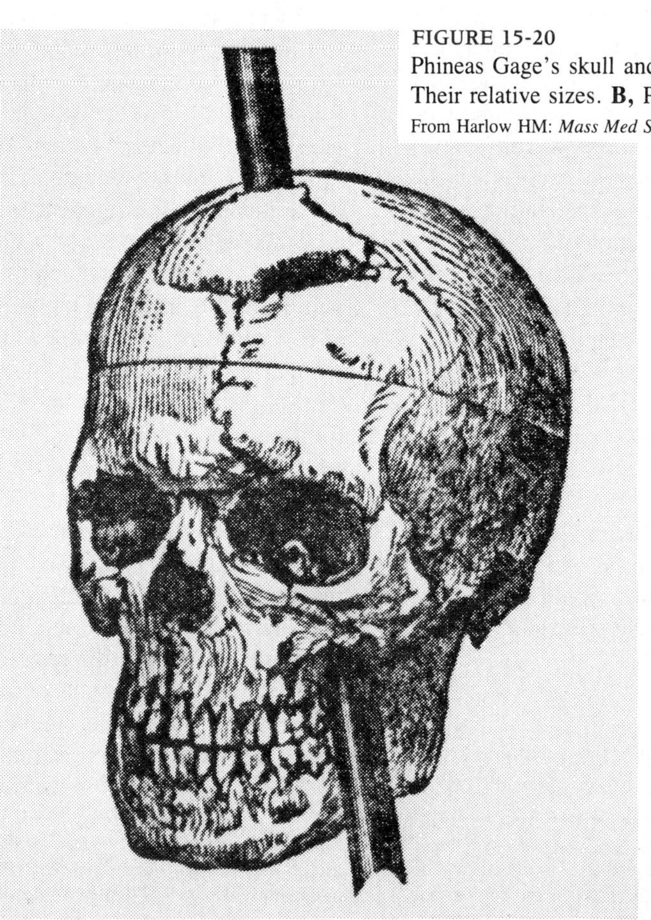

B

FIGURE 15-20
Phineas Gage's skull and the tamping iron that penetrated it. **A,** Their relative sizes. **B,** Path taken by the tamping iron.
From Harlow HM: *Mass Med Soc Publ* 2:327, 1868.

Various means of separating the prefrontal cortex from the rest of the brain (procedures called *prefrontal lobotomy* or *prefrontal leukotomy)* were used in the first half of the twentieth century as a treatment for certain severe psychoses and other conditions, but these operations have been largely abandoned in favor of therapy with drugs. The procedures were done bilaterally, but similar (though less pronounced) effects were seen after unilateral operations. There was considerable variation from one patient to another, but individuals so treated typically became carefree and often apparently euphoric, which was the beneficial effect sought; someone suffering from intractable pain, for example, would admit that there was no decrease in the pain after a prefrontal leukotomy but would no longer be bothered by it. Unfortunately, many also lost some of their capacity to do things for a delayed reward and were inclined not to observe social norms in their behavior; powers of concentration, attention span, initiative and spontaneity, and abstract reasoning all suffered.

These effects are obviously difficult to quantify or to discuss in terms of anatomical bases. Equivalent lesions in nonhuman primates produce much less complex syndromes, at least as far as can be determined by objective measurements. All we can do at this juncture is point out that the prefrontal cortex has direct access to the activity of all the other cerebral lobes (via the long association bundles mentioned earlier) (Figure 15-9) and so has abundant data at hand. The extensive interconnections between the prefrontal cortex and the dorsomedial nucleus of the thalamus also play an important role, as shown by the observation that lesions of the dorsomedial nucleus have effects in some ways similar to those of prefrontal leukotomy. Knowledge is incomplete concerning the relationship of different aspects of the prefrontal syndrome to damage in different cortical areas, but it is clear that such localization exists, at least to some extent. For example, emotional changes are more related to damage to the orbital cortex and intellectual deficits more related to damage to the lateral surface of the frontal lobe.

## CORPUS CALLOSUM

The *corpus callosum,* interconnecting the two cerebral hemispheres, is by far the largest fiber bundle in the human brain. It contains more than 300 million axons. Most of these fibers interconnect mirror-image sites, but a substantial number end in areas different from those in which they arise (for example, area 17 of one hemisphere projects to areas 18 and 19 of the contralateral hemisphere). Nearly all cortical areas receive commissural fibers (Figure 15-21), with a few notable exceptions like the hand area of the somatosensory cortex and all of area 17 not representing areas adjacent to the vertical midline. The commissural fibers to and from much of the temporal lobe, particularly the middle and inferior temporal gyri, pass through the *anterior commissure*.

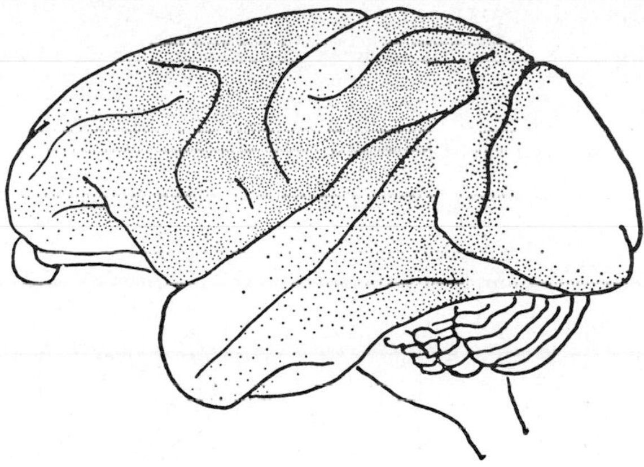

FIGURE 15-21
Distribution of degenerating axon terminals after section of the corpus callosum and anterior commissure in a rhesus monkey. Note that with a few exceptions (for example, most of the primary visual cortex—exposed here on the lateral surface of the occipital lobe—and the hand area of somatosensory cortex), the cerebral cortex is blanketed with commissural connections.

From Myers RE: Phylogenetic studies of commissural connexions. In Ettlinger EG, deReuck AVS, Porter R, editors: *Functions of the corpus callosum*, Edinburgh, 1965, J. and A. Churchill, Ltd.

We all know from common experience that something initially seen in one visual field can be identified if presented later in the contralateral visual field (for example, we can recognize a picture after it has been reversed left-to-right). The same is true for other sensory modalities such as touch*; similar transfers from one hemisphere to the other can be demonstrated easily in experimental animals. The importance of the corpus callosum for these transfers can be shown dramatically in experiments involving bisection of the optic chiasm of experimental animals. This destroys all fibers crossing from each eye to the contralateral lateral geniculate nucleus, so anything presented to one eye reaches only the ipsilateral cerebral hemisphere. Such animals, despite having bitemporal visual field deficits, continue to show normal transfer of learning from one side to the other. However, if the corpus callosum is also sectioned, the animals no longer show this transfer. It is even possible to train them to give two completely different responses to the same stimulus, depending on which eye sees the stimulus.

Section of the corpus callosum has been used as a treatment of last resort for a few human patients suffering from intractable epilepsy, to prevent seizures from spreading from one hemisphere to the other. The procedure generally

*Even though parts of the somatosensory and visual cortices receive no commissural fibers, all areas of the parietal and occipital association cortices do, so each hemisphere has access to data from the contralateral half of the body and the outside world.

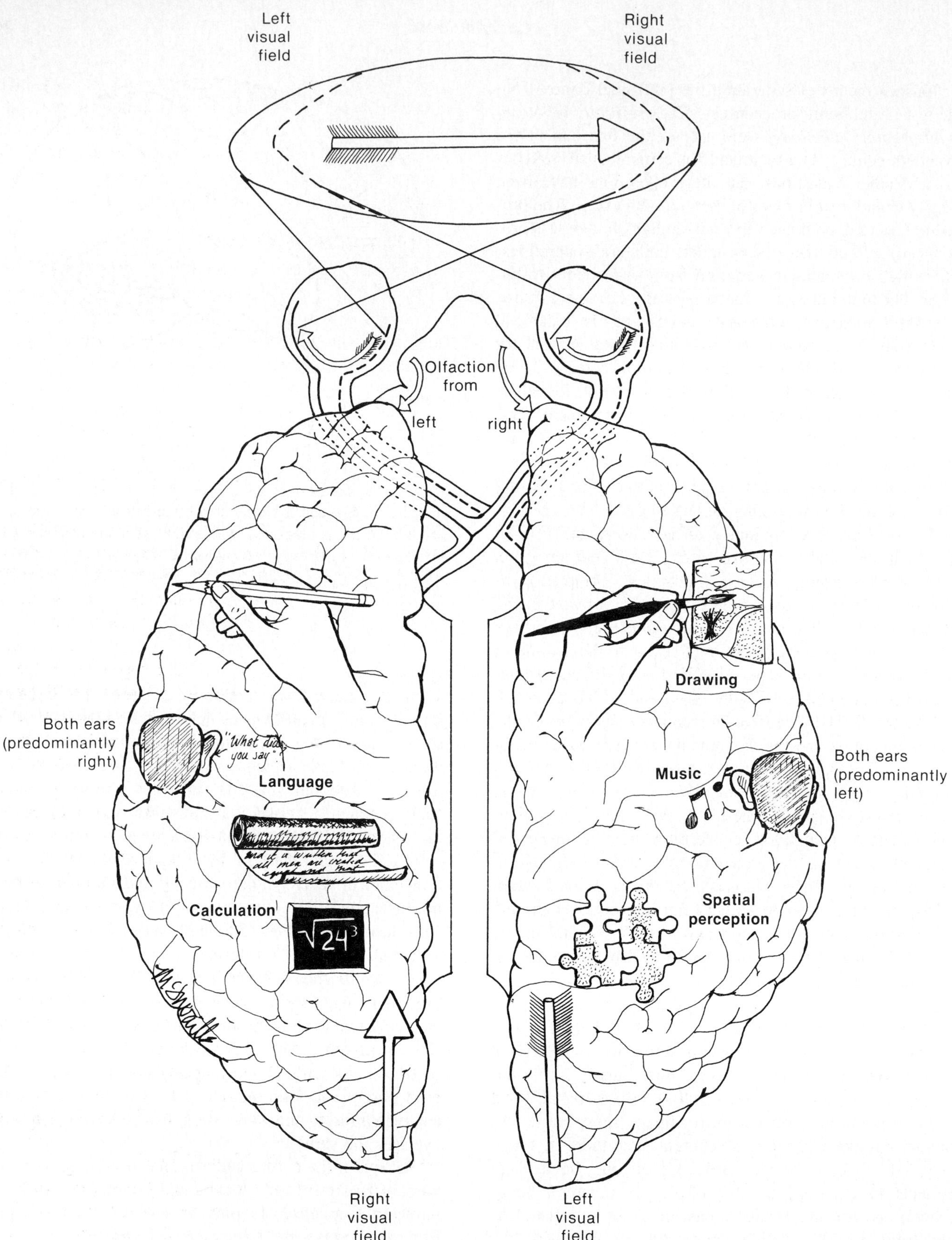


FIGURE 15-22

Schematic illustration of the different functional specializations of the two hemispheres as determined from studies of patients after callosal section.

Modified from Sperry, RW: Lateral specialization in the surgically separated hemispheres. In Schmitt, FO, Worden FG, editors. The neurosciences: third study program, Cambridge, Mass., 1974, The MIT Press.

ameliorates the epilepsy, and the patients seem otherwise more or less unchanged, but careful testing reveals some remarkable alterations. Words flashed in the right visual field can be read normally, but words flashed in the left field cannot be read, and the patient denies having seen them. As far as spoken or written responses to visual stimuli are concerned, these "split-brain" patients behave as though they have a left homonymous hemianopia. This is thoroughly consistent with the notion of dominance of the left hemisphere for language, which can organize and execute a spoken or written response; visual stimuli in the left field reach the right hemisphere, which no longer has access to the language areas. However, it is easy to show that the right hemisphere is still quite functional. For example, a picture of some object can be flashed in the left visual field and the patient asked to pick out that object manually from an assortment on a table; this can be done (usually with the left hand), even though the patient denies having seen anything. This is a clear indication that the right hemisphere has some capacity for the comprehension of language and the organization of nonverbal responses.

Continued testing of such patients has yielded some general concepts of hemisphere function that, by and large, confirm and extend the conclusions drawn from studies of patients with unilateral brain damage (Figure 15-22). The left hemisphere in most people appears to be dominant not only for language but also for mathematical ability and the ability to solve problems in a sequential, logical fashion. The right hemisphere seems to be superior in musical skills, in recognition of faces, and in tasks requiring comprehension of spatial relationships; after callosal section a patient is likely to be able to draw and copy better with the left hand than with the right hand. Problems are solved in a more comprehensive, holistic fashion by the right hemisphere. As noted previously, the right hemisphere also has some capacity for comprehension of language. The corpus callosum ordinarily welds the two hemispheres together into a unitary consciousness. After section of the corpus callosum, individuals develop close cooperation between their two hemispheres and subtle methods of cross-cuing, but nevertheless each hemisphere appears to have separate conscious experiences, creating a knotty philosophical problem.*

These same studies of split-brain patients also indicate that there is probably somewhat more bilaterality in the connections of somatic sensory and motor pathways than is commonly acknowledged. With time and practice, each hemisphere acquires not only a great deal of control over ipsilateral muscles but also considerable awareness of stimuli applied to the ipsilateral side of the body.

### Disconnection syndromes

It stands to reason that we could not reach out for a seen object unless visual information could somehow influence the activity of the motor cortex. This has been corroborated experimentally in monkeys: cuts in the parietal lobe that destroy the long association bundles connecting the frontal and occipital lobes interfere with the ability to carry out movements guided by vision in the contralateral visual field. *Disconnection syndromes* similar in principle have been proposed (and in some cases have been shown fairly convincingly) to account for some of the complex disorders that follow cerebral damage in humans.

The classic example of a disconnection syndrome is *pure word blindness,* or *alexia without agraphia*. Patients with this rare condition are able to write (thus no agraphia) but are unable to read anything (alexia)—even words they have just finished writing; they almost always have a right homonymous hemianopia as well. Alexia without agraphia occasionally follows a stroke that involves the left posterior cerebral artery if it causes destruction of the left visual cortex (hence the hemianopia) and of the splenium of the corpus callosum (Figure 15-23). As a result the language areas (in particular the left angular gyrus) are cut off from all visual input; the destroyed left visual cortex can supply none, and the intact right visual cortex can supply none, since the route through the corpus callosum is blocked. Since the language areas are undamaged and still connected to the motor cortex, verbal and written language can still be produced.

Several other disconnection syndromes have been proposed or demonstrated, and the concept is valuable in terms of understanding some disorders of higher cerebral function. Callosal section represents an ultimate example. Conduction aphasia (discussed earlier), in which Broca's and Wernicke's areas are disconnected from each other, provides another example. Disconnections of language areas from different sensory areas or from motor cortex have been invoked to explain some cases of agnosia or apraxia.

## CONSCIOUSNESS AND SLEEP

We all have an intuitive understanding of what consciousness means, but no satisfactory definition for it has yet been devised. Instead we usually settle for a listing of things that are present when consciousness is present; this list usually includes self-awareness, access to memories, and the ability to manipulate abstract ideas and to direct one's attention. Discussing the anatomical basis of consciousness is also difficult and ultimately probably impos-

---

*Everything we have seen so far indicates that the surgery has left these people with two separate minds, that is, two separate spheres of consciousness. What is experienced in the right hemisphere seems to be entirely outside the realm of awareness of the left hemisphere. This mental division has been demonstrated in regard to perception, cognition, volition, learning, and memory. One of the hemispheres, the left, dominant or major hemisphere, has speech and is normally talkative and conversant. The other, the minor hemisphere, however, is mute or dumb, being able to express itself only through nonverbal reactions." (Sperry, R.W. In Eccles, J.C., editor: Brain and conscious experience, New York, 1966, Springer-Verlag, Inc.) Not everyone agrees with Sperry's conclusion.

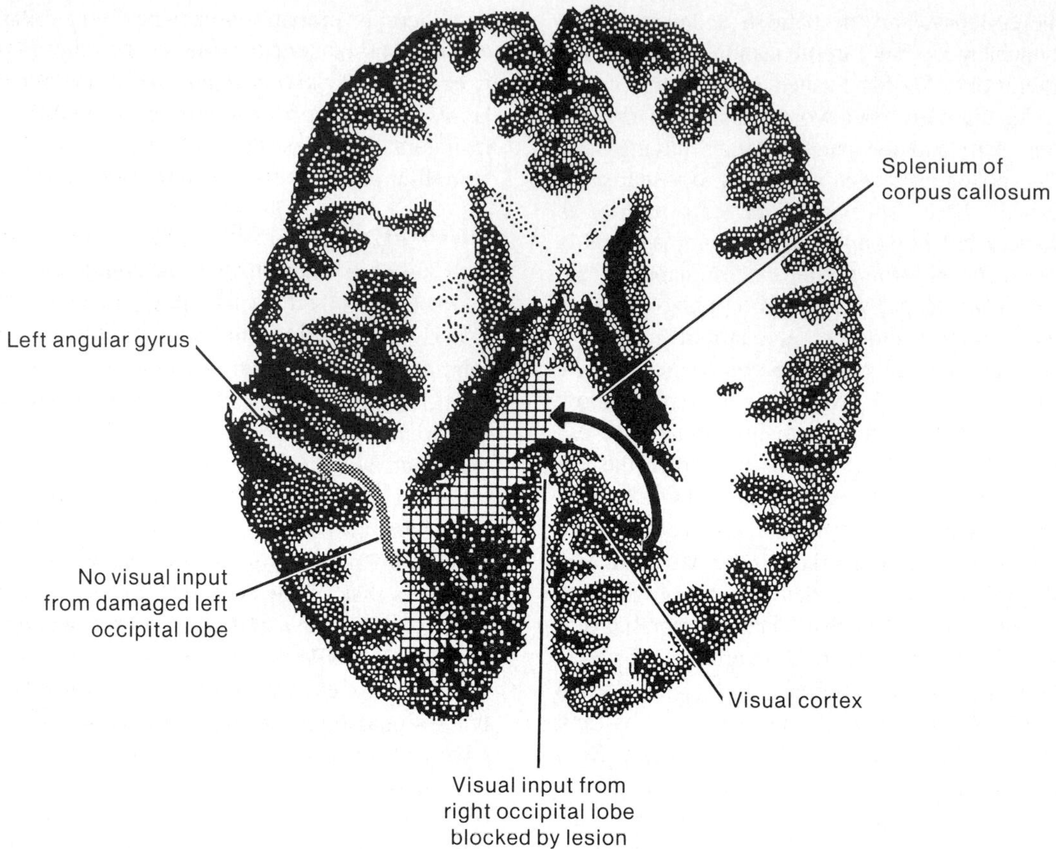


FIGURE 15-23
Diagram of a lesion that would cause pure word blindness (alexia without agraphia). Destruction of the left visual cortex prevents information from the right visual field from reaching language areas of the left hemisphere, particularly the left angular gyrus. Destruction of the splenium of the corpus callosum prevents information from the left visual fields from reaching the language areas, since the route from the right visual cortex to the left hemisphere is blocked. The language areas themselves are undamaged, so the production of language and the comprehension of speech are intact.

sible, since a complete description would require a solution to the age-old problem of the physical relationship between mind and brain. However, we can discuss anatomical structures whose well-being is important for the maintenance of consciousness. The first and most important point is that as far as we can tell, consciousness does not "reside" as a single entity in any particular part of the brain but rather arises somehow from interactions among many neural structures. Although the cerebral cortex is undoubtedly essential for many of the attributes associated with consciousness, remarkably large cortical areas can be destroyed without abolishing consciousness, and no single cortical area appears to be crucial for maintaining it. This is not to say that a fully intact cerebral cortex, all by itself, is conscious. As described in Chapter 8, the ascending reticular activating system (ARAS), part of the brainstem reticular formation, is essential for maintaining normal cortical function. The ARAS receives collaterals from virtually all sensory pathways and projects to the midline and intralaminar nuclei of the thalamus, which in turn project diffusely to widespread cortical areas. Bilateral destruction of the midbrain reticular formation or of the midline and intralaminar nuclei causes coma. (This does not imply that consciousness resides in the reticular formation; your car won't run without a battery, but when it is running, the battery is not the source of power.) Finally, there is good reason to think that other structures such as the basal ganglia, the hypothalamus and the thalamic reticular nucleus participate in the neural interactions whose result is consciousness.

Sleep is a reversible state of unconsciousness that is of great interest, not only because we spend so much time doing it but also because an understanding of the mechanisms of sleep might be expected to have a bearing on the mechanisms of consciousness in general. It was thought for a time that sleep was a passive process reflecting a decreased level of excitation of the ARAS and a consequent "shutting down" of the cerebral cortex. However, it is now apparent that active mechanisms play a major role and that specific neural structures can induce sleep by inhibiting the ARAS.

Our sleep is of two different kinds. The first, which includes several stages, is called *slow-wave* (or *synchronized*) *sleep,* because during it the electroencephalogram (EEG) is dominated by synchronous waves at various low frequencies, principally less than 4 Hz *(delta waves)*. During slow-wave sleep, muscle tone is somewhat reduced, heart rate and breathing are slowed but steady, and subjects awakened from this state seldom report elaborate dreams. Roughly every 90 to 120 minutes we shift into the second type of sleep, called *desynchronized sleep,* in which the EEG is dominated by low-voltage, high-frequency activity that is not organized into obvious waves and is remarkably similar to the activity seen in the waking state. Despite the fact that the EEG looks like that of wakefulness, an individual is harder to awaken from this stage than from slow-wave sleep; as a result, desynchronized sleep is also called *paradoxical sleep*. Desynchronized sleep is a very peculiar state, with several other distinctive properties: there is a nearly complete abolition of muscle tone, and the transmission of impulses over at least some sensory pathways is greatly decreased; blood pressure falls, and heart rate and breathing become erratic; we become lizardlike, in the sense that hypothalamic regulation of body temperature ceases. Superimposed on this background are coincident phasic events. There are bursts of inhibition of motor mechanisms, so the last vestige of muscle tone is eliminated for brief periods. Some twitching movements manage to break through the inhibition, most prominently bursts of rapid eye movements (REMs). The latter phenomenon gives rise to the most commonly used name for desynchronized sleep, which is *REM sleep*. Subjects awakened from REM sleep are likely to report that they were having a visually detailed dream.

Many aspects of the anatomical substrate of sleep have been worked out in experimental animals, and the reticular formation figures prominently in these mechanisms (Figure 15-24). Confirmation for humans is difficult to come by, since processes that damage the brainstem reticular formation to any great extent are usually fatal. The following ac-

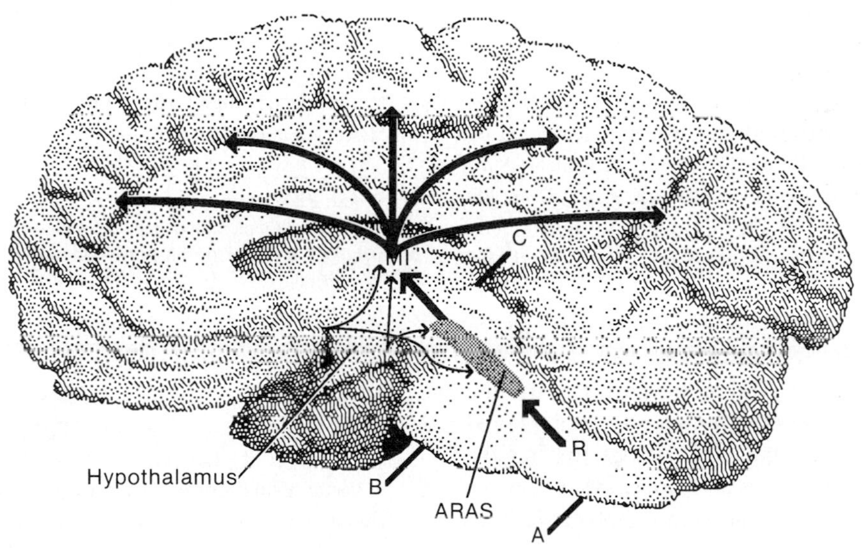


FIGURE 15-24
Summary diagram of neural structures and connections important for maintenance of the sleep-wake cycle. The ascending reticular activating system (ARAS) maintains wakefulness by acting on the cerebral cortex in a generalized manner through the midline and intralaminar nuclei of the thalamus *(MI)*. The ARAS is periodically turned off by projections from the medullary and pontine reticular formation *(R)*, inducing sleep. Diencephalic centers are also capable of inducing sleep and wakefulness via connections that are not completely understood. Separate collections of neurons in the pons are responsible for triggering periods of REM sleep. Damage caudal to point *A* causes no changes in the sleep-wakefulness cycle. Damage and point *B* disconnects sleep-inducing portions of the reticular formation from the ARAS, causing nearly constant wakefulness of the forebrain. (However, such a lesion is extremely unlikely). Damage at point *C* disconnects the ARAS from the forebrain, causing coma.

count is therefore based mainly on animal studies, but the clinical data available about humans are generally consistent with these results.

Stimulation of the midline and intralaminar nuclei at low frequencies produces sleep and synchronization of the EEG, so this part of the thalamus is considered to be a sort of final switching mechanism into which other sleep-inducing mechanisms funnel. The EEG of an animal whose brainstem has been transected in the rostral midbrain shows constant synchronized activity indicative of slow-wave sleep, at least in the acute stages after the operation. This reflects the fact that the ARAS has been disconnected from the forebrain. As long as the reticular formation is still connected to the forebrain (as, for example, after a transection of the upper cervical spinal cord), an animal shows all the standard EEG signs of cycling through wakefulness and the various stages of sleep. Some insight into what turns the ARAS off and on is provided by transecting the brainstem at a midpontine level. It might be expected that in such a case the animal would show either normal sleep and wakefulness (if this lesion leaves enough of the reticular formation attached to the forebrain) or constant sleep (if too much of the reticular formation is removed by such a lesion). Instead the animal shows signs of constant wakefulness rostral to the lesion, at least during the acute stages after the operation. This indicates not only that the parts of the ARAS crucial for wakefulness are contained in the midbrain reticular formation but also that parts of the medullary and caudal pontine reticular formation are responsible for periodically turning the ARAS off and on. No one knows where the clockwork for this mechanism in the caudal brainstem is located, but there are indications that some cells of the *raphe nuclei* of the reticular formation, which use serotonin as their neurotransmitter, are important components. One piece of evidence supporting this concept is the observation that depletion of the brain's serotonin, either by pharmacological techniques or by destruction of the raphe nuclei, causes an insomnia that can be reversed promptly by administration of serotonin. This is not a total explanation, however, because the insomnia partially resolves even if serotonin levels are not restored.

In addition to the brainstem mechanisms that regulate sleep and wakefulness, there is a second system located more rostrally. Encephalitic damage to the posterior hypothalamus of humans causes the hypersomnia of sleeping sickness, and stimulation of this area in sleeping animals causes awakening. Conversely, damage to the general region of the preoptic area and the base of the forebrain has been shown to cause insomnia, and stimulation of this area causes sleep. How this anterior "sleep center" and posterior "wakefulness center" interact with the brainstem mechanisms is not fully known. There are indications that in an intact animal the forebrain centers act in part directly on the ARAS to achieve a unified sleep-waking cycle. On the other hand, it is also known that there are direct projections from the hypothalamus and basal forebrain to the thalamus and cerebral cortex, and that 10 to 15 days after a mesencephalic transection the forebrain once again begins to cycle through the synchronized and desynchronized EEGs of apparent sleep and wakefulness.

The basic anatomical control mechanisms for REM sleep are more localized than are those for slow-wave sleep and are entirely contained in the caudal brainstem. This is shown perhaps most dramatically in the case of a cat with only those parts of its CNS up to the midpons left intact. Such an animal obviously is unable to show EEG signs of sleep and wakefulness, but at periodic intervals throughout the day and night, it does have episodes that include all the parts of REM sleep of which the spinal cord and caudal brainstem are capable. That is, there are periodic spells of decreased muscle tone and twitches of the lateral recti (the only way for REMs to be expressed in this condition).* The timing mechanism for the initiation of REM sleep is thought to be in the caudal pontine reticular formation. This timing mechanism somehow triggers neurons in various parts of the pontine and rostral medullary reticular formation, which mediate the assorted tonic processes and phasic events of REM sleep. Neurons in the vicinity of the locus ceruleus seem to be particularly important for some parts of REM sleep, notably the loss of muscle tone. Cats with bilateral damage near (but not necessarily including) the locus ceruleus have REM sleep without atonia and appear to "act out" their dreams.

REM sleep normally occurs only in the midst of periods of slow-wave sleep, so it is assumed that the REM sleep mechanisms must ordinarily be primed or triggered by the centers for slow-wave sleep.

*These REMs in the absence of cerebral hemispheres are one bit of evidence for the generally accepted conclusion that, whatever the eye movements of REM sleep are, they do not represent "looking-at-a-dream" movements.

## ADDITIONAL READINGS

Ahern GL et al.: Right hemisphere advantage for evaluating emotional facial expressions, *Cortex* 27:193, 1991.

Allen GV et al.: Organization of vesceral and limbic connections in the insular cortex in the rat, *J Comp Neurol* 311:1, 1991.

Barbas, H.: Pattern in the laminar origin of corticocortical connections, *J Comp Neurol* 252:415, 1986.

Benson DF, Zaidel E: *The dual brain; hemispheric specialization in humans,* New York, 1985, The Guilford Press.

Biemond A: The conduction of pain above the level of the thalamus opticus, *Arch Neurol Psychiatry* 75:231, 1956. *Clinical evidence for involvement of S2 in the perception of pain.*

Brinkman J, Kuypers HGJM: Cerebral control of contralateral and ipsilateral arm, hand and finger movements in the split-brain rhesus monkey, *Brain* 96:653, 1973.

Borbély AA, Tobler I: Endogenous sleep-promoting substances and sleep regulation, *Physiol Rev* 69:605, 1989.

Buser PA, Rougeul-Buser A, editors: *Cerebral correlates of con-*

*scious experience,* New York, 1978, Elsevier North-Holland, Inc.

Caramazza A, Hillis AE: Lexical organization of nouns and verbs in the brain, *Nature* 349:788, 1991.

Celesia GG: Organization of auditory cortical areas in man, *Brain* 99:403, 1976.

Critchley M: *The parietal lobes,* London, 1953, Edward Arnold (Publishers), Ltd. *The classic clinical work on the various syndromes resulting from parietal lesions.*

Damasio AR: Aphasia, *N Engl J Med* 326:531, 1992. *A recent lucid review of the various aphasic syndromes, and contemporary notions of their anatomical correlates.*

Eccles JC, editor: *Brain and conscious experience,* New York, 1966, Springer-Verlag, Inc.

Foote SL and Morrison JH: Extrathalamic modulation of cortical function, *Ann Rev Neurosci* 10:67, 1987.

Foster NL, et al: Cerebral mapping of apraxia in Alzheimer's disease by positron emission tomography. *Ann Neurol* 19:139, 1986.

Galaburda AM, et al: Right-left asymmetrics in thc brain, *Science* 199:852, 1978.

Gazzaniga M: *The social brain: discovering the networks of the mind,* New York, 1985, Basic Books, Inc. *A popularized account of left hemisphere—right hemisphere research based on callosally sectioned humans, by one of the principal workers in this field.*

Geschwind N: Disconnexion syndromes in animals and man, I and II, *Brain* 88:237 and 585, 1965. *A scholarly and influential paper arguing forcefully for the concept of complex syndromes caused by disconnections of various cerebral areas from one another.*

Geschwind N: The organization of language and the brain, *Science* 170:940, 1970.

Goldman PS, Nauta WJH: Columnar distribution of corticocortical fibers in the frontal association, limbic, and motor cortex of the developing rhesus monkey, *Brain Res* 122:393, 1977. *Pretty pictures.*

Gordon HW, Bogen JE: Hemispheric lateralization of singing after intracarotid sodium amylobarbitone, *J Neurol Neurosurg Psychiatry* 37:727, 1974.

Graff-Radford NR, Welsh K, Godersky J: Callosal apraxia, *Neurology* 37:100, 1987.

Gücer G: The effect of sleep upon the transmission of afferent activity in the somatic afferent system, *Exp Brain Res* 34:287, 1979.

Haaxma R, Kuypers HGJM: Intrahemispheric cortical connexions and visual guidance of hand and finger movements in the rhesus monkey, *Brain* 98:239, 1975. *Direct experimental demonstration of a type of disconnection syndrome.*

Heilman KM, et al: The right hemisphere: neuropsychological functions, *J Neurosurg.* 64:693, 1986.

Heilman KM, Valenstein E: *Clinical neuropsychology,* ed. 2, New York, 1985, Oxford University Press.

Heiss WD, et al: Regional cerebral glucose metabolism in man during wakefulness, sleep, and dreaming, *Brain Res* 327:362, 1985.

Herkenham M: Laminar organization of thalamic projections to thc rat ncocortcx, *Science* 207:532, 1980.

Herron J, editor: *Neuropsychology of left-handedness,* New York, 1979, Academic Press, Inc.

Hobson JA: Sleep and dreaming, *J Neurosci* 10:371, 1990. *An interesting recent review indicating simultaneously how much and how little we know about sleep.*

Jones EG: Neurotransmitters in the cerebral cortex, *J Neurosurg.* 65:135, 1986.

Jones EG, Coulter JD, Wise SP: Commissural columns in the sensory-motor cortex of monkeys, *J Comp Neurol* 188:113, 1979.

Jones EG, Powell TPS: An anatomical study of converging sensory pathways within the cerebral cortex of the monkey, *Brain* 93:793, 1970. *A study of the stepwise radiations of auditory, visual, and somatosensory information from the primary receiving areas to parts of the association cortex; done by the straightforward but clever technique of lesioning a primary area, tracing the degenerating fibers, and making lesions where the degeneration terminates.*

Jouandet ML, Gazzaniga MS: Cortical field of origin of the anterior commissure of the rhesus monkey, *Exp Neurol* 66:381, 1979.

Kenshalo DR, Jr., Isensee O: Responses of primate SI cortical neurons to noxious stimuli, *J Neurophysiol* 50:1479, 1983.

Kertesz A, Lesk D, McCabe P: Isotope localization of infarcts in aphasia, *Arch Neurol.* 34:590, 1977.

LaMotte RH, Mountcastle VB: Disorders in somesthesis following lesions of parietal lobe, *J Neurophysiol* 42: 400, 1979.

LeDoux JE, Wilson DH, Gazzaniga MS: A divided mind: observations on the conscious properties of the separated hemispheres, *Ann Neurol* 2:417, 1977. *An individual with some bilateral language representation may not give the same responses with each hemisphere after section of the corpus callosum.*

Lhermitte F: Human autonomy and the frontal lobes. II. Patient behavior in complex and social situations: the "environmental dependency syndrome," *Ann Neurol* 19:335, 1986. *Quantitative measurement of the effects of prefrontal damage is difficult, but simple observation provides fascinating insights.*

Libet B, et al: Subjective referral of the timing for a conscious sensory experience: a functional role for the somatosensory specific projection system in man, *Brain* 102:193, 1979. *How do we decide when a tactile stimulus occurs? Is it at the instant of physical contact, or when the first electrical activity reaches the postcentral gyrus, or after this activity has rattled around the cortex for awhile? A fascinating and provocative paper that addresses this question experimentally.*

Mesulam M-M: *Principles of behavioral neurology,* Philadelphia, 1985, FA Davis Co.

Morrison JH, Molliver ME, Grzanna R: Noradrenergic innervation of cerebral cortex: widespread effects of local cortical lesions, *Science* 205:313, 1979.

Mukhametov LM: Sleep in marine mammals, *Exp Brain Res Suppl* 8:227, 1984. *Porpoises appear to have evolved the novel technique of sleeping with one hemisphere at a time.*

Nauta WJH: The problem of the frontal lobe: a reinterpretation, *J Psychiatr Res* 8:167, 1971.

Pearlman AL, Birch J, Meadows JC: Cerebral color blindness: an acquired defect in hue discrimination, *Ann Neurol* 5:253, 1979.

Penfield W, Boldrey E: Somatic motor and sensory representation in the cerebral cortex of man as studied by electrical stimulation, *Brain* 60:389, 1937.

Penfield W, Rasmussen T: *The cerebral cortex of man,* New York, 1950, Macmillan, Inc. *A review of the results of cortical stimulations of a large series of patients and of the results of localized cortical excisions from these patients.*

Penfield W, Roberts L: *Speech and brain-mechanisms,* Princeton, N.J., 1959, Princeton University Press.

Plum F, Posner JB: *Diagnosis of stupor and coma,* ed 3, Philadelphia, 1980, FA Davis Company.

Powell TPS: *Certain aspects of the intrinsic organization of the cerebral cortex.* In Pompeiano O, Ajmone Marsan C: Brain mechanisms and perceptual awareness, IBRO Monograph Series, vol. 8, New York, 1981, Raven Press. *A nice review of the evidence concerning uniform organization of the cerebral cortex.*

Price BH et al: The comportmental learning disabilities of early frontal lobe damage, *Brain* 113:1383, 1990. *An important paper about two patients who had suffered extensive prefrontal damage at an early age, indicating that "In comparison with other types of brain damage which disrupt cognitive development, frontal damage acquired early in life appears to provide the neurological substrate for a special type of learning disability in the realms of insight, foresight, social judgement, empathy, and complex reasoning."*

Purpura DP: Dendritic spine "dysgenesis" and mental retardation, *Science* 186:1126, 1974.

Rechtschaffen A, et al: Physiological correlates of prolonged sleep deprivation in rats, *Science* 221:182, 1983.

Rose FC: *Progress in aphasiology,* (Adv Neurol, Vol. 42), New York, 1984, Raven Press.

Ross ED: The aprosodias: functional-anatomic organization of the affective components of language in the right hemisphere, *Arch Neurol* 38:561, 1981.

Rubens AB, Mahowald MW, Hutton JT: Asymmetry of the lateral (sylvian) fissures in man, *Neurology* 26:620, 1976.

Russell IS, Ochs S: Localization of a memory trace in one cortical hemisphere and transfer to the other hemisphere, *Brain* 86:37, 1963. *We know that inputs spread to both hemispheres under normal circumstances via the corpus callosum. This interesting paper describes what happens if one hemisphere is temporarily inactivated during acquisition of a memory.*

Sakai K: Central mechanisms of paradoxical sleep, *Exp Brain Res Suppl* 8:3, 1984.

Sallanon M et al: Long-lasting insomnia induced by preoptic neuron lesions and its transient reversal by muscimol injection into the posterior hypothalamus in the cat, *Neurosci* 32:669, 1989.

Sauerland, EK and Harper RM: The human tongue during sleep: electromyographic activity of the genioglossus muscle, *Exp. Neurol.* 51:160, 1976. *If the muscles of your tongue follow the general pattern and become flaccid during REM sleep, then why don't you get into trouble by inhaling it? Read this and find out.*

Shapiro CM, et al: Slow-wave sleep: a recovery period after exercise, *Science* 214:1253, 1981. *An old hypothesis about sleep is that we do it as some sort of "restorative" process. Our sleep patterns don't change much after ordinary exercise, but after running a marathon they do.*

Sperry RW: *Lateral specialization in the surgically separated hemispheres.* In Schmitt FO, Worden FG, editors: The neurosciences: third study program, Cambridge, Mass, 1974, The MIT Press. *A general review of results from humans with a sectioned corpus callosum by the principal figure in this type of research.*

Steriade M, McCarley RW: *Brainstem control of wakefulness and sleep*, New York, 1990, Plenum Press.

Stuss DT, Benson DF: *The frontal lobes,* New York, 1986, Raven Press.

Szentagothai J: The neuron network of the cerebral cortex: a functional interpretation, *Proc R Soc Lond* B201:219, 1978.

Talbot JD et al: Multiple representations of pain in human cerebral cortex, *Science* 251:1355, 1991. *PET scanning studies indicating that the perception of pain is accompanied by increased blood flow at least in the contralateral S1, S2, and cingulate gyrus.*

Teuber HL: *The brain and human behavior.* In Held R, Leibowitz HW, Teuber HL, editors: Handbook of sensory physiology. Vol. 8. Perception, New York, 1978, Springer-Verlag, Inc. *An interesting, scholarly, wide-ranging correlation of deficits and brain damage in humans and experimental animals.*

Van Essen DC, Anderson CH, Fellman DJ: Information processing in the primate visual system: an integrated systems perspective, *Science* 255:419, 1992. *An overview of the dozens of visual areas that have been described in primate cerebral cortex.*

Vertes RP: Brainstem control of the events of REM sleep, *Prog Neurobiol* 22:241, 1984.

Villablanca J: Behavioral and polygraphic study of "sleep" and "wakefulness" in chronic decerebrate cats, Electroencephalogr *Clin Neurophysiol* 21: 562, 1966. *In the chronic state after a rostral mesencephalic transection, the portions of the CNS both rostral and caudal to the transection are capable of some manifestations of sleep and wakefulness; amazingly enough, they do so with completely independent rhythms.*

Wada JA, Davis AE: Fundamental nature of human infant's brain asymmetry, *Can J Neurol Sci* 4:203, 1977. *We are born not only with built-in anatomical asymmetries but apparently also with built-in physiological asymmetries.*

Wada J, Rasmussen T: Intracarotid injection of sodium amytal for the lateralization of cerebral speech dominance: experimental and clinical observations, *J Neurosurg* 17:266, 1960.

Watson RT, Valenstein E, Day A, Heilman KM: Normal tactile threshold in monkeys with neglect, *Neurology* 34:917, 1984.

Whitsel BL, et al: Thalamic projections to S-I in macaque monkey, *J Comp Neurol* 178:385, 1978.

Woolsey TA, van der Loos H: The structural organization of layer IV in the somatosensory region (SI) of mouse cerebral cortex: the description of a cortical field composed of discrete cytoarchitectonic units, *Brain Res* 17:205, 1970. *A special kind of columnar organization described in a delightful paper.*

Yamadori A, et al: Preservation of singing in Broca's aphasia, *J Neurol Neurosurg Psychiatry* 40:221, 1977.

Young AW: *Functions of the right cerebral hemisphere,* New York, 1983, Academic Press.

# CHAPTER 16

## Olfactory and Limbic Systems

We seldom perceive things in a completely neutral fashion. Various sights and sounds make us happy, sad, or angry; certain odors can make some individuals positively ecstatic. There is also a two-way connection between these emotional aspects of perception on the one hand and thoughts and memories on the other: appropriate aromas can conjure up images of meals and wines consumed in the past; in addition, the remembrance of something in the past can stir the same emotions that accompanied the original event, and even thinking about something that has not happened can arouse emotions. Assuming that "thinking" depends heavily on the neocortex, it would seem likely that the anatomical substrate for feelings and emotions would at least be closely connected with the neocortex. The same system would also need to be heavily interconnected with the hypothalamus, since sensory inputs that arouse an emotion also initiate autonomic responses such as salivating and gearing up the alimentary tract or pumping adrenalin and diverting blood to skeletal muscles. Finally, the types of stimuli that elicit emotion-laden responses in us—and the responses themselves—are, in a more general sense, crucial to all animals, for these are the drive-related activities central to the preservation of individuals and their species, activities like feeding, defense, and sexual behavior.

The *limbic system* is the name given to the portions of the brain primarily concerned with such responses and behavior. As discussed in some detail later in the chapter, it includes the *cingulate* and *parahippocampal gyri* (see Figure 2-8), the *amygdala,* and the *hippocampal formation.* In view of the preceding discussion, it is not surprising that the components of the limbic system appeared early in vertebrate phylogeny and that in its connections the limbic system is interposed between the neocortex and the hypothalamus.

The olfactory nerve is the only one that projects directly to the telencephalon; as a result, the telencephalon of primitive vertebrates has been considered to be a processing station for olfactory information and the limbic system to be related to olfactory structures. Although there is some reason to think that the brains of all vertebrates are more similar to each other than had previously been suspected (so that all telencephalons play a role in the processing of all types of sensory information), the olfactory and limbic systems are still customarily discussed together. As further recognition of their phylogenetic antiquity, parts of the olfactory and limbic systems are referred to as the *paleocortex* and *archicortex*. Use of the terms varies somewhat from one author to another, but the palecortex is approximately the same thing as the olfactory cortex, and the archicortex is equivalent to the hippocampal formation. The paleocortex and archicortex, collectively called the *allocortex* or *heterogenetic cortex,* are structurally simpler than the neocortex and have fewer than six layers (in most areas, only three layers).

### OLFACTORY SYSTEM

#### Olfactory epithelium

The olfactory system begins peripherally with the *olfactory epithelium,* a pigmented, yellowish patch of cells that occupies about 2 sq cm of the roof and adjacent walls of the nasal cavity on each side. Each patch of olfactory epithelium consists of about 5 million receptor cells interspersed with supporting cells and small glands (called *Bowman's glands*). Sensory endings of the trigeminal nerve are also found in the olfactory epithelium. The trigeminal endings are responsible for the noxious sensation (not really one of smell) elicited by irritants like concentrated ammonia. The *olfactory receptors* are bipolar neurons, each with a single slender dendrite emerging

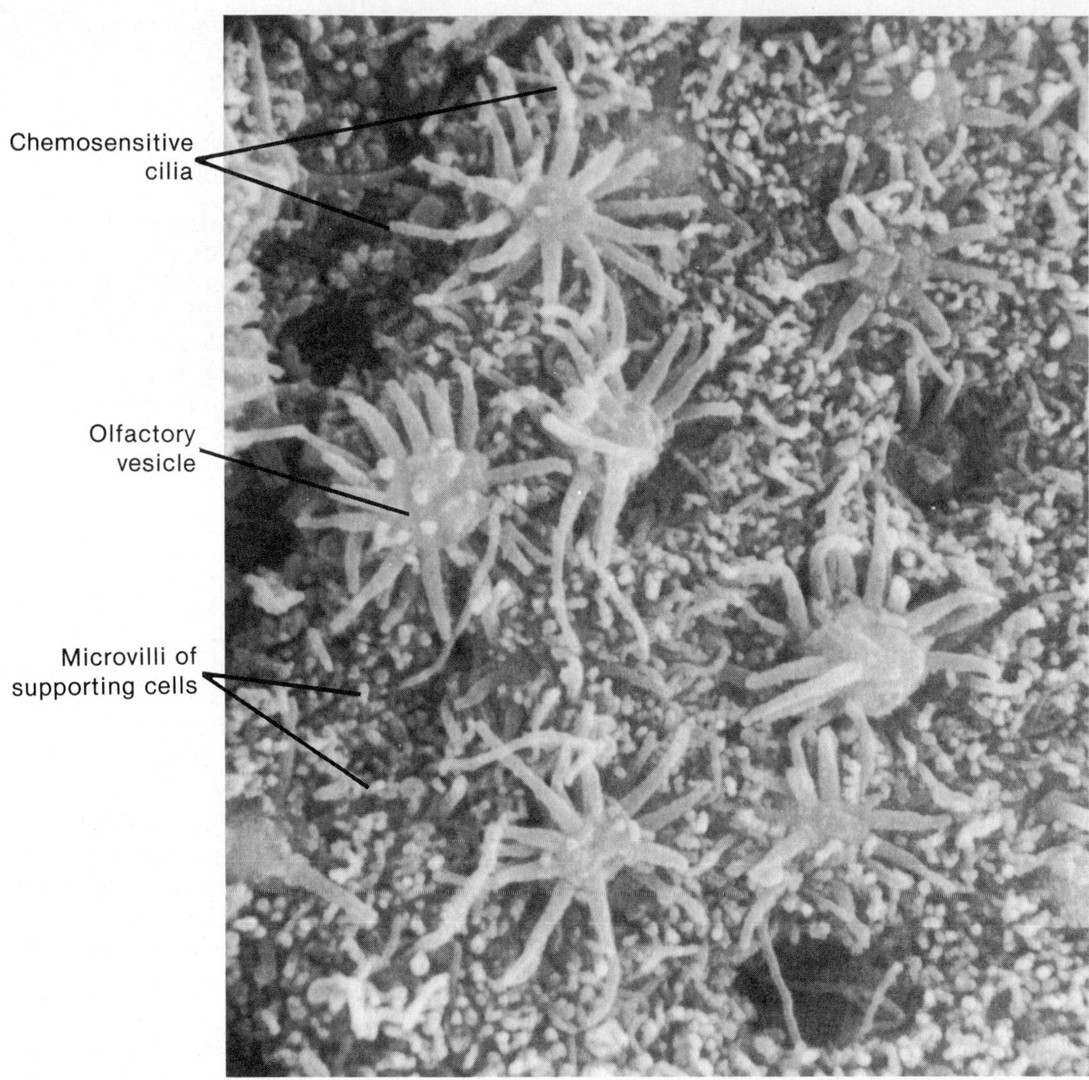


**FIGURE 16-1**
Scanning electron micrograph of the exposed surface of the olfactory epithelium: interspersed in a carpet of microvilli are olfactory vesicles, giving rise to the chemosensitive cilia of the olfactory receptors.
From Tissues and organs: a text of scanning electron microscopy by Richard G. Kessel and Randy H. Kardon. W.H. Freeman and Company. Copyright © 1979.

from one end of its cell body and an axon emerging from the other end (Figures 16-1 and 16-2). The dendrite extends to a bulbous termination, the *olfactory vesicle,* from which a series of cilia spread out over the surface of the epithelium in a layer of mucus secreted by the supporting cells and Bowman's glands. Substances to be smelled dissolve in the mucous layer and stimulate the chemosensitive cilia of the olfactory receptors.

The unmyelinated axons of the olfactory receptors are among the finest (only 0.2 μm in diameter) and most slowly conducting axons in the entire central nervous system. They collect into a series of about 20 small bundles, the *olfactory fila* (from the Latin *filum* meaning thread), which pass through the holes in the cribriform plate of the ethmoid bone and end in the *olfactory bulb.* Collectively the olfactory fila make up the first cranial nerve.

Olfactory receptors are unique among mammalian neurons in that they are replaced throughout life. Individual receptors have a life span of a month or two, and new receptors arise from undifferentiated basal cells of the olfactory epithelium. No one is quite sure how the axons of such newly formed receptors find their way to the proper synaptic sites in the olfactory bulb.

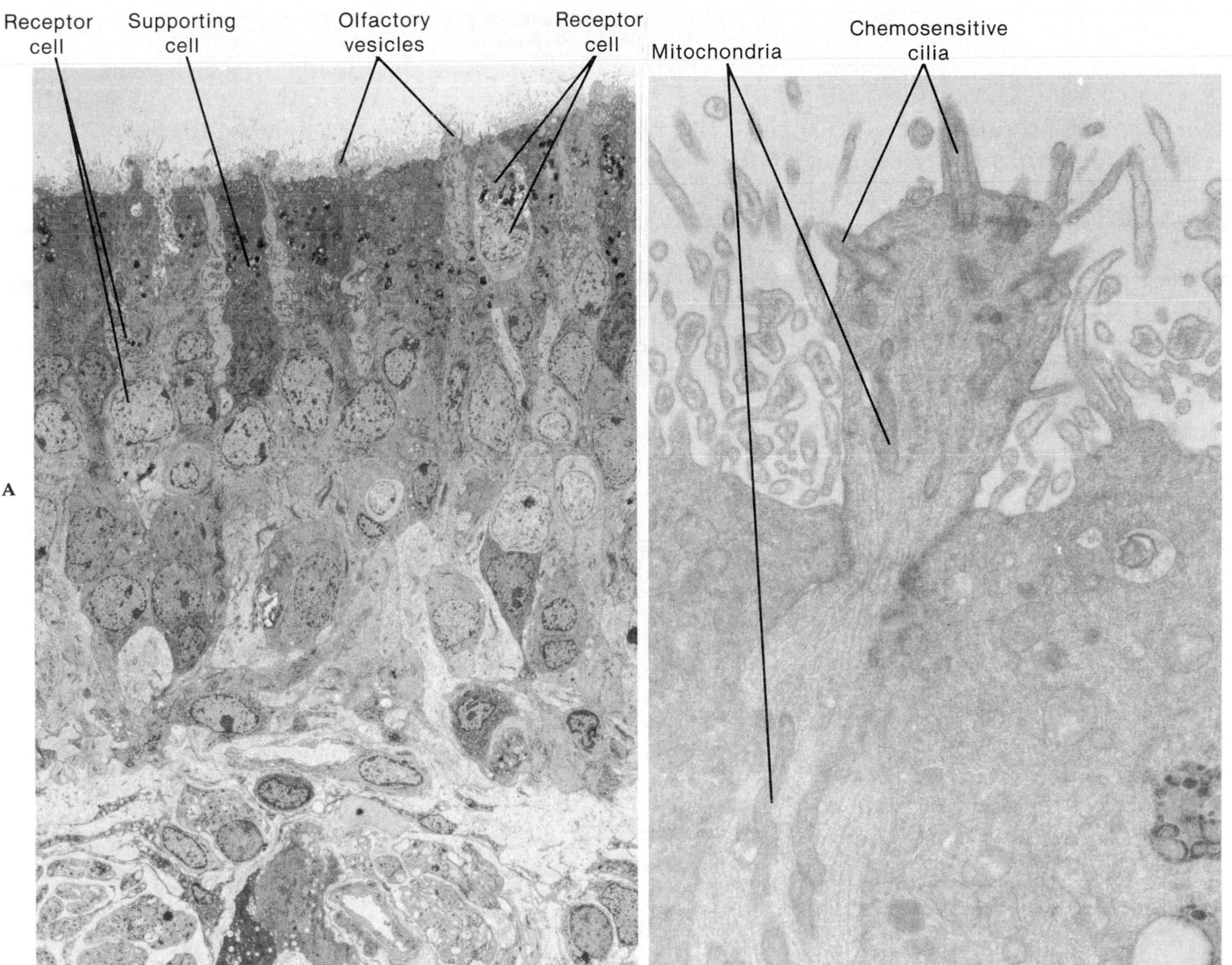


FIGURE 16-2

**A,** Transmission electron micrograph of human olfactory epithelium. Again, supporting cells and receptor cells can be seen. The receptor cell on the right is of a second, poorly understood, type that has microvillar rather than ciliary processes. **B,** Higher magnification micrograph of an olfactory vesicle.

Courtesy of Dr. David Moran and Pamela Eller, University of Colorado Health Sciences Center.

## Olfactory bulb

Animals that depend heavily on their sense of smell (called *macrosmatic* animals; from the Greek *osme* meaning odor) have a well-developed central olfactory apparatus, including a neatly laminated olfactory bulb. In *microsmatic* humans, this lamination is not as apparent, and the olfactory bulb is relatively small and poorly developed. Its most prominent cell type is the *mitral cell,* which has a triangular cell body and was named for its fancied resemblance to a bishop's miter. A mitral cell is configured like a neocortical pyramidal cell in reverse (Figure 16-3); an axon emerges from its apex and moves toward the interior of the bulb to enter the *olfactory tract,* while a dendrite emerges from its base, ascends to the surface of the bulb, and receives contacts from the incoming axons of olfactory receptors. These dendrites spread out in large spherical arborizations 100 to 200 μm in diameter called *glomeruli.* Olfactory axons terminate in these glomeruli with a great deal of convergence; it is estimated that there are 1000 olfactory receptors for each mitral cell in the rabbit. The ol-

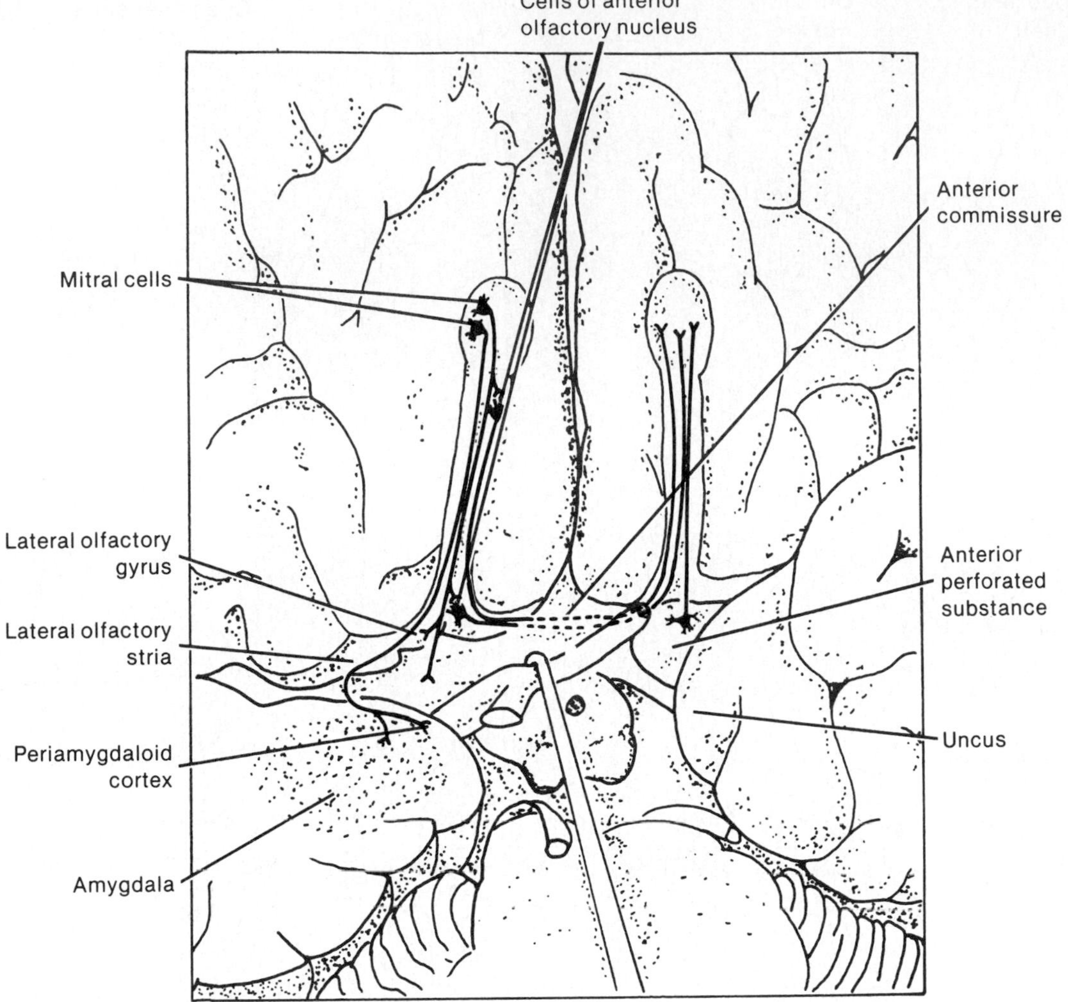


FIGURE 16-3
Olfactory bulb and initial olfactory pathways. Axons of olfactory receptors end on the dendrites of mitral and tufted cells, which in turn send their axons out through the olfactory tract. Collaterals of fibers in the olfactory tract end on cells of the anterior olfactory nucleus. Efferents to the olfactory bulb, shown on the right side of the diagram, arise in the anterior olfactory nucleus (of both sides) and in the vicinity of the anterior perforated substance. (Compare with Figure 16-4.)

factory bulb also contains interneurons (most of them called *granule cells* here as in other regions of the CNS) and a collection of *tufted cells,* which are smaller than mitral cells but also send their dendrites into the glomeruli and their axons into the olfactory tract. The olfactory bulb, like other sensory relays in the CNS, also receives a contingent of efferent fibers that are assumed to regulate or tune its sensitivity in some way. Some of these efferents arise in the vicinity of the *anterior perforated substance.* Others arise from the *anterior olfactory nucleus,* a collective name for clusters of cells scattered all along the olfactory tract.

Axons of mitral and tufted cells proceed caudally in the olfactory tract, giving off collaterals to cells of the anterior olfactory nucleus along the way. Fibers from the anterior olfactory nucleus then project to both olfactory bulbs (Figure 16-3). At the junction between the orbital frontal cortex and the anterior perforated substance, the olfactory tract diverges to form the *olfactory trigone* (Figure 16-4). The two sides of this triangle are formed by the *medial* and *lateral olfactory striae,* and its base merges with the anterior perforated substance. Fibers from the anterior olfactory nucleus enter the medial olfactory stria, cross the midline through the anterior part of the anterior commissure, and project to the contralateral olfactory bulb. Some fibers from the olfactory bulb continue straight back through the

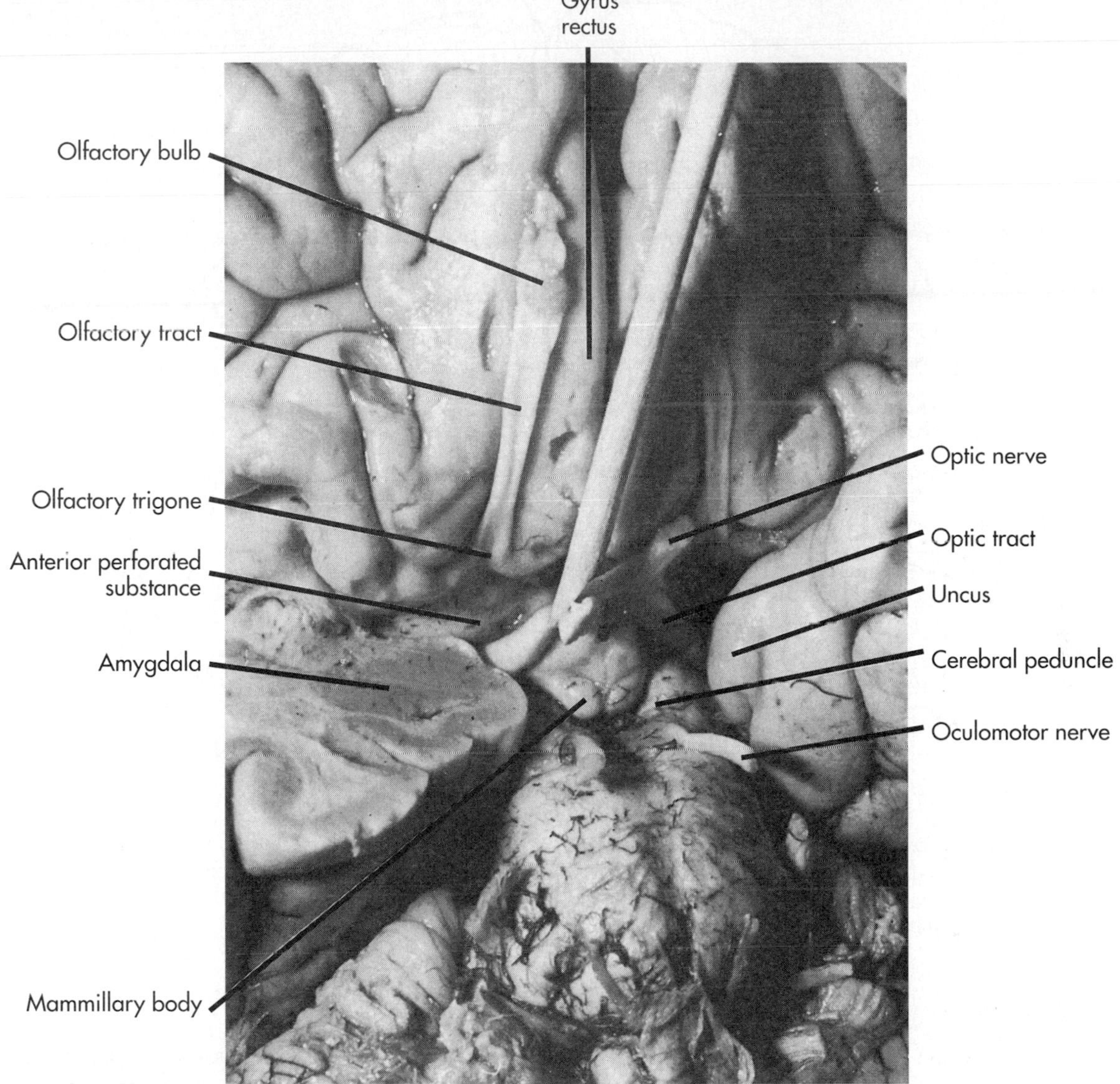


FIGURE 16-4
Olfactory and other structures at the base of the brain. The right temporal pole has been removed and the optic chiasm retracted.

olfactory trigone and end in the adjacent portion of the anterior perforated substance, but most of them enter the lateral olfactory stria. The lateral stria is therefore the principal central projection pathway for the olfactory system.

## Central connections

The lateral olfactory stria travels along the lateral edge of the anterior perforated substance covered by a thin layer of gray matter called the *lateral olfactory gyrus*. When it reaches the posterior border of the anterior perforated substance, it curves up onto the surface of the temporal lobe in the vicinity of the uncus and disappears. Along this course it terminates in two places (Figure 16-5): the *primary olfactory cortex* and a portion of the amygdala.* The primary olfactory cortex consists of the lateral olfactory gyrus and part of the uncus and is itself subdivided into two portions. The lateral olfactory gyrus, together with part of the olfactory region of the uncus, is called the *piriform cortex*. The remainder of the olfactory region of the

*Hence the olfactory system is unique in that no thalamic relay is interposed between receptors and cerebral cortex. However, in this case the cortical destination is paleocortex and the thalamus does become involved in the pathway from olfactory cortex to neocortex.

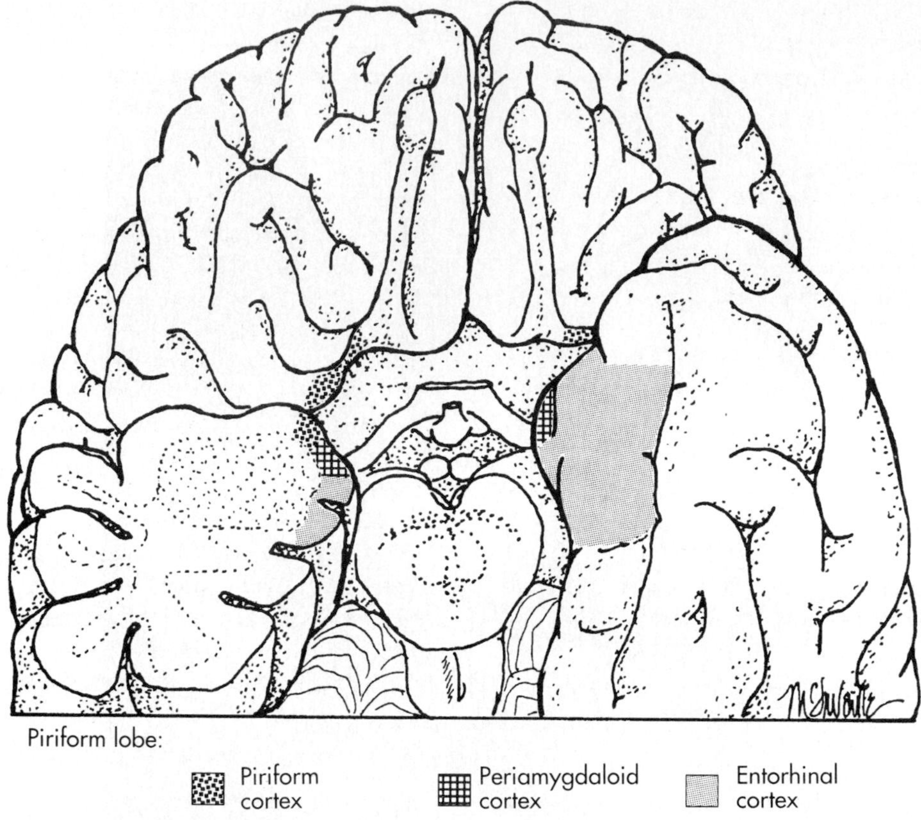


FIGURE 16-5
Diagram of the base of the brain showing the location of the primary olfactory cortex. (Olfactory tract fibers only end in a small, rostral portion of the entorhinal cortex. Most of the entorhinal area serves as part of the olfactory association cortex.) Fibers of the olfactory tract also terminate directly in a portion of the amygdala.

uncus is called the *periamygdaloid cortex,* since it is continuous with the underlying amygdala.

These primary receiving sites for olfactory information project in turn to the hypothalamus and the rest of the amygdala and to the *olfactory association cortex,* part of which occupies the anterior part of the parahippocampal gyrus and corresponds to Brodmann's area 28 (see Figure 15-12). This area, commonly referred to as the *entorhinal cortex,* lies adjacent to the primary olfactory cortex and receives projections directly from the olfactory tract, in addition to projections from the primary olfactory cortex. As is shown later in this chapter, however, the entorhinal cortex does considerably more than serve as the olfactory association cortex. The piriform, periamygdaloid, and entorhinal cortices taken together are sometimes referred to as the *piriform lobe* because this portion of the telencephalon in some vertebrates is relatively large and pear shaped.

Like other sensory systems, the olfactory system has an area of neocortex associated with it. This olfactory cortical area is located posteriorly on the orbital surface of the frontal lobe, extending onto the anterior insula (adjacent to gustatory cortex). The primary olfactory cortex sends information to this neocortical area through a relay in the dorsomedial nucleus of the thalamus, as well as through direct projections.

The olfactory system is unusual in a number of respects. It has already been noted that it is the only sensory system that projects directly to the telencephalon without a thalamic relay. You also may have noticed that central olfactory projections, at least up to the level of the association cortex, are uncrossed.* This implies a strange state of affairs in which each cerebral hemisphere is concerned with the contralateral visual field, the contralateral half of the body, and substances entering the *ipsilateral* nostril. That this is indeed the case has been shown in experiments with patients who had undergone section of the corpus callosum as described in Chapter 15. Although such patients can only name (that is, speak about) things in the right vi-

*While just the opposite of the pattern of connections in most other sensory systems, this uncrossed pathway is reminiscent of that found for gustation, another chemical sense (see Chapter 9). Both senses are represented in adjacent areas of orbital and anterior insular cortex, and both are primarily uncrossed.

sual field or the right hand, they can only name odors presented to the left nostril. Furthermore, if an identifiable odor is presented to one nostril, they can pick out the corresponding object by feeling around with the contralateral, but not the ipsilateral, hand.

### Some functional aspects of the olfactory system

Although our sense of smell is exquisitely sensitive and allows some remarkable discriminations, it is less well developed in humans (and less important in everyday life) than in many other species. As a consequence of some head injuries, the olfactory fila may be torn loose from the olfactory bulb. Someone deprived of the sense of smell (that is, rendered *anosmatic*) by this or some other means is likely to complain less of loss of olfaction than of the fact that food tastes bland. (Much of what we attribute to our sense of taste actually depends on the aromas of what we eat and drink.) However, testing olfaction can sometimes provide useful diagnostic clues. For example, tumors growing at the base of the skull beneath the orbital surface of the frontal lobe can become quite large before they cause any symptoms other than unilateral anosmia.

Piriform cortex has been directly identified as functionally important olfactory cortex in humans, since electrical stimulation there causes olfactory sensations. Clues pointing in the same direction were provided in the nineteenth century by the British neurologist Hughlings Jackson, who noted that seizures originating in the vicinity of the uncus may begin with an illusion of smell or taste, most often an unpleasant one. The seizure may go on to include motor phenomena such as chewing movements or smacking of the lips and alterations of consciousness such as a "dreamy state" or a feeling of déjà vu. Seizures of this type are still known as *uncinate fits*.

## LIMBIC SYSTEM

In 1878 Broca pointed out that a general feature of mammalian brains is a great horseshoe-shaped rim of cortex surrounding the junction between the diencephalon and each cerebral hemisphere (Figure 2-8). The ends of the arc are joined by olfactory areas at the base of the brain so that a complete loop is formed, with the olfactory tract and bulb extending anteriorly like the handle of a tennis racket. He referred to this ring of cortex at the margin of the hemisphere as the *limbic lobe* (from the Latin *limbus* meaning border) and suggested that the entire lobe might be concerned with the sense of smell. However, the limbic lobe includes the cingulate and parahippocampal gyri and the hippocampal formation, and it soon became apparent that olfaction is not the primary responsibility of these areas. For example, although dolphins have no olfactory bulbs and are thought to be completely anosmatic, they nevertheless have well-developed hippocampi. A few rare cases have been reported of humans with congenital absence of the olfactory bulb and tracts but with apparently normal limbic lobes. Finally, more recent anatomical and physiological experiments have shown that, aside from the already mentioned olfactory areas at the base of the brain, the limbic lobe does not receive a particularly large amount of olfactory input.

The limbic lobe does, however, fit many of the previously described criteria for an anatomical substrate for drive-related and emotional behavior. As is shown in the remainder of this chapter, the limbic cortex is connected in one direction with widespread neocortical areas and in another direction with the hypothalamus. Physiological evidence has supported this view, and the conglomerate of the limbic lobe, its connections, and a few additional structures has come to be referred to as the *limbic system*. There is, unfortunately, no universal agreement on the total list of structures that should be included in the term "limbic system," but the concept should be clear by the end of this chapter. All authors would include the cingulate and parahippocampal gyri,* the hippocampal formation, the amygdala, and the *sepal area* (located at the base of the septum pellucidum) (Figure 16-6); most would include the hypothalamus, parts of the midbrain reticular formation, and the olfactory areas. Beyond that, the boundaries get fuzzy; some authors include various of the thalamic and neocortical regions interconnected with undisputed limbic components, whereas others do not.

The interconnections of limbic components are numerous and complex, but the overall concept of the system is not. The output end (in terms of programming or triggering behavioral outputs) is a continuous core of neural tissue extending from the septal area through the hypothalamus and into the midbrain reticular formation. The *medial forebrain bundle* (Figures 10-17 and 10-18) is its principal longitudinal fiber pathway.† Two major limbic subsystems feed into this common output. The first (Figure 16-7) is centered around the hippocampal formation, utilizes the

*Some authors consider the cingulate and parahippocampal gyri to be intermediate in structure between the archicortex and paleocortex on the one hand and the neocortex on the other; they refer to these two gyri as the *mesocortex* or *juxtallocortex*.

†Activation of these output structures is also apparently responsible for triggering some of the feelings that are one object of drive-related behavior. Animals with electrodes implanted in certain CNS locations, if given control of the button that turns on stimulation through these electrodes, will push the button with great zest. Electrode locations that elicit self-stimulation are widespread in the limbic system, but the most effective sites are in the septal area and along the medial forebrain bundle; animals with electrodes there will stimulate themselves at great rates for long periods and may be willing to forego food or sleep or to endure painful stimuli to press the button. Sites with the opposite effect (that is, sites at which animals will try hard to avoid being stimulated) are fewer and are principally located in the vicinity of the periaqueductal gray matter of the midbrain. These results have been generally confirmed for humans. Direct stimulation of the septal area, as an experimental treatment for certain psychiatric disorders, often yields a feeling of well-being, which is diffuse and hard to define but definitely pleasant. Stimulation near the periaqueductal gray matter sometimes causes unbearable feelings of horror and pain—an indication of the complexity of this region, since stimulation at very nearby sites can cause analgesia (see Chapter 8).

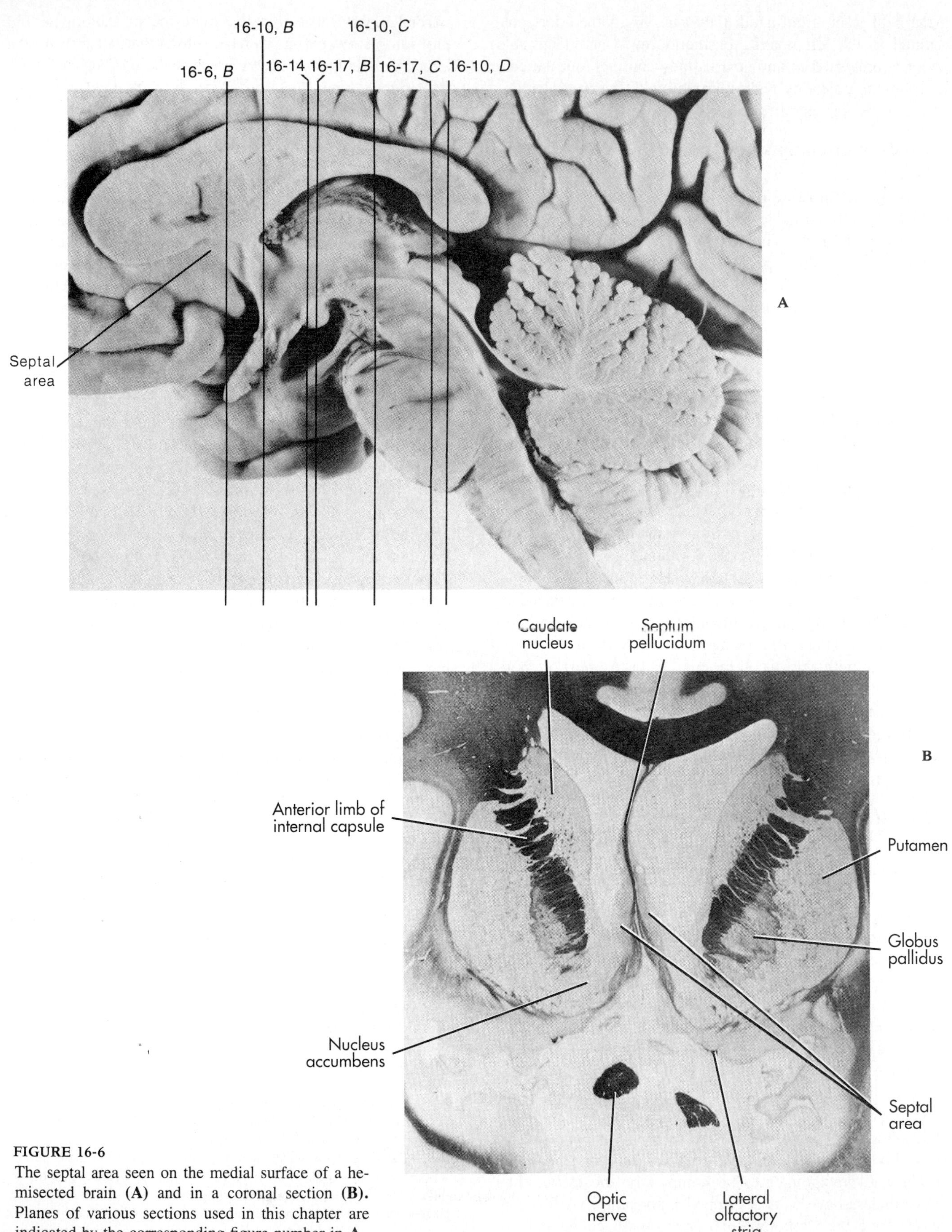


**FIGURE 16-6**
The septal area seen on the medial surface of a hemisected brain **(A)** and in a coronal section **(B)**. Planes of various sections used in this chapter are indicated by the corresponding figure number in **A.**

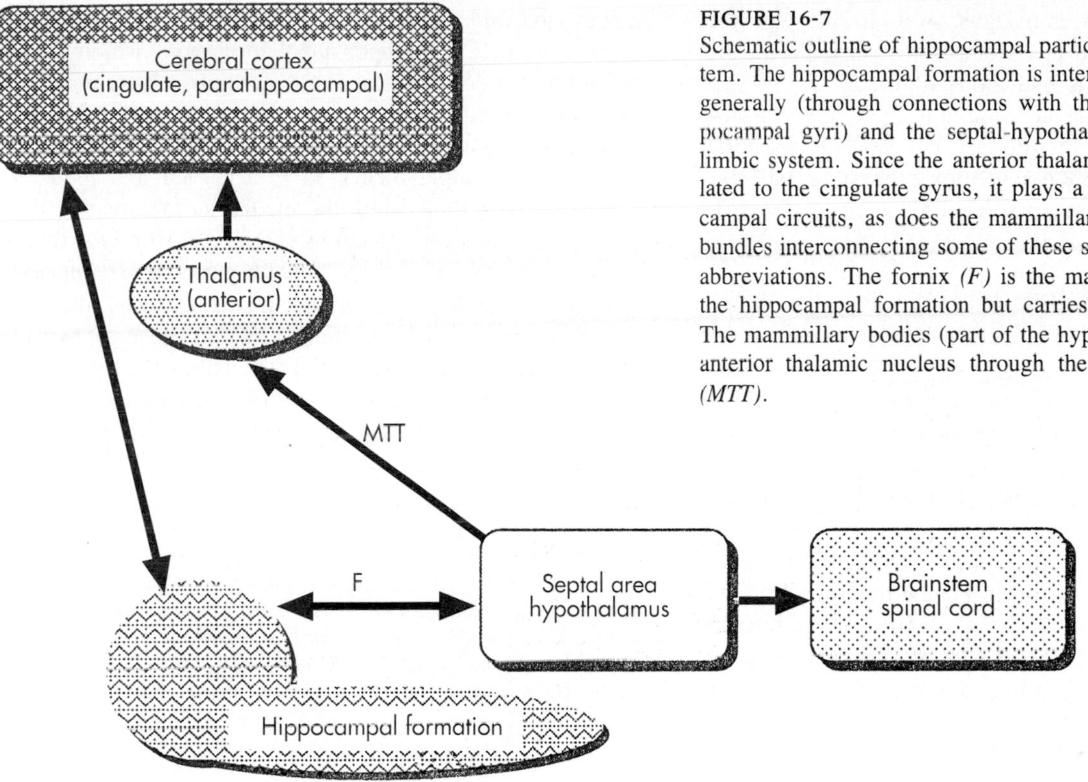


**FIGURE 16-7**
Schematic outline of hippocampal participation in the limbic system. The hippocampal formation is interposed between neocortex generally (through connections with the cingulate and parahippocampal gyri) and the septal-hypothalamic output core of the limbic system. Since the anterior thalamic nucleus is closely related to the cingulate gyrus, it plays a prominent role in hippocampal circuits, as does the mammillary body. The major fiber bundles interconnecting some of these structures are indicated by abbreviations. The fornix *(F)* is the major output pathway from the hippocampal formation but carries some afferents as well. The mammillary bodies (part of the hypothalamus) project to the anterior thalamic nucleus through the mammillothalamic tract *(MTT)*.

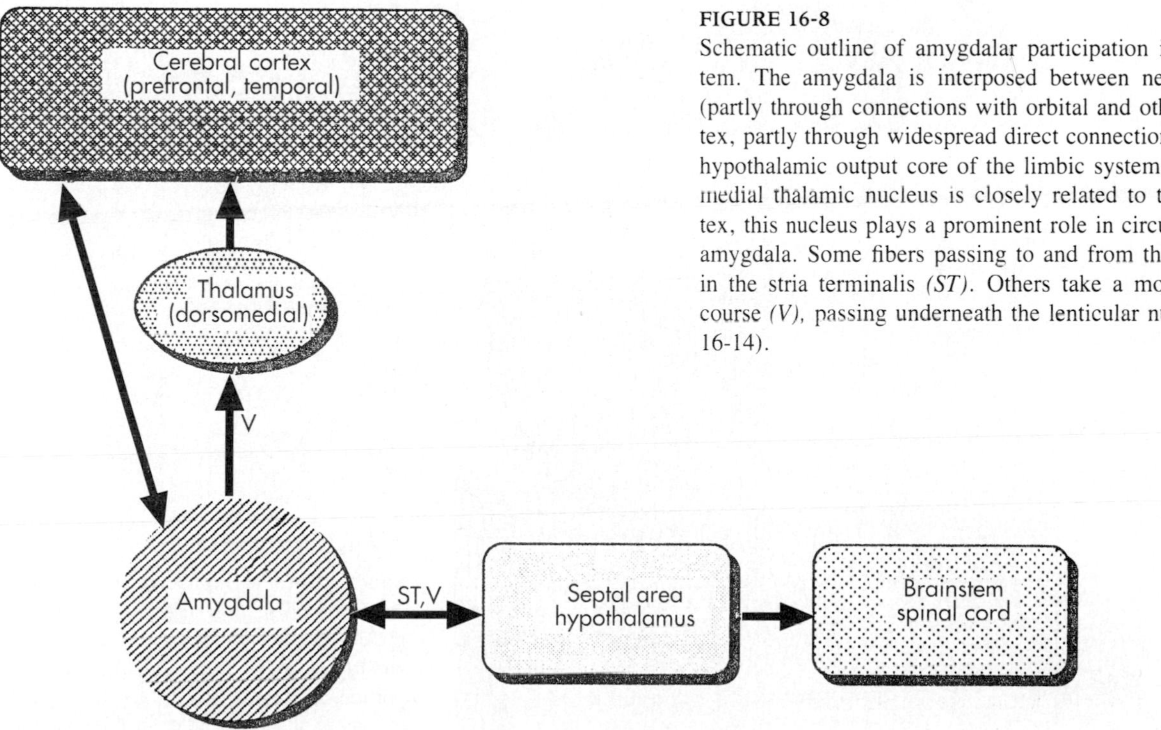


**FIGURE 16-8**
Schematic outline of amygdalar participation in the limbic system. The amygdala is interposed between neocortex generally (partly through connections with orbital and other prefrontal cortex, partly through widespread direct connections) and the septal-hypothalamic output core of the limbic system. Since the dorsomedial thalamic nucleus is closely related to the prefrontal cortex, this nucleus plays a prominent role in circuits formed by the amygdala. Some fibers passing to and from the amygdala travel in the stria terminalis *(ST)*. Others take a more diffuse ventral course *(V)*, passing underneath the lenticular nucleus (see Figure 16-14).

cingulate and parahippocampal gyri as its liaison with the neocortex generally, and has a close relationship with the anterior thalamic nucleus and the mammillary body. The second (Figure 16-8) is centered around the amygdala, utilizes prefrontal (especially orbital) and anterior temporal cortex as its liaison with the neocortex generally, and has a close relationship with the dorsomedial nucleus of the thalamus.

## Hippocampal formation

The paleocortex and archicortex occupy most of the surface of each cerebral hemisphere in lower vertebrates. As the area devoted to the neocortex expands through phylogeny, the archicortex moves dorsally and then rolls around onto the medial surface of the hemisphere, whereas the paleocortex moves ventrally onto the base of the brain. With the continued expansion of the hemisphere in primates, the hippocampal formation becomes one more structure that is carried around in a great arc—in this case ending up in the temporal lobe as the floor of the inferior horn of the lateral ventricle (Figure 16-9). Traces of its heritage are revealed by a thin strand of rudimentary gray matter (the *hippocampal rudiment* or *indusium griseum*), continuous with the hippocampal formation, which is left behind on the dorsal surface of the corpus callosum and by the long, curved course of the fornix, the most prominent hippocampal output pathway (Figure 16-10).

The hippocampal formation is a curved and recurved sheet of cortex folded into the medial surface of the temporal lobe. Transverse sections (Figure 16-9) reveal that it has three distinct zones: the *dentate gyrus,* the *hippocampus* proper,* and the *subiculum.* In such sections, the dentate gyrus and the hippocampus have the form of two interlocking Cs. The subiculum is a transitional zone continuous with the hippocampus at one of its edges and with the cortex of the parahippocampal gyrus at the other edge. The entire hippocampal formation has a length of about 5 cm

*Also called *Ammon's horn* (or *cornu ammonis,* after an Egyptian deity with ram's horns) because of the way the hippocampi curve downward and outward from the hippocampal rudiment into the temporal lobes. Hippocampal nomenclature has a long, colorful, and not entirely logical history, as discussed by F.T. Lewis in "The significance of the term *hippocampus*" (J Comp Neurol 35:213, 1923-1924). Many authors now use the term "hippocampus" to refer to the entire hippocampal formation.

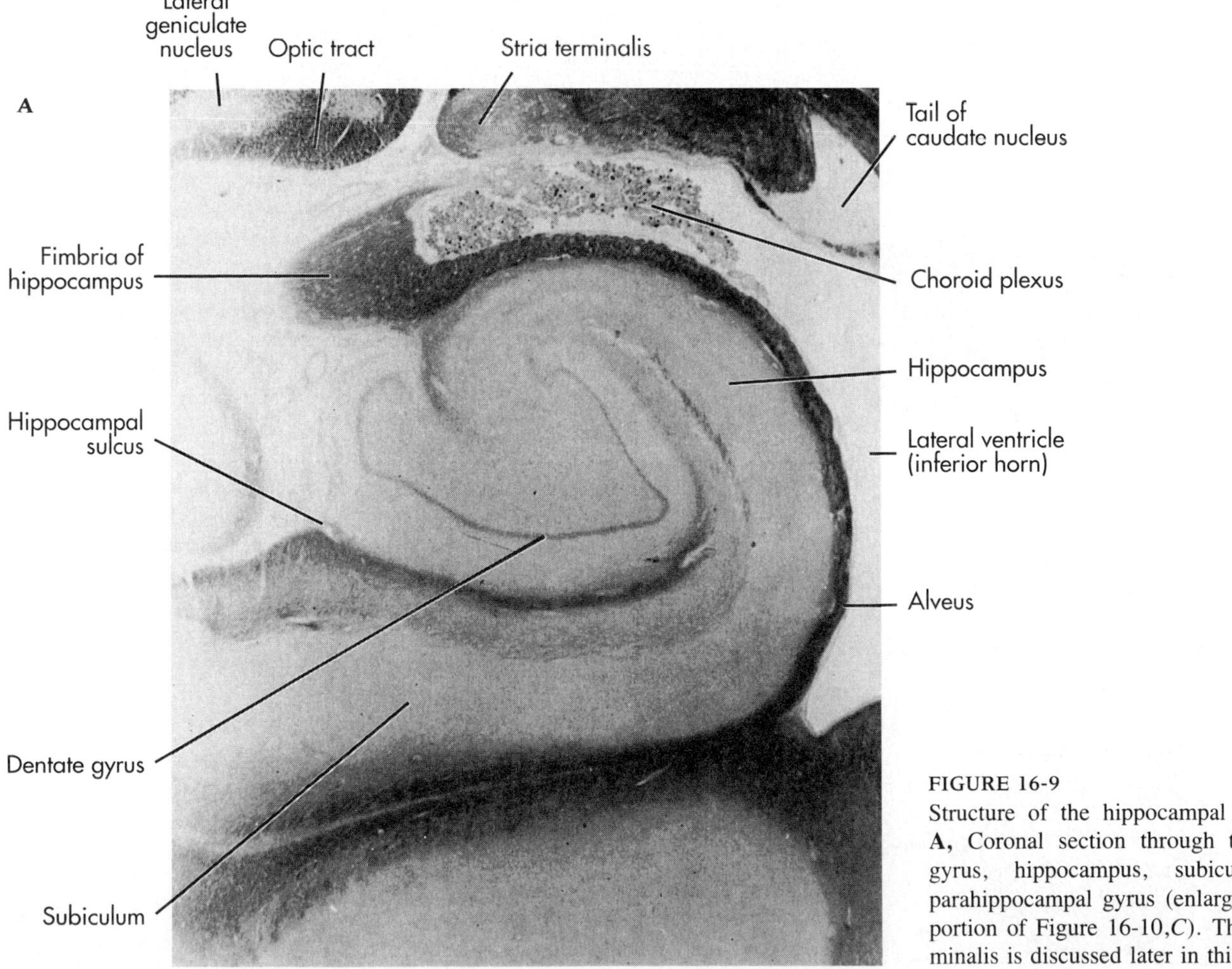


FIGURE 16-9
Structure of the hippocampal formation. **A,** Coronal section through the dentate gyrus, hippocampus, subiculum, and parahippocampal gyrus (enlargement of a portion of Figure 16-10,*C*). The stria terminalis is discussed later in this chapter.

in the inferior horn from its anterior end at the amygdala to its tapering posterior end near the splenium of the corpus callosum. Along this course numerous small blood vessels enter the hippocampal formation from the adjacent subarachnoid space by penetrating the dentate gyrus, thus giving this gyrus the beaded or toothed appearance for which it was named.

### *Histology*

The hippocampus and the dentate gyrus are three-layered, with a superficial *molecular layer* and a deep *polymorphic layer,* both similar to the layers of the same name in the neocortex. The intermediate stratum is a *granule cell layer* in the dentate gyrus and a *pyramidal cell layer* in the hippocampus. The molecular layer of the hippocampus faces the dentate gyrus, and the hippocampal equivalent of subcortical white matter is a layer of fibers called the *alveus* that lies just beneath the ependymal lining of the ventricle (Figure 16-9). The molecular layer of the dentate gyrus faces the subarachnoid space, and its output fibers, which do not leave the hippocampal formation, project directly into the hippocampus. The subiculum, as mentioned previously, is the zone of transition from the hippocampus to the parahippocampal gyrus and changes gradually from a three-layered to a six-layered cortex.

The alveus contains both afferents to and efferents from the hippocampal formation (primarily the latter). These fibers collect into a bundle called the *fimbria* (Latin for fringe) *of the hippocampus* at the edge of the choroid fissure (Figure 16-9). When the hippocampal formation ends near the splenium of the corpus callosum, the fimbria becomes a detached bundle called the *crus of the fornix*. The two crura converge and join in the midline to form the *body of the fornix,* which travels forward at the inferior edge of the septum pellucidum (Figure 16-10). At the interventricular foramen, the fornix turns inferiorly and posteriorly, diverging into the *columns of the fornix,* which then pass through the middle of the hypothalamus toward the mammillary bodies (see Figures 10-11 and 10-16).

The connections of the hippocampal formation have

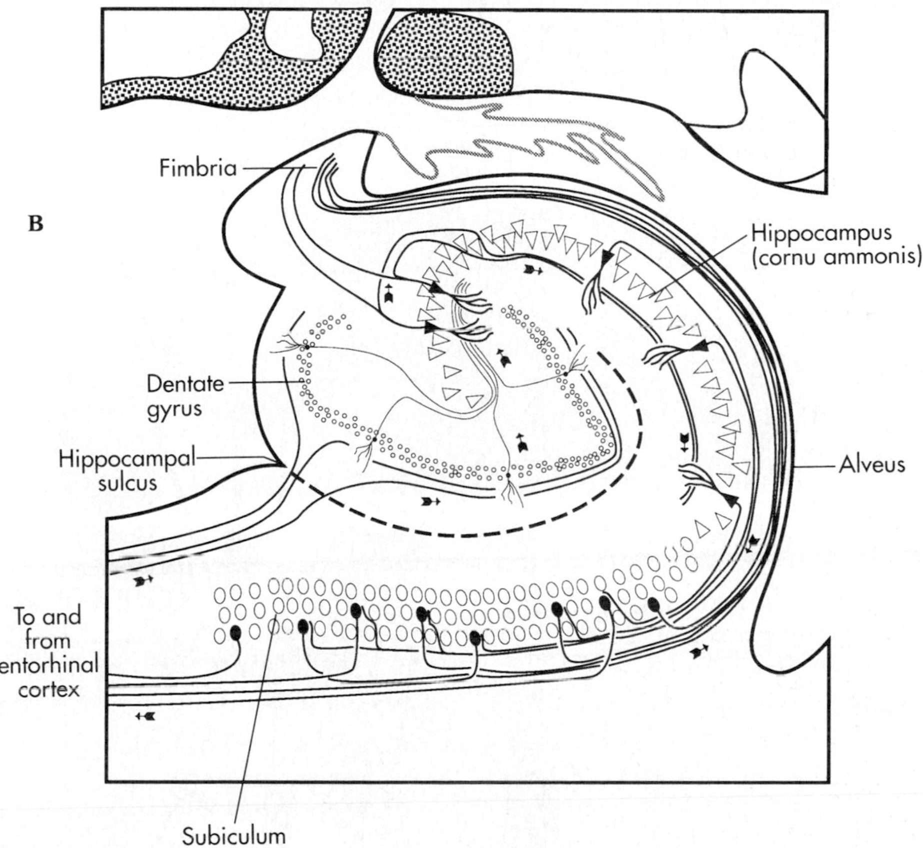


FIGURE 16-9 cont'd

**B,** Schematic diagram showing the general arrangements of cells and fibers in the hippocampal formation. A few hippocampal efferents arise from pyramidal cells of the hippocampus itself, but most, as indicated, are now known to arise from the subiculum. Note that the major route of information flow through the hippocampal formation is a one-way circuit, starting with inputs from entorhinal cortex and then passing successively through the dentate gyrus, two sectors of hippocampal pyramidal cells, and the subiculum. Finally, subicular neurons project either through the fornix or directly back to cerebral cortex.

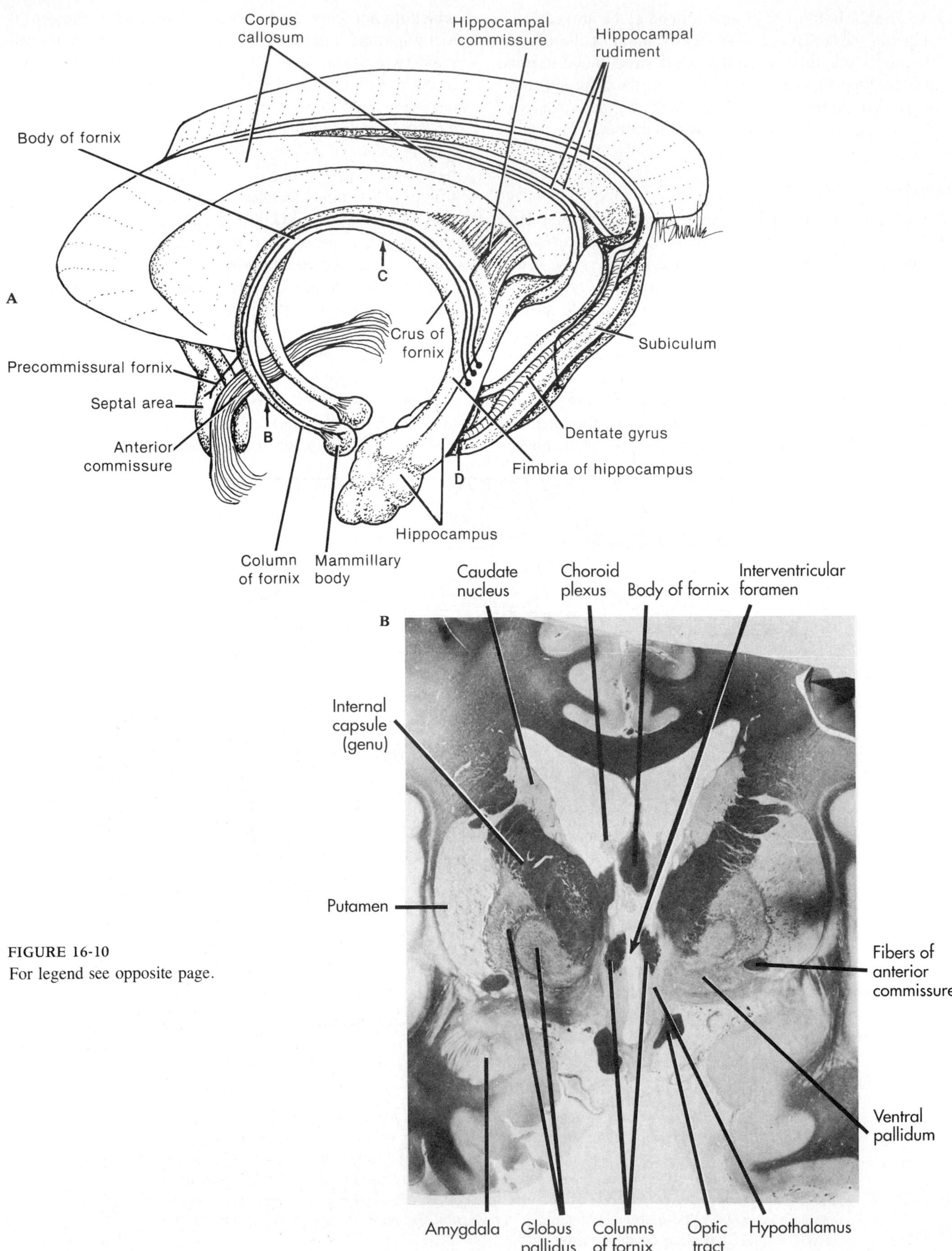


FIGURE 16-10
For legend see opposite page.

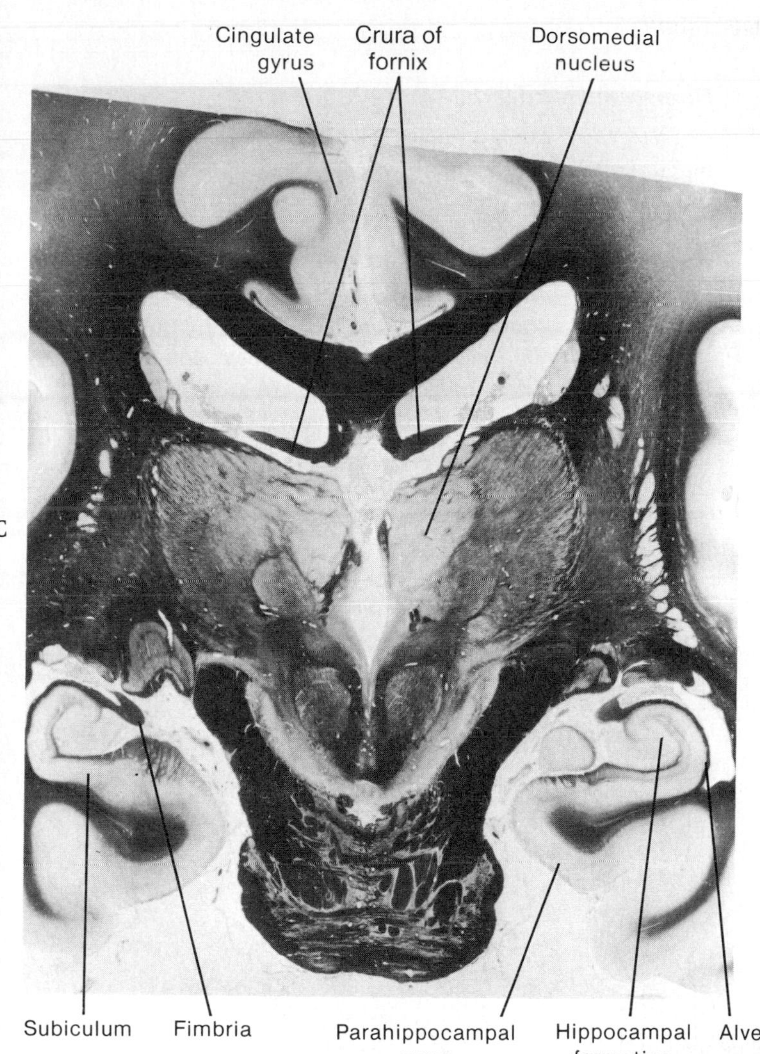


FIGURE 16-10
Origin and course of the fornix. This bundle, mostly efferent fibers from the hippocampal formation, begins as fibers that collect on the ventricular surface of the hippocampus as the alveus. The fibers then move medially to form the fimbria of the hippocampus and then part company with the hippocampal formation near the splenium to become the crus of the fornix. The two crura converge on the midline, forming the body of the fornix; as they do so, a few fibers are exchanged between the two crura in the hippocampal commissure. The body of the fornix diverges again near the anterior commissure and interventricular foramen into the columns of the fornix. Most of these fibers continue on through the hypothalamus as the postcommissural fornix, ending primarily in the mammillary bodies. Some, however, split off in front of the anterior commissure as the precommissural fornix, ending primarily in the septal area. **A** shows this course in a dissection of the fornix and neighboring structures. **B, C,** and **D** are coronal sections at the levels indicated in **A.**

A modified from Nieuwenhuys R, et al: The human central nervous system, New York, 1978, Springer-Verlag, Inc.

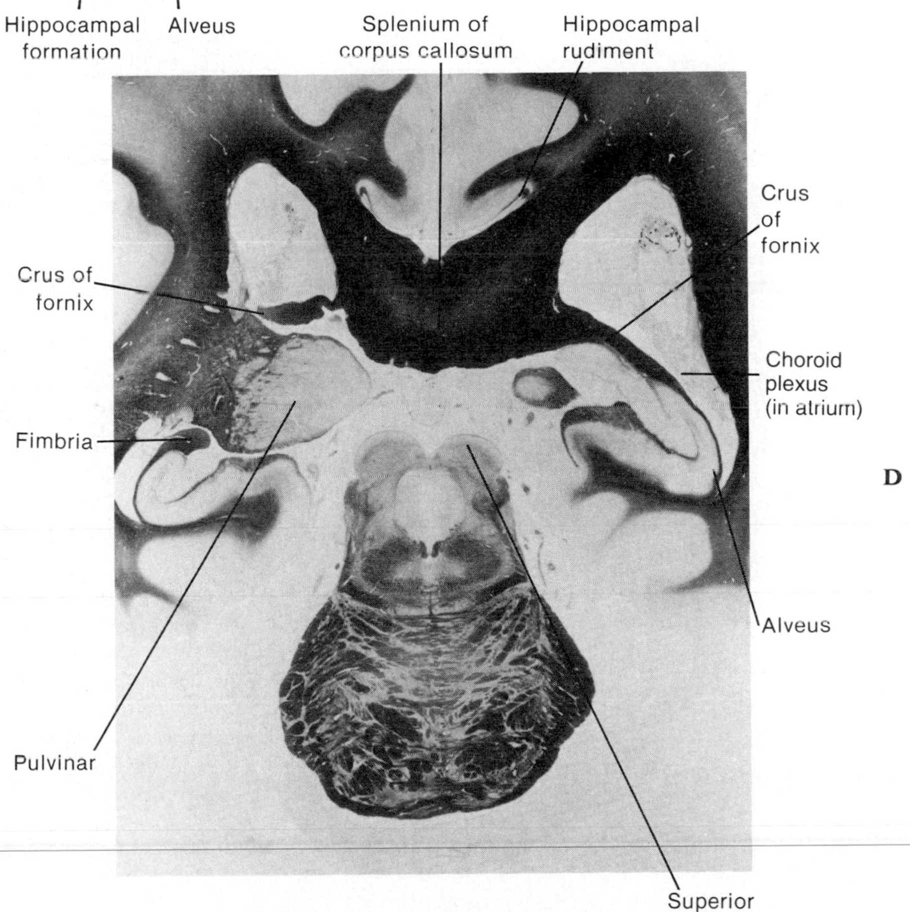

been mapped in ruthless detail and in three dimensions. Proceeding around its C shape (as seen in transverse sections), the hippocampus has been divided into several zones,* all of whose connections differ somewhat from one another and from those of the subiculum and dentate gyrus. Along the course of the hippocampal formation through the temporal lobe, its connections change. Finally, afferents from different sources end at different levels on the apical dendrites of hippocampal pyramidal cells. The high degree of order has made the hippocampal formation very attractive for anatomical and physiological research, particularly in studies of neural plasticity and regeneration. However, to keep matters manageable the following account treats the hippocampal formation, by and large, as a uniform structure.

*These zones, each a narrow longitudinal strip of hippocampus, are commonly referred to as *CA fields* (derived from CA as an abbreviation for cornu ammonis). Hence neurons of the dentate gyrus project primarily to CA3 pyramidal cells, whose axon collaterals project to CA1 pyramidal cells. CA1 in turn projects to the subiculum, where most of the output from the hippocampal formation arises (see Figure 16-9,*B*).

### *Hippocampal afferents*

By far the most prominent source of afferents to the hippocampal formation is the adjacent entorhinal cortex (Figures 16-5 and 16-11). If the entorhinal cortex received only olfactory inputs, this would not be very impressive, but it also receives projections from the cingulate gyrus (via the cingulum), from the orbital cortex (via the uncinate fasciculus), and from the amygdala and other areas of the temporal lobe. Through these additional connections the hippocampal formation has access to virtually all types of sensory information. In addition, some septal and hypothalamic fibers reach the hippocampal formation through the fornix. Finally, a few fibers arrive from the contralateral hippocampal formation by passing from one crus of the fornix to the other beneath the splenium of the corpus callosum in the *hippocampal commissure* (Figure 16-10).

### *Hippocampal efferents*

The hippocampal formation sends many fibers directly back to the entorhinal cortex and also to other cortical areas, but its most anatomically prominent output pathway is

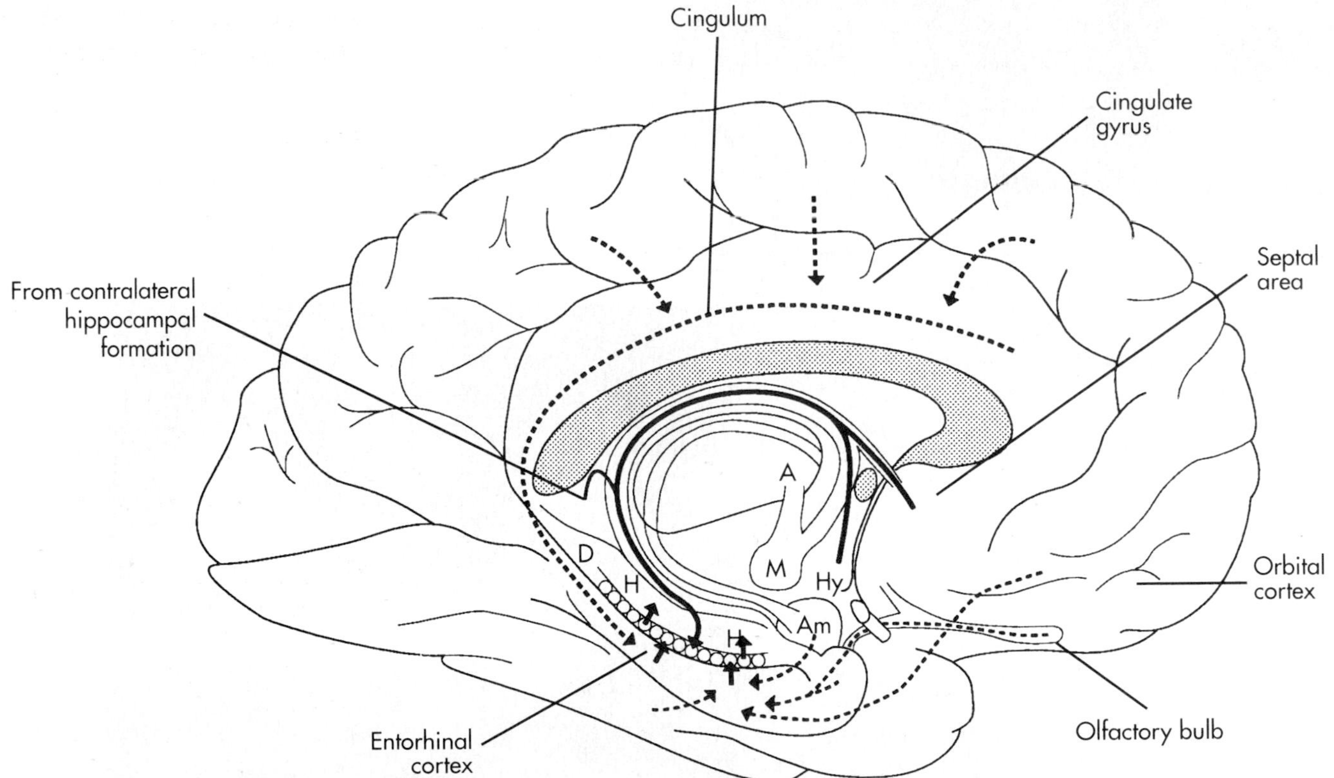


FIGURE 16-11
Afferents to the hippocampal formation *(H)*. The major source is the entorhinal cortex, which in turn collects inputs from cingulate, temporal, and orbital cortices and from the amygdala *(A)* and olfactory cortex. Other hippocampal inputs arrive from the septal area and hypothalamus *(Hy)* and from the contralateral hippocampal formation, all via the fornix. Indirect inputs are indicated by dashed pathways. This is a simplified diagram and other connections, such as inputs from the locus ceruleus and direct inputs from the amygdala, are not indicated. Other abbreviations: *A*, anterior thalamic nucleus; *D*, dentate gyrus; *M*, mammillary body.

The drawing of the brain in this and similar figures in this chapter was adapted from an illustration in Warwick R, Williams PL: Gray's anatomy, 35th British ed., Philadelphia, 1973, W.B. Saunders Co.

the fornix (Figure 16-12).* Fornix fibers arch forward under the corpus callosum along the path depicted in Figure 16-10 (except for the few that cross in the hippocampal commissure). At the level of the interventricular foramen, some fibers split off in front of the anterior commissure as the *precommissural fornix*. Most of these end nearby in the septal and preoptic areas, but some continue on to reach orbital and anterior cingulate cortex. The remaining fibers of the fornix (the *postcommissural fornix*) do one of two things; some turn sharply posteriorly and end in the anterior thalamic nucleus, whereas the rest travel through the hypothalamus in the column of the fornix and end mainly in the mammillary body (although some end in other hypothalamic areas or in the midbrain reticular formation). Since the mammillothalamic tract ends in the anterior nucleus, the hippocampal formation can influence this part of the thalamus both directly and indirectly.

*It was a long-standing anatomical tenet that the efferent fibers in the fornix are the axons of the prominent pyramidal cells of the hippocampus. However, recent work has shown that most of these axons actually end locally in the subiculum. The hippocampus proper provides part of the output to the septal area, but the bulk of the output from the hippocampal formation arises in the subiculum.

The anterior thalamic nucleus projects to the cingulate gyrus, thus completing a great loop through the diencephalon and telencephalon (Figure 16-13). Beginning in the hippocampal formation, the pathway proceeds through the fornix to the mammillary body, from there in sequence to the anterior thalamic nucleus, the cingulate gyrus, and part of the parahippocampal gyrus (the entorhinal cortex), and finally back to the hippocampal formation. James Papez pointed out in 1937 that this loop provided for interactions among the neocortex, limbic structures, and the hypothalamus and proposed that it might be the anatomical substrate of emotional experience. While undoubtedly a great oversimplification (for one thing, hippocampal connections are considerably more complex than this loop would indicate), this idea provided the impetus for a great deal of research into the structure and function of the limbic system; the loop is still known as the *Papez circuit*.

### *Hippocampal function*

A variety of changes in autonomic and endocrine function have been described as resulting from hippocampal stimulation or damage in experimental animals, consistent with the connections between the hippocampal formation and the septal nuclei and hypothalamus; a number of be-

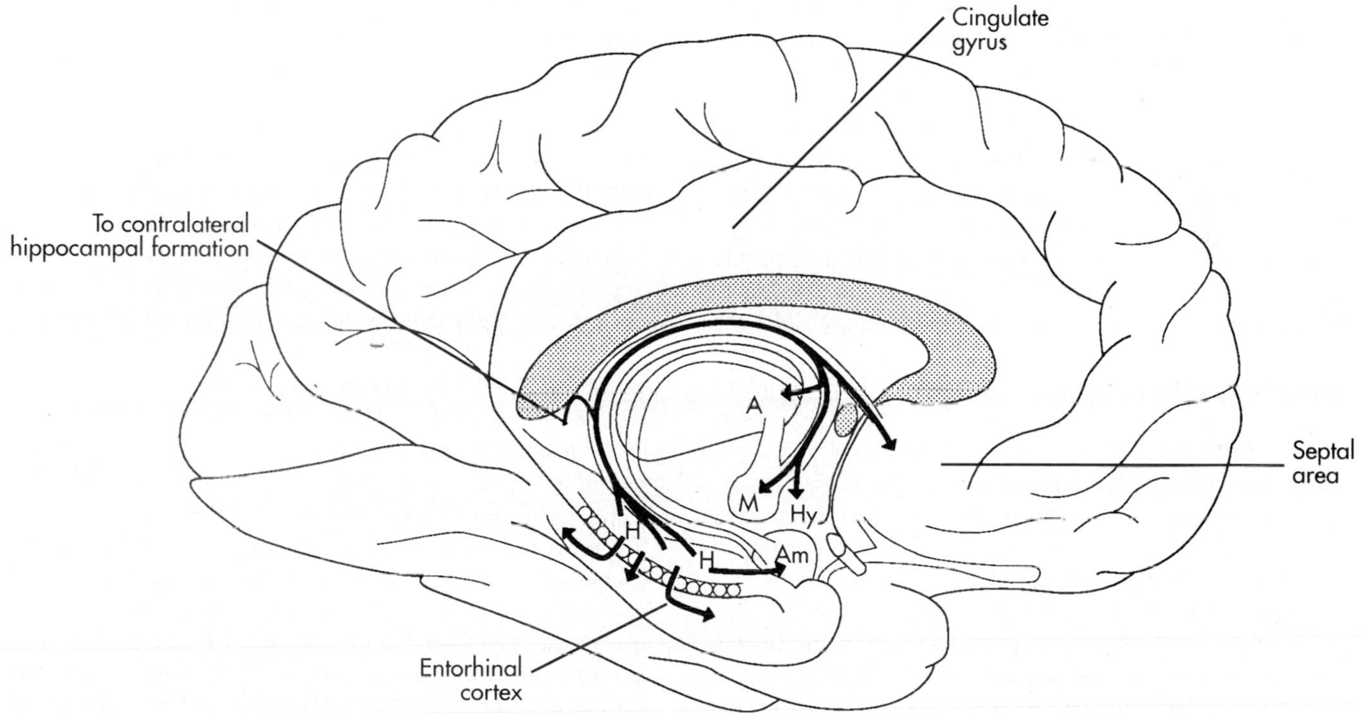


**FIGURE 16-12**
Efferents from the hippocampal formation *(H)*. One major efferent pathway is the fornix, through which fibers reach an assortment of anteriorly situated forebrain structures. In addition, many fibers pass directly from the subiculum to the entorhinal cortex, to the amygdala *(Am)*, or backward along the cingulum to the cingulate gyrus. Some fibers of the precommissural fornix spread beyond the septal area and reach orbital and anterior cingulate cortices. *A*, Anterior thalamic nucleus; *Hy*, nonmammillary regions of the hypothalamus; *M*, mammillary body.

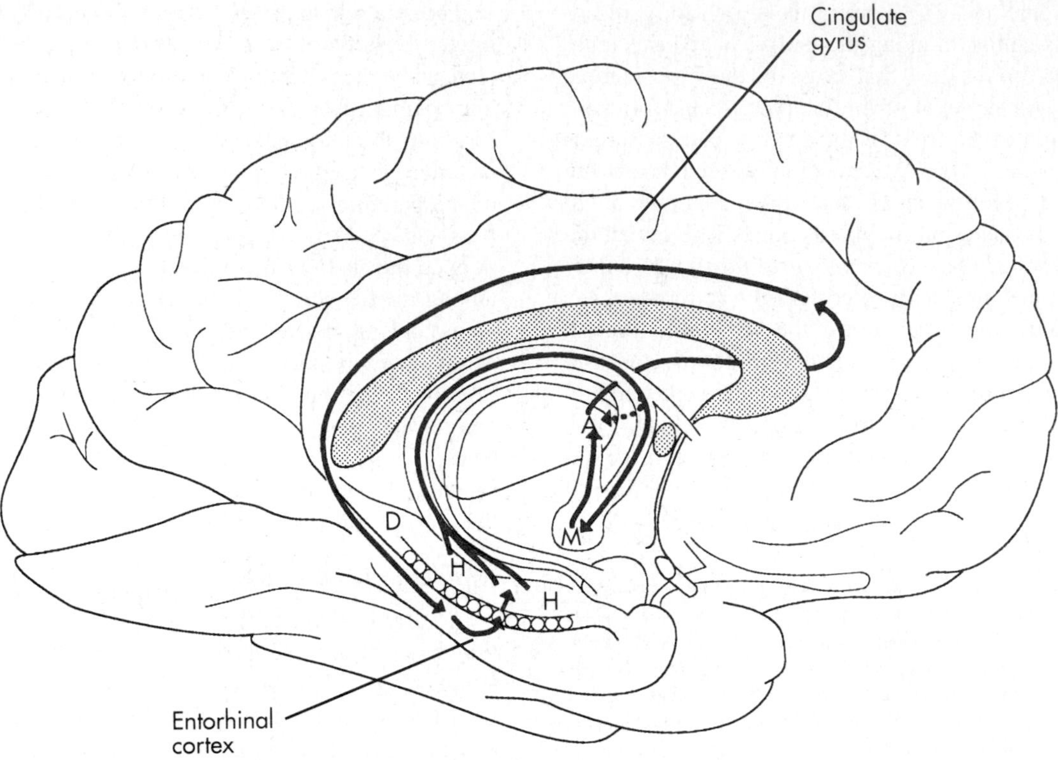


FIGURE 16-13
The Papez circuit. The shortcut from the hippocampal formation directly to the anterior thalamic nucleus, not part of the circuit as originally proposed, is indicated by a dashed line. *A,* Anterior thalamic nucleus; *D,* dentate gyrus; *H,* hippocampal formation; *M,* mammillary body.

havioral changes have been described as well. Despite this, however, it has not yet been possible to derive one general function or set of functions for the hippocampal formation. The most prominent role ascribed to it in humans has to do with learning and memory. Neurosurgeons discovered (by accident) in the early 1950s that after bilateral removal of the medial parts of the temporal lobe (or after unilateral removal from patients with preexisting damage on the other side), humans have a striking memory deficit. After such surgery, patients are unable to form new memories of facts and events. There is typically some retrograde amnesia for events that occurred before the surgery, but beyond some point in the past, early memories are intact. However, a new item such as a list of numbers or a dictated phrase disappears at the first distraction, although it can be retained for a little while if the patient has nothing else to do but concentrate on that item. Intelligence is more or less undisturbed, but nevertheless, this is an enormously debilitating problem. Imagine being perpetually unable to remember new acquaintances; unable to keep track of events in the lives of relatives and old friends; unable to complete simple tasks because of the inability to remember why they were begun; unable to read a story because there is no memory of sentences preceding the current one. Interestingly, this amnesia applies only to specific facts and events and not to the learning of new skills. Such a patient could, for example, learn in repeated attempts how to assemble a jigsaw puzzle more and more skillfully, at the same rate as a normal individual, despite never remembering having seen the puzzle before.

Since the hippocampal formation is a major part of the medial temporal lobe and since a memory deficit occurs in cases where little appears to be damaged other than the two hippocampal formations, the function of laying down or consolidating new memories has been attributed to this portion of the limbic system. (Memories themselves must reside elsewhere in the CNS—presumably as distributed sets of neocortical connections—since old memories can still be retrieved after medial temporal damage.)

Damage to the mammillary bodies (which occurs in the course of widespread damage to the periaqueductal and periventricular gray matter as a result of chronic alcoholism) is correlated with a similar memory deficit. The condition is called *Korsakoff's psychosis*. Patients so afflicted may have relatively intact intelligence but an inability to form new memories. They typically make up answers as they go along, concealing to some extent the memory loss (hence a wonderful alternate name for Korsakoff's psychosis: the *amnestic confabulatory syndrome*). This led to the appealing notion that the entire Papez circuit is involved in learning and memory. Unfortunately, things are rarely as simple as they seem, and acceptance of the hippocampal

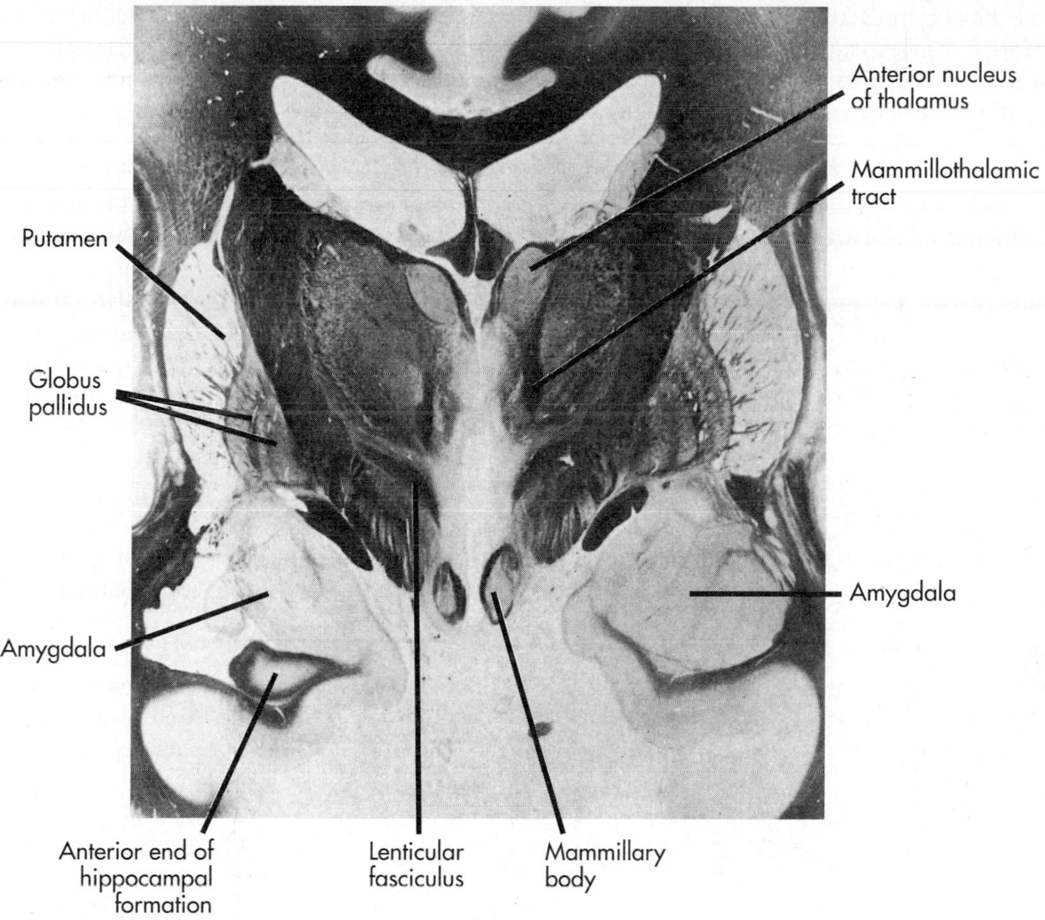


FIGURE 16-14
Coronal section through the amygdala. Note the fairly direct route beneath the lenticular nucleus that is available for fibers interconnecting the amygdala and various diencephalic and telencephalic structures (the ventral amygdalofugal pathway).

role in memory has developed slowly. For example, bilateral destruction of the cingulum causes no particular memory loss,* and destruction of the fornix does not cause a memory deficit comparable in magnitude to that seen after medial temporal damage. In addition, there have been cases in which reported destruction of the mammillary bodies was not accompanied by memory loss. Some investigators claim that the only common factor in all cases of Korsakoff's psychosis is bilateral damage to the medial thalamus (that is, the dorsomedial nuclei). Finally, it seemed for a long time that careful, selective damage to the hippocampal formations of experimental animals paradoxically did not produce the same severe memory deficit found in humans.

*Interestingly, bilateral section of the cingulum causes emotional changes similar to those seen after prefront leukotomy—a type of change that might be expected after damage to the limbic system. This operation has been used on an experimental basis as a treatment for intractable pain and for certain psychiatric disorders.

Explanations for these apparent discrepancies have come from the realization that there are multiple kinds of memory systems working in parallel with each other, and from increased knowledge of hippocampal anatomy. As mentioned previously, humans with amnesia can still learn new motor skills, indicating that this form of learning does not require an intact hippocampal formation. In general, it now appears that varieties of learning and memory like pattern recognition, habits, conditioned autonomic reactions to stimuli, and motor skills—memories not built around the conscious recall of specific items—do not depend on the hippocampal formation. Rather, the hippocampal formation and nearby cortical areas (such as entorhinal cortex) play a crucial role, one that slowly diminishes over months or even years, in consolidating explicit memories of facts and events. Since the hippocampal formation has substantial outputs that do not travel through the fornix (Figure 16-12), damage to the fornix does not cause a major impairment of memory. Similarly, damage restricted to the hippocampal formation and sparing entorhinal and nearby cortices causes only partial amnesia. The critical structure whose damage causes Korsakoff's psychosis has still not been determined with certainty.

## Amygdala

The amygdala is a collection of nuclei lying beneath the uncus of the temporal lobe at the anterior end of the hippocampal formation and the inferior horn of the lateral ventricle (Figure 16-14). It merges with the periamygdaloid cortex, which forms part of the surface of the uncus. The amygdala also abuts the tail of the caudate nucleus as the latter ends in the temporal lobe (Figure 13-4) and was considered at one time to be one of the basal ganglia, which by definition comprised all subcortical gray masses of the telencephalon. The amygdala does have some connections with the striatum (see Figure 16-18), but the overall pattern of its connections is typical of the limbic system.

### *Afferents to the amygdala*

The amygdala receives a great deal of sensory input in a highly processed form. Single amygdalar cells may be selective or may respond to various combinations of many different sensory modalities, including somatosensory, visual, auditory, and all types of visceral inputs. The afferents carrying this information arise in several locations (Figure 16-15) and reach the amygdala by traveling in the reverse direction along the paths followed by amygdalar efferents (described in the next section).

Visceral inputs, particularly olfactory inputs, are especially prominent. Some olfactory tract fibers end in part of the amygdala, and this part in turn projects to the rest of the amygdala; olfactory inputs also arise in the piriform cortex. Additional visceral information reaches the amygdala indirectly from the hypothalamus, septal area, orbital and insular cortex, and also by more direct routes; for example, the parabrochial nucleus projects to the amygdala, and it seems likely that the same may be true of other visceral nuclei in the brainstem. The temporal and anterior cingulate cortices also project to the amygdala and are probably responsible for most of the auditory, visual, and somatosensory information that reaches this structure.

### *Efferents from the amygdala*

Fibers leave the amygdala through two major pathways to reach many of the same areas that send afferents to it (Figure 16-16). The first pathway is the *stria terminalis,*

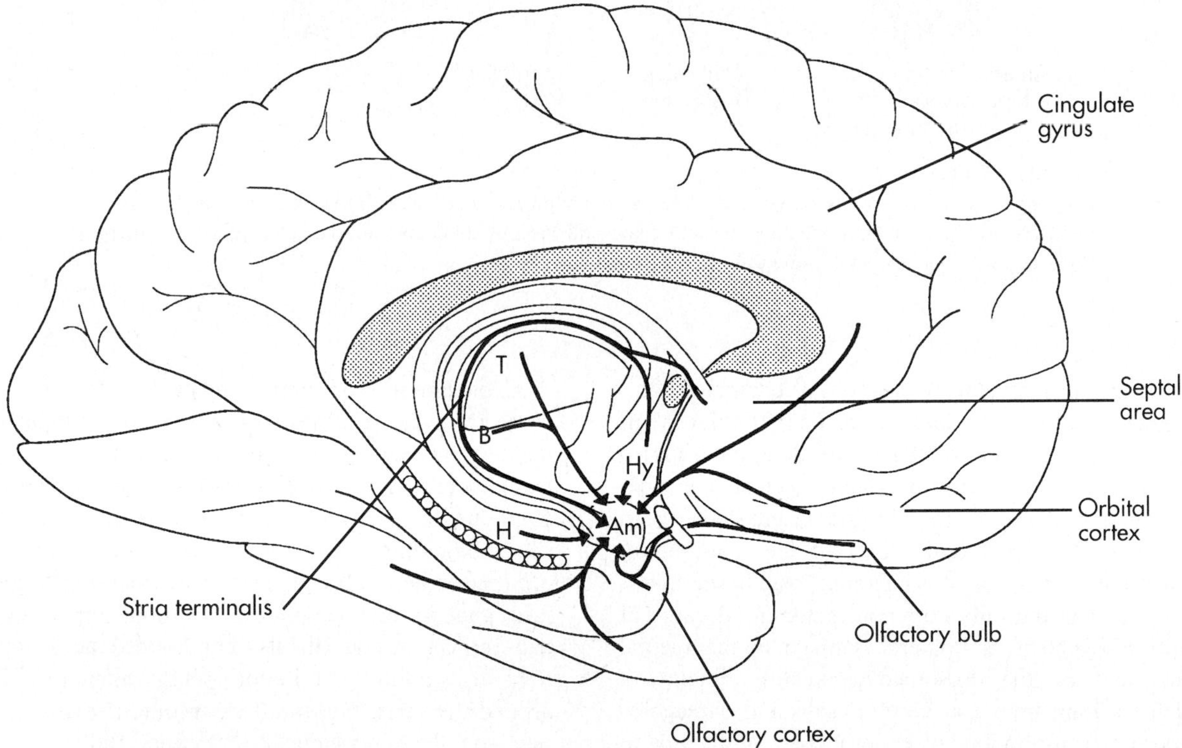


FIGURE 16-15

Afferents to the amygdala *(Am)*. These arrive via four routes: (1) from the hypothalamus *(Hy)* and septal area through the stria terminalis; (2) from the thalamus *(T)* and hypothalamus *(Hy),* and from orbital and anterior cingulate cortex, through the ventral pathway; (3) from the olfactory bulb and olfactory cortex through the lateral olfactory stria; and (4) directly from temporal lobe structures such as neocortical areas and the hippocampal formation *(H)*. Additional inputs reach the amygdala from brainstem sites *(B)* like the parabrachial nucleus.

which arches around from the temporal lobe toward the interventricular foramen in company with the caudate nucleus and the thalamostriate (or terminal) vein. In the body of the lateral ventricle, the stria terminalis lies in the groove between the caudate nucleus and the thalamus (Figure 16-17). Fibers of the stria terminalis distribute mainly to the septal area and the hypothalamus.

The second efferent route goes by the awkward name of the *ventral amygdalofugal pathway* (particularly awkward since it also contains many afferents to the amygdala). These fibers pass underneath the lenticular nucleus (Figure 16-14) and spread out to blanket the base of the brain, ending in the septal area and the hypothalamus, in olfactory regions like the anterior olfactory nucleus, the anterior perforated substance, the piriform cortex, and in the orbital and anterior cingulate cortices. Some reach the *ventral striatum,* which includes the area of fusion of the putamen and the head of the caudate nucleus (the *nucleus accumbens,* Figure 16-6,*B*) as well as adjacent portions of the striatum. The ventral striatum in turn projects to an extension of the globus pallidus, the *ventral pallidum,* beneath the anterior commissure (Figure 16-10,*B*). The ventral striatum and pallidum are links in a basal ganglia circuit similar to that involved in motor functions (Figure 16-18). In this case, however, the inputs to the basal ganglia are from limbic structures like the amygdala and hippocampal formation; the outputs relay in the dorsomedial nucleus of the thalamus rather than the VA/VL complex and influence prefrontal and orbital frontal cortex. The functional significance of this recently discovered limbic connection with the basal ganglia is not yet clear, but it does provide one more indication that the basal ganglia are not wholly motor in function. Many ventral amygdalofugal fibers turn dorsally in the diencephalon and reach the dorsomedial nucleus of the thalamus. Finally, some amygdalar efferents enter neither the stria terminalis nor the ventral pathway but rather pass directly to entorhinal cortex and other cortical areas in the temporal lobe and beyond.

### *Amygdalar function*

As complex as the connections of the amygdala appear, they are dominated by extensive interconnections with the septal area and hypothalamus on the one hand and with prefrontal cortex, both directly and indirectly (via the dorsomedial nucleus), on the other. This puts it in a position to influence both drive-related behavior patterns and the

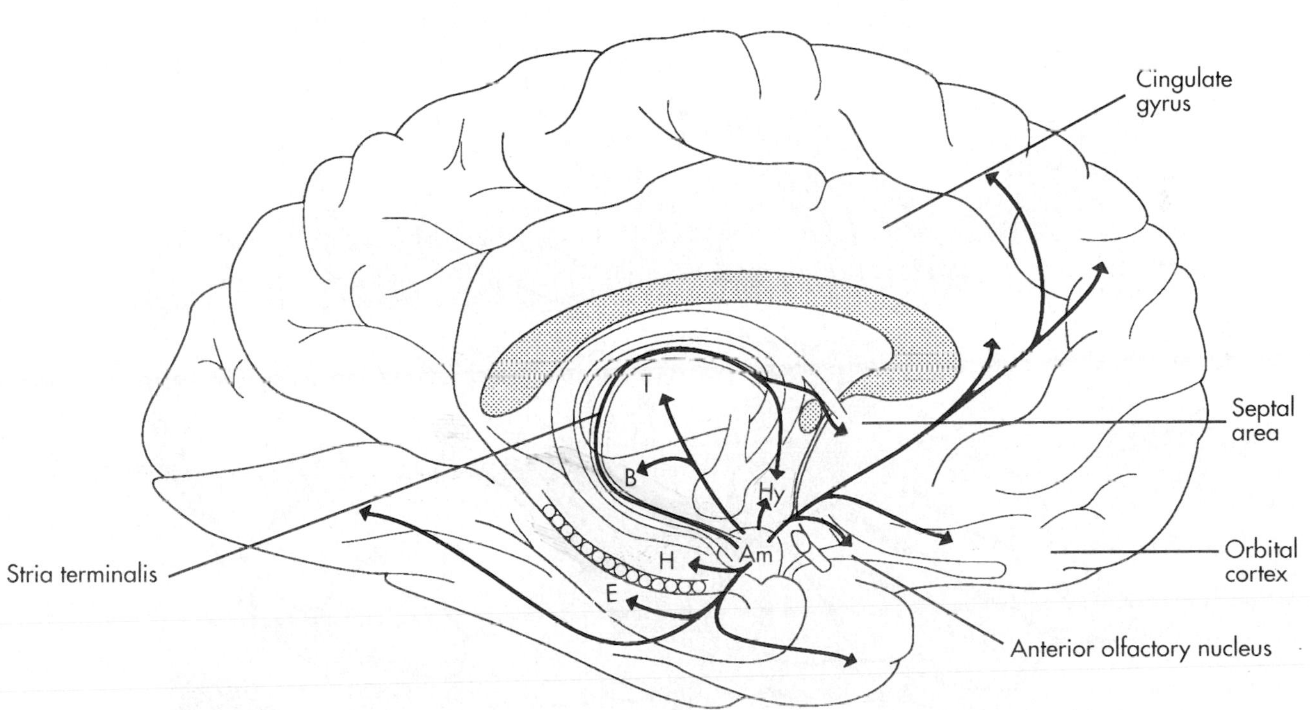


FIGURE 16-16
Efferents from the amygdala. These take three routes: (1) the stria terminalis, which reaches the septal area and hypothalamus *(Hy);* (2) the ventral amygdalofugal pathway to the hypothalamus *(Hy),* thalamus *(T),* widespread areas of frontal and insular cortex, olfactory structures and various brainstem sites *(B);* and (3) direct projections to the hippocampal formation *(H),* entorhinal cortex *(E)* and temporal and other neocortical areas.

subjective feelings that accompany these activities. In the first of these two roles, the amygdala can be considered a sort of higher order modulating influence on the hypothalamus. Almost any visceral or somatic activity that can be elicited by stimulating the hypothalamus (including such things as feeding or cardiovascular and respiratory changes) can also be elicited by stimulating some point in the amygdala. The responses to amygdalar stimulation tend to be more "natural" than those to hypothalamic stimulation, building up gradually and then decaying slowly at the end of the stimulus. Conversely, syndromes such as the aphagia or hyperphagia that follow selective lesions of parts of the hypothalamus can also be caused by amygdalar lesions, although in this case the syndromes are less severe.

The role of the amygdala in subjective feelings (presumably involving interactions with both the prefrontal cortex and the hypothalamus) has also been indicated in electrical studies. When an animal's amygdala is stimulated, it most often stops whatever it was doing and becomes very attentive. This may be followed by responses of defense, raging aggression, or fleeing. Amygdalar stimulation in humans can cause a variety of emotions, but the most common is fear accompanied by all its normal autonomic manifestations (for instance, dilation of the pupils, release of adrenalin, and increased heart rate). Conversely, bilateral destruction of the amygdala causes a great decrease in aggression, and as a result the animals are tame and placid. This is part of a different kind of memory deficit, one that impairs the ability to learn or remember the appropriate emotional and autonomic responses to stimuli.

### Some functional aspects of the limbic system

One classic technique for studying the function of a structure is to remove it or destroy it and then see what happens. Removing the temporal lobe back to the level of the primary auditory cortex should certainly incapacitate the limbic system to a great extent, since the amygdala and

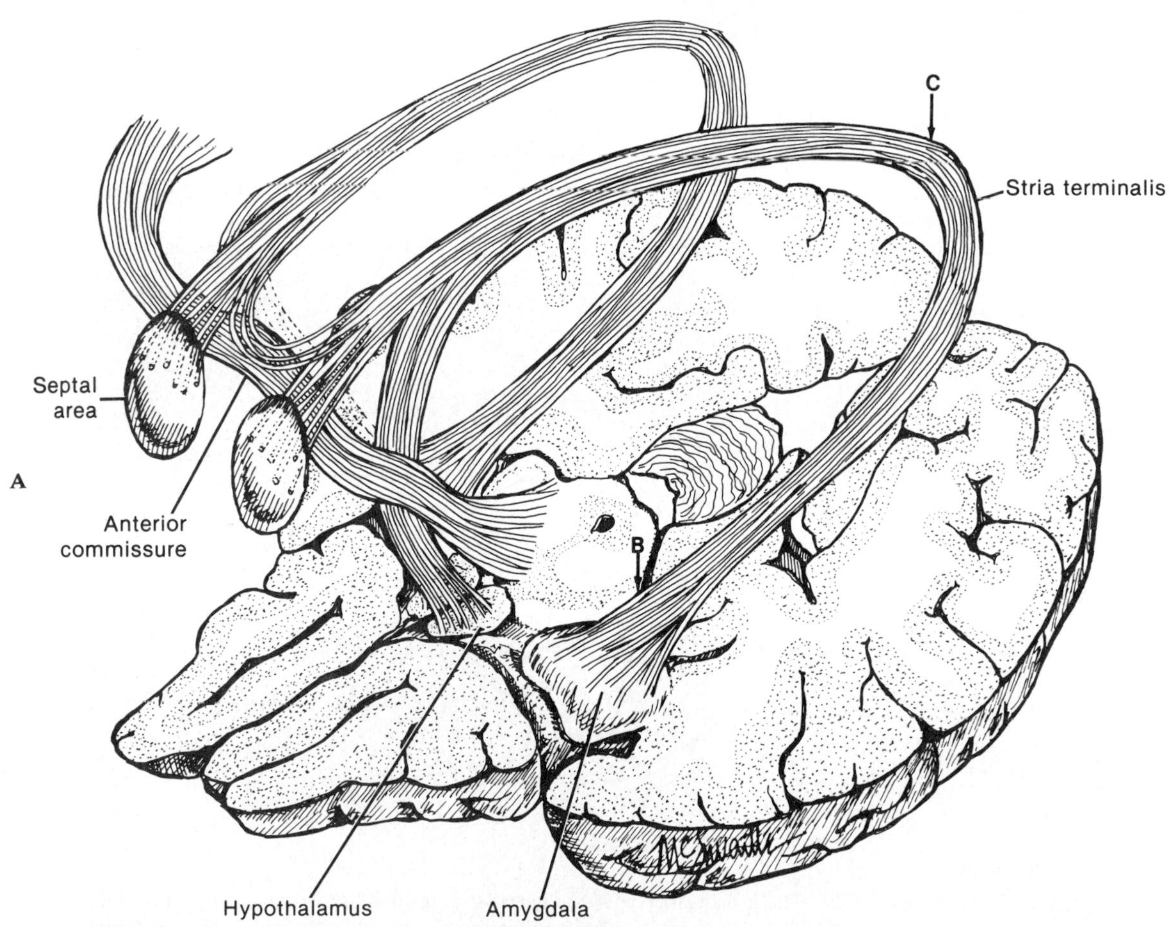


FIGURE 16-17
Origin and course of the stria terminalis. **A,** Dissection of the stria terminalis and neighboring structures indicating the course of some of its fibers.

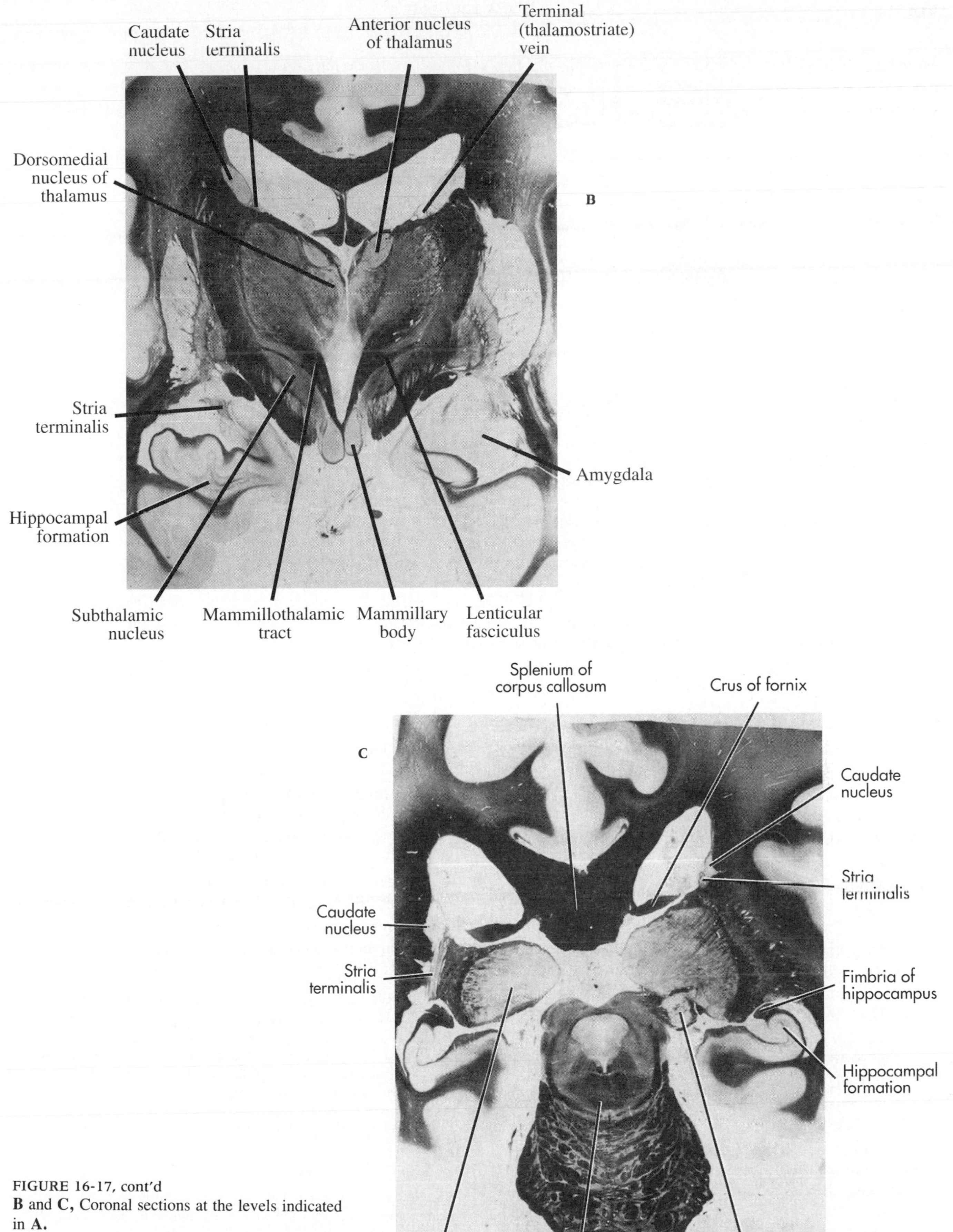


FIGURE 16-17, cont'd
**B** and **C,** Coronal sections at the levels indicated in **A.**

**A** suggested by a drawing in Isaacson RL: The limbic system, New York, 1974, Plenum Press.

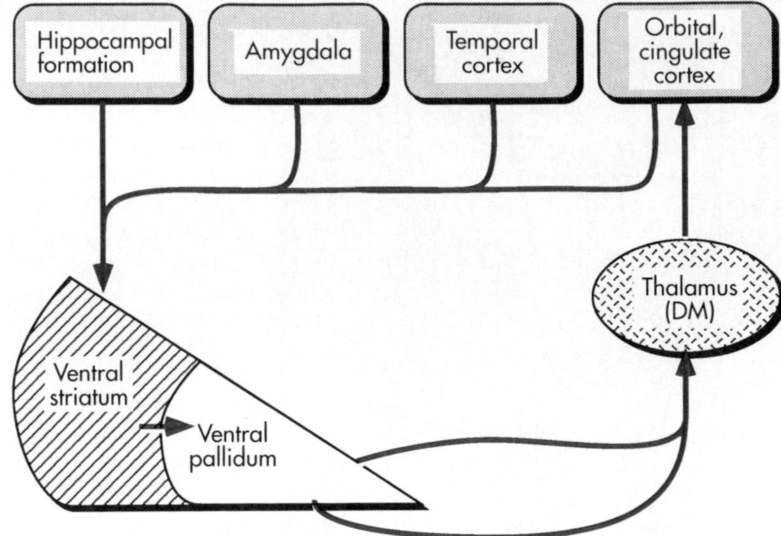


FIGURE 16-18
Schematic diagram of the limbic connections of the basal ganglia, which are similar in principle to basal ganglia connections previously discussed (compare to Figure 13-5,*B*). In this case, separate parts of the striatum (Figure 16-6,*B*) and globus pallidus (Figure 16-10,*B*) are involved, with inputs from the hippocampal formation and amygdala and outputs through the dorsomedial nucleus to prefrontal cortex. (The ventral striatum includes the nucleus accumbens as well as restricted ventral portions of the putamen and caudate nucleus.) In addition, the ventral striatum, like the rest of the striatum, receives a dopaminergic input; in this case, the fibers arise just medial to the substantia nigra in the *ventral tegmental area*. The total extent of the parallelism between limbic and nonlimbic parts of the basal ganglia, such as all the fiber bundles used and all the nuclei contacted, is not yet known.

most of the hippocampal formation and parahippocampal gyrus would be lost. When this is done to animals bilaterally, a constellation of deficits results called the *Klüver-Bucy syndrome* for the investigators who first described it.

1. The animals are fearless and placid, showing an absence of emotional reactions. They do not respond to threats, to social gestures by other animals, or to objects they would normally flee from or attack.
2. Male animals become hypersexual and are impressively indiscriminate in their choice of sex partners. They are likely to mount other animals of the same sex, animals of whatever species may be available, or inanimate objects.
3. They show an inordinate degree of attention to all sensory stimuli, as though ceaselessly curious. They respond to every object within sight or reach by sniffing it and examining it orally. If the object can in any sense be considered edible, they eat it. Partly because of this, they eat much more than normal animals.
4. Although they incessantly examine all objects in sight, they recognize nothing and may pick up the same thing over and over. This was called "psychic blindness" by Klüver and Bucy and would now be called visual agnosia.

The Klüver-Bucy syndrome has been fractionated to some extent, and different parts of it can be attributed to the loss of different structures. Thus the placidity results from destruction of the amygdala, the hypersexuality from loss of the piriform cortex, and the visual agnosia from damage to visual association areas on the inferior surface of the temporal lobe. The composite syndrome is tremendously detrimental.* Leaving aside the visual agnosia, it is as though the animal still had intact all the behavior patterns central to satisfying basic drives but could no longer tell when and in what context to use them.

*"A monkey which approaches every enemy to examine it orally will conceivably not survive longer than a few hours if turned loose in a region with a plentiful supply of enemies. We doubt that a monkey would be seriously hampered under natural conditions, in the wild, by a loss of its prefrontal region, its parietal lobes or its occipital lobes, as long as small portions of the striate cortex remained intact." (Klüver H, Bucy PC: Preliminary analysis of functions of the temporal lobes in monkeys, *Arch Neurol Psychiatry* 42:979, 1939.)

## ADDITIONAL READINGS

Aggleton J.P. (editor): The amygdala: neurobiological aspects of emotion, memory, and mental dysfunction, New York, 1992, Wiley-Liss.

Amaral DG, Insausti R: Hippocampal formation. In Paxinos, G., editor: *The human nervous system,* San Diego, 1990, Academic Press.

Andy OJ, Stephan H: The septum in the human brain, *J Comp Neurol* 133:383, 1968. *There is a tendency to think of the septal area as small and rudimentary in humans, but this paper argues that in fact it reaches its highest development in us.*

DeFrance JF, editor: *The septal nuclei, advances in behavioral biology,* vol. 20, New York, 1976, Plenum Press.

Duvernoy HM: *The human hippocampus: an atlas of applied anatomy,* Munich, 1988, J.F. Bergmann Verlag.

Gaffan D, Murray EA: Amygdalar interaction with the mediodorsal nucleus of the thalamus and the ventromedial prefrontal cortex in stimulus-reward associative learning in the monkey, *J Neurosci* 10:3479, 1990.

Gordon HW, Sperry RW: Lateralization of olfactory perception in the surgically separated hemispheres of man, *Neuropsychologia* 7:111, 1969.

Graziadei PPC, et al: Neurogenesis of sensory neurons in the primate olfactory system after section of the fila olfactoria, *Brain Res* 186:289, 1980. *Olfactory receptor neurons can be replaced after injury, which makes them highly unusual neurons.*

Holmes EJ, et al: Ablations of the mammillary nuclei in monkeys: effects on postoperative memory, *Exp Neurol* 81:97, 1983.

Isaacson RL: *The limbic system,* ed 2, New York, 1982, Plenum Press.

Kaada BR: *Stimulation and regional ablation of the amygdaloid complex with reference to functional representations.* In Eleftheriou, BE, editor: The neurobiology of the amygdala, New York, 1972, Plenum Press.

Klüver H, Bucy PC: Preliminary analysis of functions of the temporal lobes in monkeys, *Arch Neurol Psychiatry* 42:979, 1939. *Still interesting reading.*

LeDoux JE, Romanski L, Xagoraris A: Indelibility of subcortical emotional memories, *J Cog Neurosci* 1:238, 1989. *Recent work on the role of the amygdala in learning the emotional significance of stimuli.*

Lewis FT: The significance of the term *hippocampus, J Comp Neurol* 35:213, 1923-24. *A caustic but interesting paper concerning "the flight of fancy which led Arantius, in 1587, to introduce the term 'hippocampus'. . . .recorded in what is perhaps the worst anatomical description extant. It has left its readers in doubt whether the elevations of cerebral substance were being compared with fish or beast, and no one could be sure which end was the head."*

Lilly R et al.: The human Klüver-Bucy syndrome, *Neurol* 33:1141, 1983.

Machne X, Segundo JP: Unitary responses to afferent volleys in amygdaloid complex, *J Neurophysiol* 19:232, 1956. *Single cells that respond equally well to a brief shock to the sciatic nerve and to a whiff of something.*

Malamud N: Psychiatric disorder with intracranial tumors of limbic system, *Arch Neurol* 17:113, 1967.

Norgren R: Taste pathways to hypothalamus and amygdala, *J Comp Neurol* 166:17, 1976.

Olton DS, Gamzu E, Corkin S: Memory dysfunctions: an integration of animal and human research from preclinical and clinical perspectives, *Ann NY Acad Sci* 444, 1985.

Papez JW: A proposed mechanism of emotion, *Arch Neurol Psychiatry* 38:725, 1937. *The evidence wasn't very strong by today's standards, but the idea has been extremely influential anyway.*

Penfield W, Mathieson G: Memory: autopsy findings and comments on the role of hippocampus in experiential recall, *Arch Neurol* 31:145, 1974. *The conventional hippocampus-memory hypothesis in a well-written account by one of the neurosurgeons who made the unfortunate discovery.*

Price JL: Olfactory system. In Paxinos, G., editor: *The human nervous system,* San Diego, 1990, Academic Press.

Reiman EM et al.: Neuroanatomical correlates of anticipatory anxiety, *Science* 243:1071, 1989. *PET scanning studies implicating the anterior ends of the temporal lobes in the neural circuitry underlying feelings of fear and anxiety.*

Rosene DL, van Hoesen GW: Hippocampal efferents reach widespread areas of cerebral cortex and amygdala in the rhesus monkey, *Science* 198:315, 1977.

Seifert W: *Neurobiology of the hippocampus,* New York, 1983, Academic Press.

Shepherd GM: *The synaptic organization of the brain,* ed. 3, New York, 1990, Oxford University Press. *Chapter 5, olfactory bulb; Chapter 10, olfactory cortex; Chapter 11, hippocampus.*

Sims KS, Williams RS: The human amygdaloid complex: a cytologic and histochemical atlas using Nissl, myelin, acetylcholinesterase and nicotinamide adenine dinucleotide phosphate diaphorase staining, *Neurosci* 36:449, 1990.

Slotnick BM, Kaneko N: Role of mediodorsal thalamic nucleus in olfactory discrimination learning in rats, *Science* 214:91, 1981.

Squire LR: Memory and the hippocampus: a synthesis from findings with rats, monkeys, and humans, *Psychol Rev* 99:195, 1992.

Squire LR, Zola-Morgan S: The medial temporal lobe memory system, *Science* 253:1380, 1991. *A brief history of recent thinking about the role of the hippocampus, nearby cortical areas, and the amygdala in explicit memory for facts and events.*

Swanson LW, Cowan WM: Hippocampo-hypothalamic connections: origin in subicular cortex, not Ammon's horn, *Science* 189:303, 1975.

Van Hoesen GW, Pandya DP: Some connections of the entorhinal (area 28) and perirhinal (area 35) cortices of the rhesus monkey. III. Efferent connections, *Brain Res* 95:39, 1975.

Victor M, Adams RD, Collins GH: *The Wernicke-Korsakoff syndrome: a clinical and pathological study of 245 patients, 82 with post-mortem examination,* Philadelphia, 1971, F.A. Davis Co.

Zola-Morgan S, et al: Human amnesia and the medial temporal region: enduring memory impairment following a bilateral lesion limited to field CA1 of the hippocampus, *J Neurosci* 6:2950, 1986. *Partial amnesia in a rare human case with anatomically verified damage more or less restricted to a portion of the hippocampal formation.*

# CHAPTER 17

# *Chemical Neuroanatomy*

Early in this century, Ramon y Cajal and others used the Golgi stain to demonstrate that the nervous system is a collection of individual neurons (e.g., Figure 1-1) rather than a vast syncytial network, as some had alleged. An obvious corollary of this demonstration is that neurons must have mechanisms by which they communicate with each other. While there are some instances in which neurons are directly coupled, allowing ionic currents to flow from one into another, we now know that in most cases neurons communicate with each other by releasing neuroactive chemical transmitters, typically at specialized sites called *synapses*.*

The first insights into how synapses between neurons might work came from studies of the neuromuscular junction. Here the endings of motor neurons release a small-molecule transmitter *(acetylcholine),* which diffuses across the cleft between neuronal ending and muscle fiber, attaches to receptor molecules in the muscle fiber membrane, and initiates permeability changes and consequent depolarization (Figure 17-1). The depolarization is short-lived because an enzyme (acetylcholinesterase) simultaneously competes for acetylcholine and hydrolyzes it. It is now apparent that the neuromuscular junction is representative of only one type of synaptic interaction. Dozens of neurotransmitters have been described to date. Some are small molecules like acetylcholine (see Figures 17-2 to 17-5), while others are larger peptide molecules; some produce brief changes in membrane potential, while others produce prolonged potential changes or changes in membrane properties that last days or longer.*

The discovery that Parkinson's disease, with its characteristic set of neurological abnormalities, is associated with a defect in a particular neurotransmitter system ignited intense interest in trying to understand the relationship between neuroanatomical structures and neurotransmitters. A given neuron contains no more than a few of the known neurotransmitters, and methods are now available to define the neurotransmitter content of individual neurons or groups of neurons (see Plates 6 and 10). While we are far from a detailed understanding of the localization and function of all neurotransmitters, enormous progress has been made in the last 30 years. This chapter presents a brief overview of the various kinds of transmitters and the nuclei and pathways associated with some of them.

## TYPES OF NEUROTRANSMITTERS

Nearly all of the known or suspected neurotransmitters fall into one of two general categories: some are small amine molecules and the others are peptides. The small-molecule transmitters are synthesized by cytoplasmic enzymes and can therefore be manufactured and packaged for release in individual synaptic endings (like the transmitter shown schematically in Figure 17-1). Peptide transmitters, in contrast, are manufactured in the neuronal cell body, where they are cleaved from larger precursor proteins, packaged for release, and dispatched by axonal

*"Synapse" stared out as a noun, derived from a Greek word meaning a point of contact. It is now also used commonly as a verb referring to one neuron making a synaptic contact on another.

*Alternate terms like *neuromodulator* or *neurohormone* are used by many authors to refer to neuroactive substances that have long-lasting effects or diffuse from sites that are not typical synapses. For the sake of simplicity, however, all such molecules are referred to as *neurotransmitters* in this chapter.

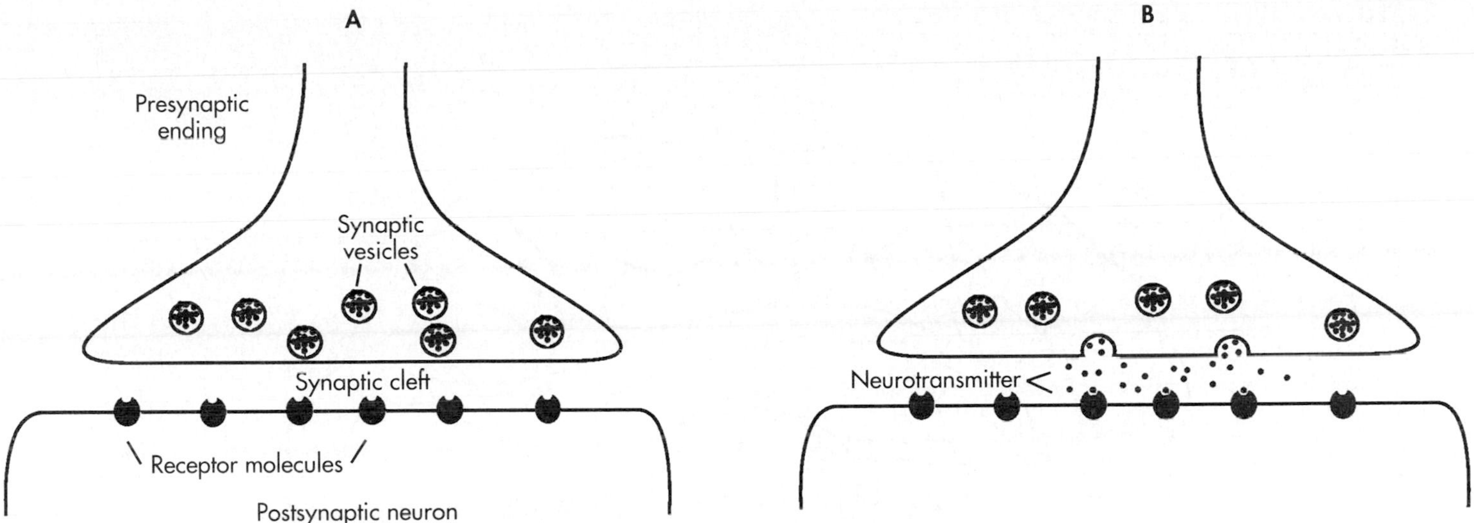


FIGURE 17-1
Schematic diagram of a "typical" synapse, both at rest (A) and caught in action (B). The presynaptic ending contains neurotransmitter molecules prepackaged in synaptic vesicles for release; a specialized area of the postsynaptic neuron, containing an array of receptor molecules specific for that neurotransmitter, is apposed to the presynaptic ending. Depolarization of the presynaptic ending causes some of its vesicles to merge with the presynaptic membrane and dump their contents into the synaptic cleft. Neurotransmitter molecules then diffuse across the synaptic cleft and some of them bind to postsynaptic receptor molecules. Transmitter-receptor binding causes some change in the postsynaptic neuron, such as rapid opening of an ion channel or a slower cascade of biochemical events that culminates in an electrical or other change. Effects of the neurotransmitter are limited in time either by degradative enzymes that destroy the transmitter or by transport systems that shuttle it back into the presynaptic ending or into neighboring glial cells.

transport to synaptic endings. There are only about 10 known small-molecule transmitters (of which six are particularly prominent—see Table 11), whereas there are dozens of neuroactive peptides.

In addition to acetylcholine, there are two other kinds of small-molecule transmitters. Some are amines called *monoamines* (or *biogenic amines*) derived metabolically from amino acids (see Figures 17-4 and 17-5). Others are themselves amino acids (see Figure 17-9).

## ACETYLCHOLINE

Acetylcholine (Figure 17-2) was the first neurotransmitter to be discovered. It plays an especially prominent role in the peripheral nervous system, as the transmitter released by alpha and gamma motor neurons, by preganglionic autonomic neurons, and by postganglionic parasympathetic neurons. It was thought for a time that acetylcholine might be similarly widespread in the central nervous system, but we know now that its distribution there is more restricted. *Cholinergic* neurons (Figure 17-3) are concentrated in parts of the reticular formation and in the *basal forebrain,* and are also found in the striatum, where they account for some of its large interneurons. The physiological action of acetylcholine is different at central and peripheral endings. It typically mediates excitatory events in the periphery that are brief and spatially precise, whereas its actions in the CNS are slower and more diffuse.

$$CH_3-\overset{\overset{\displaystyle O}{\|}}{C}-O-CH_2-CH_2-\underset{\underset{\displaystyle CH_3}{|}}{\overset{\overset{\displaystyle CH_3}{|}}{N^+}}-CH_3$$

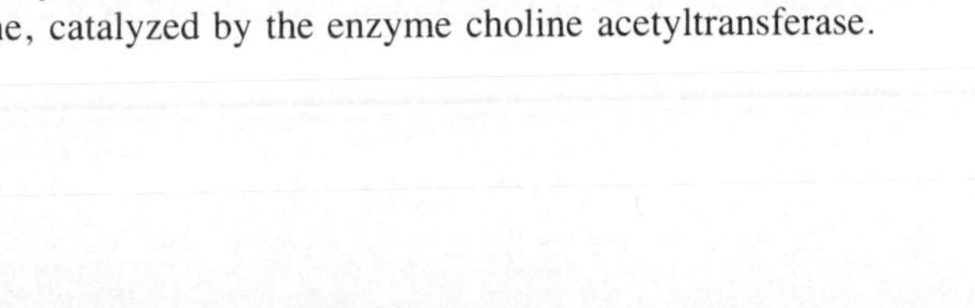

FIGURE 17-2
Acetylcholine, which is manufactured by the acetylation of choline, catalyzed by the enzyme choline acetyltransferase.

"Basal forebrain" is a loosely used term that refers approximately to the area at and near the inferior surface of the telencephalon, between the hypothalamus and the orbital cortex. The basal forebrain reaches the surface of the brain in the anterior perforated substance and extends superiorly into the septal area (see Figures 16-4 and 16-6). The connections and function of this portion of the telencephalon have been notoriously difficult to unravel; partly as a result of this difficulty, the area beneath the anterior commissure has long been referred to somewhat oxymoronically as the *substantia innominata* (literally, the "stuff

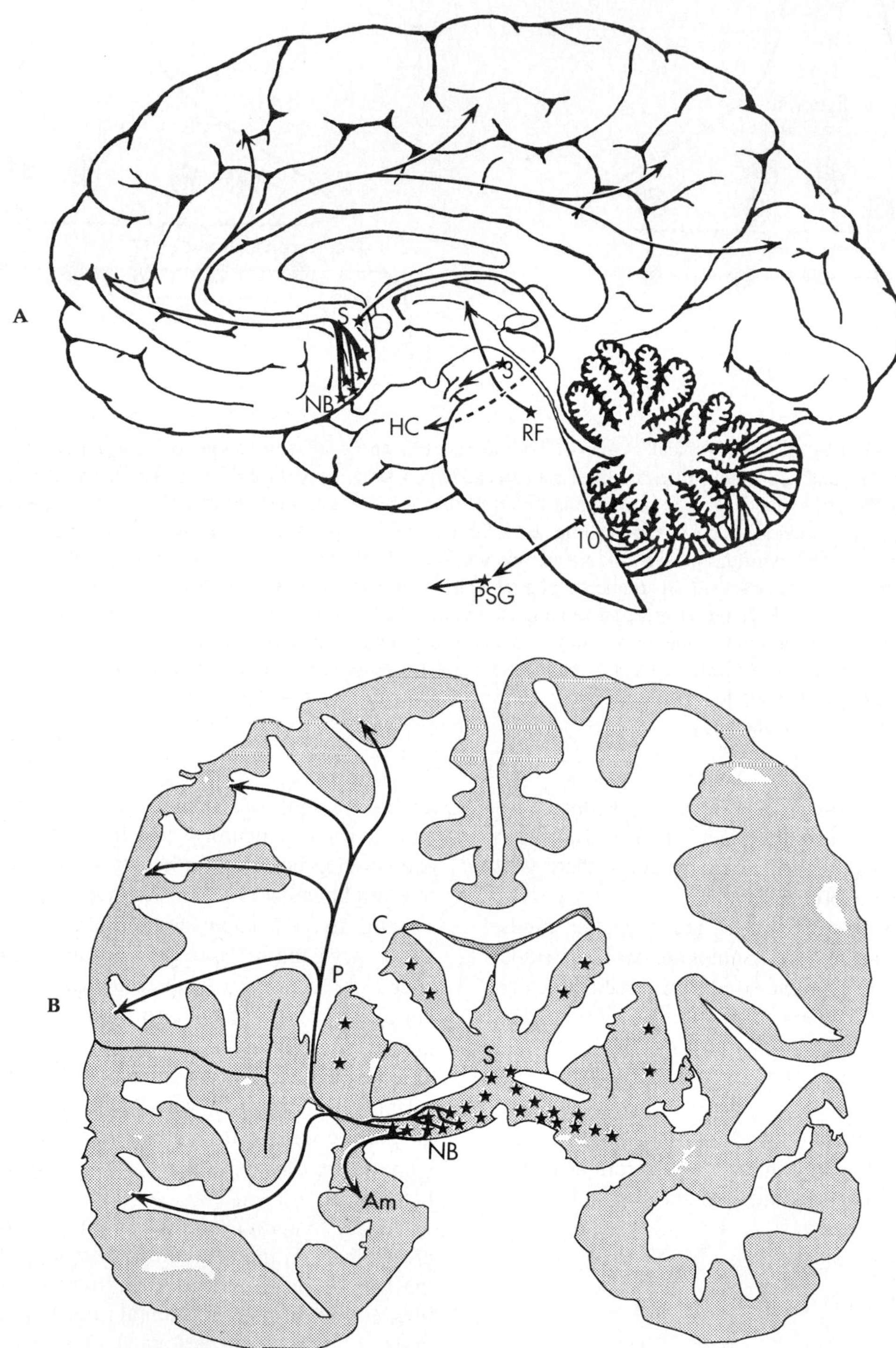


FIGURE 17-3
Principal locations of cholinergic cell bodies and pathways. Abbreviations: *3,* oculomotor nucleus (representing lower motor neurons generally); *10,* dorsal motor nucleus of the vagus nerve (representing preganglionic autonomic neurons generally); *PSG,* parasympathetic ganglion; *Am,* amygdala; *C,* caudate nucleus; *HC,* hippocampal formation; *NB,* nucleus basalis; *P,* putamen; *RF,* reticular formation; *S,* septal area.

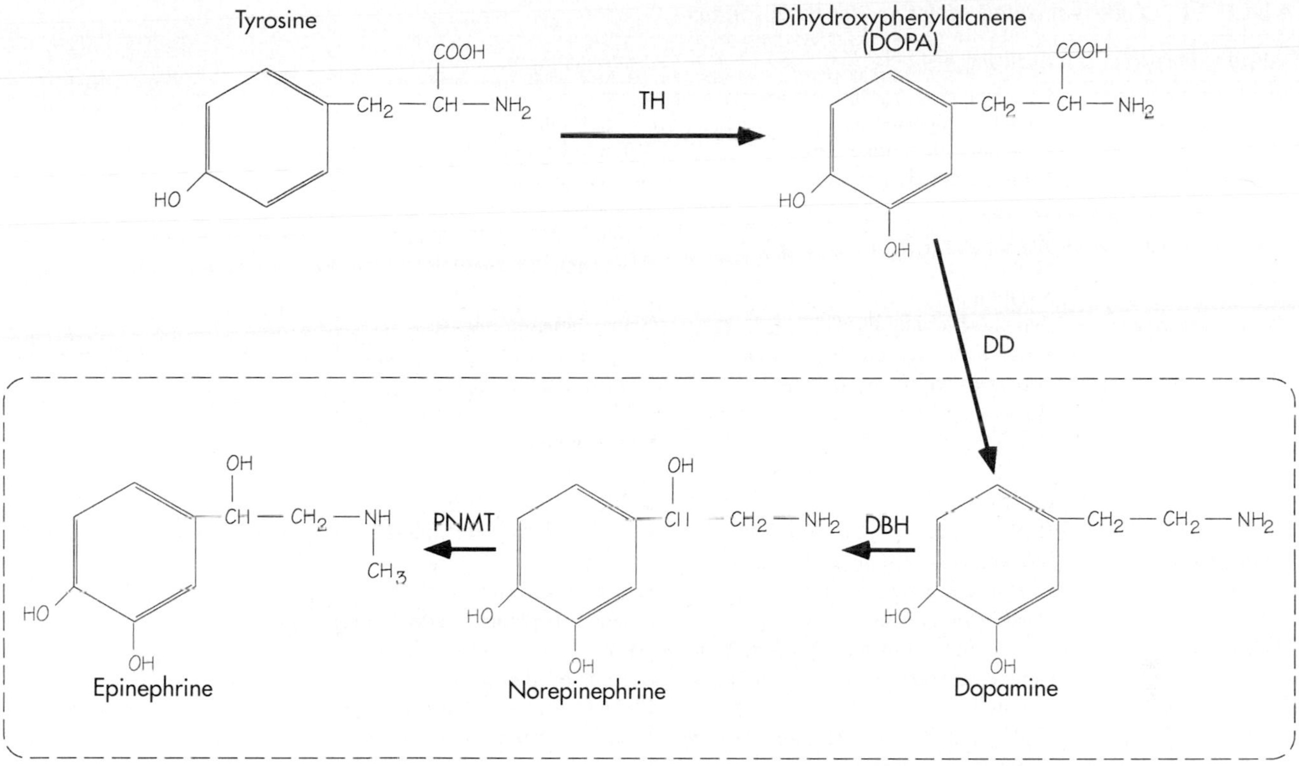

Tyrosine
COOH
CH2 — CH — NH2
HO
TH
Dihydroxyphenylalanene
(DOPA)
COOH
CH2 — CH — NH2
HO
OH
DD
OH
CH — CH2 — NH
CH3
PNMT
HO
OH
Epinephrine
OH
CH — CH2 — NH2
DBH
HO
OH
Norepinephrine
CH2 — CH2 — NH2
HO
OH
Dopamine

FIGURE 17-4
The catecholamine neurotransmitters (enclosed in the dashed box), so named because each includes a catechol group, which is the substituted benzene ring shown in color. These neurotransmitters are synthesized in a series of reactions that starts with the amino acid tyrosine. Epinephrine plays a relatively minor role as a neurotransmitter in the human brain, but dopamine and norepinephrine are widely distributed. Abbreviations for enzymes: *DBH*, dopamine-β-hydroxylase; *DD*, DOPA decarboxylase; *PNMT*, phenylethanolamine-*N*-methyltransferase; *TH*, tyrosine hydroxylase (the rate-limiting enzyme for the whole pathway).

Tryptophan
TrH
5HTD
HO
CH2 — CH2 — NH2
N
H
Serotonin
(5-Hydroxytryptamine)

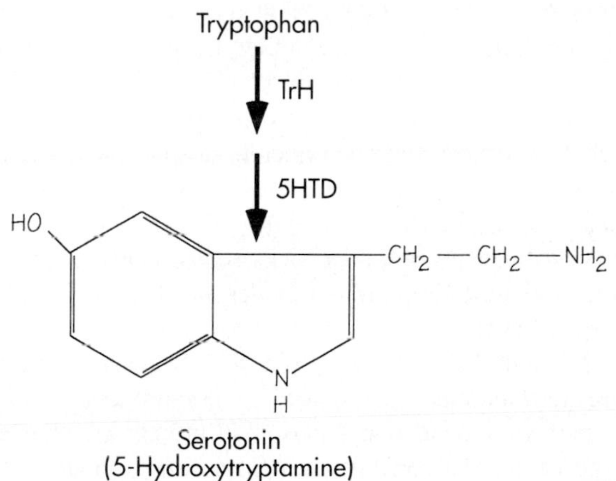

FIGURE 17-5
Structure and synthesis of serotonin. The pathway begins with the amino acid tryptophan, which is hydroxylated in a rate-limiting step catalyzed by tryptophan hydroxylase *(TrH)*. The resulting 5-hydroxytryptophan is decarboxylated in a reaction catalyzed by 5-hydroxytryptophan carboxylase *(5HDT)*, resulting in serotonin.

with no name"). Recent work has demonstrated that a prominent component of the substantia innominata, the *nucleus basalis* (or *basal nucleus of Meynert*) is the major collection of forebrain cholinergic neurons. Neurons of the nucleus basalis, together with some from related nuclei in and near the septal area, blanket the neocortex, hippocampal formation, and amygdala with cholinergic endings. These widespread projections suggest that the nucleus basalis is involved in general regulation of the level of forebrain activity, and there is considerable evidence that these cholinergic neurons (together with the cholinergic projections from the reticular formation to the thalamus) play a critical role in the sleep-wakefulness cycle.

## MONOAMINES

The monoamine transmitters are derived fairly directly from amino acids. Two of the three most prominent of these molecules, *norepinephrine* and *dopamine* (Figure 17-4), are derived from tyrosine. (They are also referred to as *catecholamines* because of the catechol nucleus that forms part of each.) The third major monoamine transmitter, *serotonin* (Figure 17-5), is derived from tryptophan.

**TABLE 11** *Principal Small-Molecule Neurotransmitters*

| *Neurotransmitter* | *Location of neurons* | *Location of terminals* |
|---|---|---|
| Acetylcholine | Lower motor neurons | Skeletal muscle |
| | Preganglionic autonomics | Autonomic ganglia |
| | Parasympathetic ganglia | Glands, smooth muscle |
| | Reticular formation | Thalamus |
| | Nucleus basalis | Cerebral cortex, amygdala |
| | Septal area | Hippocampal formation |
| | Striatum | Local |
| Norepinephrine*† | Sympathetic ganglia | Glands, smooth muscle |
| | Locus ceruleus, reticular formation | Widespread areas of forebrain, cerebellum, brainstem, spinal cord |
| Dopamine*† | Substantia nigra (compact part) | Caudate nucleus, putamen |
| | Ventral tegmental area | Limbic structures, cerebral cortex |
| | Hypothalamus | Infundibulum |
| | Retina (some amacrine cells) | Local |
| | Olfactory bulb | Local |
| Serotonin* | Raphe nuclei | Widespread areas of forebrain, cerebellum, brainstem, spinal cord |
| Glutamate | Interneurons in many CNS sites | Local |
| | Dorsal root ganglion cells | Spinal gray matter |
| | Cortical pyramidal cells | Striatum, thalamus, motor neurons, etc. |
| GABA** | Interneurons in many CNS sites | Local |
| | Cerebellar cortex (Purkinje cells) | Deep cerebellar nuclei |
| | Striatum | Globus pallidus, substantia nigra |
| | Globus pallidus, substantia nigra | Thalamus, subthalamic nucleus |
| | Thalamic reticular nucleus | Thalamus |

*Monoamines; †catecholamines; **gamma-aminobutyric acid

Monoamine-containing neurons, for the most part, are found only in the brainstem (although there are a few dopaminergic neurons in the forebrain). Despite this restricted distribution, these neurons, like those of the nucleus basalis, have far-flung connections (see Figures 17-6 to 17-8), suggesting that they too are involved in regulating or tuning the activity of large portions of the central nervous system. Nevertheless, there are characteristic differences between the termination patterns of fibers containing acetylcholine, norepinephrine, dopamine, and serotonin. This, together with consistent associations between certain transmitter systems and neurological syndromes (for example, dopamine and Parkinson's disease), suggests strongly that each of these four transmitters plays a distinctive role in the central nervous system.

## Norepinephrine

Neurons containing norepinephrine (called *noradrenergic* neurons from the synonym *noradrenaline* for norepinephrine) are found only in the pons and medulla. Half or more are located in the *locus ceruleus* (see Figure 8-12), and the remainder in lateral parts of the medullary reticular formation, in the solitary nucleus and the dorsal motor nucleus of the vagus, and in a few other sites (Figure 17-6). Collectively, these noradrenergic neurons project to most of the central nervous system. Ascending fibers traverse the dorsal longitudinal fasciculus or travel through the central tegmental tract to the medial forebrain bundle, and then diverge to reach the thalamus, hypothalamus, limbic forebrain structures, and the cerebral cortex (Figure 17-6). All areas of the cerebral cortex appear to receive some noradrenergic innervation, but that to somatosensory cortex is particularly dense. Descending fibers project to other parts of the brainstem and to all spinal levels, and some travel through the superior cerebellar peduncle to reach the cerebellar cortex* and deep nuclei. Despite the diverse nature of these projections, there is some anatomical specificity in their pattern. For example, the locus ceruleus provides most of the output to the cerebral cortex, while the lateral reticular formation provides most of the output to the spinal cord.

As might be expected from the extensive pattern of these terminations, activation of noradrenergic neurons and pathways results in widespread effects in other areas of the central nervous system. Some hints about possible functions of this system are provided by the response patterns of neurons in the locus ceruleus. These cells are

*Just as noradrenergic and some other fibers "break the rules" by circumventing the thalamus on their way to the cerebral cortex, so too are they atypical in reaching the cerebellum not as mossy or climbing fibers, but rather as diffuse projections.

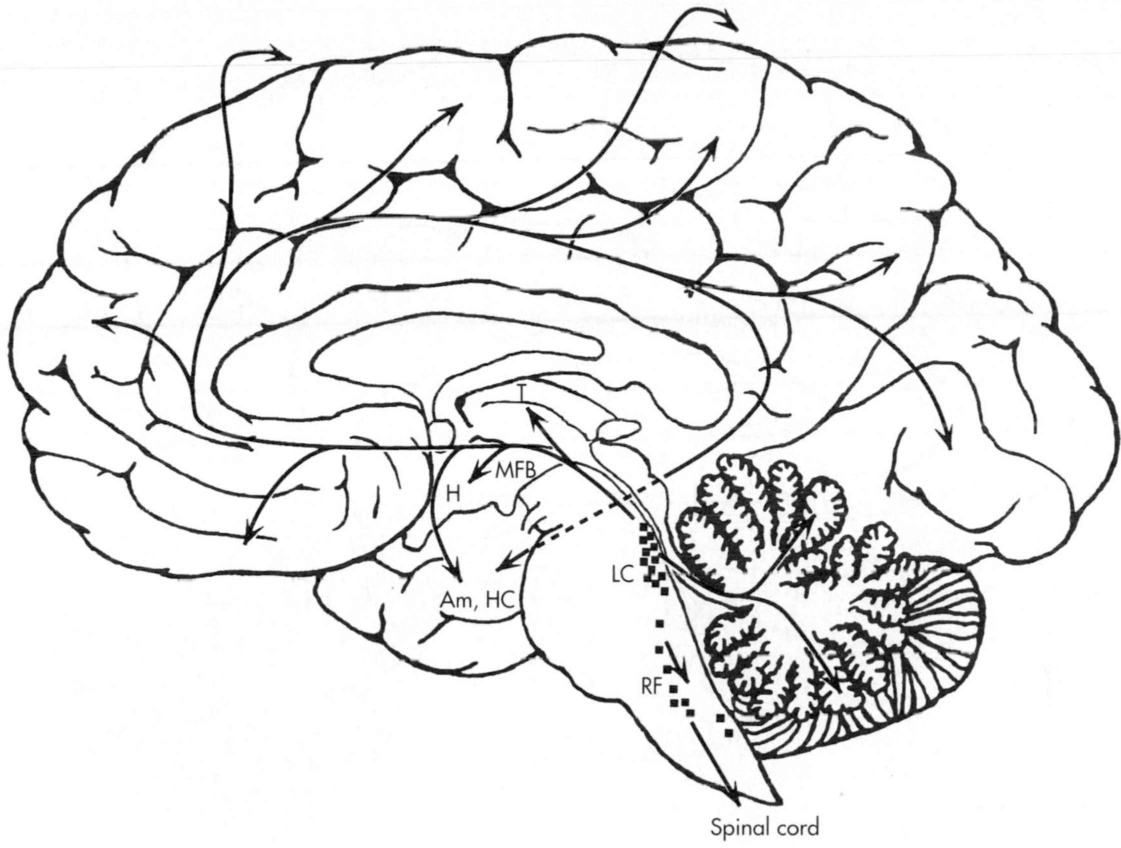


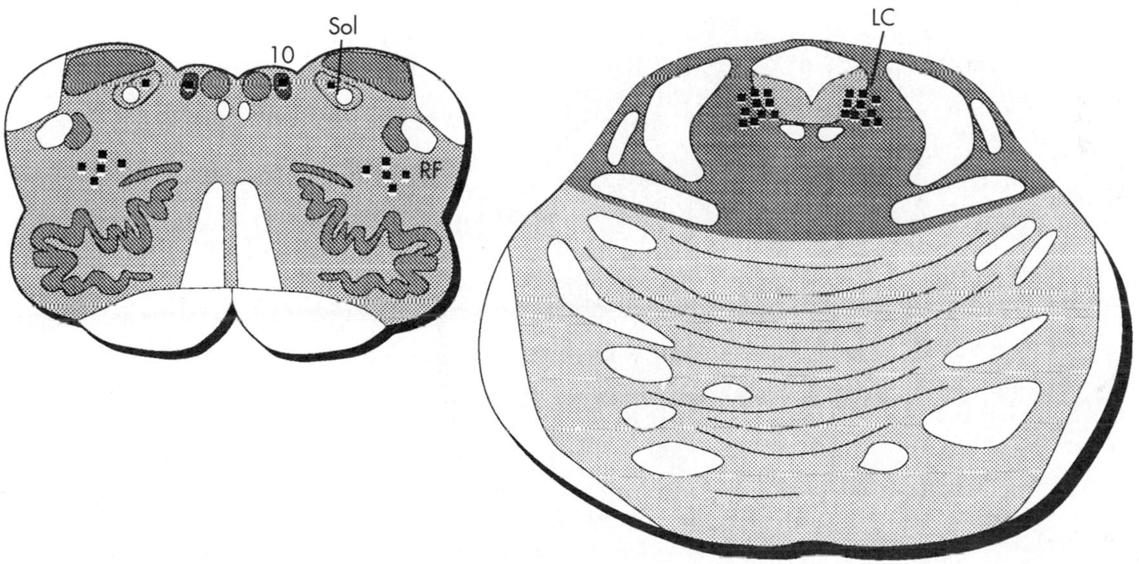


FIGURE 17-6
Principal locations of noradrenergic cell bodies and pathways. Noradrenergic fibers project from the locus ceruleus *(LC)* via the medial forebrain bundle *(MFB)* to the thalamus *(T)*, hypothalamus *(H)*, amygdala *(Am)*, hippocampal formation *(HC)*, to widespread additional areas of the forebrain, and to the cerebellum (via the superior cerebellar peduncle). More noradrenergic fibers, mostly in the rostral medullary reticular formation, project to the brainstem and spinal cord. The actual situation is more complicated than this: there are noradrenergic neurons in a few other places, such as the dorsal motor nucleus of the vagus *(10)* and the solitary nucleus *(Sol)*; the projections of the locus ceruleus and of reticular noradrenergic neurons overlap with each other; and additional pathways are used.

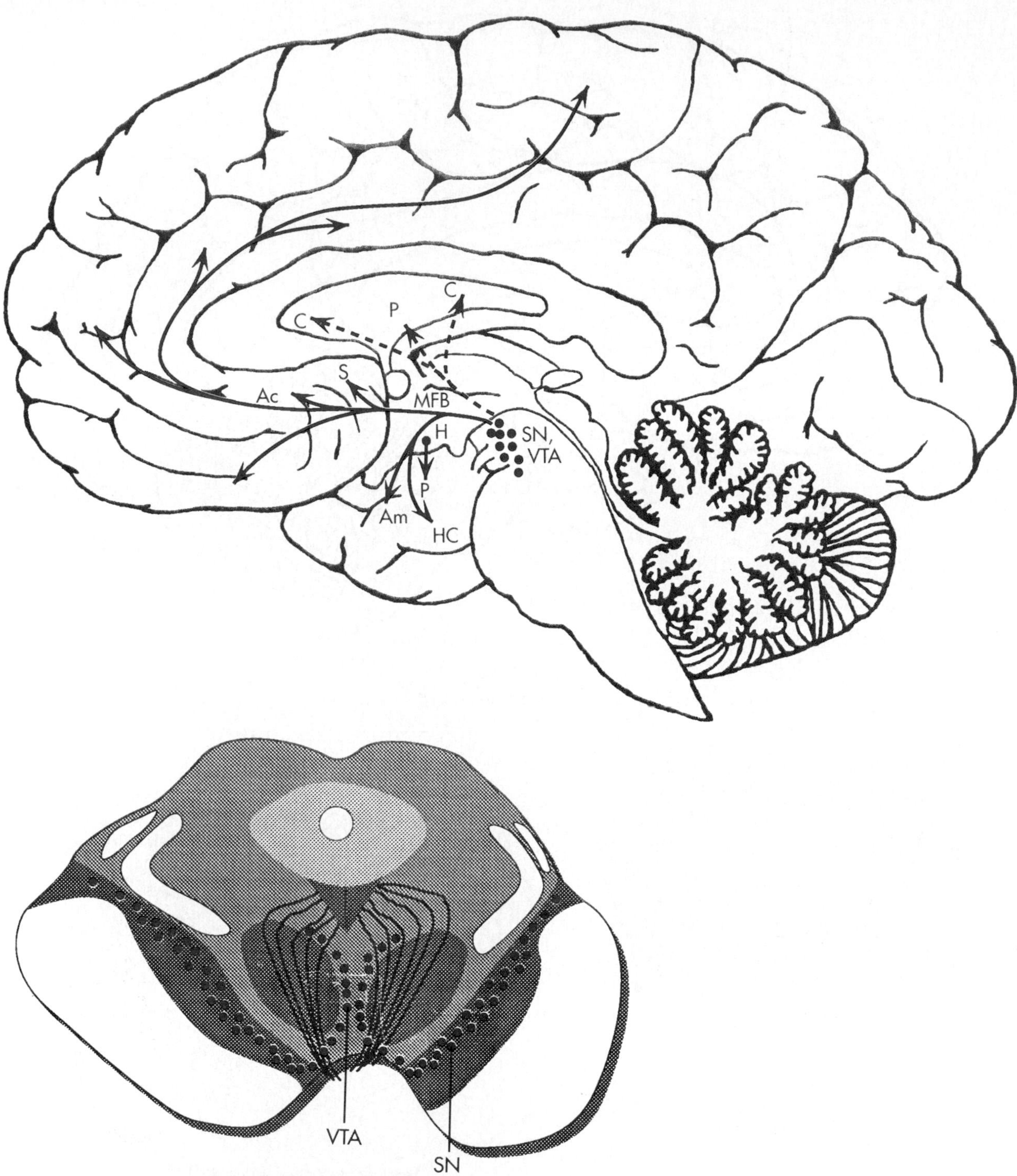


FIGURE 17-7
Principal locations of dopaminergic cell bodies and pathways. The nigrostriatal projection (dashed lines) from the compact part of the substantia nigra *(SN)* to the caudate nucleus *(C)* and putamen *(P)* is particularly prominent. In addition, the mesolimbic and mesocortical projections from the ventral tegmental area *(VTA)* travel through the medial forebrain bundle *(MFB)* to reach the septal area *(S)*, nucleus accumbens *(Ac)*, parts of the amygdala and hippocampal formation *(Am, HC)*, and neocortical areas. Finally, there are dopaminergic neurons in the hypothalamus *(H)* that project to the infundibular stalk of the pituitary *(P)*.

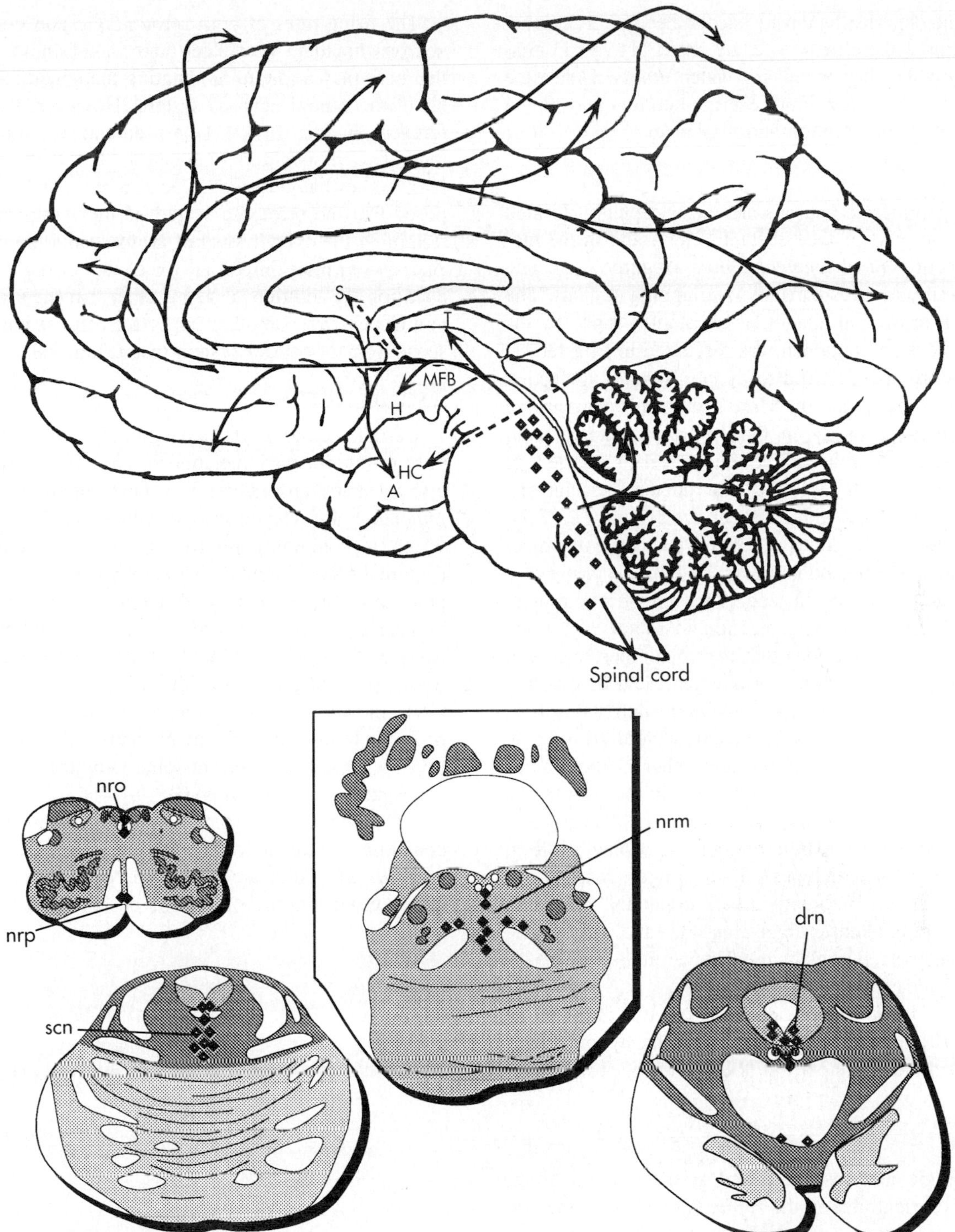


FIGURE 17-8
Principal locations of serotonergic cell bodies and pathways; these neurons and fibers are the most numerous and extensively distributed of the monoaminergic systems. The cell bodies are located in the raphe nuclei of the brainstem. Rostral raphe nuclei project, mainly through the medial forebrain bundle *(MFB)*, to virtually every part of the forebrain, including the thalamus *(T)*, hypothalamus *(H)*, striatum *(St)*, amygdala *(Am)*, hippocampal formation *(HC)*, and all neocortical areas. Caudal raphe nuclei project to the brainstem, cerebellum, and spinal cord; as in the case of noradrenergic neurons, the projections of rostrally and caudally situated cells actually overlap to some extent. The most commonly used terms for some prominent raphe nuclei are indicated in the lower half of the figure: *drn*, dorsal raphe nucleus; *nrm*, nucleus raphe magnus; *nro*, nucleus raphe obscurus; *nrp*, nucleus raphe pallidus; *scn*, superior central nucleus.

nearly silent electrically during sleep, become somewhat active during wakefulness, and are most active in situations that are startling or call for watchfulness. Hence the locus ceruleus and other noradrenergic neurons may play a role in maintaining attention and vigilance.

### Dopamine

Most dopaminergic neurons are mesencephalic, located in the compact part of the substantia nigra and in the medially adjacent *ventral tegmental area* (Figure 17-7), and project rostrally in three partially overlapping streams. The nigrostriatal projection from the substantia nigra to the caudate nucleus and putamen was discussed in Chapter 13; these fibers are also referred to as *mesostriatal,* reflecting their origin in the midbrain. *Mesolimbic* and *mesocortical* fibers originate primarily in the ventral tegmental area, join the medial forebrain bundle, and travel to a variety of forebrain destinations including the nucleus accumbens, septal area, amygdala, and cerebral cortex (Figure 17-7). As in the case of the locus ceruleus, the cortical projections are extensive but nonuniform; in this instance motor and limbic areas are emphasized. The nigrostriatal projection and the mesocortical projection to motor cortex are both consistent with the idea that the dopaminergic system is involved in the initiation of movement, and that its disruption is instrumental in the movement deficits seen in Parkinson's disease. However, the extensive dopaminergic projections to limbic structures and other cortical areas suggest that this system is also involved in motivation and cognition. Consistent with this, there is evidence (mentioned later) that the dopamine system may play a role in certain forms of mental illness. Interestingly, many drugs of abuse directly or indirectly cause dopamine release in the nucleus accumbens, suggesting that the mesolimbic projection may be involved in whatever it is that makes some things pleasurable.

Additional dopaminergic neurons are found in the retina (see Plate 10), the olfactory bulb, and the hypothalamus (where dopamine participates in the control of prolactin secretion).

### Serotonin

Serotonergic neurons are found at most levels of the brainstem, concentrated in the *raphe nuclei.** Like the noradrenergic neurons described above, they innervate virtually all parts of the central nervous system (Figure 17-8); the serotonergic innervation is in fact even more extensive and profuse. Projections from the rostral raphe nuclei join the medial forebrain bundle and the dorsal longitudinal fasciculus and reach the forebrain. The cortical innervation is most dense in sensory and limbic areas. Caudal raphe nuclei provide most of the projection to the brainstem and spinal cord.

*The Greek word *rhaphe* means "seam," and is used in this case to refer to the midline seam between the two halves of the brainstem.

The firing rates of both serotonergic and noradrenergic neurons fluctuate with sleep and wakefulness, suggesting that both play a role in modulating the general activity levels of the central nervous system. However, there are differences in the cortical layers and areas emphasized by these two transmitters, indicating that their roles are at least somewhat different. For example, it has been proposed that the serotonin system is more important for determining the overall level of arousal, and the norepinephrine system more important for phasic changes in level of attention. In addition, it seems clear that the serotonin system has at least one other important role, as part of the descending pain-control system (see Chapter 8).

## AMINO ACIDS

Certain amino acids serve double duty, involved not only in intermediary metabolism and protein synthesis but also as neurotransmitters. The most important of these are *glutamate* and its derivative *gamma-aminobutyric acid,* which is commonly referred to by its acronym GABA (Figure 17-9). Glutamate is the major transmitter for brief, point-to-point, excitatory synaptic events in the CNS, playing a role analogous to that of acetylcholine in the periphery. Conversely, GABA is the major transmitter for brief, point-to-point, inhibitory synaptic events in the CNS. In addition to these two amino acids, aspartate is the probable transmitter at some excitatory CNS synapses, and glycine is the transmitter at some inhibitory CNS synapses (especially in the spinal cord).

As might be expected from these roles, interneurons containing glutamate or GABA are widespread in the nervous system. There are also prominent examples of projection neurons that use one or the other. For example, corti-

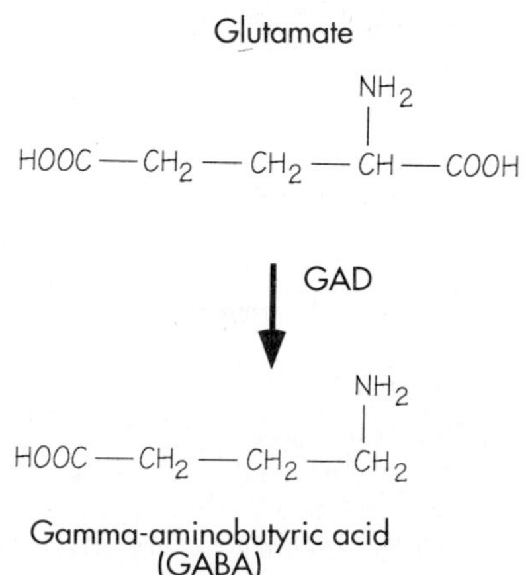


FIGURE 17-9
The two most prominent amino acid neurotransmitters, glutamate and gamma-aminobutyric acid (GABA). GABA is synthesized from glutamate via a decarboxylation catalyzed by glutamic acid decarboxylase *(GAD).*

cal pyramidal cells are rich in glutamate and the myriad cortical outputs are thought to use this amino acid as a transmitter; the endings of primary afferents in the spinal cord and the endings of ascending pathways in thalamic relay nuclei also use glutamate. The inhibitory projections from Purkinje cells to the deep cerebellar nuclei, from the striatum to the globus pallidus and substantia nigra, and from the globus pallidus and substantia nigra to the thalamus all use GABA as a transmitter, as does the regulatory input to the thalamus from its reticular nucleus.

## PEPTIDES

There were demonstrations more than half a century ago that some neurons secrete hormones, as in the cases of the magnocellular neurosecretory neurons of the hypothalamus that produce oxytocin and vasopressin. These observations were extended when, beginning in the early 1970s, the hypothalamic releasing and inhibiting factors were isolated and characterized as short chains of amino acids, or peptides. Work since that time, using recently available experimental techniques, has fundamentally transformed our view of the relationship between peptides and the function of the nervous system. It is now apparent that there are far more kinds of neuroactive peptides (or *neuropeptides*) in the brain than previously imagined—the number now stands at more than 50—and that most or all of them can function as neurotransmitters or neuromodulators (like the enkephalins mentioned in Chapter 8). For example, the 14-amino-acid peptide *somatostatin* was originally described as the hypothalamic inhibiting factor that controls the secretion of growth hormone by the anterior pituitary. It was subsequently found that hormonally released somatostatin accounts for only about 10% of the somatostatin in the brain, and that this peptide is localized primarily in the synaptic endings of neurons in many different CNS locations. Another example is the 11-amino-acid peptide *substance P*, originally described as a smooth muscle relaxant isolated from gut, which has been localized in the synaptic endings of striatal projection neurons, some dorsal root ganglion cells, and other neurons.

Some neuropeptides are widely distributed, and presumably have multiple or general functions. Others have a more restricted distribution, and may be associated with a specific function. For example, the octapeptide *angiotensin II* is a blood-borne hormone produced as part of the kidney's response to dehydration; it acts in the kidney and elsewhere outside the nervous system to promote water retention. Blood-borne angiotensin II also acts as a neurohormone by entering the CNS in the wall of the third ventricle and activating neurons in the subfornical organ (Figure 5-14). Finally, a system of neurons (including those of the subfornical organ) that apparently use angiotensin II as a transmitter orchestrate vasopressin secretion, blood pressure adjustments, and a search for water.

Most or all neurons that contain a neuropeptide also contain one of the "classical" small-molecule transmitters described earlier. This means that there are often separate subpopulations of neurons in a CNS area, each with its own chemical signature. For example, the GABAergic striatal neurons that project to the external pallidal segment also contain enkephalin, while those that project to the internal pallidal segment also contain substance P. The functional consequences of this coexistence of transmitter substances are unknown in most cases, but it seems clear that single synapses can mediate multiple effects with different time courses and sensitivities.

## SOME FUNCTIONAL ASPECTS OF NEUROTRANSMITTER ANATOMY

Many of the drugs used to treat neurological and psychiatric disorders are known to have effects at synapses involving particular neurotransmitters. For example, phenothiazine derivatives (e.g., Thorazine) and related drugs used as antipsychotics in the treatment of schizophrenia block dopamine receptors, suggesting that the mesolimbic and mesocortical projections may be involved in this disorder. Similarly, drugs commonly used as antidepressants enhance the effectiveness of transmission at norepinephrine and serotonin synapses. Finally, the benzodiazepines (e.g., Valium, Librium) often used as tranquilizers bind to GABA receptors and increase the effects of transmitter released at GABA synapses. Observations like these, coupled with our recent ability to map out the cells, axons, and synaptic endings that use a neurotransmitter, have raised hopes of being able to better understand these disorders and to develop more effective drugs for their treatment. Although there are few disorders in which malfunction of a single neurotransmitter system accounts for all findings, there is a growing number of examples in which one transmitter plays a major role.

Alzheimer's disease is a devastating and sadly common illness characterized by extensive neuronal atrophy (particularly in the neocortex and hippocampal formation), memory loss, personality change, and ultimately, profound dementia. There is a dramatic loss of acetylcholine in the cortex and hippocampal formation of Alzheimer's patients, and a corresponding loss of neurons in the nucleus basalis and nearby cholinergic cell groups. This led to the hope that an acetylcholine replacement therapy, analogous to the use of *l*-dopa in Parkinson's disease, might help Alzheimer's patients. Unfortunately such attempts were unsuccessful, and it has since been found that multiple transmitter systems are affected in Alzheimer's disease. For example, cortical somatostatin-containing interneurons are affected as much as cholinergic neurons. Although acetylcholine deficiency is still thought to be important in the pathogenesis of Alzheimer's disease, the fundamental basis of the neuronal degeneration is still unknown.

Most neurons have receptors for glutamate, the principal excitatory neurotransmitter, and this amino acid is available in high concentrations in excitatory synaptic terminals. Ordinarily, glutamate released at synapses is taken back up rapidly into the presynaptic terminal or surrounding glial cells, so that postsynaptic membranes are exposed to this amino acid only briefly. This is important, because more than a brief dose is toxic—prolonged exposure to glutamate triggers a sequence of events that can injure or even kill neurons, a phenomenon called *excitotoxicity*. Overexposure to glutamate could arise either from excessive release or from deficient reuptake, and both mechanisms are now thought to play a role in some forms of neuropathology. Part of the mechanism of brain damage in stroke may be centered around the release of toxic amounts of glutamate in response to anoxia, and some degenerative diseases of the nervous system (including Huntington's disease) may result from localized defects in glutamate reuptake.

## ADDITIONAL READINGS


Baker KG et al: The human locus coeruleus complex: an immunohistochemical and three-dimensional reconstruction study, *Exp Brain Res* 77:257, 1989.

Beal MF, Martin JB: Neuropeptides in neurological disease, *Ann Neurol* 20:547, 1986.

Brozoski TJ et al: Cognitive deficit caused by regional depletion of dopamine in prefrontal cortex of rhesus monkey, *Science* 205:929, 1979.

Carlsson A, Falck B, Hillarp N-A: Cellular localization of brain monoamines, *Acta Physiol Scand* 56, Suppl. 196, 1962. *The first systematic mapping of monoamine-containing neurons in the CNS, using a histochemical technique that makes them fluorescent.*

Choi DW, Rothman SM: The role of glutamate neurotoxicity in hypoxic-ischemic neuronal death, *Ann Rev Neurosci* 13:171, 1990.

Cooper JR, Bloom FE, Roth RH: *The biochemical basis of neuropharmacology,* ed 6, New York, 1991, Oxford University Press.

von Euler US, Gaddum JH: An unidentified depressor substance in certain tissue extracts, *J Physiol* 72:74, 1931. *The original description of the isolation of substance P from intestine and brain. Unbeknownst to the authors, this was the first recorded isolation of a neuropeptide.*

Fibiger HC: Cholinergic mechanisms in learning, memory and dementia: a review of recent evidence, *Trends Neurosci* 14:220, 1991.

Fillenz M: *Noradrenergic neurons,* New York, 1990, Cambridge University Press.

Foote SL, Morrison JH: Extrathalamic modulation of cortical function, *Ann Rev Neurosci* 10:67, 1987. *A review of direct cortical input from fiber systems containing norepinephrine, dopamine, serotonin, and acetylcholine.*

Gaspar P et al: Catecholamine innervation of the human cerebral cortex as revealed by comparative immunohistochemistry of tyrosine hydroxylase and dopamine-beta-hydroxylase, *J Comp Neurol* 279:249, 1989.

Grant SJ, Aston-Jones G, Redmond DE Jr.: Responses of primate locus coeruleus neurons to simple and complex sensory stimuli, *Brain Res Bull* 21:401, 1988.

Guillemin R: Peptides in the brain: the new endocrinology of the neuron, *Science* 202:390, 1978.

Jacobs BL, Azmitia EC: Structure and function of the brain serotonin system, *Physiol Rev* 72:165, 1992.

Jones EG: Neurotransmitters in the cerebral cortex, *J Neurosurg* 65:135, 1986.

Koob GF: Drugs of abuse: anatomy, pharmacology, and function of reward pathways, *Trends Pharmacol Sci* 13:177, 1992.

Le Moal M, Simon H: Mesocorticolimbic dopaminergic network: functional and regulatory roles, *Physiol Rev* 71:155, 1991.

Lundberg JM, Hökfelt T: Coexistence of peptides and classical neurotransmitters, *Trends Neurosci* 6:325, 1983.

Mesulam M-M, Geula C: Nucleus basalis (Ch 4) and cortical cholinergic innervation in the human brain: Observations based on the distribution of acetylcholinesterase and choline acetyltransferase, *J Comp Neurol* 275:216, 1988.

Mesulam M-M et al: Human reticular formation: cholinergic neurons of the pedunculopontine and laterodorsal tegmental nuclei and some cytochemical comparisons to forebrain cholinergic neurons, *J Comp Neurol* 281:611, 1989.

Napier TC, Kalivas PW, Hanin I: *The basal forebrain. Anatomy to function* (*Adv Exp Med Biol,* vol. 295), New York, 1991, Plenum Press.

Nieuwenhuys R: *Chemoarchitecture of the brain,* Berlin, 1985, Springer-Verlag.

Olney JW: Inciting excitotoxic cytocide among central neurons. In Schwartz RW, Ben-Ari Y: *Excitatory amino acids and epilepsy (Adv Exp Med Biol,* vol. 203), New York, 1986, Plenum Press. *"One of my major research goals in recent years has been to answer a simple question: 'Can one CNS neuron excite another CNS neuron to death?' "*

Paxinos G: *The human nervous system,* San Diego, 1990, Academic Press.

Pearson J et al: Human brainstem catecholamine neuronal anatomy as indicated by immunocytochemistry with antibodies to tyrosine hydroxylase, *Neurosci* 8:3, 1983.

Perry TL, Hansen S: What excitotoxin kills striatal neurons in Huntington's disease? Clues from neurochemical studies, *Neurol* 40:20, 1990. *The implication from these studies is that it's glutamate.*

Reiner A, Anderson KD: The patterns of neurotransmitter and neuropeptide co-occurrence among striatal projection neurons: conclusions based on recent findings, *Brain Res Rev* 15:251, 1990.

Saper CB, Chelimsky TC: A cytoarchitectonic and histochemical study of nucleus basalis and associated cell groups in the normal human brain, *Neurosci* 13:1023, 1984.

Schwartz J-C et al: Histaminergic transmission in the mammalian brain, *Physiol Rev* 71:1, 1991. *One more amine neurotransmitter, this one prominent in hypothalamic neurons.*

Smith Y, Séguéla, Parent A: Distribution of GABA-immunoreactive neurons in the thalamus of the squirrel monkey *(Saimiri sciureus), Neurosci* 22:579, 1987.

Smith Y et al: Distribution of GABA-immunoreactive neurons in the basal ganglia of the squirrel monkey *(Saimiri sciureus), J Comp Neurol* 259:50, 1987.

Torack RM, Morris JC: The association of ventral tegmental area histopathology with adult dementia, *Arch Neurol* 45:497, 1988.

Whitehouse PJ et al: Alzheimer's disease and senile dementia: loss of neurons in the basal forebrain, *Science* 215:1237, 1982.

Willner P, Scheel-Kruger J: *The mesolimbic dopamine system: from motivation to action,* New York, 1991, John Wiley and Sons.

Woolf NJ: Cholinergic systems in mammalian brain and spinal cord, *Prog Neurobiol* 37:475, 1991.

# APPENDIX

## Coronal sections of the forebrain

When the nervous system is discussed in terms of functional subsections, as in the preceding chapters, it is sometimes difficult to envision how the various parts are related to the whole. Therefore, an appendix is provided here in the same philosophy as that at the end of Chapter 9, with a wide variety of forebrain and brainstem structures labeled. The appendix is a series of nine photographs of brain sections cut in the coronal planes indicated in Figure A-1. The sections were provided to the University of Arizona in 1966 by the late Dr. Paul I. Yakovlev and appear here through the courtesy of Dr. Jay B. Angevine, Jr., Professor of Anatomy, The University of Arizona College of Medicine.

Only major structures that were mentioned prominently in this book are indicated. In addition, in order to keep the number of labels manageable, cerebral sulci were in general left unlabeled and a number of structures that appear in each section (e.g., the corpus callosum) were not labeled every time they appeared. Very abbreviated descriptions of labeled structures are provided; additional details can be found elsewhere in the text.

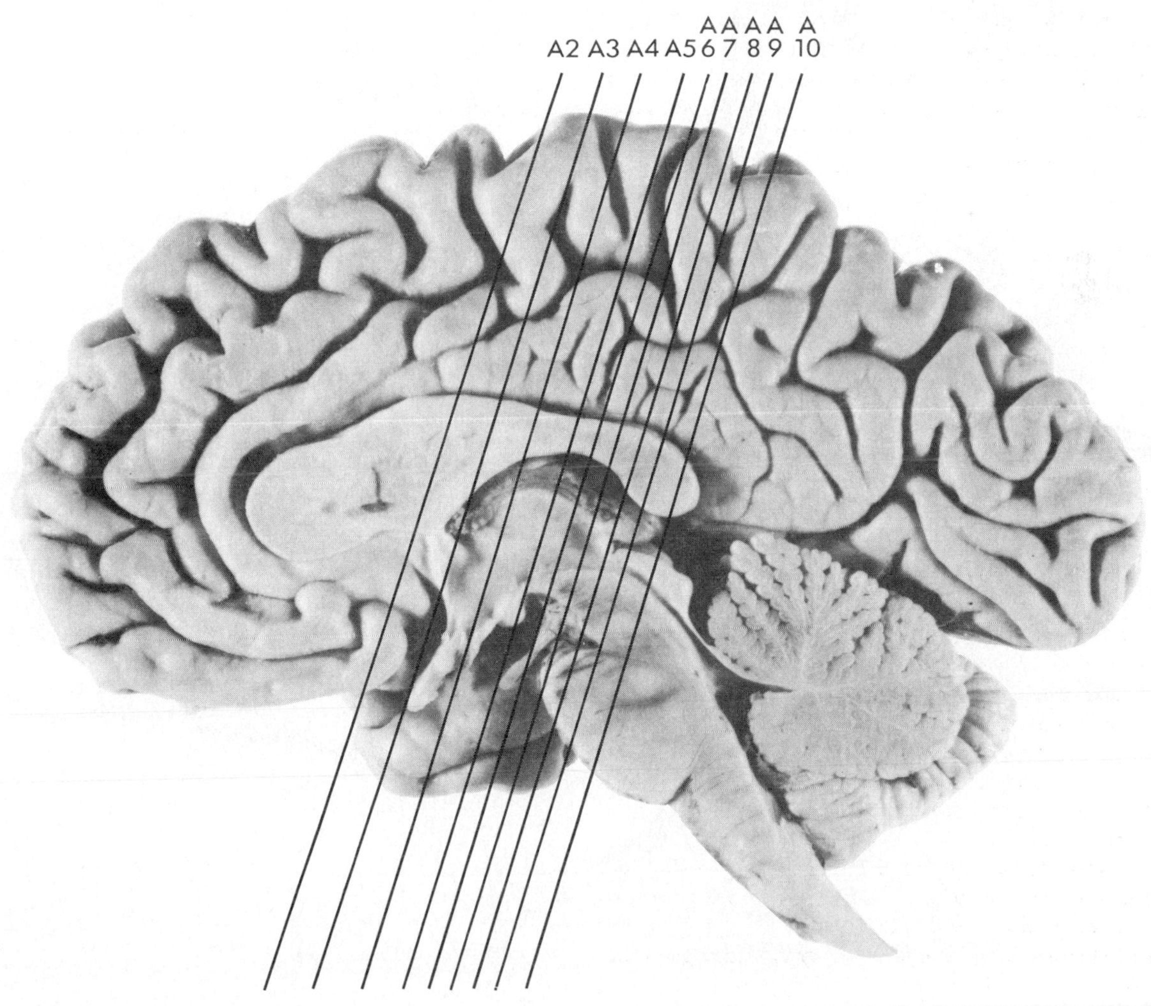


FIGURE A-1

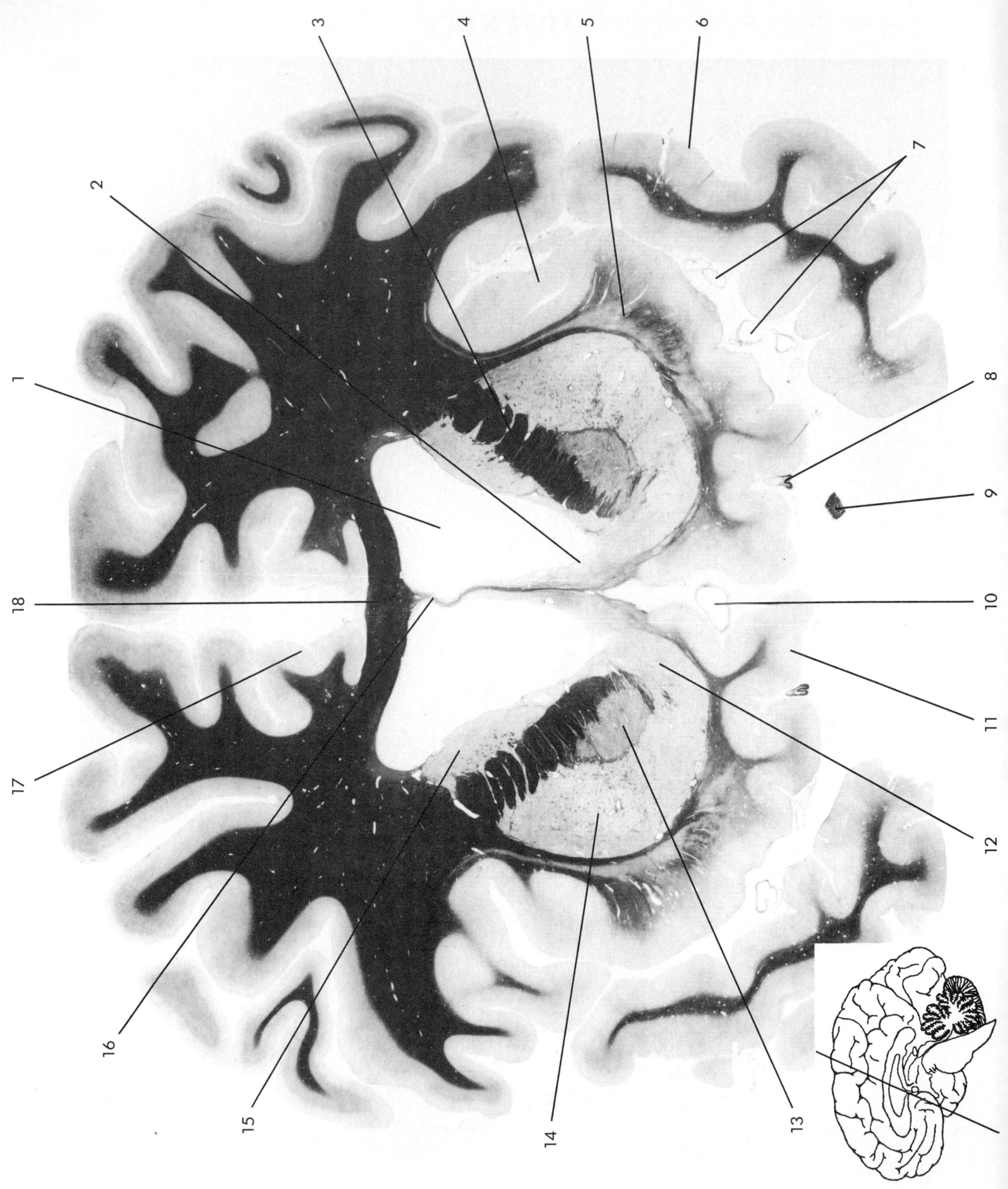
1
2
3
4
5
6
7
8
9
10
11
12
13
14
15
16
17
18

*Figure A-2 Anterior horn of the lateral ventricle*

1. Anterior horn of the lateral ventricle.
2. Septal nuclei. Reciprocally connected with the amygdala, hippocampal formation, hypothalamus, and other limbic structures.
3. Anterior limb of the internal capsule. Contains projections to and from prefrontal and anterior cingulate cortex, including those from the dorsomedial and anterior nuclei.
4. Insula. Includes gustatory and autonomic areas.
5. Claustrum. Reciprocal connections with cerebral cortex, poorly understood function.
6. Anterior end of the temporal lobe (temporal pole). Limbic cortex.
7. Branches of the middle cerebral artery. Will emerge from the lateral sulcus and supply the lateral surface of the cerebral hemisphere.
8. Olfactory tract. Projections from the olfactory bulb to the piriform cortex and amygdala.
9. Optic nerve. Axons of retinal ganglion cells on their way to the lateral geniculate nucleus, superior colliculus, and a few other sites.
10. Anterior cerebral artery. Branches parallel the corpus callosum and supply the medial surface of the frontal and parietal lobes.
11. Gyrus rectus. Part of orbital frontal cortex; extensive limbic connections, particularly in circuits involving the amygdala.
12. Nucleus accumbens. The part of the striatum with predominantly limbic connections.
13. Globus pallidus (lateral or external segment). Afferents from the caudate nucleus and putamen, efferents to the subthalamic nucleus.
14. Putamen. The part of the striatum with predominantly motor connections.
15. Head of the caudate nucleus, the part of the striatum predominantly connected with association cortex.
16. Septum pellucidum. Paired membrane separating the two lateral ventricles.
17. Cingulate gyrus. Extensive limbic connections, particularly in circuits involving the hippocampal formation.
18. Corpus callosum. Commissural fibers interconnecting most cortical areas.

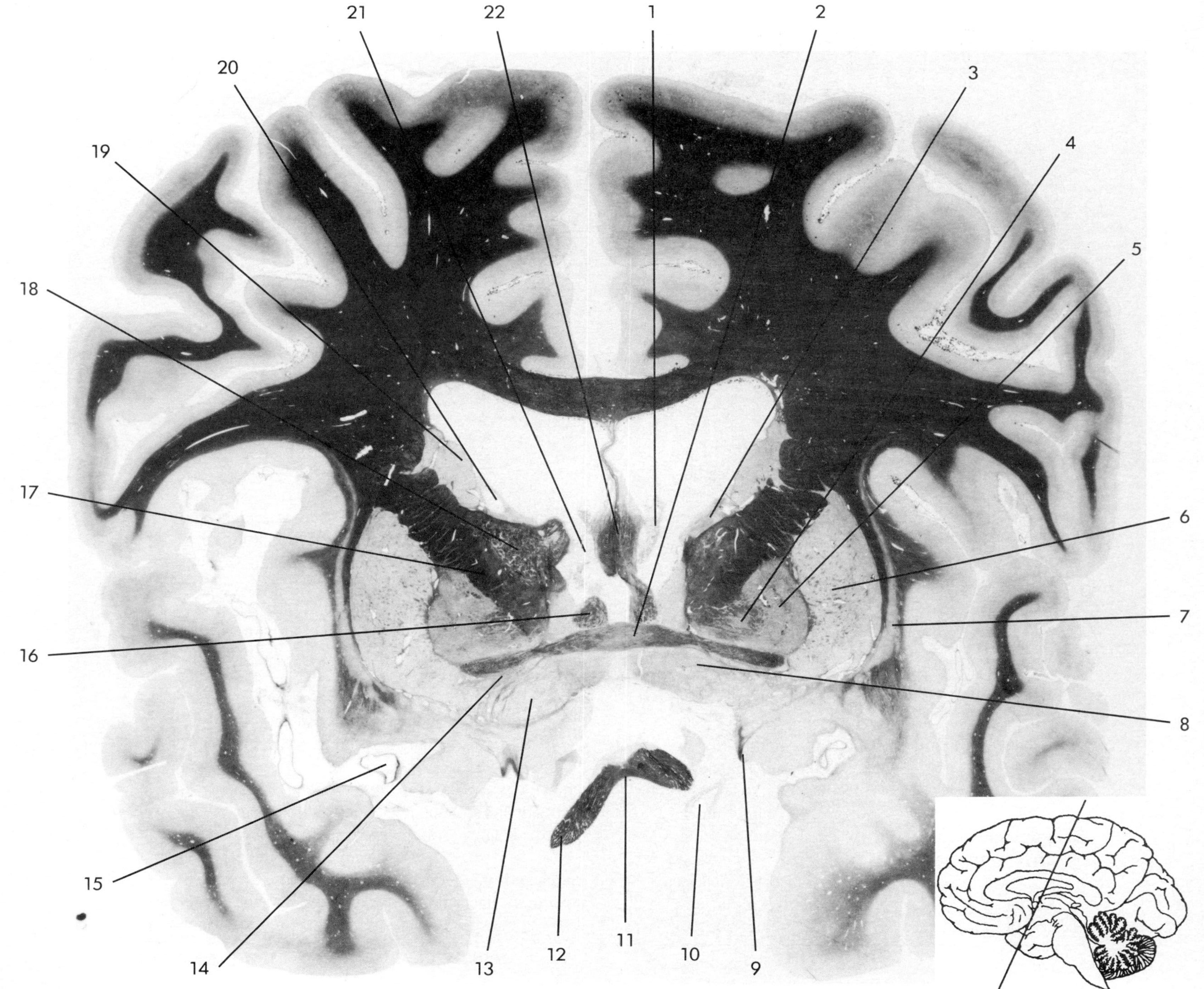
21
22
1
2
20
3
19
4
5
18
17
6
7
16
8
15
14
13
12
11
10
9

*Figure A-3 Anterior commissure*

1. Choroid plexus adjacent to the interventricular foramen.
2. Anterior commissure. Commissural fibers interconnecting the temporal lobes, together with a few crossing olfactory fibers.
3. Stria terminalis. Efferents from the amygdala to the septal area and hypothalamus.
4. Globus pallidus (medial or internal segment). Afferents from the caudate nucleus, putamen, and subthalamic nucleus, efferents to the thalamus.
5. Globus pallidus (lateral or external segment). Afferents from the caudate nucleus and putamen, efferents to the subthalamic nucleus.
6. Putamen. The part of the striatum with predominantly motor connections.
7. Claustrum. Reciprocal connections with cerebral cortex, poorly understood function.
8. Location of the nucleus basalis (of Meynert). Groups of large cholinergic neurons, situated in the substantia innominata, that innervate most forebrain areas.
9. Olfactory tract. Projections from the olfactory bulb to the piriform cortex and amygdala.
10. Internal carotid artery, just before it bifurcates into the anterior and middle cerebral arteries.
11. Optic chiasm, where optic nerve fibers from the nasal half of each retina decussate.
12. Optic nerve. Axons of retinal ganglion cells on their way to the lateral geniculate nucleus, superior colliculus, and a few other sites.
13. Nucleus accumbens. The part of the striatum with predominantly limbic connections.
14. Ventral pallidum. Limbic extension of the globus pallidus, with inputs from the nucleus accumbens.
15. Middle cerebral artery.
16. Column of the fornix. Efferents from the hippocampal formation to the septal area and mammillary bodies.
17. Genu of the internal capsule. Contains projections to and from frontal cortex.
18. Reticular nucleus, covering the anterior (and lateral) surface of the thalamus. Afferents from the thalamus and cerebral cortex, GABAergic efferents to the thalamus.
19. Junction between the head and body of the caudate nucleus, the part of the striatum predominantly connected with association cortex.
20. Terminal (thalamostriate) vein.
21. Interventricular foramen.
22. Body of the fornix. Efferents from the hippocampal formation to the septal area and mammillary bodies.

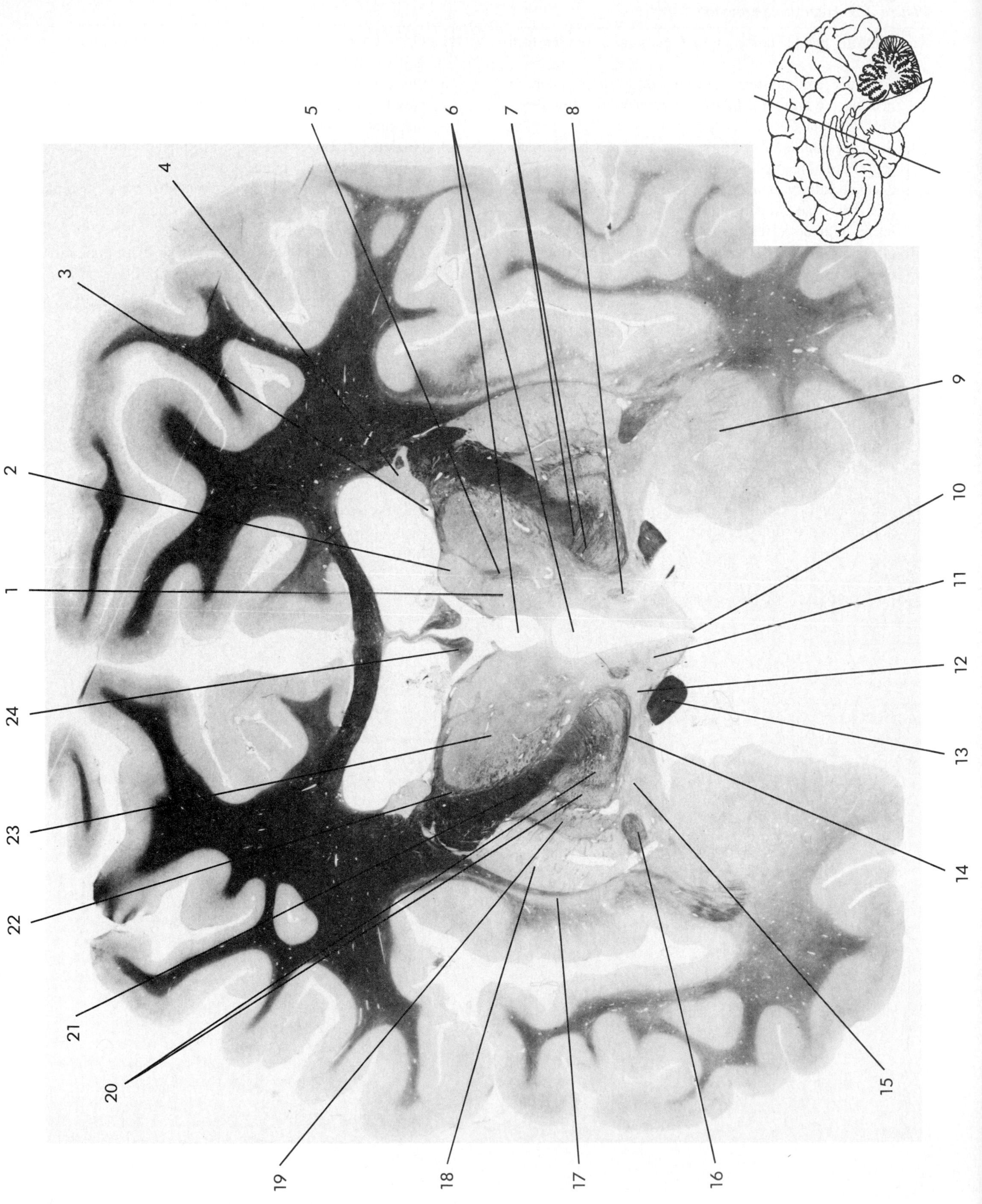
1
2
3
4
5
6
7
8
9
10
11
12
13
14
15
16
17
18
19
20
21
22
23
24

*Figure A-4 Anterior thalamus*

1. Dorsomedial nucleus. Connections with prefrontal association cortex.
2. Anterior nucleus. Afferents from the mammillary body (via the mammillothalamic tract), efferents to the cingulate gyrus.
3. Terminal (thalamostriate) vein.
4. Body of the caudate nucleus, the part of the striatum predominantly connected with association cortex.
5. Mammillothalamic tract. Projection from the mammillary body to the anterior nucleus of the thalamus. Part of the Papez circuit.
6. Third ventricle. The two portions indicated are separated by the interthalamic adhesion (massa intermedia).
7. Lenticular fasciculus (passing through internal capsule). Part of the projection from the globus pallidus to the thalamus.
8. Column of the fornix. Efferents from the hippocampal formation to the septal area and mammillary bodies.
9. Amygdala. A collection of nuclei forming the core of one of the two major limbic circuits.
10. Median eminence of the hypothalamus. Former attachment point of the infundibular stalk.
11. Medial zone of the hypothalamus. At this level, includes the ventromedial and dorsomedial nuclei.
12. Lateral hypothalamic nucleus.
13. Optic tract. Axons of ganglion cells from half of each retina, on their way to the lateral geniculate nucleus, superior colliculus, and a few other sites.
14. Ansa lenticularis. Part of the projection from the globus pallidus to the thalamus.
15. Location of the nucleus basalis (of Meynert). Groups of large cholinergic neurons, situated in the substantia innominata, that innervate most forebrain areas.
16. Fibers that will cross in the anterior commissure, interconnecting the temporal lobes.
17. Claustrum. Reciprocal connections with cerebral cortex, poorly understood function.
18. Putamen. The part of the striatum with predominantly motor connections.
19. Globus pallidus (lateral or external segment). Afferents from the caudate nucleus and putamen, efferents to the subthalamic nucleus.
20. Globus pallidus (medial or internal segment). Afferents from the caudate nucleus, putamen, and subthalamic nucleus, efferents to the thalamus.
21. Posterior limb of the internal capsule. Contains projections to and from sensorimotor and parietal cortex, including corticospinal fibers and the somatosensory radiation.
22. Reticular nucleus of the thalamus. Afferents from the thalamus and cerebral cortex, GABAergic efferents to the thalamus.
23. Ventral anterior and ventral lateral nuclei (VA/VL). Afferents from the cerebellum and basal ganglia, efferents to motor areas of cortex.
24. Body of the fornix. Efferents from the hippocampal formation to the septal area and mammillary bodies.

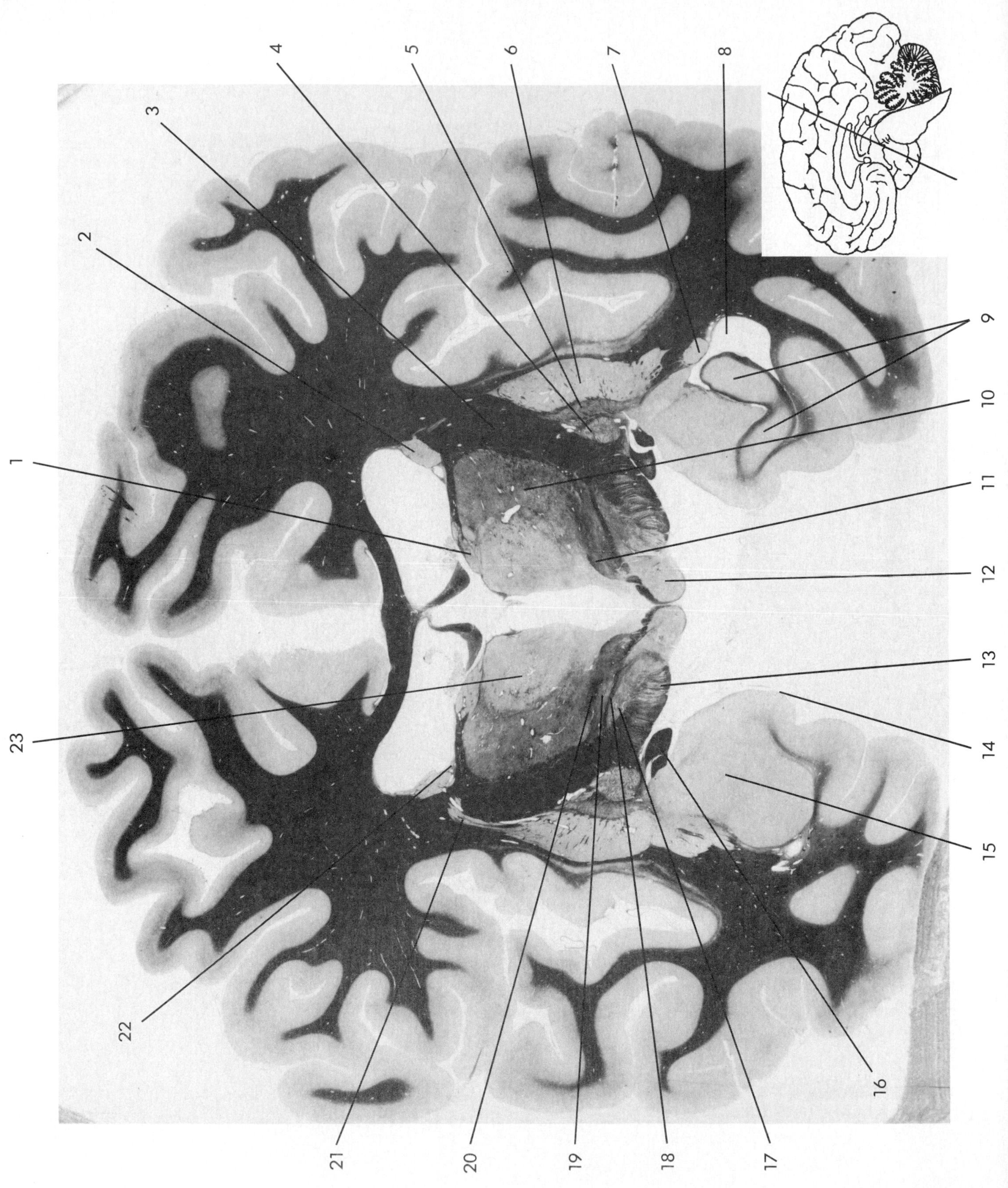
1
2
3
4
5
6
7
8
9
10
11
12
13
14
15
16
17
18
19
20
21
22
23

*Figure A-5 Midthalamus; mammillary bodies*

1. Lateral dorsal nucleus. Efferents to the cingulate gyrus.
2. Body of the caudate nucleus, the part of the striatum predominantly connected with association cortex.
3. Posterior limb of the internal capsule. Contains projections to and from sensorimotor and parietal cortex, including corticospinal fibers and the somatosensory radiation.
4. Globus pallidus (medial or internal segment). Afferents from the caudate nucleus, putamen, and subthalamic nucleus, efferents to the thalamus.
5. Globus pallidus (lateral or external segment). Afferents from the caudate nucleus and putamen, efferents to the subthalamic nucleus.
6. Putamen. The part of the striatum with predominantly motor connections.
7. Tail of the caudate nucleus, the part of the striatum predominantly connected with association cortex.
8. Inferior horn of the lateral ventricle.
9. Anterior end of the hippocampal formation, the core of one of the two major limbic circuits.
10. Ventral lateral nucleus (VL). Afferents from the cerebellum and basal ganglia (primarily the former), efferents to motor areas of cortex.
11. Mammillothalamic tract. Projection from the mammillary body to the anterior nucleus of the thalamus. Part of the Papez circuit.
12. Mammillary body. Afferents from the hippocampal formation, efferents to the anterior nucleus of the thalamus. Part of the Papez circuit.
13. Substantia nigra. The reticular part receives inputs from the striatum and projects to the thalamus; the compact part contains pigmented, dopaminergic neurons that project to the striatum.
14. Uncus. The proximity of the surface of the uncus to the cerebral peduncle can cause clinical problems.
15. Amygdala. A collection of nuclei forming the core of one of the two major limbic circuits.
16. Optic tract. Axons of ganglion cells from half of each retina, on their way to the lateral geniculate nucleus, superior colliculus, and a few other sites.
17. Subthalamic nucleus. Afferents from and efferents to the globus pallidus.
18. Lenticular fasciculus. Part of the projection from the globus pallidus to the thalamus.
19. Zona incerta. One more source of direct inputs to the cerebral cortex; function unknown.
20. Thalamic fasciculus. Projections from the cerebellum and basal ganglia to the ventral anterior and ventral lateral nuclei (VA/VL).
21. Gray bridge between putamen and caudate nucleus; part of the reason the striatum got its name.
22. Stria terminalis. Efferents from the amygdala to the septal area and hypothalamus.
23. Dorsomedial nucleus. Connections with prefrontal association cortex.

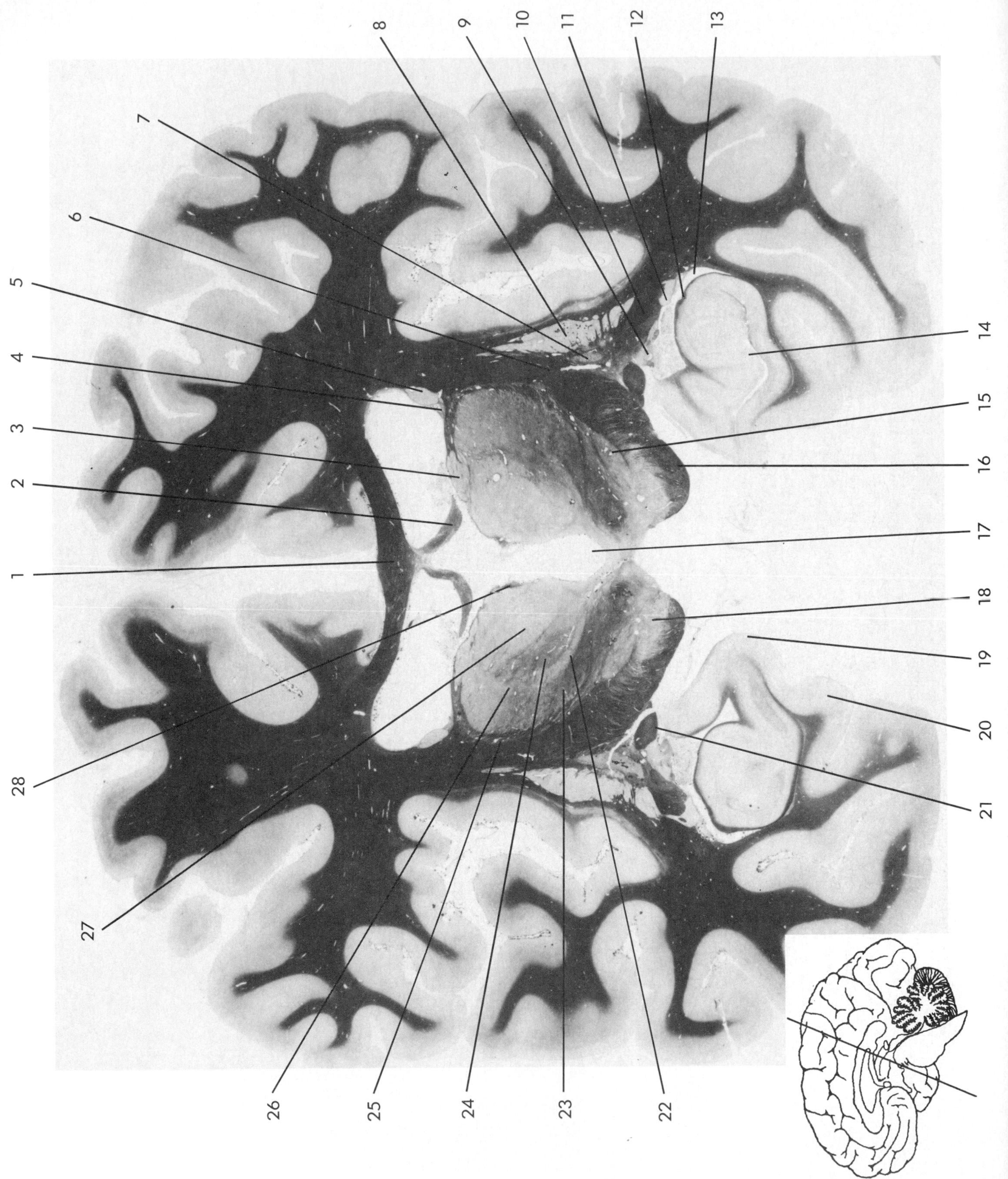
1
2
3
4
5
6
7
8
9
10
11
12
13
14
15
16
17
18
19
20
21
22
23
24
25
26
27
28

*Figure A-6 Midthalamus*

1. Corpus callosum. Commissural fibers interconnecting most cortical areas.
2. Body of the fornix. Efferents from the hippocampal formation to the septal area and mammillary bodies.
3. Lateral dorsal nucleus. Efferents to the cingulate gyrus.
4. Terminal (thalamostriate) vein, with adjacent stria terminalis.
5. Body of the caudate nucleus, the part of the striatum predominantly connected with association cortex.
6. Posterior limb of the internal capsule. Contains projections to and from sensorimotor and parietal cortex, including corticospinal fibers and the somatosensory radiation.
7. Globus pallidus (lateral or external segment). Afferents from the caudate nucleus and putamen, efferents to the subthalamic nucleus.
8. Putamen. The part of the striatum with predominantly motor connections.
9. Stria terminalis, which has now emerged from the posterior surface of the amygdala. Efferents from the amygdala to the septal area and hypothalamus.
10. Sublenticular part of the internal capsule. Contains projections to and from temporal and some other cortical areas, including the auditory radiation and part of the optic radiation.
11. Tail of the caudate nucleus, the part of the striatum predominantly connected with association cortex.
12. Alveus. Hippocampal efferents on the ventricular surface of the hippocampal formation.
13. Inferior horn of the lateral ventricle.
14. Hippocampal formation, the core of one of the two major limbic circuits.
15. Subthalamic nucleus. Afferents from and efferents to the globus pallidus.
16. Basis pedunculi (of the cerebral peduncle). Corticospinal, corticobulbar, and corticopontine fibers.
17. Third ventricle.
18. Substantia nigra. The reticular part receives inputs from the striatum and projects to the thalamus; the compact part contains pigmented, dopaminergic neurons that project to the striatum.
19. Uncus. The proximity of the surface of the uncus to the cerebral peduncle can cause clinical problems.
20. Parahippocampal gyrus. This anterior level is entorhinal cortex, source of most afferents to the hippocampal formation.
21. Optic tract. Axons of ganglion cells from half of each retina, on their way to the lateral geniculate nucleus, superior colliculus, and a few other sites.
22. Ventral posteromedial nucleus (VPM). Afferents from trigeminal and solitary nuclei, efferents to somatosensory and gustatory cortex.
23. Ventral posterolateral nucleus (VPL). Afferents from the spinal cord (spinothalamic tract) and posterior column nuclei, efferents to somatosensory cortex.
24. Centromedian nucleus, the largest of the intralaminar nuclei. Afferents from the globus pallidus, efferents to the striatum.
25. Reticular nucleus of the thalamus. Afferents from the thalamus and cerebral cortex, GABAergic efferents to the thalamus.
26. Ventral lateral nucleus (VL). Afferents from the cerebellum and basal ganglia (primarily the former), efferents to motor areas of cortex.
27. Dorsomedial nucleus. Connections with prefrontal association cortex.
28. Stria medullaris of the thalamus. Site of attachment of the roof of the third ventricle, and a route through which septal efferents reach the habenula.

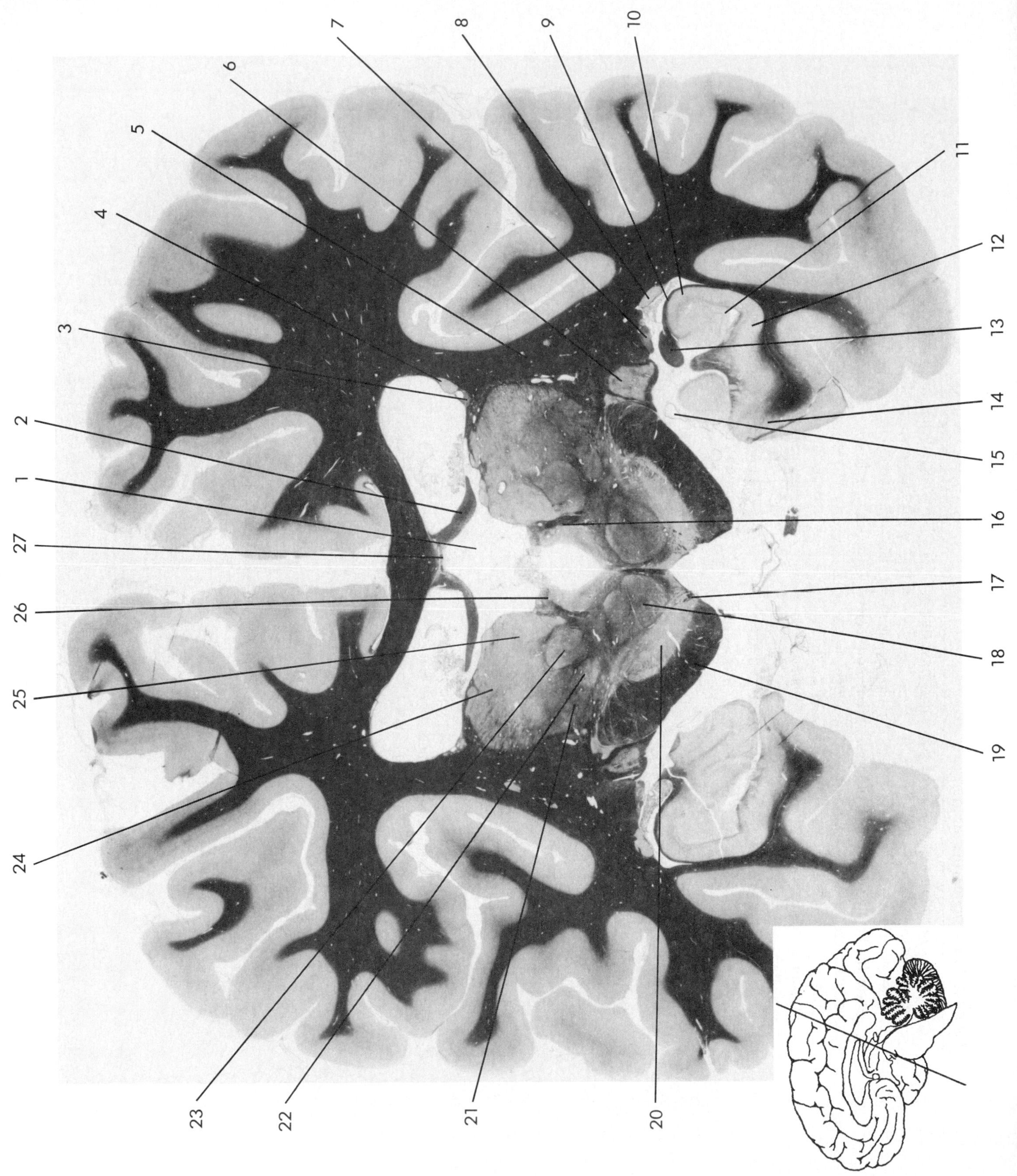
1
2
3
4
5
6
7
8
9
10
11
12
13
14
15
16
17
18
19
20
21
22
23
24
25
26
27

*Figure A-7 Posterior thalamus; habenula*

1. Transverse cerebral fissure. An extension of subarachnoid space, situated above the roof of the third ventricle and containing the internal cerebral veins.
2. Body of the fornix. Efferents from the hippocampal formation to the septal area and mammillary bodies.
3. Stria terminalis (adjacent to terminal vein). Efferents from the amygdala to the septal area and hypothalamus.
4. Body of the caudate nucleus, the part of the striatum predominantly connected with association cortex.
5. Retrolenticular part of the internal capsule. Contains projections to and from the parietal and occipital lobes, including part of the optic radiation.
6. Lateral geniculate nucleus. Afferents from the retina, efferents to visual cortex.
7. Stria terminalis. Efferents from the amygdala to the septal area and hypothalamus.
8. Tail of the caudate nucleus, the part of the striatum predominantly connected with association cortex.
9. Alveus. Hippocampal efferents on the ventricular surface of the hippocampal formation.
10. Hippocampus (cornu ammonis), a subdivision of the hippocampal formation. Afferents from the dentate gyrus, efferents to the subiculum and septal area.
11. Dentate gyrus, a subdivision of the hippocampal formation. Afferents from entorhinal cortex, efferents to hippocampal pyramidal cells.
12. Subiculum, a subdivision of the hippocampal formation and its principal source of efferents. Afferents from the hippocampus proper.
13. Fimbria of the hippocampus. Hippocampal efferents that have assembled from the alveus, on their way into the fornix.
14. Parahippocampal gyrus. This anterior level is entorhinal cortex, source of most afferents to the hippocampal formation.
15. Posterior cerebral artery.
16. Fasciculus retroflexus (=habenulointerpeduncular tract!). Conveys limbic output from the habenula to the midbrain reticular formation.
17. Oculomotor nerve, just emerging from the midbrain.
18. Red nucleus. Afferents from the cerebellum, efferents to the inferior olivary nucleus and spinal cord.
19. Basis pedunculi (of the cerebral peduncle). Corticospinal, corticobulbar, and corticopontine fibers.
20. Substantia nigra. The reticular part receives inputs from the striatum and projects to the thalamus; the compact part contains pigmented, dopaminergic neurons that project to the striatum.
21. Ventral posterolateral nucleus (VPL). Afferents from the spinal cord (spinothalamic tract) and posterior column nuclei, efferents to somatosensory cortex.
22. Ventral posteromedial nucleus (VPM). Afferents from trigeminal and solitary nuclei, efferents to somatosensory and gustatory cortex.
23. Centromedian nucleus, the largest of the intralaminar nuclei. Afferents from the globus pallidus, efferents to the striatum.
24. Lateral posterior nucleus. Connections, similar to those of the pulvinar, with parietal-occipital-temporal association cortex.
25. Dorsomedial nucleus. Connections with prefrontal association cortex.
26. Habenula, a relay in caudally directed limbic projections. Afferents from the septal area, efferents to the midbrain reticular formation.
27. Hippocampal commissure. Fibers interconnecting the two hippocampal formations.

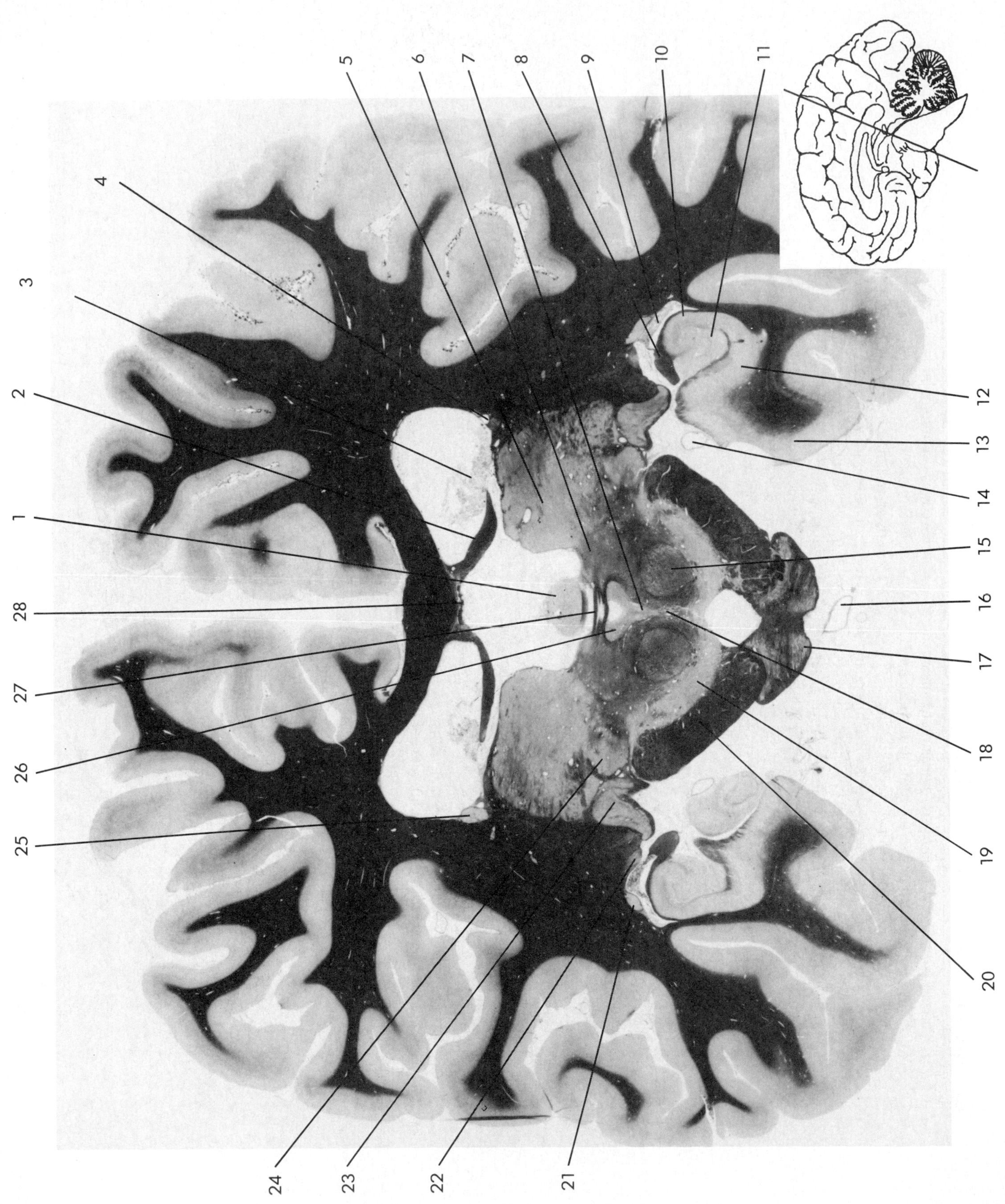
1
2
3
4
5
6
7
8
9
10
11
12
13
14
15
16
17
18
19
20
21
22
23
24
25
26
27
28

*Figure A-8 Posterior commissure*

1. Pineal gland. An endocrine gland important in seasonal cycles of some animals; function unclear in humans.
2. Body of the fornix. Efferents from the hippocampal formation to the septal area and mammillary bodies.
3. Choroid plexus in the body of the lateral ventricle.
4. Stria terminalis (adjacent to terminal vein). Efferents from the amygdala to the septal area and hypothalamus.
5. Pulvinar. Connections with parietal-occipital-temporal association cortex.
6. Pretectal area. Part of the pupillary light reflex pathway; afferents from retinal ganglion cells, efferents to the Edinger-Westphal nucleus.
7. Oculomotor nucleus. Lower motor neurons for extraocular muscles and the levator palpebrae, preganglionic parasympathetic neurons for the ciliary muscle and pupillary sphincter.
8. Fimbria of the hippocampus. Hippocampal efferents that have assembled from the alveus, on their way into the fornix.
9. Choroid plexus in the inferior horn of the lateral ventricle.
10. Hippocampus (cornu ammonis), a subdivision of the hippocampal formation. Afferents from the dentate gyrus, efferents to the subiculum and septal area.
11. Dentate gyrus, a subdivision of the hippocampal formation. Afferents from entorhinal cortex, efferents to hippocampal pyramidal cells.
12. Subiculum, a subdivision of the hippocampal formation and its principal source of efferents. Afferents from the hippocampus proper.
13. Parahippocampal gyrus. This anterior level is entorhinal cortex, source of most afferents to the hippocampal formation.
14. Posterior cerebral artery.
15. Red nucleus. Afferents from the cerebellum, efferents to the inferior olivary nucleus and spinal cord.
16. Basilar artery.
17. Most rostral pontine nuclei. Afferents from cerebral cortex (via the cerebral peduncle), efferents to contralateral cerebellar cortex (via the middle cerebellar peduncle).
18. Ventral tegmental area. Contains dopaminergic neurons that project to a variety of limbic and neocortical areas.
19. Substantia nigra. The reticular part receives inputs from the striatum and projects to the thalamus; the compact part contains pigmented, dopaminergic neurons that project to the striatum.
20. Basis pedunculi (of the cerebral peduncle). Corticospinal, corticobulbar, and corticopontine fibers.
21. Tail of the caudate nucleus, the part of the striatum predominantly connected with association cortex.
22. Stria terminalis. Efferents from the amygdala to the septal area and hypothalamus.
23. Lateral geniculate nucleus. Afferents from the retina, efferents to visual cortex.
24. Medial geniculate nucleus. Auditory afferents via the inferior brachium, efferents to auditory cortex.
25. Body of the caudate nucleus, the part of the striatum predominantly connected with association cortex.
26. Periaqueductal gray. Part of a descending pain-control pathway.
27. Posterior commissure. Crossing fibers dealing with vertical eye movements and the pupillary light reflex.
28. Hippocampal commissure. Fibers interconnecting the two hippocampal formations.

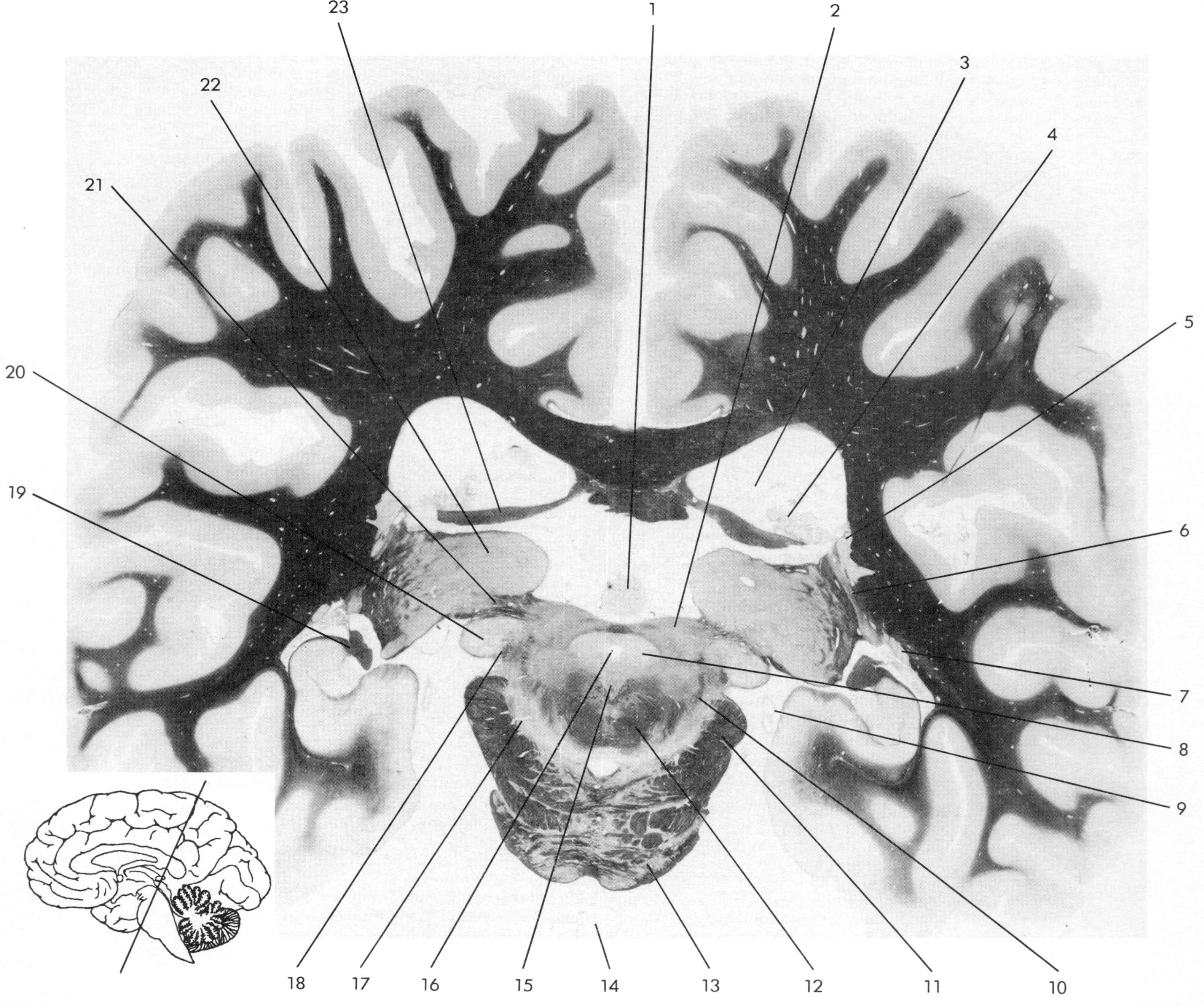
1
2
3
4
5
6
7
8
9
10
11
12
13
14
15
16
17
18
19
20
21
22
23

*Figure A-9 Posterior thalamus; midbrain*

1. Pineal gland. An endocrine gland important in seasonal cycles of some animals; function unclear in humans.
2. Rostral end of the superior colliculus. Afferents from the retina and visual cortex, efferents to the pulvinar and other structures; functions in visual attention and eye movements.
3. Choroidal vein, draining the choroid plexus of the lateral ventricle.
4. Choroid plexus in the body of the lateral ventricle.
5. Body of the caudate nucleus, the part of the striatum predominantly connected with association cortex.
6. Stria terminalis cut tangentially as it curves around with the lateral ventricle. Efferents from the amygdala to the septal area and hypothalamus.
7. Tail of the caudate nucleus, the part of the striatum predominantly connected with association cortex.
8. Periaqueductal gray. Part of a descending pain-control pathway.
9. Posterior cerebral artery.
10. Medial lemniscus. Somatosensory afferents from the posterior column nuclei and trigeminal main sensory nucleus, on their way to the VPL/VPM.
11. Basis pedunculi (of the cerebral peduncle). Corticospinal, corticobulbar, and corticopontine fibers.
12. Superior cerebellar peduncle. Efferents from the deep cerebellar nuclei, on their way to the red nucleus and VL.
13. Pontine nuclei. Afferents from cerebral cortex (via the cerebral peduncle), efferents to contralateral cerebellar cortex (via the middle cerebellar peduncle).
14. Basilar artery.
15. Oculomotor nucleus. Lower motor neurons for extraocular muscles and the levator palpebrae, preganglionic parasympathetic neurons for the ciliary muscle and pupillary sphincter.
16. Cerebral aqueduct, the connection between the third and fourth ventricles.
17. Substantia nigra. The reticular part receives inputs from the striatum and projects to the thalamus; the compact part contains pigmented, dopaminergic neurons that project to the striatum.
18. Inferior brachium (brachium of the inferior colliculus). Auditory afferents from the inferior colliculus on their way to the medial geniculate nucleus.
19. Fimbria of the hippocampus. Hippocampal efferents that have assembled from the alveus, on their way into the fornix.
20. Medial geniculate nucleus. Auditory afferents via the inferior brachium, efferents to auditory cortex.
21. Superior brachium (brachium of the superior colliculus). Contains afferents from the retina to the superior colliculus and pretectal area.
22. Pulvinar. Connections with parietal-occipital-temporal association cortex.
23. Crus of the fornix. Efferents from the hippocampal formation to the septal area and mammillary bodies.

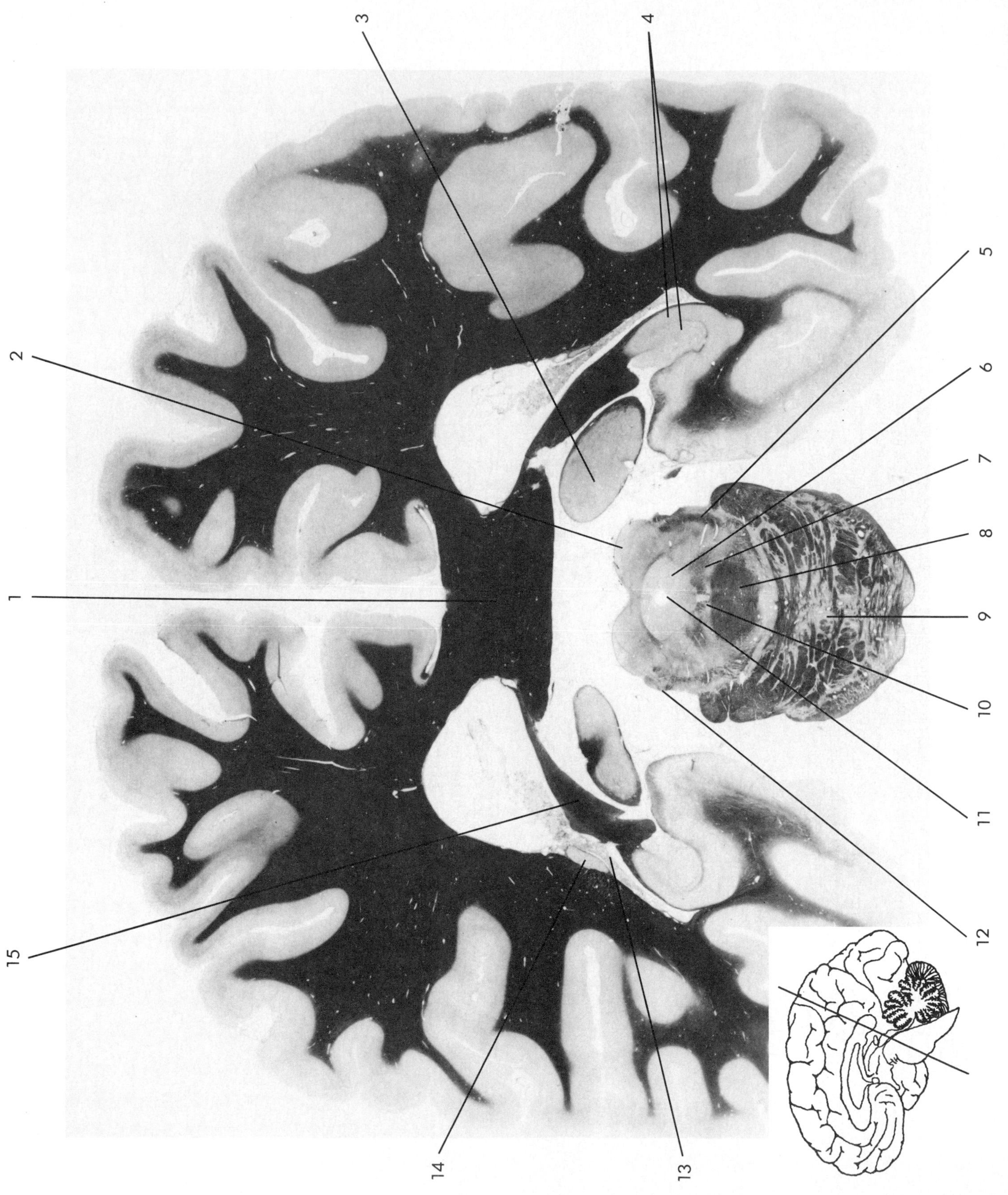
1
2
3
4
5
6
7
8
9
10
11
12
13
14
15

*Figure A-10 Atrium of the lateral ventricle*

1. Splenium of the corpus callosum. Commissural fibers interconnecting posterior cortical areas.
2. Superior colliculus. Afferents from the retina and visual cortex, efferents to the pulvinar and other structures; functions in visual attention and eye movements.
3. Pulvinar. Connections with parietal-occipital-temporal association cortex.
4. Posterior end of the hippocampal formation, the core of one of the two major limbic circuits.
5. Medial lemniscus. Somatosensory afferents from the posterior column nuclei and trigeminal main sensory nucleus, on their way to the VPL/VPM.
6. Periaqueductal gray. Part of a descending pain-control pathway.
7. Central tegmental tract. A complex bundle that contains fibers descending from the red nucleus to the inferior olivary nucleus, as well as ascending monoaminergic fibers.
8. Decussation of the superior cerebellar peduncles. Efferents from the deep cerebellar nuclei, on their way to the red nucleus and VL.
9. Pontine nuclei. Afferents from cerebral cortex (via the cerebral peduncle), efferents to contralateral cerebellar cortex (via the middle cerebellar peduncle).
10. Medial longitudinal fasciculus (MLF). Involved in coordinating horizontal eye movements; includes fibers from contralateral abducens interneurons on their way to medial rectus motor neurons.
11. Cerebral aqueduct, the connection between the third and fourth ventricles.
12. Inferior brachium (brachium of the inferior colliculus). Auditory afferents from the inferior colliculus on their way to the medial geniculate nucleus.
13. Choroid plexus, cut tangentially as it curves through the atrium of the lateral ventricle.
14. Caudate nucleus, cut tangentially as it curves around with the lateral ventricle.
15. Hippocampal efferent fibers passing from the fimbria of the hippocampus to the crus of the fornix.

# Index

**H**

## I